Psychosocial Occupational Therapy:

A Clinical Practice

D1507831

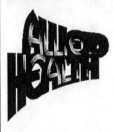

Psychosocial Occupational Therapy:
A Clinical Practice

Elizabeth Cara, MA, OTR, MFCC

Assistant Professor, San Jose State University

San Jose, California

Anne MacRae, Ph.D., OTR

Professor, San Jose State University

San Jose, California

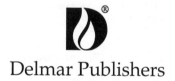

Delmar Publishers

DELMAR

™

THOMSON LEARNING

Africa • Australia • Canada • Denmark • Japan • Mexico • New Zealand • Philippines
Puerto Rico • Singapore • Spain • United Kingdom • United States

Cover Design: Vincent S. Berger

Delmar Staff

Acquisitions Editor: Dawn Gerrain
Marketing Manager: Darryl Caron
Project/Development Editor: Coreen Rogers

Production Coordinator: John Mickelbank
Art and Design Coordinator: Vincent S. Berger
Editorial Assistant: Donna L. Leto

COPYRIGHT © 1998
Delmar is a division of Thomson Learning. The Thomson Learning logo is a registered trademark used herein under license.

Printed in the United States of America
8 9 10 XXX 03 02 01

For more information, contact Delmar, 3 Columbia Circle, PO Box 15015, Albany, NY 12212-0515; or find us on the World Wide Web at http://www.delmar.com

International Division List

Japan:
Thomson Learning
Palaceside Building 5F
1-1-1 Hitotsubashi, Chiyoda-ku
Tokyo 100 0003 Japan
Tel: 813 5218 6544
Fax: 813 5218 6551

Australia/New Zealand
Nelson/Thomson Learning
102 Dodds Street
South Melbourne, Victoria 3205
Australia
Tel: 61 39 685 4111
Fax: 61 39 685 4199

UK/Europe/Middle East:
Thomson Learning
Berkshire House
168-173 High Holborn
London
WC1V 7AA United Kingdom
Tel: 44 171 497 1422
Fax: 44 171 497 1426

Latin America:
Thomson Learning
Seneca, 53
Colonia Polanco
11560 Mexico D.F. Mexico
Tel: 525-281-2906
Fax: 525-281-2656

Canada:
Nelson/Thomson Learning
1120 Birchmount Road
Scarborough, Ontario
Canada M1K 5G4
Tel: 416-752-9100
Fax: 416-752-8102

Asia:
Thomson Learning
60 Albert Street, #15-01
Albert Complex
Singapore 189969
Tel: 65 336 6411
Fax: 65 336 7411

Library of Congress Cataloging-in-Publication Data: 97-21044

ISBN: 0-8273-6283-8

Contents

Preface

In 1954, Wade and Franciscus wrote:

> The attitude of the occupational therapist toward the mental disease and the approach which he makes to the patient determine to a great extent the quality of the therapy he administers and the results he obtains. Opportunities for the development of a therapeutic approach and a healthy mental attitude toward this group of patients should hold the highest priority in the educational plan of the student therapist (p. 77).

This is not an outdated notion but rather the principle that guides our teaching and clinical work. It is our hope that through the chapters of this book, the occupational therapy student and the practicing occupational therapist will develop or enhance, not only their knowledge of mental health care, but also their respect for, and understanding of, people with mental illness.

Health care—specifically, mental health care—is a dynamic field, with new ideas being introduced and old ones being discarded at sometimes-unpredictable rates. This is one of the inherent problems in writing a textbook on this topic. The editors and contributing authors have made every effort to provide the most up-to-date information available, but it is up to the readers to study with a critical view and supplement the information as appropriate.

As of the writing of this text, there were several unresolved issues that are addressed in individual chapters and one controversy that applies to all the chapters: the use of terminology. What is the best word to describe the role of the person receiving services or treatment? This may seem like a relatively simple, even trivial, issue, but it is not. A word can be a label with subtle emotional, often derogatory, meanings attached to it. If one doubts the power of a label, consider that it was not long ago that terms such as *idiot* and *moron* were considered accurate medical terminology. Finding the best word to describe the people involved in a therapeutic relationship has been an ongoing debate for some time, and it is unlikely to be resolved with a simple answer.

It is the editors' opinion that finding a single, universal term for this role is not possible at this time. Rather, the term's meaning does, and should, vary depending on the setting where treatment is given as well as the philosophy guiding the treatment. For example, the term *patient* still seems appropriate when discussing people hospitalized for acute disorders. Client is the preferred term for a person accessing ongoing contractual services, such as those found in the case management relationship. Currently, the term *consumer* seems to be favored, as it implies that the receivers of service have freedom of choice and control over their own lives. However, no one term is ideal, and the reader should be aware of the limitations of language. For example, when using the term *consumer*, one needs to ask, "What exactly is being consumed?" If the person is clearly using a specific service, such as a prevocational assessment package, then the term makes sense, but in ongoing supportive services, the most valuable commodity offered is the therapeutic relationship (and, obviously, the therapist is not for consumption). The term *participant* would be more accurate in such a relationship, but since it is not a widely used or recognized term, it may be confusing when used in documentation. In summary, the reader is cautioned about the limitations of language and encouraged to think about the nuances of terms and be particularly aware of their context. Although labels are sometimes necessary for the sake of clarity, it is recommended that every effort be made to maintain human dignity and identity by using such terms as *person* or *individual* whenever possible.

Another controversial use of terminology applies to all the chapters of this book. What is the best word to describe the specific area of service that we are targeting? As with words applied to people, words used to describe a specific arena in which we practice can have subtle meanings attached to them. For some time the term *psychosocial* has been applied very broadly in occupational therapy practice. *The Random House College Dictionary* (1973) defines psychosocial as "pertaining to or caused by both psychological and social factors." It is a useful term that implies treating the psyche, or mind, and social factors, as distinguished somehow from bodily, physical factors (though we all recognize how mind and body, as embedded in a social context, are interconnected and that you cannot possibly treat one without treating the other).

However, *psychosocial* could be applied to everyone, whether able or disabled in body and/or mind. A term that more specifically elucidates and distinguishes this text is *psychiatry*, "the practice or the science of treating mental disorders" (*Random House College Dictionary*, 1973). "Mental disorders" encompasses psychosocial causes and problems; however, the term is even richer, encompassing biology, chemistry, cognition and perception, linguistic, interpersonal, environmental, and cultural factors and the manifestations of each. Although the techniques discussed in the chapters are directed toward the amelioration of "psyche," or mental, problems as they manifest in the social or interpersonal realm, the techniques are applied specifically in the treatment of mental disorders.

Again, it is our opinion that there is not yet one universal term that adequately describes our practice. Instead, the term will vary throughout chapters; *mental health, mental health arena, psychiatric,* and *psychosocial* are used somewhat interchangeably according to each author's bias. The reader is encouraged to think about the various terms in the continuing quest to clarify practice in the mental health arena and, hopefully, to discover a universal term that does justice to our complex treatment for mental disorders.

In the past two decades, different models of occupational therapy have been delineated and expanded on. There has also been a focus on developing assessments specifically for occupational therapy. The historical roots of our profession have vibrantly infused and broadened our sense of ourselves as professionals. We recognize the importance of models, assessments, and history; however, the purpose of this text is to fill what we perceive as a gap in the information for the clinician practicing in mental health. It is intended to inform students and beginning therapists of the basic and rich forms of occupational therapy that are practiced in mental health. We have included overviews of theories, evaluation and treatment, and the occupational therapy process, but our primary purpose is not theoretical but rather clinical. We aim to provide sound information regarding treatment specifically for practice in psychiatry. To that end we employed clinicians as chapter authors and encouraged them to discuss what they actually do in their practice. We also provided an understanding of mental disorders, as they are currently defined in the *Diagnostic and Statistical Manual of Mental Disorders, Fourth Edition* (DSM-IV) (APA, 1994). Our goal is to provide students and beginning clinicians with information they will need to adequately practice as a psychiatric occupational therapy clinician.

Because we wanted the text to be clinical in its focus and, therefore, encouraged our chapter authors to write about their practice, we have allowed for differing styles and opinions. In fact, throughout the book you may find that the authors disagree. You may also realize that some chapters vary in depth or breadth of scope or focus, either more on understanding a disorder or more on providing treatment. The chapters include a resource list and also a list of suggested readings. For example, Chapter 18, on vocational programming, encourages a psychosocial community approach, whereas Chapter 2, on personal effects of mental illness, focuses on family and national support groups. All chapters include case illustrations, some of which are brief illustrations of particular points made in the chapter while others are long illustrations of treatment. We have allowed for a variety of authorship styles, which, we think, appeals to our various readers' styles and helps to enhance learning.

Information on treatment for one population in one chapter can easily translate into treatment for another population. For example, the relaxation exercises for anxiety disorders described in Chapter 12 can also be helpful for many other people, particularly those with agitated depression, personality disorders, or HIV, due to the symptoms of anxiety that they may experience. In fact, due to the recent explosion of information concerning stress in everyday life, there are probably very few people who would not find them beneficial. Hopefully, readers can extrapolate and adapt treatment suggestions for various populations and settings.

You will find that the length of chapters varies depending on how much information is in the literature. For example, Chapter 10, on mood disorders, is shorter than Chapter 12, on anxiety disorders. There is much information, particularly in occupational therapy, about depression, but less about generalized anxiety disorder. We encourage you to be analytical in your reading, to interact with the material in a critical way, and to freely use this volume as a base from which to create your clinical practice.

We do not know what the mental health arena will look like in the near future. It is changing rapidly and being strongly influenced by managed care. Treatment is becoming more acute and is being dictated by cost-efficiency, while at the same time it seems that more people are in need of services. In this book, we have attempted to provide a broad base of information that includes what we know of "mental disease" and its treatment through occupational therapy to date. This text provides the infrastructure on which daily life in psychiatric occupational therapy exists. We believe that this knowledge will not change but rather can only be added to, and we invite the reader to take this underlying structure and build on it.

SUSTAINING PROFESSIONAL IDENTITY IN MENTAL HEALTH—PERSONAL PATHS

We often hear comments predicting the demise of psychiatric occupational therapy, but occupational therapists are a diverse group of people in a multifaceted profession. The occupational therapy (OT) philosophy and process is not fully articulated in the literature; however, despite diverse paths into the field and in practice, there are common threads of a belief system that is enculturated in the profession. Historically, this belief system was not separate from the practice in mental health, and we believe it will sustain our unique contribution in the psychosocial arena.

Throughout the text we present case illustrations to make concepts, ideas and people with various diagnoses and problems "come alive" and, hopefully, be remembered. In keeping with that, and in the wish that psychosocial occupational therapists and practitioners could be sustaining mentors, we present here some case illustrations of people's personal paths into the profession, excerpted from personal statements they provided. We highlight the interests, joys, rewards and challenges of occupational therapists who work in mental health. While these therapists represent the vast differences of our paths, it is also clear that there is a unifying passion and an identity. It is our hope that the passion infuses this text, and that threads of a common belief system and identity will be recognized throughout. The first two are our own.

LIZ CARA

College Faculty, San Jose, CA

I graduated from college with a BA in history, moved to Pennsylvania and began working in business. Although I was very successful, becoming a manager by the age of 24, I felt that administration was dry and that I was not doing anything to benefit people. I literally went to the library and researched careers. Health care careers matched my requirements—working with and benefiting people, available jobs, and the flexibility to move to other states and countries.

I had never heard of occupational therapy until a physiatrist (an MD who specializes in physical rehabilitation) steered me to it. I talked with people from several departments at the University of Pennsylvania before enrolling, but it seemed that the occupational therapists were the most animated, lively, interesting people, and they discussed their job as if it were fun.

OT school offered me a combination of learning that I loved—science, psychology and crafts. I thought then and still do that it is the perfect course; it integrated all of the things I want to know about. I originally wanted to work with people with arthritis, but during my fieldworks, I realized that I really liked the opportunity for creativity, unpredictability, and up-close relationships in mental health. I looked forward to the non-sameness of every day and I felt that indeed, I had an effect on people.

Since entering the field, I have had the opportunity to work in a variety of settings and roles on both coasts; with teenagers on an in-patient locked unit, at an in-patient psychiatric facility exclusively for women, at one of the oldest private psychiatric hospitals that based treatment on moral treatment. Also, my experience in community settings includes developing an agency known as Community Vocational Enterprises, specializing in vocational rehabilitation for people with serious mental illness, working in a clubhouse model program called Townehouse Creative Living Center, and coordinating vocational treatment for a large community residential organization.

Practicing occupational therapy in the mental health area has fit who I am as a person. It satisfies my values, particularly my very deep belief that the essence of life is relationship. I am thrilled that I now have the opportunity to be an educator and continue to impart my knowledge and values.

ANNE MACRAE

College Faculty, San Jose, CA

My first degree was in education, and although I loved teaching (and still do!), I felt there was something else I wanted to do. I spent several years exploring possibilities, taking courses, and working as a program leader in a recreation center for people with disabilities, and developed a special fascination for the workings of the brain. I found that cognitive, affective and perceptual dysfunctions were evident in a wide variety of developmental, physical and psychiatric conditions but I was still resistant to pursuing a medically oriented career. I also wanted to pursue my creative, artistic, and social interests that seemingly didn't fit into a health care profession. A friend of mine who is a physical therapist told me about OT and said it would be a perfect match for me. She was right! I returned to graduate school for a master's degree in occupational therapy and I never regretted that choice.

My first couple of years in practice, I worked in the home health care arena. This experience led me to the strong belief that mental health is essential to address in any treatment plan. The primary diagnostic categories seen in home health care are cardiovascular, neurological, orthopedic and oncologic, but I often felt that the real issues behind dysfunction were more related to problems with adjustment, depression, substance abuse, and various cognitive and perceptual dysfunctions.

As part of my teaching responsibilities, I currently supervise an on-campus occupational therapy mental health clinic which allows me a wonderful blend of clinical practice, teaching and supervision. In addition, I maintain a limited practice at San Francisco General Hospital, a large county facility serving a very diverse and often disenfranchised population. Most of the clients that I see in both of these settings have serious and persistent mental illnesses. I consider this group to be one of the most stigmatized in the western world, consequently, a necessary part of my work is being involved in community education to increase awareness about the plight of people with mental illness.

JUDY PRITCHETT

Clinical director and program developer, community outreach agency, New York City

I was very interested in schizophrenia because I had relatives with that disorder, but my first occupational exposure to mental illness was as a mental health aide in a day treatment center. It became apparent to me that the activities done at this center—crafts, cooking, outings, artwork and clerical groups—were more meaningful and therapeutic than the group or individual talking therapies. After two years working for this program in the Riverdale Mental Health Association, I decided to go to graduate school for a degree in occupational therapy.

I had felt strongly that I always wanted to work in mental health, but somehow my first job out of OT school was in a school for multiply handicapped children. In this setting I clearly saw the relevance of sensory integration theory and perceptual motor development, and could relate this information easily to the processing deficits seen with schizophrenia. I also developed programs related to sex education and career exploration which are examples of what I think is OT at its best: focusing on areas of human occupation that are in themselves important and meaningful while developing specific competencies and providing activities that improve psychosocial adjustment in many other ways, including improved self esteem, reality testing and social skills.

For the last ten years I worked at Project Reachout, a program for the mentally ill homeless population. I liked this setting most of all, because it allowed me to have fun addressing a serious social problem and because I could see people who had been outcasts become part of a community which we created and which in turn connected them to a broader community from which they had become estranged. We enabled them to learn the skills they lacked in order to make this connection, and we enabled them to access and value the supports they needed in order to stay connected.

ANITA MARYE NELSON

Clinician & program developer, home health agency, Colorado Springs

I was originally a COTA (Certified Occupational Therapy Assistant) in the military, and a "die hard" physical disabilities clinician with little or no interest in practicing in mental health. After a job relocation, I was reassigned to work in mental health. The organization at that base was such that the OTR's (Occupational Therapists, Registered) treated patients with physical disabilities and the COTA's treated patients with psychiatric disabilities. Actually, it was a negative experience because I didn't feel competent. But the experience did lead me to pursue further education.

I returned to school to become an OTR and developed an appreciation for the generalist perspective of occupational therapy and a greater understanding of the underlying theory. My psychiatric internship at the Kettering Medical Center in Ohio opened my eyes to the richness of mental health OT. This experience was positive because of excellent role modeling, communication, and supervision.

My present practice is in home care where the primary caseload consists of patients needing physical rehabilitation. When the agency decided to expand to include a psychiatric caseload, they initially did not consider including occupational therapy, but at my persuasion, OT has been made an integral part of the mental health team. Home care provides me the opportunity to work in an interdisciplinary team, in a 'real-life' setting, with a mixed caseload that allows me to put the generalist OT concepts into practice.

SUSAN LANG

Private practice, San Francisco

I was initially attracted to the physical disabilities area of OT because it seemed more organized, concrete, and easier to follow. I was especially interested in neuroanatomy and that interest has persisted. But my internship in physical dysfunction was very negative—I almost left OT altogether. Fortunately, my internship experience in psychiatry was extremely positive, and I ended up being hired there afterward. Langley Porter Institute is part of a large teaching hospital at University of California Medical Center in San Francisco. It was a very supportive learning environment that used an excellent multidisciplinary approach. It was here that I felt I was able to develop my expertise and my skills. But this was also my most "traditional" job setting.

Another unique setting in which I worked was the Indian Hospital in Santa Fe, New Mexico. It was an incredible experience for me because I have always been fascinated by cross cultural issues, but it was also here that I think I became most aware of what clients had to offer me, rather than the other way around. In this setting, there was a bit of irony in that I was using non-verbal interventions among a cultural group whom I consider to be masters at nonverbal communication.

My respect for the diversity of clients and what they bring to the therapeutic relationship led me to my favorite treatment arena, which is private practice. Most occupational therapists who engage in private practice do so through the use of contracts with particular agencies. Another way to do private practice is to provide direct services to clients. There are limitations in reimbursement but I prefer this approach because it allows me the greatest autonomy and flexibility.

Mental health care has changed so much that occupational therapists have become more central; in terms of the overall goals of mental health, the whole functional arena has become central to treatment. Although the problems in mental health care are very real, I have no doubt that we have a valuable service to offer and there are many avenues for occupational therapists in mental health to explore and pursue.

VIRGINIA STOEFFEL

College Faculty, Milwaukee, WI

I wanted to be an occupational therapist since I was 13. At that time my mother had cancer and indeed died. One of my sisters was hospitalized with major depression and a suicide attempt. I was aware that people had feelings around illness. My perception was that people might be able to deal with their feelings through activities.

I was shaped by and formed by my supervisor on my level I fieldwork. She told me that I had very good interpersonal skills, even more advanced than those expected of level II students; she urged me to develop my skills in mental health. I also benefited from an excellent professor in mental health . . . she knew how to bring out the best in me . . . she felt that I was self-actualized!

I was hired onto a pilot project for those with substance abuse. This broadened into addictive disorders, such as eating disorders. This began a long and fruitful career as the program developed into long-term, outpatient, wellness and prevention programs. I was fortunate to move into different management jobs. Eventually I worked on a research program implementing cognitive behavioral programs for people, and I realized how substance abuse interfered with people carrying out performance roles.

I am sustained in my career because I am continually amazed at the strengths and resiliency people bring with them. I have always been interested in what makes people tick, what drives them and I have good observation and interpersonal skills. I know how to be human with people; that includes being flexible, adaptive, open, vulnerable to others, confident in myself. . . . People have remarked that I pay attention to them.

What is rewarding? to see that people can make changes in a supportive and trusting, consistent relationship. It makes me really aware, too, as a parent what needs to be done and how to be with my family, and how to keep myself grounded.

I want to say that I don't see psychosocial practice as a dying art. What we have to offer is a package that helps people best in a fairly economical way—they get the most bang for their buck by having an occupational therapist as part of their health care system.

It is not uncommon for people to enter occupational therapy as a second career, or not to know at first their choice of an OT practice area. One of the themes of these illustrations is that people often thought that they wanted to practice in a different area, until they discovered mental heath. Although they do not articulate exactly how mental health captured them, the choice to practice is not necessarily a conscious decision, of the head only, but clearly includes an unconscious process of the heart. One of the themes is the significance of key people in our lives or role models who help us discover our paths, whether serendipitous or logical. This is especially important during clinical internships, a concept that is further elaborated in Chapter 20, Fieldwork Supervision in a Mental Health Setting.

Another theme of these vignettes is the idea that occupational therapy is a career that, while not without its challenges, can provide deep personal satisfaction, and that there is a shared belief in the efficacy and practicality of what we do. All of the occupational therapists interviewed worked at one time or another in what would be considered traditional settings. They also explored and developed programs in nontraditional settings—community agencies, schools, outreach programs, homeless shelters, university-based collaborative programs, private practice, clubhouse model programs, and home health care agencies. This diversity in occupational therapy practice settings sometimes makes it difficult to define our scope, but it also provides us with remarkable flexibility. The generalist nature of occupational therapy practice provides opportunities in a broadly described mental health arena, even within the tremendous changes going on in health care delivery today. Chapter 7, The

Psychosocial Issues of Physical Illness and Disability, and all of Part 5, address diverse and nontraditional practice settings in psychosocial practice.

A theme touched on by the illustrators was becoming aware of mental illness and psychosocial problems in relatives' lives. This awareness developed into a desire to be an occupational therapist who could assist one in daily occupations or into an understanding and interpersonal facility in working with people with mental illnesses. This theme is discussed from the family viewpoint in Chapter 2, The Social and Personal Effects of Mental Illness.

"Creativity," "unpredictability," "flexibility," "non-sameness," "have fun"— all describe the work of occupational therapy in psychiatry. Although there are no specific chapters that address these intangible and more elusive qualities, each chapter author was asked to convey what they felt was unique, important, and perhaps not written about in their personal clinical experience, and these terms were their answers.

In the prefatory illustrations, a theme of relationship, an awareness of what clients had to offer in a reciprocal connection, and a yen for knowledge of what is happening to a person was evident throughout. People speak of being interested in what makes others tick, being able to support them in their daily lives, being accepting and embracing the whole person for where and who they are. At the same time they speak of being interested in neurology and in special conditions and sustaining that interest throughout their careers. We hope the reader will recognize that these themes are implicit in all of the chapters of the book.

Although we can specify certain themes through different paths, we are still not able to state definitively what attracts a person to the practice of occupational therapy in the mental health arena. We believe that this is as it should be in a diverse, eclectic profession in which beliefs are historically based on complex and broad concepts of adaptation and occupation. We also believe it's as it should be because diverse practitioners create their practice in mental health even as they practice this occupation daily in varied contexts.

We hope that this text will evoke a desire to know more about this rich field and the people in it, and we hope that you will follow the spirit of these occupational therapist case illustrations and practice with seriousness, passion, fun, intelligence, clarity, and creativity.

References

American Psychiatric Association. (1994). *Diagnostic and Statistical Manual of Mental Disorders* (4th ed.). Washington, DC: Author.

Wade, B. & Franciscus, M. L. (1954). *Occupational therapy for the mentally ill.* In H. Willard and C. Spackman, *Principles of occupational therapy* (2nd ed.). Philadelphia: Lippincott, pp. 76–116.

Acknowledgments

We are pleased that our individual authors, many of whom are not primarily writers, agreed that a comprehensive text in psychiatric occupational therapy needed to be written. We thank them for their valuable contributions and their willingness to take a great deal of time and work through many revisions, which represent the depth of their commitment to their work and to the profession.

As educators we have been graced with many students who have contributed their ideas, challenged our thinking, offered coffee when we most needed it, and continually encouraged us with their spirit. Gwyneth Owen, a recent graduate of the San Jose State Occupational Therapy master's program, provided much needed—and always willing—investigative, clerical, general, and soul support. Sandy Wu-Feng, a recent graduate of the San Jose State Occupational Therapy baccalaureate program, supplied timely clerical and Web information, as well as enthusiasm. We appreciated as well their consistent responsibility and intelligence.

As clinicians we have been graced with many patients and clients who allowed us to work with them and validated the success of our treatment approaches. Through their willingness to be vulnerable and their demonstrated resiliency they have inspired us. We hope that, even if indirectly, this text will serve them.

We also enjoyed the voluntary contributions of an advisory board of occupational therapists, psychologists, pharmacists, psychiatrists, nurses, marriage and family counselors, and educators who were gracious and willing to be involved early on in this project in the trust that it would become a useful book.

ADVISORY BOARD

Mary Brinson, MA, OTR
Director of Program Development
Department of Occupational Therapy
Butler Hospital, Providence

Roxanne Castaneda, MS, OTR/L
Director, Community Forensic
  Evaluation Program and Resource
  Development
Clifton T. Perkins Hospital Center
Jessup, MD

Phyllis Connolly, PhD, RN, CS
Professor
San Jose State University

Joseph Cosgrove, MD
Formerly, Department of Psychiatry
San Francisco General Hospital

Patricia Crist, PhD, OTR
Chair and Professor
Department of Occupational Therapy
Duquesne University, Pittsburgh

Charles E. Gallagher, MA, OTR/L
Occupational Therapist
Delaware County Intermediate Unit
Media, PA
Clinical Assistant Professor
Thomas Jefferson University, Philadelphia

Linda Gutterman, OTR
Director of Rehabilitation and
  Wholistic Health Service
Village Center for Care
AIDS Day Treatment Program
New York City

Susan Haiman, MPS, OTR/L, FAOTA
Assistant Professor and Academic
  Coordinator of Clinical Education
Philadelphia College of Pharmacy and
  Science

Vivian Imperiale, MA
Client Services Manager
Community Vocational Enterprises
San Francisco
Past President of the California
  Alliance for the Mentally Ill (CAMI)

Mark Leary
Deputy Chief of Psychiatry
San Francisco General Hospital
Assistant Clinical Professor
University of California at San Francisco

Lela Llorens, PhD, OTR, FAOTA
Professor Emerita
San Jose State University
Consultant, Occupational Therapy and
  Gerontology

Ardath McDermott, MS, OTR
Lecturer
San Jose State University

Julie McGruder, BS, MA, MSED, OTR
Professor
The University of Puget Sound
Tacoma, WA

Christina A. Peterson, MLIS
Life Sciences Librarian
San Jose State University

Annette Pinto, OTR
Staff Therapist
San Francisco General Hospital
Gay, Lesbian and HIV Focus Unit

Judy Polito, OTR
Occupational Therapist
Conditional Release Program
San Bernadino County Behavioral
  Health
San Bernadino, CA

Victoria Schindler, MA, OTR
Director of Rehabilitation Services
Forensic Psychiatric Hospital
West Trenton, NJ

Linda Schmieder, PhD
Consultant/Private Practice
Prescott, AZ

Patricia Scott, MA, OTR/L
Assistant Professor
University of Florida

Susan Stark, MSOT, OTR/C
Washington University Medical School
St. Louis

Mary Stowell, PhD, CMHC, OTR
Private Practice
Bainbridge Island, WA

Gary Viale, PharmD, BCPD
Assistant Director of Pharmacy
Santa Clara Valley Health and Hospital
  System
Assistant Clinical Professor
University of California at San Francisco

PART I

The Mental Health Arena

The Occupational Therapy Process in Mental Health

Anne MacRae and Elizabeth Cara

Key Terms

culture

occupation

temporality

third-party reimbursement

Chapter Outline

Introduction
The Philosophy of Occupational Therapy
The Occupational Therapy Process
    Relationship
    Activity
    Environment
    Additional Methods
    Outcomes
Considerations in the Process
    Culture
    Temporality
Summary

Introduction

Occupational therapy (OT) is a generalist field with a number of specialty areas. The core concepts of the profession bind OT practitioners together and provide a unique professional identity, regardless of practice setting. Nevertheless, within practice settings and specialty areas there are varying representations of the occupational therapy practice and different aspects of the OT process may take priority. This chapter describes the authors' interpretation of the occupational therapy process in the mental health arena. While the concepts discussed here are relevant to occupational therapy practice in any setting, emphasis is placed on the psychosocial considerations of the OT process.

THE PHILOSOPHY OF OCCUPATIONAL THERAPY

As with other health professionals, occupational therapists adhere to different schools of thought for the planning of treatment. There are, however, basic philosophical premises underlying occupational therapy, which foster a sense of professional identity and guide practice. In order to understand the occupational therapy process, it is important to have some consensus on the underlying philosophy of occupational therapy, which is the unifying force of the profession.

The Representative Assembly of the American Occupational Therapy Association (AOTA) outlined the philosophical base of occupational therapy as follows:

> Using their capacity for intrinsic motivation, human beings are able to influence their physical and mental health and their social and physical environment through purposeful activity. Human life includes a process

of continuous adaptation. Adaptation is a change in function that promotes survival and self-actualization. (Cited in Hopkins, 1988, p. 38)

The concept of **occupation** is central to occupational therapy. Nevertheless,
the term itself has been used in the literature in various, sometimes ambiguous, ways. We concur with the position of the AOTA (1995) that occupations
involve mental abilities and skills but do not always include an associated observable or physical behavior. In the OT process, one of the ultimate goals of
treatment is the developing, nurturing, and restoring of occupations.

> As the patient executes and fulfills his or her choice, the therapist learns
> about the healing power of occupation. Occupational choice rekindles
> the will to live, and mobilizes the mind to discipline the body, in enact-
> ing the creative processes associated with reversing disability. (Rogers,
> 1983, p. 609)

It is the performance aspects of occupation that have most often been discussed in the OT literature, but these are more accurately described as "activities."

Three major, closely related themes are prevalent in the occupational therapy literature. The first is the use of purposeful activity that includes activities that have personal and cultural meaning and provide a basis for
"exploration and learning, practicing and achieving mastery" (Hopkins &
Tiffany, 1988, p. 94). Yerxa, following a humanistic-phenomenologic perspective, stated, "Occupational therapy's use of 'meaningful' and 'purposeful'
activity places value upon the *patient's* view of meaning" (1979, p. 27).

A second theme of occupational therapy is the premise of occupational performance, which is the "accomplishment of tasks related to self-care/self-main-
tenance, work/education, play/leisure, and rest/relaxation" (Christiansen &
Baum, 1991, p. 855). The relationship between purposeful activity and occupational performance is both practical and philosophical. On a practical level,
occupational therapists use purposeful activities as treatment methods to improve a patient's performance of self-care, work, and leisure skills. On a philosophical level, there is a belief that purposeful activities positively influence
an individual's occupational performance. This was expressed by Reilly, who
stated that "man, through the use of his hands as they are energized by mind
and will, can influence the state of his own health" (1962, p. 2), and rephrased
by Barris, Kielhofner, and Watts: "The fundamental occupational therapy hypothesis is that people can become competent and confident through what
they do" (1988, p. 107).

Central to both purposeful activity and occupational performance is the
concept of "doing." In their seminal article, "Doing and Becoming: Purposeful Action and Self-Actualization," Fidler and Fidler stated:

The word doing is selected to convey the sense of performing, producing or causing. It is purposeful action in contrast to random activity in that the action is directed toward the intrapersonal (testing a skill), the interpersonal (clarifying a relationship), or the nonhuman (creating an end product). (1978, p. 305)

The third major theme in occupational therapy is interaction with the environment. The conceptualization of the environment as significant in the OT process can be found in the historical writings of the profession and in every major frame of reference used in occupational therapy.

The concept of environment used in this chapter is limited to the nonhuman elements of space and objects and their influence on human interaction. This is conceptually different than the definitions currently found in the OT literature. Based on systems thinking and the extensive influence of the model of human occupation, the term *environment* is usually described as everything external to the individual. For example, Christiansen and Baum (1991) include the concepts of space and associated objects, cultural influences, social relationships, and resources as part of a prescribed environmental assessment. Our concern with this kind of taxonomy of the environment is that it dilutes the significance of the individual and the relationships of the individual. Although systems theory specifically dictates that all aspects of a system are connected and related, our preference is to highlight and focus the interrelationships of the occupational therapy process by differentiating relationships from environment.

THE OCCUPATIONAL THERAPY PROCESS

The process described in this chapter has several facets that are unique to occupational therapy, but we freely acknowledge that ideas from several disciplines, including psychology, sociology, and education, have contributed to the development of the occupational therapy process. Nevertheless, a discipline can retain its unique identity by grounding a multitude of different ideas in its common philosophy.

Figure 1-1 describes the elements of the occupational therapy process specific to mental health practice, including its initiation, methods, and outcomes.[1] We identify the core methods of occupational therapy as relationship, activity, and environment. However, it should be emphasized that these methods are not necessarily distinct entities — all affect each other and all overlap.

The initiation of the OT process has traditionally been considered to be the referral to occupational therapy. In the professions' early history, occu-

---

[1]In presenting figure 1-1, the authors wish to acknowledge Lela Llorens, Ph.D., O.T.R., F.A.O.T.A., who greatly influenced our thinking about this process through her writings and teachings.

INITIATION

Referral and case finding

Determination of services required

Identification of strengths and deficits

Goal setting

METHODS/PROCEDURES

Core methods

    Therapist-Client Relationship

    Selected Activity to facilitate occupational performance

    Environmental manipulation and adaptation

Additional methods

    Psychoeducation

    Home programs

    Family instruction

    Specialized technologies

OUTCOME

Development and restoration of occupations

Improvement or maintenance of occupational function (rehabilitation)

Improvement or maintenance of quality of life

Stabilization and prevention

Figure 1-1. Elements of the Occupational Therapy Process

pational therapy was initiated by a medical prescription (Dunton & Licht, 1950), and referrals by physicians are still generally considered necessary for **third-party reimbursement.** However, occupational therapists have achieved some level of autonomy from medicine and often actively seek cases rather than depending on the passive process of referrals. This trend, coupled with increasing consumer involvement and patient activism, has opened many avenues for the initiation of the OT process. For example, in the OT psychosocial clinic at San Jose State University, over half of the clients are self-referred. Prospective clients hear about the clinic through friends or a variety of community- or hospital-based programs, but the initial contact with the clinic and the request for services come from the individual client. Moreover, clients who self-initiate the process often have a higher level of investment in its success.

After the referral, it is still necessary for the occupational therapist to determine if the individual is a candidate for occupational therapy. In other words, does occupational therapy have anything to offer this client? The determination of needed services will vary depending on the setting, but it is accomplished through a combination of data-gathering techniques. These may include a review of the client's psychiatric history from a medical chart or other health care records, formal and informal conversations with other clinicians, a family interview, an initial client interview, and formal evaluations conducted by the occupational therapist. The result of this determination must show the specific need for occupational therapy by identifying real or potential deficits in occupational performance and not merely provide information on diagnosis and symptoms. Another facet of the occupational therapy process is the need to identify and utilize a patient's strengths rather than only deficits. In her Eleanor Clark Slagle Lecture, Joan Rogers explained: "After gleaning a clear perception of the patient's problems, the therapist then begins to search for cues indicative of the health of the patient as avidly as the search was conducted to identify dysfunction" (1983, p. 604). This is one characteristic of OT that differentiates it from medical practice (Devereaux, 1984).

Goal setting is then undertaken in conjunction with the client and accomplished as part of the treatment-planning process. This is also a facet of the OT process that has changed because of increased patient activism and involvement. Goals should primarily be identified by the individual client or patient as much as possible, with facilitation by the occupational therapist. The investment and involvement on the part of the client increases the possibility that the goals will be personally meaningful. In the authoritarian model of OT, the occupational therapist determined the goals and administered the therapy accordingly. This concept of the therapist as expert — who knows what is best for the client — is considered archaic and can be counterproductive. This does not mean that the occupational therapist does not have expert knowledge or insights that the client might lack. It simply means that goal setting is a cooperative venture that needs to identify the patient's personal goals.

Relationship

Themes of relationship in occupational therapy are found embedded in various concepts, such as the therapeutic use of self, use of the self in relationship, and clinical reasoning (Fleming, 1991; Kielhofner, 1995; Mattingly, 1991b; Peloquin, 1990; Schwartz, 1991). The emphasis implied in the therapeutic use of self in relationship is on the self and the skills of the occupational therapist. The emphasis implied in clinical reasoning is on understanding the client and, to a lesser extent, the dynamic interplay in the here and now between therapist and client. Being conscious of self is considered a skill, along with other personal attributes and communication skills, that is utilized in the interaction between patient and therapist. Although the emphasis is on awareness in the relationship with the client, the therapist is emphasized; that is, the accumulated and learned skills of the therapist are carefully applied to the client.

In *Willard and Spackman's Occupational Therapy* (Hopkins & Smith, 1993), Gibson and Richert discuss the personal/professional self and the importance of the relationship to the treatment (1993, pp. 557–565). They focus on the awareness of the therapist in developing a trusting relationship and also mention interpersonal issues of the client and the therapist that may challenge a therapeutic relationship. In another chapter, Schwartzberg elaborates on the therapeutic, or conscious, use of self and adds the importance of being aware of subjective responses as useful for understanding how the therapist or others may be responding to the client (1993, pp. 269–274). However, she declares that one's subjective responses (which are usually unconscious) may not be in the client's best interest. We take the view that subjective responses are central to any relationship, and therefore, unconscious, subjective thoughts and feelings (as realized through the process of self-reflection) should always be considered important, and particularly in psychiatric occupational therapy. Our thinking is supported by contemporary thought from different fields, as well as from early literature in psychiatric occupational therapy.

Christiansen and Baum, in a useful analysis of the form of a relationship, discuss a sociological view (1991, p. 153). The dimensions of a relationship are content, form, availability, strength, and symmetry. Also discussed are the setting and the person's characteristics, presumably both those of the patient and client. This analysis of the form of a relationship describes group norms and roles but not a relationship as experienced by two separate people who bring to it their separate, subjective worldviews.

Mosey discusses the conscious use of self as "the manipulation of one's responses to assist a client" (1986, p. 200). She, too, emphasizes the important qualities of the therapist, including self-awareness, empathy, flexibility, humor, honesty, compassion, and humility. The relationship is considered to be a collaborative process, and some issues that may arise are considered. We support the efficacy of these attitudes of the therapist in the relationship, and we would expand the emphasis to encompass the impact of the client and the dyadic exchange on the therapist's attitudes.

Denton perhaps comes closest to our concept of relationship in describing the impact of the therapist on the patient. She describes the conscious use of self as "the deliberate use of one's own responses to the patient as part of the treatment process" (1987, p. 148). Therapists are said to help restore patients' self-esteem through an attitude of respect and acceptance that they convey to the patients. Self-esteem is also enhanced through the way in which a task or activity is presented to the patient. In addition, successful use of the self in the relationship is attributed to therapists modeling (providing a model of) a "mature, competent and admirable person" (1987, p. 150).

More recently, OT literature has shifted its emphasis from the use of self to understanding the meanings that clients present. For example, Kielhofner (1995) and Mattingly (1991a, 1991b) focus on understanding and paying careful attention to the narratives, or metaphors, of the client. Peloquin defines the vision of the therapeutic relationship as one of competence and caring, involving equal emphasis on the clients' visions. "Recommitment to regarding the patient as a vital partner . . . can lead to exchanges marked by mutuality, caring and competence" (1990, p. 21). Fleming (1991) and Schwartz (1991) discuss clinical reasoning based on images that one holds of the client and can project for the client's future. Occupational therapy reflects other clinical professions that increasingly focus on the perspective of the patient/client (Cottrell, 1993). Mattingly (1991a) suggests that therapists use narrative to hear the clients' stories and understand their ways of dealing with disability. Mattingly further states that "a narrative model of reasoning, as opposed to scientific reasoning in the traditional sense, is fundamental to the thinking of occupational therapists" (1991a, p. 998). Frank (1996) advocates for the use of various methods of life history to understand the patient's perspective:

> Broadly defined, the life history is a narrative approach in which empirical methods are used to reconstruct and interpret the lives of ordinary persons. Life histories, as a genre, can include case histories, life-charts, life stories, hermeneutic case reconstruction, therapeutic emplotment, and other biographical methods. (1996, p. 252)

In summary, the relationship in occupational therapy has been defined in terms of:

— the therapist and the conscious use of self as a tool,

— the collaborative, interactive process and the therapist's communication skills,

— challenges brought up by the attitudes and personality qualities in the client, and

— understanding of the client's world and the meanings clients convey to us.

The Relationship as Core Process.   Until recently, the OT literature has failed to emphasize the responsibility of the therapist as a reflective person who is impacted by, and reactive to, the client. Not only should therapists strive to understand their clients' meaning and subjective world, but at the same time, they should strive to understand their own subjective world as it is impacted by their clients. In other words, therapists should understand that the clients' meanings are filtered through their own subjective world in the here and now interaction. Additionally, as hinted at by Peloquin (1990), the therapist may represent a specific type of person for the client, who represents client's needs or desires (in Peloquin's example, competence and caring). Therapists should attempt to understand what they represent for their clients. So, ultimately, the needs, desires, hopes, and meanings — the subjective worlds — of the client and the therapist contribute to the therapeutic relationship.

Both worlds, and what is continually being created, should be acknowledged. The relationship, the environment, and the activity are equally important and together constitute the occupational therapy process in psychiatry.

> Historically relationship was included as a core method along with occupation and environment specifically in mental health practice. Perhaps the most important key in treatment implementation is the therapeutic relationship between you and the patient. This relationship is frequently conceived of as the most important ingredient regardless of the type of therapy employed. . . . The conscious use of self, or deliberate use of one's own response to the patient as part of the treatment process, is regarded as a legitimate tool of OT, and is embraced, in some form, by all OT frames of reference. (Denton, 1987, p. 148)

The proceedings of the 1956 Allenberry Conference on the Function and Preparation of the Psychiatric Occupational Therapist were published in 1959 (West, 1959). Throughout these proceedings the emphasis is on therapeutic use of self and connection in the relationship. The occupational therapists emphasized the importance of the initial contact with the patient and believed that the first contact would determine day-to-day work and also the final results of treatment (West, 1959, p. 3).

Much of the proceedings discussed the use of self as a tension reduction or need satisfying object, as found in the then popular psychological theories of motivation, ego psychology, and object relations. This is not the case today, though there continues to be an emphasis on therapists' self-awareness, ability to differentiate their own needs from those of the client, and ability to bring warmth, understanding, flexibility, and objectivity to the treatment situation (West, 1959, p. 27). The participants defined clearly the difference between a professional and a friendship relationship. They also went so far as to define activities as a means to an end, which is quite an opposite viewpoint from the context of occupational therapy today.

We do not advocate a return to the emphasis on relationship over activity. We do, however, advocate that an elevation of relationship be included along with activity and environment in the occupational therapy process. Our emphasis on interpersonal or empathic skills is in addition to, not instead of, activity. It is based on earlier philosophy in psychiatric occupational therapy that recognized the importance of knowing oneself as one aspect of the interpersonal relationship.

Contemporary Related Trends in Psychology.   The movement in occupational therapy toward understanding the worlds of clients through their narratives is mirrored in other fields. In psychology it is called constructivism (Neimeyer & Mahoney, 1995) or social constructionism (Gergen, 1985).

> [Constructivism] is a panoply of perspectives cutting across the human sciences and humanities whose common threads include an acknowledgment of divergent realities, socially constituted and historically situated. . . . Language, in this view actually constitutes the structures of social reality, requiring the cultivation of new approaches [such as narrative]. (Neimeyer & Mahoney, 1995, p. 13)

Constructivism in psychology includes a family of theories and therapies emphasizing that human beings are active in constructing their own experience, that the processes responsible for the construction of their own experience (perception and memory) operate at unconscious levels of awareness, and that development and experience reflect an ongoing operation of self-organizing.

The social constructionist movement is an aspect of constructivism in psychology that explains a way of thinking about how professionals in different disciplines acquire knowledge of, or understand, the world. It acknowledges the constraints of language and the fact that understanding is an active, cooperative effort of persons in relationship. In other words, understanding is mutually and socially constructed, not the product of empirical research of a separate object on a separate subject, which means that "rather than looking toward natural sciences and experimental psychology for kinship, an affinity is rapidly sensed with a range of what may be termed interpretive disciplines, that is, disciplines chiefly concerned with rendering accounts of human meaning systems" (Gergen, 1985, p. 270). Occupational therapy can thus be included with non-experimental psychology, sociology, anthropology, history, philosophy, and literary studies.

Contemporary trends in psychoanalysis and psychoanalytical psychology also acknowledge the mutuality of meaning: the interpretation of meaning for clients is a mutual process including both the client and the therapist. Kohut (1971, 1977; Kohut & Wolfe, 1978) and his colleagues recognize the importance of the client's narratives as understood through empathy and introspection by the therapist. They emphasize empathy with the other person as a basis for understanding and enhanced interpersonal communication. They discuss the importance of listening and understanding and explain how the process leads to an enhanced self-concept and further positive communication. The interpersonal approach required in all interactions, whether individual, group, or evaluative, is to maintain empathy and respond in an empathic way. This means always striving to understand the needs of the client. This is in line with recent occupational therapy emphases on the client and his or her meaning systems. This theoretical approach also recognizes the impact of the therapist on the client in here-and-now interactions. In this approach the function of the therapist for the client is also delineated.

Stolorow and his collaborators (Atwood & Stolorow, 1984; Stolorow, Atwood, & Brandchaft, 1994) acknowledge and investigate the importance of both the client and therapist in a reciprocal and mutual system and consider all meaning arising in a dynamic intersubjective context. The intersubjective process emphasizes the interplay between the personal universes of the client and the therapist. Meaning arises at the intersection of the two worlds. In this context, all aspects of meaning are consistently contributed by both people, who thus influence each other. The intersubjective process, then, necessitates the critical element of ongoing self-reflection by the therapist on how he or she is affected by the subjective meanings of the client and how this in turn leads to his or her ability to influence the client.

CASE ILLUSTRATION: JULIA — THE IMPORTANCE OF THE RELATIONSHIP IN THE CONTEXT OF OCCUPATION

Julia was expecting to be discharged from the partial hospitalization program in anticipation of returning to her job in marketing management. In occupational therapy (OT) groups her behavior became more demanding, and she became insistent on getting help and answers from the therapist right away. In addition , she began to ask for extra materials for her projects, as well as extra time from the occupational therapist outside the OT groups for help in completing her projects. She began to brashly demand praise for projects that had been finished rather haphazardly. At the same time, in the occupational therapy "transitioning" group, she refused to take credit for her insightful comments regarding herself and others and instead attributed her ability to the skill of the occupational therapist, who was also the group leader.

The therapist was puzzled by Julia's behavior, as she had enjoyed a warm relationship with her. She liked Julia and believed she had been helpful to her and that Julia had had a similarly satisfying experience. She thought that naturally Julia might have some fears of leaving and possibly was asking for help in recognizing that she could indeed function "outside." Therefore, the occupational therapist set limits on extra demands for time and material. While recognizing that Julia had worked hard on her project, she attempted to assist her in reasoning and to go over the step-by-step planning that Julia had used while working on the project. The occupational therapist also downplayed her own group skills, thus attributing all treatment gains to Julia. She hoped to help Julia recognize that indeed she was ready to leave and had the skills and resources to function independently.

Julia became increasingly demanding regarding projects and time, haphazard in the way she completed projects, and unwilling to admit her insightful abilities, while increasingly praising the therapist's group skills. Her behavior became more arrogant and impulsive, while she also seemed increasingly distant and somewhat surly. The occupational therapist concentrated on understanding Julia's words and actions. She reflected on her own thoughts and feelings and what her own words and behaviors might convey to Julia. The therapist considered what she might mean to Julia. She realized that perhaps Julia's projects were symbols of her stay at the partial hospitalization and served as a connection to the people there. Julia knew that she could function independently but wanted to make sure she kept something that she had personally fabricated when she left. The goal was to finish. In addition, perhaps making demands on the therapist's time and offering lavish praise while denying her own positive attributes were Julia's way of conveying her gratitude and sense of connection. If Julia were too independent or competent, perhaps, she feared, the therapist would cease to think of her with warmth and caring.

Based on her self-reflection and empathy, the occupational therapist changed her responses. She let Julia know that she understood the urgency of finishing projects and acceded to some of her extra demands. She also began to graciously accept Julia's compliments regarding her group skills. Julia became less demanding and calmer. Now she was able to assess her stay at the program positively and looked forward to discharge based on the knowledge that the staff would remain caring, responsive, and interested in her.

Discussion

When the OTR thought about her function for Julia and attempted to empathize with Julia's experience, she responded in a way that helped Julia transition from the hospital. The case illustrates the mutual influence of the therapist and client on each other and the importance of understanding the meanings conveyed by each other's actions.

Activity

Occupational therapists have historically used activities as a primary method of intervention beginning with the guiding principles of Adolph Meyer (1922). Although there seems to be consensus among occupational therapists about the profession's role in promoting occupation, through the years the interest in the use of activity as a primary method of treatment has waxed and waned. It is our view that activity is an essential part of the OT process, especially in mental health practice. In 1954, Misbach Edgerton stated, "In an age that is becoming increasingly mechanized, it is a healthy thing to retain the time-honored hand skills for their value in mental hygiene and as hobbies, if for no other reason" (1954, p. 48). These words ring even more true as we approach the millennium. Cynkin and Mazur Robinson concur and add, "Today, we still affirm, in our professional documents, our theoretical and philosophical speculations, and our legal definitions that activities are the distinctive hallmark of occupational therapy. . . . [This] commitment . . . implicitly assumes that *dysfunction is reversible through engagement in activities*" (1990, p. 3, emphasis in original). Leary explains:

Activities are the essence of human existence. Through activity people establish their values and goals. Activity-based programmes have a role in all levels of health care; promoting wellness and personal growth, preventing health problems, meeting health needs, in rehabilitation, and in maintaining abilities and management. At most levels they can play a part in helping people find new directions for their lives. (1994, p. 3)

Understanding the characteristics of activity allows the therapist to generate new ideas and adapt old ones and make the therapeutic process fun, useful, and meaningful for clients. The following is a discussion of these characteristics and how activities can be used to best meet therapeutic goals.

Passive versus Active. Examples of passive activities include movies, lectures, listening to music, spectator events, and guest speakers. Active tasks imply "doing" or participating and include arts and crafts, games, and engagement in a variety of activities of daily living such as grooming and cooking. Passive occupations usually do not hinder participation because of limitations. They are nonthreatening and may appeal to various particular interests or learning styles. They may be enjoyed at a symbolic level and often have a shared social function. On the other hand, many clients need more stimulation in order to attend to a task. Passive occupations generally do not address deficits of motor or sensory problems. Moreover, because there is no experiential (tactile) component, people with cognitive impairment or tactile learners may not derive much benefit from passive occupation.

Fabricated versus Prefabricated. Examples of fabricated activities are games designed by the therapist and crafts to be made from raw materials. Prefabricated activities include board games and crafts to be made from kits. Fabricated activities are usually less expensive and can be tailored to the individual. These activities also have the potential of being more creative, because of their inherent adaptability. One limitation of fabricated activities, particularly in crafts, is that the end product may not look as pleasing to the patient as a prefabricated craft. This is significant because the intrinsic motivation and satisfaction, as well as the experience of success, are very important to the therapeutic process. The most serious limitation of fabricated activities is the amount of the therapist's time that is needed for construction. As occupational therapists experience greater levels of economic pressure to increase productivity and contain costs, it is likely that fabrication will become a diminished art in the field. Ideally, the choice of fabricated or prefabricated activity is based on the specific therapeutic needs of the client.

Simple versus Complex. Simple tasks may increase a client's self-esteem because of the increased likelihood that the task can be completed. Complex tasks may be too frustrating for some clients, causing them to give up. Simple tasks are commonly used in OT clinics because of limited resources of time and space. However, they have the potential of being viewed as boring or childish, and of providing insufficient opportunity to learn and grow. The more complex the task, the more pride a client will have in being able to do it (providing he or she has the ability to complete the task). Occupational therapists are specifically trained in grading activities to achieve the proper degree of complexity.

Structured versus Unstructured.   Some activities are, by definition, more structured then others. For example, finger painting is very unstructured, and games with rules are generally structured. Unstructured activities are usually more creative, but many people with behavioral difficulties, poor motivation, or limited functional ability need structure in order to complete an activity. Regardless of the activity, the primary responsibility for the structure comes from the therapist. It is a mistake to assume that the nature of the activity itself will provide sufficient structure.

CASE ILLUSTRATION: ARLENE — THE STRUCTURED ACTIVITY

Arlene is a 27-year-old woman currently experiencing a manic episode. Her first two days in the hospital were spent in seclusion, but the treatment team now feels that she is sufficiently stable to attend the occupational therapy groups.

The occupational therapy intern decided to provide Arlene with a ceramic slip mold to create a cup. Arlene's response was: "Great! I want to make a 144-piece Queen Anne's dining set!" She proceeded to open every cabinet in the clinic to find supplies. When Arlene found some metal used for jewelry making, she decided she also wanted to make silverware for her dining set.

Initially, the occupational therapy intern tried to follow Arlene around the clinic and limit the amount of supplies she was taking. When it became clear that the limits were not enough, the intern changed the activity for the day. After coaxing Arlene to sit down, she provided her with an 11 by 14 inch piece of drawing paper and colored markers. Her instructions to Arlene were, "You can draw whatever you want, but stay within the boundaries of the paper."

Discussion

A craft such as pouring ceramic slip into a mold would generally be considered highly structured, but in this case, the lack of specific guidelines and instructions at the beginning of the activity created a potentially chaotic situation. Moreover, the process does not give immediate gratification, which is important for this client. On the other hand, free-hand drawing is quite unstructured and potentially creative, but the activity was given structure by the provision of clear expectations.

Long Term versus Short Term.   A project may be considered long term if it is going to take more than four or five sessions to complete. The advantages of long-term projects are that they give clients something to look forward to in clinic, the end products are usually more complex, and there may be more investment in them. Limitations of long-term projects include the possibility that clients will lose interest or become frustrated by the complexity and lack of immediate gratification. Storage space for long-term projects is also a problem in many clinics. Another significant limitation of the long-term project in the current health care environment is that in the case of many clients, it is likely that they will be discharged before the project is completed. As a result, occupational therapists often feel that they have no choice but to present short-term projects. One solution is to have a long-term task as an ongoing backup project or select an ongoing task that has short-term components and contributes to the community nature of the clinic. The ownership would be credited to the clinic rather than individual client. For example, in the OT psychosocial clinic at San Jose State University, the group has been working on a large latch-hook mural for three years. It is rarely used in a planned group activity; rather, the latch hook is left out on the table every clinic day during the free social time. It is the expectation that ongoing clients will instruct new clients and new student therapists in latch-hook technique.

CASE ILLUSTRATION: DARRYL — THE OT PROJECTS

Darryl has a diagnosis of schizophrenia and a history of recurrent hospitalizations at the county general hospital. During acute episodes, he typically has a short attention span and has difficulty completing projects. Nevertheless, Darryl reports that he enjoys the activities, and he always reminds the occupational therapist which projects he did during his prior hospitalization.

During one of Darryl's recent hospitalizations, the occupational therapist introduced an activity called the diversity quilt. Each group participant was instructed to create a 6 by 6 inch square for the quilt that represented a cultural idea that he or she valued. Various media were provided, including felt, markers, fabric scraps, and sequins. The occupational therapist helped clients identify ideas for the quilt square and suggested techniques for each participant in order to facilitate the completion of a successful project. Some clients finished a square in 15 minutes while others took the entire hour session to finish their project. Darryl worked on his quilt square for about 20 minutes, making a felt representation of the flag of Kenya. The therapist requested that the quilt squares remain in the clinic and explained that eventually they would be sewn together and displayed in the clinic.

Darryl was readmitted to the hospital three months later. He noticed the displayed quilt as soon as he came into the clinic room and proceeded to examine every square until he found the one he had completed. He also pointed out his completed quilt square to all the staff and patients on the unit.

Discussion

This illustrates how a traditional long-term project can also be used in a short-term way and how clients can become invested in an ongoing project that symbolizes a community and their valued part in it.

Process versus Product.   It is possible to use the same material for very different kinds of results and therapeutic goals, depending on the goal of the project. For example, clay can be very free form or structured with molds. Similarly, playing in the water is a process, while swimming in a race is a product. A process-oriented group can be less threatening because clients do not feel that their work is being judged. Moreover, the therapist can present the activity in a way that emphasizes its purpose as for their immediate enjoyment. Clients may feel freer to experiment if there will be no visible end product. Process-oriented activities can also be used for very specific therapeutic goals such as using scented massage oils for tactile and olfactory stimulation. Product-oriented activities often provide an experience of success for patients. The product can fulfil some roles that some people with disabilities find difficult to fill otherwise. For example, clients may make presents for significant others, which allows them to take the role of provider even if unemployed or living on limited income. In some cases, the end product may simply be a personal statement of accomplishment.

CASE ILLUSTRATION: SOPHIA — THE CHRISTMAS ACTIVITIES

Sophia, a 36-year-old Latina woman with a history of recurrent depression, is an active member of a clubhouse model treatment center. The OT group decided to sponsor a Christmas party for the members of the clubhouse, staff, and clubhouse supporters. Initially, Sophia was reluctant to participate in any of the planning activities and would not discuss her reticence.

At the beginning of one of the clubhouse sessions, the occupational therapist conducted a process-oriented group as a prelude to a group discussion. This particular group provided sensory stimulation using scented oils with a winter holiday theme, such as cinnamon, pine, and peppermint. Each participant was requested to identify the scent in several opaque bottles and share a memory elicited by it. The feelings described in the shared memories of the group were varied, including happy, funny, sad, tragic, and angry. Sophia told the group that she had many happy memories of cooking with her mother during the Christmas season and felt it was an important holiday to celebrate as part of her Catholic heritage. Toward the end of the group session, Sophia began crying and related a story about her drunken father beating her mother on a Christmas Eve. The group was very supportive of her and she was encouraged to further explore the issues that had been raised with her psychotherapist.

Later the same day, Sophia volunteered to chair the decorating committee for the Christmas party and began work with the occupational therapist on planning a series of product-oriented groups, including craft sessions to make table centerpieces and ornaments for the tree.

Discussion

In this illustration, a group with products — various scents — was used to stimulate a process of remembering and symbolizing. It led Sophia to feel more interested in holiday activities and to become an initiator and planner, roles she had previously rejected.

Individual versus Group (and Variations).   Although most occupational therapists in mental health settings run groups, that does not necessarily mean that they always employ group projects. For example, an arts and crafts group may actually be a group of people working on individual projects, each of a completely different nature, whereas a team sport is a true group activity. Individual activities provide for more independence and choice; therefore, they may be more motivating for some individuals than group activities, but care must be taken to avoid isolation. Individual activities may be a prelude to group involvement for particularly vulnerable clients or those with acute psychosis.

CASE ILLUSTRATION: INDIVIDUAL AND GROUP TREATMENT

Thomas is a 22-year-old man hospitalized for the first time with a severe psychotic episode. Upon admission, Thomas was extremely delusional, frightened, and paranoid. He refused to come out of his room and paced the floor incessantly. The next day, he appeared to be calmer but continued to refuse all participation in the therapeutic milieu. The occupational therapist learned from the man's mother that he was quite a good artist. Thomas barely tolerated the staffs' initial attempts to talk with him, but he did allow the occupational therapist to leave some art supplies in his room, which he used. Over the next several days, the therapist checked in with Thomas several times a day and discussed his current drawings. He was regularly invited to the OT groups, which he continued to shun. On his fifth day of hospitalization, Thomas wandered into the OT clinic room to look for more supplies; he stayed and observed the group for 15 minutes. Gradually over the next several days, Thomas attended the groups for longer periods of time and began to participate in the activities, although he remained withdrawn and passive when in groups, preferring to work alone on his artwork. Occupational therapy treatment goals included: instruction in symptom management techniques, increasing reality orientation, and structured use of time, as well as the development of socialization and communication skills.

Discussion

The intervention with Thomas showed a gradation from solitary activities to tolerating group activities. (An unmet goal is participation in socially interactive groups.) However, this gradation does not imply that group involvement is necessarily superior to individual activity or is even always desirable. The ability to occupy oneself with activity when alone is very important for many individuals with mental illness, and the variations of individual and group activities have therapeutic potential for differing goals.

Internal versus External Motivators.   How an activity is presented often makes a difference in the clients' motivation level. External motivation may include participation in a token economy or the earning of privileges by attending activities. Sometimes, however, there is a fine line between what is intrinsically and what is extrinsically motivating. For example, clients with major depression may not want to do anything positive for themselves, so starting out by having them do things for others and then modifying the activities to have them do something for themselves may be appropriate. Moreover, doing something positive for someone else often allows a client to maintain a sense of usefulness and allows him or her to have fun participating in activities without feeling childish.

CASE ILLUSTRATION: THE MOTIVATION OF ARTHUR JONES

Arthur Jones, who is 72, is currently being treated for major depression and has been in a geriatric day treatment center for the past three weeks. He has consistently refused to actively participate in occupational therapy, although he does attend the groups to "watch." The occupational therapist arranged to have a group of young school children visit the center and perform a harvest festival pageant. Prior to their visit the occupational therapist suggested that the client group make thank-you presents for the children. Since it was near Halloween, it was decided to bake cookies and package them in cloth "ghosts." The preparations took three sessions. With the therapist's encouragement, Arthur begrudgingly started to participate halfway through the first session. By the third session, however, he was initiating parts of the task and socializing with other clients. After the children's performance, Arthur took charge of distributing the presents. His affect brightened considerably during the interaction with the children and his overall participation in subsequent OT groups improved.

Discussion

It is unlikely that Arthur would have engaged in this activity on his own. Doing something for another, in this case children, provided a sense of purpose and meaning otherwise lacking in his mind. In the process, Arthur was able to experience joy and productivity, which had a sustained effect. It is possible that the changes noted in Arthur's affect and behavior are at least partially attributed to medication and spontaneous recovery. Nevertheless, this activity provided the catalyst for Arthur to experience satisfaction in occupational roles.

Environment

Occupational therapy is provided in a wide variety of treatment settings. Among the most common are inpatient hospitals with both locked and unlocked units, outpatient clinics, day treatment programs, and partial hospitalization programs. In addition, occupational therapists specializing in mental health are currently developing programs in many so called nontraditional sites, including home health care, vocational and community programs, jails and prisons, and homeless shelters. Many of these sites are discussed in chapters throughout this book, and although divergent in appearance, all are appropriate venues for occupational therapy services. For the purposes of this section, the treatment environment is described as "the clinic," but obviously, adaptations must be made in some settings. Regardless of the treatment setting and, in many cases, despite some of its limitations, occupational therapists place great importance on the environment in the OT process. This has been documented since the early writings of the profession. For example, in 1954, Wade and Franciscus stated that:

> An orderly, well-kept, attractive unit is good mental hygiene in itself and is important for the morale of patient and therapist alike. It gives to the patient a feeling of order and direction rather than one of chaos and indirection. All supplies and equipment should have a given place in which to be kept when not in use, and the therapist must assume the responsibility of seeing that each item is returned to its proper place, not merely pushed aside in a heap on a shelf until it is impossible to locate desired items as they are needed. In addition, a working area need not be drab and depressing, for with ingenuity, some inexpensive material and paint, any room can be made inviting and attractive, and many patients would enjoy working on a project, taking pride in the end result. These latter considerations are an important part of the therapist's responsibility in creating a therapeutic atmosphere. (1954, p. 83)

When arranging the clinic, an awareness of the environmental impact on occupational performance is essential. Figure 1-2 (on the next page) outlines the environmental considerations in relation to the occupational performance components, as well as a "relational" component. Although this component is not part of the occupational performance model, we added it to emphasize its significance in the OT process. It is our view that relationships are inade-

COMPONENT	ENVIRONMENTAL CONSIDERATIONS
Motor/Physical	Are all supplies in the clinic physically accessible to the clients? Is there sufficient space to engage in tasks? Are all pieces of furniture and equipment ergonomically correct for maximum health benefits? Is there outside space available for physical pursuits? Is there adequate ventilation? Is there access to rest rooms and areas for clean up? Is drinking water available for hydration?
Sensory	Is there adequate light for the tasks? Are there opportunities for multi-sensory stimulation? Are the auditory and visual stimuli balanced to prevent sensory overload? Are there safety features in place to prevent burns, cuts, etc.?
Cognitive	Are supplies presented in an orderly and familiar way? Are instructions provided at the level of the individual clients? Are there age-appropriate methods established to provide cues for clients as necessary?
Psychological	Does the environment invite safe exploration of issues? Is there space for groups to be arranged? Is the clinic seen as a pleasant and calm place to be?
Sociocultural	Is there opportunity for spontaneous interaction with others? Is there evidence that there is sensitivity to the potential diversity of the client group? Will clients be able to identify with images presented?
Spiritual	Is the clinic environment conducive to the exploration of personal meaning? Is there an atmosphere of trust and openness? Is there a sense of celebrating the specialness of humanity?
Relational	Is the therapist a model for genuineness, authenticity, humanness, responsibility and respect? Is the therapist able to engender respect and convey a sense of competence?

Figure 1-2. Occupational Performance Components and Their Environmental Considerations.

quately addressed with the sociocultural component of the occupational performance model.

An occupational therapy clinic should be a warm, inviting, and safe place. All aspects of each individual client's humanity should be recognized and acknowledged. What may seem like trivial details on the surface can greatly affect the overall "feel" of the clinic. For example, it is optimum if fresh water is available at all times. This is a gesture of courtesy and should stem from a desire to have clients in the clinic feel comfortable. It is also an acknowledgment of the problems of dehydration commonly found in people on psychotropic medication. It is therefore a tool to educate clients about symptom and side effect management, as well as for role modeling healthy nutritional habits.

Determining the level of sensory stimulation in the clinic can be difficult, especially in regard to auditory stimulation. People have very different thresholds of tolerance to sound. For some individuals, it is necessary to have a quiet room for them to engage in any task. It is especially important for the therapist to provide a quiet place to which some clients can retreat if others are engaging in a particularly noisy activity such as a project involving hammering. On the other hand, if used judiciously and carefully, sound (as in music) can enhance the therapeutic effect of an activity and the clinic environment. "Music can facilitate mood changes, alter states of awareness, modify one's consciousness and increase affective response. . . . [M]usic can be effectively used to shift a person's attention, soothe agitation and as an aid with visualization techniques" (MacRae, 1992, p. 275).

Additional Methods

We consider relationship, activity, and environment to be the core principles of the occupational therapy process. However, it is evident in the literature that OT practice is not limited to these methods. Llorens stated that "purposeful activity or occupation is not the totality of intervention that is offered by occupational therapy[;] . . . intervention include[s] counseling, educating, and providing home programs for parents and other family members" (1984, p. 33). In a mental health setting, some methods used by occupational therapists, such as psychoeducational groups, are shared by other disciplines. These include groups on symptom management, coping, and communication skills, as well as a variety of practical life-management skills. Regardless of shared responsibilities or superficial similarities, occupational therapy methods are grounded in a unique philosophical perspective.

Specialized technologies are common additional methods in practice focused on physical disabilities, but they also exist in mental health practice. These may include the use of specific computer training for the amelioration of cognitive-perceptual dysfunctions or specialized sensory integration or body work techniques, as well as a variety of alternative or nontraditional health care techniques. Because the methods that fall into this category are often not unique to occupational therapy, concern is sometimes voiced about their place in OT practice. It is our position that OT intervention must include the identified core methods, but the broad philosophy of occupational therapy, coupled with the specific needs of the individual clients, dictates the appropriateness of the use of additional methods. For example, many of the additional methods used by occupational therapists are viewed as *enabling*, meaning that they are necessary precursors to specific occupational behaviors.

The fact that occupational therapy is a generalist profession precludes the idea that all of the methods will be unique. Overlap with other professions is inevitable, and it is up to all professionals on a treatment team to not only provide their unique contributions, but in cases where there is overlap, to collaborate in a responsible way to provide quality comprehensive service in a cost-efficient manner.

Outcome

The foremost outcome of occupational therapy services is the development, improvement, or restoration of occupation. In mental health settings, the specific functional outcomes encompass the entire range of performance areas, including activities of daily living and productive and leisure activities. Many people, even those with serious and persistent mental illness, can accomplish substantial goals within these areas, with observable behavioral change. However, in some cases the outcome of occupational therapy is subtle and may take considerable time. In this era of cost containment, it is essential that occupational therapists be able to articulate such outcomes and demonstrate the need for skilled interventions. For example, in acute psychiatric settings, it is often not possible to achieve substantial change in functional performance. However, occupational therapy facilitates the stabilization process of acute episodes, allowing the patient to benefit from follow-up treatment. Activities in acute care are often enabling precursors to improved function. In some cases, acute care treatment must be viewed as part of a treatment continuum, where the outcome of the treatment only constitutes the initial part of the process, including evaluation. Because a knowledge of functional ability is crucial for appropriate discharge planning, occupational therapists are vital on an in-patient unit. Establishing lines of communication between occupational therapists treating the same client in different treatment settings allows the entire OT process to be completed.

The documentation of functional outcomes in mental health OT is also problematic because of the cyclical and sometimes chronic nature of many mental illnesses. Continued structure and support provided by occupational therapy contributes to the prevention of relapse and maintenance of function, particularly in the community. There is a current perception that it is not cost-efficient for the occupational therapist to be directly involved with clinical treatment on a long-term basis. However, the skills and experience of an occupational therapist can be invaluable in developing programs and training and supervising nonprofessionals. Although consultation and supervision are important, viable roles for OT in mental health, it is our view that occupational therapists should also retain their role as clinicians. Our specific clinical training has been shown to be effective in preventing relapse and maintaining function even within long-term settings (Lynn, Caffey, Klett, Hogarty, & Lamb, 1979), but more research is needed to verify the cost-efficiency of preventative approaches.

CONSIDERATIONS IN THE PROCESS

The two prime considerations presented in this section, culture and temporality, have been conceptualized in various ways in the OT literature, but we prefer to view these concepts as considerations in the overall OT process rather than distinct phenomena. The occupational therapy process flows in a logical sequence, but these considerations involve all aspects of the process from the initiation of services through expected outcomes.

Culture

Recent rehabilitation research has advocated the perspective that appropriate provision of services can only occur when the cultural diversity of patients, the interaction of patient culture with the culture of the provider, and the professional orientation of the western medical model are taken into consideration. (Pope-Davis, Prieto, Whitaker, & Pope-Davis, 1993, p. 838)

Cultural awareness is necessary for the delivery of all quality health care, but it has particular significance for the mental health field because of the nature of practice. Concepts of normal and abnormal behavior are the basis for psychiatric diagnosis. The definition of normality, however, can differ cross-culturally. Thus, what is normal to one culture can be abnormal to another. Since the concept of normality is undoubtedly value laden, the issue of **culture** must be addressed, not only in the treatment process, but in evaluation and diagnosis as well.

Embedded in one's culture are beliefs and attitudes regarding spirituality, family structure, gender roles, and health care, all of which affect relationships, the choice of activity, and the preferred environment. In addition, cultural values vary tremendously and must be taken into account when planning any aspect of intervention. For example, grooming in European-American culture is considered a private activity, which is usually undertaken in the bedroom or bath, but in other cultures, such as among Latina women, grooming can be a highly social activity, whereby helping each other with hair styles and makeup is considered highly desirable (Dillard et al., 1992). Figure 1-3 lists the spectrum of cultural values to be taken into consideration in the OT process. It is the responsibility of occupational therapists to educate themselves about the particular values of the cultural groups who may be the recipients of OT services.

Temporality

Temporality has been discussed in the occupational therapy literature since the inception of the profession. Indeed, Barris et al. state that the theme of time is one of the early and central concepts of occupational therapy (1988).

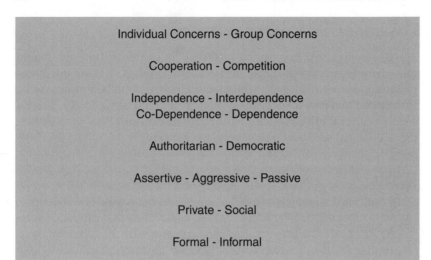

Figure 1-3.   The Spectrum of Cultural Values.

Most of the occupational therapy models and frames of reference address time in some form, as either a parameter, component, or subsystem. However, time is pervasive and does not fit neatly in any of the designed structures of OT theory. Rather than view time as a specific substructure of the OT process, we suggest that time sense be considered at every stage of the process. Although the importance of temporality has been recognized in the OT literature, it must be acknowledged that, particularly in the profession's early writings, the concept of time sense was firmly imbedded in a Western, industrialized society's concept of time. A culturally competent therapist will first determine if a client's time sense is culturally different from what is usually expected in Western society. Otherwise it is possible to erroneously assume the presence of a pathology or dysfunction when actually encountering a norm within the individual's cultural world.

Besides cultural differences, time sense varies with age and developmental stages. The conventional concept of time is based on the time sense of young to middle-age adults. However, children and the elderly, who comprise a large percentage of occupational therapy recipients, have quite a different time sense. Children tend to operate very much in the "here and now," with little appreciation or understanding of the future. The elderly also tend not to be future oriented; rather, their time sense tends to be retrospective. All aspects of the OT process must be adjusted accordingly to meet the specific needs of these populations.

Certain disorders can also markedly change a person's sense of time. Among these conditions are acute and chronic pain as well as disorders causing organic changes in the brain such as traumatic brain injury, tumors, and dementia. People with schizophrenia also show marked temporal distortion, especially in the ability to plan for the future. There is a very strong sense of being stuck in present time and living only in the moment, unable to process the events of the past or determine a future course (MacRae, 1993; Suto & Frank, 1994) . Neville (1980) also stated that the ability to project into the future is often deficient in persons with psychiatric disorders.

There are many implications for treatment in cases where the therapist has a different time sense than the person receiving services. The trends toward managed care and increased productivity in the workplace have placed a high value on a minute-increment therapy model, in which the quantity of therapy minutes is equated with the quality of the intervention. These trends must somehow be reconciled with the trends toward incorporating multicultural and individual client perspectives and needs.

Summary

This chapter describes the process of occupational therapy in mental health practice. The core methods of the occupational therapy process are relationship, activity, and environment. However, additional methods are also used, which at times overlap with those of other professions. Consideration must be given to temporality and culture in all aspects of the process.

In today's rapidly changing health care system, therapists must continue to be resourceful in order to deliver quality care. Priorities, technologies, and modes of service delivery will almost certainly change, but occupational therapists have a unique philosophy and process with which to guide changing practice and respond to current trends.

Review Questions

1. What are the unifying beliefs of occupational therapists?
2. What are unique methods of occupational therapy? What are methods that may be shared with other disciplines?
3. What is the difference between an occupation and an activity?
4. What are the desired outcomes of occupational therapy in mental health settings?
5. Describe why temporality and culture are important considerations in all aspects of the OT process.

Learning Activities

1. Look through several supply catalogs and develop inexpensive ways to create similar products. Adapt an activity designed for one purpose to the needs of a different client population.

2. Start a collection of ideas for potential OT activities. Try out a system for filing or for composing lesson plans.
3. Conduct two role-plays presenting an activity to someone acting as a client. In each play, act in the different ways listed below. Notice how the client responds in each situation.

	Situation # 1	Situation #2
Body	Slumped	Lively, open
Voice	Mumbled, low	Direct, clear
Eye contact	None	Direct
Language	Apologetic	Confident, direct
Affect	Depressed	Excited
Activity	Not prepared, delayed start	Prepared, easy to start

4. Attend an event with people of a different cultural group from your own. What value differences do you notice? How would these differences affect treatment planning in occupational therapy?

References

American Occupational Therapy Association. (1995). Position paper: Occupation. *American Journal of Occupational Therapy, 49*(10), 1015–1018.

Atwood, G., & Stolorow, R. (1984). *Structures of subjectivity: Explorations in psychoanalytic phenomenology.* Hillsdale, NJ.: Analytic Press.

Barris, R. , Kielhofner, G., & Watts, J. (1988). *Occupational therapy in psychosocial practice.* Thorofare, NJ: Slack.

Christiansen, C., & Baum, C. (1991). *Occupational therapy: Overcoming human performance deficits.* Thorofare, NJ: Slack.

Cottrell, R. F. (Ed.). (1993). *Psychosocial occupational therapy: Proactive approaches.* Rockville, MD.: American Occupational Therapy Association.

Cynkin, S., & Mazur Robinson, A. (1990). *Occupational therapy and activities health: Toward health through activities.* Boston: Little, Brown & Co.

Denton, P. (1987). *Psychiatric occupational therapy: A workbook of practical skills.* Boston: Little, Brown & Co.

Devereaux, E. (1984). Occupational therapy's challenge: The caring relationship. *American Journal of Occupational Therapy, 38,* 791–798.

Dillard, M., Andonian, L., Flores, O., Lai, L., MacRae, A., & Shakir, M. (1992). Culturally competent occupational therapy in a diversely populated mental health setting. *American Journal of Occupational Therapy, 46,* 721–726.

Dunton, W. R., & Licht, S. (Eds.) (1950). *Occupational therapy: Principles and practice.* Springfield, IL: Thomas.

Fidler, G., & Fidler, J. (1978). Doing and becoming: Purposeful action and self-actualization. *American Journal of Occupational Therapy, 32,* 305–310.

Fleming, M. H. (1991). The therapist with the three track mind. *American Journal of Occupational Therapy, 45*(11), 1007–1014.

Frank, G. (1996). Life histories in occupational therapy clinical practice. *American Journal of Occupational Therapy, 50,* 251–264.

Gergen, K. (1985). The social constructionist movement in modern psychology. *American Psychologist, 40,* 266–275.

Gibson, D., & Richert, G. (1993). The therapeutic process. In H. Hopkins & H. Smith (Eds.), *Willard and Spackman's occupational therapy* (8th ed., pp. 557–565). Philadelphia: Lippincott.

Hopkins, H. (1988). Current basis for theory and philosophy of occupational therapy. In H. Hopkins & H. Smith (Eds.), *Willard and Spackman's occupational therapy* (7th ed., pp. 38–42). Philadelphia: Lippincott.

Hopkins, H., & H. Smith (Eds.). (1993). *Willard and Spackman's occupational therapy* (8th ed.). Philadelphia: Lippincott.

Hopkins, H., & Tiffany, E. (1988). Occupational therapy — Base in activity. In H. Hopkins and H. Smith (Eds.), *Willard and Spackman's occupational therapy* (7th ed., pp. 93–101). Philadelphia: Lippincott.

Kielhofner, G. (1995). *A model of human occupation: Theory and application* (2nd ed.). Baltimore, MD: Williams & Wilkins.

Kohut, H. (1971). *The analysis of the self.* New York: International University Press.

Kohut, H. (1977). *The restoration of the self.* New York: International University Press.

Kohut, H., & Wolfe, E. (1978). The disorders of the self and their treatment: An outline. *International Journal of Psycho-Analysis, 59,* 413.

Leary, S. (1994). *Activities for personal growth.* Sydney: Maclennan & Petty.

Llorens, L. (1984). Changing balance: Environment and individual. *American Journal of Occupational Therapy, 38*(1), 29–34.

Lynn, M. W., Caffey, E. M., Klett, C. J., Hogarty, G. E., & Lamb, R. (1979). Day treatment and psychotropic drugs in the aftercare of schizophrenic patients. *Archives of General Psychiatry, 36,* 1055–1066.

MacRae, A. (1992). The issue is: Should music be used therapeutically by occupational therapists? *American Journal of Occupational Therapy, 46,* 275–277.

MacRae, A. (1993). *Coping with hallucinations: A phenomenological study of the everyday lived experience of people with hallucinatory psychosis.* [CD-ROM]. Abstract from Dissertation Abstracts International: 53/12, p. 6562.

Mattingly, C. (1991a). The narrative nature of clinical reasoning. *American Journal of Occupational Therapy, 45*(11), 998–1005.

Mattingly, C. (1991b). What is clinical reasoning? *American Journal of Occupational Therapy, 45*(11), 979–986.

Meyer, A. (1922). The philosophy of occupational therapy. *Archives of Occupational Therapy, 1,* 1–10.

Misbach Edgerton, W. (1954). Activities in occupational therapy. In H. Willard & C. Spackman (Eds.), *Principles of occupational therapy* (2nd ed.). Philadelphia: Lippincott.

Mosey, A. C. (1986). *Psychosocial components of occupational therapy.* New York: Raven.

Neimeyer, R., & Mahoney, M. (1995). *Constructivism in psychotherapy.* Washington, D.C.: American Psychological Association.

Neville, A. (1980). Temporal adaptation: Application with short-term psychiatric patients. *American Journal of Occupational Therapy, 34*(5), 328–331.

Peloquin, S. (1990). The patient-therapist relationship in occupational therapy: Understanding visions and images. *American Journal of Occupational Therapy, 44,* 13–21.

Pope-Davis, D., Prieto, L., Whitaker, C., & Pope-Davis, S. (1993). Exploring multicultural competencies of occupational therapists: Implications for education and training. *American Journal of Occupational Therapy, 47*(9), 838–844.

Reilly, M. (1962). Occupational therapy can be one of the great ideas of 20th century medicine. *American Journal of Occupational Therapy, 16,* 1–9.

Rogers, J. (1983). Eleanor Clark Slagle Lectureship — 1983. Clinical reasoning: The ethics, science, and art. *American Journal of Occupational Therapy, 37*(1), 601–611.

Schwartz, K. B. (1991). Clinical reasoning and new ideas on intelligence: Implications for teaching and learning. *American Journal of Occupational Therapy, 45*(11), 1033–1037.

Schwartzberg, S. L. (1993). Tools of practice: Therapeutic use of self. In H. Hopkins and H. Smith (Eds.), *Willard and Spackman's occupational therapy* (8th ed., pp. 269–274). Philadelphia: Lippincott.

Stolorow, R., Atwood, G., & Brandchaft, B. (Ed.). (1994). *The intersubjective perspective.* Northvale, NJ: Jason Aronson.

Suto, M., & Frank, G. (1994). Future time perspective and daily occupations of persons with chronic schizophrenia in a board and care home. *American Journal of Occupational Therapy, 48*(1), 7–18.

Wade, B., & Franciscus, M. L. (1954). Occupational therapy for the mentally ill. In H. Willard & C. Spackman (Eds.), *Principles of occupational therapy* (2nd ed.). Philadelphia: Lippincott.

West, W. (Ed.). (1959). *Psychiatric occupational therapy.* Rockville, MD: American Occupational Therapy Association.

Yerxa, E. (1979). The philosophical base of occupational therapy. In *Occupational therapy — 2001.* Rockville, MD: American Occupational Therapy Association.

Suggested Reading

Cottrell, R. P. (1996). *Perspectives on purposeful activity: Foundations and future of occupational therapy.* Bethesda, MD: American Occupational Therapy Association.

Hall, E. T. (1976). *Beyond culture.* Garden City, NY: Anchor Press/Double-day.

Kielhofner, G. (1977). Temporal adaptation: A conceptual framework for occupational therapy. *American Journal of Occupational Therapy, 31*(4), 235–242.

Neville, A., Kreisberg, A., & Kielhofner, G. (1985). Temporal dysfunction in schizophrenia. *Occupational Therapy in Mental Health, 5,* 1–19.

Peloquin, S. (1991). Time as commodity: Reflections and implications. *American Journal of Occupational Therapy, 45*(2), 147–154.

Reed, K. (1984). *Models of practice in occupational therapy.* Baltimore: Williams & Wilkins.

Spadone, R. A. (1992). Internal-external control and temporal orientation among Southeast Asians and white Americans. *American Journal of Occupational Therapy, 46*(8), 713–719.

Stolorow, R. (1994). The intersubjective context of intrapsychic experience. In R. Stolorow, G. Atwood, & B. Brandchaft (Eds.), *The intersubjective perspective* (pp. 3–14). Northvale, NJ: Jason Aronson.

Stolorow, R., & Atwood, G. (1992). *Contexts of being: The intersubjective foundations of psychological life.* Hillsdale, NJ: Analytic Press.

CHAPTER 2

The Social and Personal Effects of Mental Illness

Carole Calkins, MA
Director of Interships and Volunteers
Diretor of Housing Resources
ALLIANCE for Community Care, San Jose, California

Sharon Roth, RN, BSN, MA
Cash Management Liaison
Kaiser Permanente, Oakland, California

Key Terms

Alliance for the Mentally Ill (AMI)
client-driven services
consumers' movement

decompensation
schizophrenogenic mother
treatment team

Chapter Outline

Introduction

This chapter was developed from first-hand accounts and experiences of serious and persistent mental illness. While material has been changed to protect confidentiality, the case vignettes found throughout the chapter reflect universal experiences of both individuals with serious mental illness and their family members, who are equally affected. Both authors have personal experience as parents — and one also as a sibling — of individuals with serious mental illness. Perceptions of serious mental illness vary from individual to individual among those who have contact with it. Figure 2-1 offers some of the many impressions that serious mental illness imprints on those who deal with it.

THE FAMILY PERSPECTIVE—WHO IS THE PATIENT?

We generally think of the person with a mental illness as the patient. However, mental illness reaches beyond the individual, affecting the other family members and the person's significant relationships. Because so much focus falls on the symptoms or behaviors of the ill family member, the (increasing) needs of the family are generally minimized or overlooked. Considering the severe disruption that accompanies mental illness, it is amazing how many families have been able to cope without the benefit of professional help or education.

The illness often comes on so suddenly that the family is caught off guard. This results in confusion, fear, denial, isolation, and a myriad of responses, as one might expect when a loved one becomes ill and there is little information given as to the cause. At other times, there is a gradual change in the individual that is difficult to understand, which, in adolescents, is often thought

Mental Illness — What's it Like?

It: is emotionally and physically painful.
      is frustrating.
      is confusing.
      is costly.
      makes you poor and unable to pay bills.
      means you are overly dependent on others.
      is time consuming.
      means you're angry at yourself and others.
      means you hate yourself and others
      means you don't trust yourself.
      is a lot of hard work.
      means losing control.
      means feeling guilty.
      means being lonely.
      means you are often a failure.
      means you are treated differently from "normal" people.
      means people won't let you be normal.

Mothers:
feel judged before I'm known, and stigmatized.
feel outraged and silenced at the same time - outraged by being blamed again, silenced by the fact that if I express my rage at this new person who blames me, it will be used against me as proof that I am unstable.
feel healed and able to move ahead.
sometimes get overwhelmed.
feel such pain for her/him. It is so unfair.
believe she has a right to take her own life if that is what she decides and feel sad.
believe I will never give up hoping for a cure.

Fathers:
I feel devastated by knowing my child has this illness.
The stress is getting to me.
I'm damned bewildered and confused. I don't know where to go or what to do.
I worry that he will end up on the streets or in jail.
We often fight about what is best to do. This illness is dividing us.

Siblings:
I'm afraid it will happen to me someday - or to my children, if I have any.
I love my brother but resent him and the time he takes.
I don't feel I can talk about my problems to my parents, they have so much to worry about already.
I learned to not feel guilty that she got the illness and not me.
I became a social worker.

(continues)

Figure 2-1. A Sampling of Impressions of Mental Illness from Philadelphia Community Access

Psychiatrist:
> I am expected to "cure" my patients, but sometimes I truly don't know what else to do.
> I'm afraid I'll be sued.
> I'm isolated, there is so little coordination with other programs.

Social Worker:
> I feel effective when I can help a client tap into his or her talents and strengths.
> There are not enough resources.
> I feel let down by my client's failures.
> I like the challenge and enjoy many of my clients, though the work is difficult.

Emergency Worker:
> I feel frustrated when I can't do what I feel is the best for the client.
> All I ever see is people in crisis; I never get to see improvement.
> Sometimes there are no doctors, beds or meds available; what should I do then?
> A lot of crisis situations could be averted, but family members wait until the last minute.
> At times I deal with other people's mistakes.

Figure 2-1.   (continued)

to be teenage rebellion. Sometimes the change in the individual is partially due to substance abuse, which may evoke other family responses. Unless a diagnosis is made, support and education are provided, and the family is included in the consultation about treatment and care, relief may be denied the family, yet often treatment is not sought for months or even years.

Until that time, the family members may be at odds with one another about what is really wrong and how to respond to the individual's puzzling behaviors. They begin to experience a totally new set of relationships as exacted by the effects of the illness and their lack of understanding about what to do. When this happens, the family members, or each of the members in differing ways, may need their own professional intervention. In addition, for parents, the fear of having done something to cause this in a son or daughter is often reinforced by insensitive treatment professionals who do not interact with the parents in a positive or empathic manner. Some therapists even continue to believe in the concept of the **schizophrenogenic mother**. This old theory has been refuted but still lingers in outdated textbooks and can be heard in discussions by uninformed professionals, as described in the following illustration.

CASE ILLUSTRATION

One parent remembers her son at 11 years of age. He had been on medication for attention deficit disorder for five years without improvement. As he reached puberty, his pediatrician stated that the mother was neurotic and that if she simply left the boy alone and stopped worrying, he would outgrow the behaviors. By 12 years of age, he was already using street drugs and committing petty theft, for which he was arrested. He spent the next six years in the criminal justice system. At 18 years of age his probation officer observed that there was something wrong with the boy and referred him for assessment. The diagnosis was schizophrenia. The mother states that she felt a profound sense of relief in knowing that the mental illness she had suspected for years had finally been confirmed and would now be treated.

Discussion

One can certainly understand the need for a mother coping with the long-standing difficult behavior of her child to benefit from an early referral. To label her neurotic hardly addresses the stresses of her situation. It is more likely that this mother was depressed, overanxious, and aware of the risk of having her marriage fail. In addition, other siblings might have been equally affected and in need of some treatment interventions. In fact, the entire family would probably have benefited from occasional therapy in the course of dealing with such traumatic issues as having a child who abused drugs and alcohol, committed theft, and was incarcerated, and for managing the resultant feelings of guilt and stigma.

Family Roles

In healthy families, there are roles and rules that typically define how each member behaves. The parents provide the basic needs of food, clothing, and shelter; give guidelines for behavior; and offer nurturance and support during difficult times in their children's development. How these basic needs are provided and how roles are assigned may differ from one culture to another. In most cultures in the United States, the children are expected to abide by the rules, while being given opportunities to learn by experience. When a member becomes ill, consultation within the family is the usual first step. If this is unsuccessful, the family may look outside to paraprofessionals, teachers, clergy, or health care providers. For most cultures this is not easy, as there is a great deal of shame and blame related to mental problems. Ideally, a careful assessment is made with the family fully involved in the process; and a diagnosis is then given, along with treatment plans, a prognosis, and referrals for services. Everyone is helped to understand the illness and course of treatment, including the expected outcome.

Few families deal with mental illness easily. The family roles may be changed for a number of reasons, but lack of information and poor guidelines for coping are the major reasons why problems occur. Even the most well-adjusted family will be forced to adapt. If they do this through gaining information and education about how best to deal with the ill member, they will become a successfully coping family. For example, their roles may shift as members take on new responsibilities, resulting in parents becoming more involved with the ill member due to increased behavioral demands. Other changes will include finding support from other families, losing friends who cannot cope or are frightened by the ill member, getting time off from work to deal with crisis, and finding ways to maintain stable relationships with each of the other members.

Siblings will be faced with fears of becoming ill, too. They also must face the stigma of having a brother or sister who is "crazy." In addition, they receive less attention from their parents because of the demands of the ill member. Coping involves giving up a lot without getting angry. There is often confusion as to what is the illness and what is simply bad manners, so that expectations of the ill member are sometimes unrealistic. Later, as the family members learn more about managing mental illness, they may feel guilty about earlier demands they made and may even worry that their emotional reactions may have caused the individual to get worse (Bernheim, Lewine, & Beale, 1982).

The family that does not know how to reach out for help may actually be so affected by the ill family member that they all become dysfunctional. There may also be a history of mental illness in the family, as in the following illustration.

CASE ILLUSTRATION

When I was 12, my aunt told me that my mother had been hospitalized when I was 3 years old. She thought my mother had told me. Well, she hadn't. My mother and I had a very close relationship, and I was devastated to think that she had kept this major secret from me. I alternated between feeling anger toward her, for hiding this from me, and anger toward my father, for fighting with my mother all the time. My feelings for my mother changed from thinking of her as my capable parent to feeling very protective of her, like with a doll that could break. For the most part, this was my overriding perception of her, which would now stick with me always.

Discussion

In this case, mental illness became a devastating family secret. When the secret was revealed, it altered a child's perception of his parent.

Crisis and the Family

Because of their close proximity and long history with the individual, family members are more likely than treatment team members to recognize an individual's decompensating mental health. The signs of decompensation, as described by Meinhardt (1988), are listed in Table 2-1. Families are encouraged to watch for these signs and be able to report them; conversely, clinicians are encouraged to listen to the families' stories in order to understand the current crisis.

Mentally ill persons have crises that are often difficult to predict and manage. Moreover, people respond to crisis differently. Certainly, mental illness can represent a crisis for a family. What is important to remember is that the ideal family response to the crisis of mental illness is rarely the typical response. Figure 2-2 provides guidelines for families to reduce and prepare for the incidence of crisis. While each experience may differ from one family or individual to another, there are some things that families can do.

People are not taught how to be a family. Each partner brings unique experiences to the marriage. Hopefully, these are shared and blended as the couple evolves into a family. Both partners bring strengths and weaknesses to the new unit. It is critical for the professional to assess the family from two perspectives, as individuals and as a group. The strengths, coping skills, typical defenses, responses to past crisis, personality variables, cultural backgrounds, stages in the life cycle, levels of education, understanding and acceptance of mental illness, and levels of personal guilt and feelings of stigma are only a few of the areas to be assessed (Marsh, 1993). It is of utmost importance to take care of each member of the family so that they remain healthy and can serve as a continued support to the ill member. The rules on learning to take care of oneself can increase each family member's tolerance for the stress and salvage the family's caring relationship.

As the clinician encourages the family members to develop internal resources, both individually and as a group, they will become more independent, capable, resourceful, and, most of all, accepting of mental illness as a fact of life for them. Crisis management becomes a part of this. No family wants to be in a state of crises all the time, so there is great motivation to learn to reduce the incidence of crises.

Table 2-1. Signs of Decompensation

Early symptoms	Middle symptoms	Late symptoms
Mood shifts	Drops usual routine	Extreme change in behavior
Poor concentration	Develops erratic sleep pattern	
Preoccupation		Assaultive or destructive
Mild depression	Stops caring for self	
Fears	Loses interest in almost everything	Suicidal thoughts or actions
Altered sleep patterns		
Change in appetite	Depression deepens	Requires hospital stay
Loss of energy	Denial or poor insight	
Withdrawal into isolation	Stops taking medications	

Source: Meinhardt (1988).

1. Get to know the members of the treatment team. Know how to contact them for regular questions as well as emergencies, and how to alert them of increased symptoms.
2. Keep a journal, using a loose leaf notebook. Section it into Health History, Psychiatric History, Medications, Placements, What Works and What Makes Things Worse, Resources. Add any other sections you personally feel are important.
3. Document what is most successful in the journal. This might be having only one or two visitors for dinner rather than a party.
4. Rely on experience with the mentally ill person to tell you when there is subtle, but significant change that might indicate future problems.
5. Do not argue with someone who is mentally ill. It is better to state your thoughts in simple language and then "back off" to allow time for the message to sink in. Keep calm and in control, using a lowered voice.
6. Give the individual time to calm down if upset. Suggest a walk, a nap, listening to music in another part of the house.
7. Call for help if the situation begins to get out of hand. This may be to another family member, or someone on the treatment team. It may also be to the police.
8. Invite a local police officer to your home to meet the ill family member and to get some history regarding past problems and potential help you might need. Establishing a relationship of cooperation and trust may avoid unnecessary stress if they are needed in the future.
9. Don't slip into denial about what is happening. Delaying an intervention may only make things worse. Whenever possible discuss your concerns with the ill member.
10. Remember that when your family member is becoming out of control, he/she needs you to be in control.

Figure 2-2. Crisis Management Guidelines

Guiding the family from the present situation to healthy coping should be a goal for the clinician. The family can be an important support system for the ill family member. Generally, there are many strengths that can be reinforced among individual members. New roles can be defined that balance the burden, and opportunities to grieve can be provided. Mental illness is a loss — a great loss to the individual, but also a loss to the relatives and friends who lose the person they knew to the effects of the illness.

RESPONSES TO MENTAL ILLNESS

The Individual

What is it like to be mentally ill? The following illustrations include examples of how mental illness has affected individuals differently. Among the responses there are basic categories that emerge: denial, blame, substance use/abuse, isolation, suicidal ideation, and fear. All these areas can benefit from treatment. The most difficult is denial, because if the individual refuses to acknowledge that something is wrong, there is little chance of beginning treatment unless he or she is committed or incarcerated. Even then, if the patient refuses treatment, there are laws that prevent it.

CASE ILLUSTRATIONS

My family seemed to be a pretty intense bunch — my parents alternated between being very loving toward each other and arguing loudly. I grew up feeling different from most of the people around me. Later, I was diagnosed as having bipolar illness.

I started using drugs and alcohol as a teenager. I always thought that caused me to become mentally ill. Now I know it was more complicated than that. I used drugs to be like everyone else, but it also made me feel better. I didn't hear the voices as much. The drugs I take now help with that, too, but I don't like the other ways they make me feel.

I have schizophrenia. I guess I'll never find a girlfriend and I'd like to have someone to be close to, to hug.

My family says I have mental illness. But I think I have special powers. I can hear things they can't. Like the traffic outside sometimes has hidden messages in the noise the tires make on the road. Or the music I listen to can do that. Sometimes it tells me bad things, over and over, like, "You're no good, you're no good." Then I feel worthless and want to die. That can be scary.

I hate this illness. It is so hard. And there is nothing I can do about it. Sometimes I just want to die and get it over. The only reason I don't kill myself is because I believe I'll have to come back and live this life all over again if I commit suicide, and I couldn't stand that.

Once in treatment, the individual must deal with other issues, of which the most common is compliance with medications. Because of the many side effects, medications are often a problem. Helping the individual to experience the benefits during the early stages of treatment is difficult because during this phase, the medications are still being tried to see what benefits they provide. It may take months or years to find the best combination for the presenting symptoms. In addition, the diagnosis may not be clearly understood due to the symptoms' complexity.

Some individuals will continue to use alcohol or other substances in spite of being told they should not. Even when they know that this can be extremely dangerous, the addiction is often too great for them to manage. This presents problems in terms of what issues should be given priority. Generally, it is thought that unless the substance abuse is controlled, there is little that one can do about the mental illness. It is too risky to treat the individual with medications when there is substance abuse. The combination can be deadly. Getting them into twelve-step programs will be difficult if there is also a denial about being mentally ill (see Chapter 8 on substance abuse). These individuals often are seen in homeless shelters or on the streets. They present a great challenge for the treatment professionals as well as the family.

Once the ill person is on medications and stable, other symptoms may present. One of these is isolation. This may be due to a paranoid fear that is not based on reality or to chronic symptoms such as poor motivation. It is very difficult for people on major tranquilizers to get up and out of bed. Depression has a similar effect. The social world collapses and friends are lost. People remember having had a much different life before the illness, but cannot regain it. The resulting sense of loss is great. With it comes a fear of what the future holds. How will they live on limited resources? Where will they go and who can they trust? Sometimes suicide looks like the best alternative.

There are many questions that face a person with a mental illness. They form the tip of an iceberg that contains a myriad of devastating realities for the individual. Some of these realities are too painful to accept. Moving from disability to ability will surely be an important focus of treatment, as discussed in the following illustration.

CASE ILLUSTRATION

It wasn't until I accepted all of the labels as being conditions that I have (not who I am), that I could begin to get well. I started reading up on manic depression and attending AA [Alcoholics Anonymous] meetings. I took charge of my own wellness. Doctors and therapists weren't going to heal me (though some have been invaluable). Medication alone couldn't do it either. Until I felt the need to remain clean and sober for myself and to stay on medication and monitor my own symptoms, I did not improve. Today, I haven't been hospitalized for five years. I have remarried, have one of my children living with me, and see the other regularly. I have been working full time for four years, and I accept who I am in a way that I was never able to before.

Discussion

Moving to ability meant acceptance of having a disease, learning about it, remaining clean and sober and generally "taking charge" of one's own life.

Family Members

Emotions reported by relatives coping with ill family members have been described as including feelings of anxiety, anger, frustration, depression, exhaustion, and helplessness. There are both objective and subjective burdens. *Objective* refers to the demands of the illness on the family; *subjective* refers to the personal suffering of each member due to having a family member with mental illness (Marsh, 1993). The objective burden is substantial and well documented (see, e.g., Hatfield & Lefley, 1993; Marsh, 1993).

Denial is usually a first reaction. One parent can remember hoping that her son was "on drugs" so that he would be better when he stopped using. This same reaction is often stated time and again in the "Caring and Sharing" support groups, sponsored by the **Alliance for the Mentally Ill (AMI).** Friends who do not understand the ramifications of the illness believe that the proper discipline of the behaviors would stop them. This makes it difficult to differentiate between denial and stigma. Either one is the product of a basic lack of education about mental illnesses.

Grief comes after acceptance of the diagnosis and with the realization that the hopes and dreams one had for one's child are no longer possible. The individual has grown and developed into someone who may physically appear the same but has changed dramatically in personality and behavior, often leaving the family mourning the loss of what might have been. This is further complicated during any remissions or periods of stabilization, when there may be the hope that a cure has been effected. The family is thrown back into the grieving process with each subsequent episode. Unlike grief from death, this grieving process can be as cyclic as the illness, undergoing no resolution. It will be important to work with the family to develop coping skills and an understanding of this process (Bernheim & Lehman, 1985).

Guilt can be as devastating as any of the other emotions. To believe that one has caused the mental illness in a loved one can make the family burden even greater. Without education about the possible genetic and viral causes of mental illness, each family member may think it was caused by something he or she said or did to the ill person. Mothers are especially vulnerable to this situation, which in the past was the main focus of blame, especially by professionals. The term *schizophrenogenic mother,* coined in the early 1950s, refers to a parenting style that is cold, rejecting, distant, aloof, and yet dominating. This might also be the style of the father, but the mother was the primary target because of the relatively longer time the children spent with the nonworking mother in those days. In addition, siblings who feel thankfulness that they did not get the disease often experience a form of survivor guilt.

Questions asked of family members by insensitive clinicians, such as, "What did you do to cause this break?" or "What was going on at home?" contribute to the guilt. The family must be aided in understanding that they were responding to bizarre behavior and did the best they could. They did not cause the illness. A genetic predisposition may have been present, and for some, the symptoms simply manifest themselves when an environmental stressor was introduced, such as the death of a parent, experimental drug use, a heavy work or school schedule, moving from home, or the breakup of a relationship. Only more research will allow a true understanding of this process.

Fear can destroy a family. For example, the siblings may fear that they will become ill, too. A very real physical fear can also exist because the ill relative may be frightening and sometimes threatening. Often parents relate that they are afraid of their children because of the anger displayed. Many families have used restraining orders to control the angry mentally ill member from attacking them. One mother was forced to use a gun in self-defense when her son ran toward her in anger. She fired the gun to stop him and accidentally killed him, causing a tragedy no parent should have to experience.

While those with a mental illness are no more violent than the normal population, the family is often the target of their anger. There are any number of reasons for their rage and frustration. The ill member may be aware that the siblings are getting on with their lives while he or she is, in effect, on a treadmill, or even becoming worse. They may feel that the parents should be giving them money or material goods and are out of touch with reality. Their symptoms may result in cognitive impairment and poor judgment affecting their relationships with family members. The frustration and anger expressed by the ill person can be very frightening to the family and creates an added burden.

Diminished socialization from the stigma and embarrassment evoked by an ill relative affects the entire family. Large family get-togethers become a thing of the past, either because of the behavior of the ill person and avoidance of other family members or because of protective feelings for that person. Family holiday celebrations become too difficult for siblings and their friends or extended family and, over a period of time, may even cease to happen. "Can we take a chance and invite the Joneses to the wedding or will their mentally ill son be too disruptive?" "Will the stress of attempting to control my behavior be too much and cause an embarrassing episode?" "How can a family be included when one of the members always causes embarrassment or chaos?" Typically, the entire family will become excluded from the social events.

CONFLICTS

The confidentiality of patient information and the involvement of the family in treatment decisions does, at times, create conflict between families and the mental health system. The following sections describe some of the issues related to these conflicts as perceived by family members.

Confidentiality Issues

A mother recently expressed her frustration with the health care system because her adult son, who resides with her, was hospitalized after he stopped taking his medication and **decompensated.** When she called the hospital she could not get confirmation that he was there, due to confidentiality laws in her state. (Each state has such laws, which vary somewhat but effectively protect the adult psychiatric patient from any information being given out without his or her express written consent.) The mother, as the primary caregiver, was not informed about medication changes, treatment, or discharge plans. The son was over eighteen years of age; thus, the treatment professionals were bound by the laws of confidentiality. There had been no release-of-information form signed by the son to give permission to talk with his mother. She asked that they do this, but it did not happen until she and her husband went to the hospital with the forms and made the request in person. Even then, it was only with the son's persistence that the forms were signed.

The confidentiality laws are so protective of individual rights that they can interfere with continuity of care. When the family caregivers are not included, the continuity of care is greatly diminished. Often the family has the best record of effective medications and treatment over the years and can be invaluable as a resource in the treatment planning. It is seldom likely that ill persons can give accurate information at times when they have decompensated. Records are not conveyed easily from one place to another, so medications are often changed or interrupted, delaying stabilization. Often the parent or another family caregiver — who may be the only person who knows what works — is the last person asked because of the confidentiality laws.

Many family members now understand the law and have found ways of sharing information in times of crisis that will not violate the rules of confidentiality or the rights of the ill individual. In particular, families are permitted to share information with professionals even though the professional is not permitted to share information with them. Providing a history of the course of the illness and a list of helpful medications can aid in the treatment. Many professionals recognize the value of the family as a part of the **treatment team.** Sometimes everyone can work through a case manager who has a signed release form on file.

Treatment Issues

Information about medications can be critical to the timely care of a patient, but past history about experiences with medication is often necessary in order to prescribe the most useful drug or prevent serious complications. One family member may explain: "We know that our son is extremely sensitive to certain medications. There is one in particular that has immediate, extreme side effects. One of the reasons our son refuses medications is the fear of experiencing these side effects again." Without the family input, this individual is at risk of being given a medication that has had poor results in the past, thus further reinforcing the belief that medicines are bad.

In addition, there may be other kinds of family information that can be helpful. For example, one family told of their son relapsing for seemingly no apparent reason. On further inquiry, the mother suggested that the death of his grandfather and, six months later, the death of one of the family dogs were the triggering events that caused the man to become confused and stop taking prescribed medications. She stated that he showed no emotion and was unable to cry or mourn. Obviously there was sadness, but it was unexpressed, and his inability to know how to deal with the deaths was a critical factor in the relapse.

Many treating professionals want to hear about the significant events that are stressors for their patients, but the time constraints of managed care often do not permit this. This man's doctor had no way of knowing about the deaths without the parents sharing that information. Because the man had schizophrenia, he was not considered a good candidate for insight-oriented therapy and was not being seen by a therapist who might have discussed these losses with him (see Chapter 9 on schizophrenia). People with psychosis are often discounted when it comes to therapy needs, even as it relates to the normal events for which one might be expected to have difficulty in coping. By regular check-ins with the family, such stressors can be identified and worked through.

Another treatment issue is the value of having the family monitor any medication side effects while the individual is living at home. It is important that the family understand the medications, their use, possible side effects, and what to do if there are problems. Education generally covers this, but the family that is excluded from treatment will not be given this information, as is shown in the next case illustration.

CASE ILLUSTRATION

One mother remembers how her son visited for the weekend. After noticing him becoming increasingly agitated and confused, she called his residential facility to report her observations and was told that the cause was probably the reduced dosage of medicine he was on. His medications had been decreased the day before he was to go home, yet the family was not advised of this. The mother just remembers that she was terrified that there would be a crisis again and the police would need to be called. Her anxiety could have been avoided had the family been told about the reduced medications.

There are, of course, times when the ill individual does not wish to have the family involved. This presents additional problems for the continuity of care. One of the recent outcomes of grass-roots support is the **consumers' movement.** The voice of the mentally ill grows stronger as more individuals come "out of the closet" to speak of their experiences and complain about treatment. This has resulted in **client-driven services** in most states, such as California, New York, and Minnesota. As the individual with a mental illness gains a voice in his or her own care, the family may be less involved. This presents a problem when there is a crisis because it is helpful to have all members of the support/treatment team involved in the intervention. Establishing healthy relationships prior to a crisis will help maintain involvement.

Education and careful mediation between members by the health professional are important. After establishing a trusting relationship among members, setting rules and roles about communication may be possible, with contracts written about how this will work. A treatment team that includes all the caregivers and the individual with the mental illness can generally work out solutions to potential problems and include the perspective of both the mentally ill family member and the family.

INVOLVEMENT OF FAMILY IN THE TREATMENT REGIME

Because of the prevailing attitude toward parents, and especially mothers, during the 1950s and 1960s, families of the seriously mentally ill were generally considered dysfunctional. When psychiatric hospitals were closed in the early 1960s, people with mental illness were forced into communities across the nation. The result was an increase of persons in other institutions, such as nursing homes and the criminal justice system (Talbot, 1988), more homeless (Bachrach, 1988), and more families taking in a mentally ill son or daughter.

Recent research showing that many mental illnesses are neurobiological diseases with a genetic base has gone far in changing the attitudes of professionals toward parents. Today, there is less blaming, more openness, and a greater willingness to work with families. Advocacy work by the AMI has also helped to change attitudes toward families with a mentally ill member.

AMI support groups began to spring up across the country 20 years ago. At one time, there was a new group forming every 15 minutes. Families were so hungry for information and help in dealing with mental illness. The stigma that kept these diseases in the closet came under attack as conferences and workshops sprang up. Mental illness still carries tremendous stigma, but with families receiving grass-roots support, the pain and suffering are being reduced. One outcome of this is the inclusion of the family on the treatment team. The typical treatment team has many different players and each has a role in contributing to the care of the individual with a mental illness, including the mentally ill individual (Woolis, 1992). Throughout this text, the concept of team is discussed. Depending on the setting, the disciplines represented may vary, but it is always optimum to include both the client and interested family when possible.

Family Education

Often the family members have been so immersed in meeting one crisis after another that they have had little or no information about the illness itself. If they have been given a diagnosis, they will usually make every effort to learn about the disorder. It is not unusual for health professionals to provide a list of reading material for family members, but the most important help is information presented in a clear format with an opportunity for questions and answers. This is provided in classes and workshops across the country. Mental health professionals who offer these classes generally are impressed with the level of insight, interest, and commitment on the part of the families in attendance. Our own experience in working with family support groups confirms this.

The course outline generally follows a historical perspective of mental illness, including myths, diagnostic criteria for mood disorders, thought disorders and anxiety disorders, treatment therapies in common usage, medications and side effects, legal aspects, community supports, symptom management, and communication skill building. Often a support group will evolve from these courses, providing ongoing information sharing among members and consultation with the mental health professional.

One of the most important outcomes of these courses and workshops is a growing appreciation of the family in coping with difficult to treat symptoms. This has resulted in a paradigm shift away from blame and pathologizing the family. Instead, the family is seen as competent and capable. Given the tools, family members can be excellent team partners. The competency paradigm (Marsh, 1993) offers many advantages. While the competency model has long been used in education, when applied to the mentally ill, it offers a more positive approach for working with the family. Accordingly, the mental health professional focuses on competencies and competence deficits rather than on functional and dysfunctional family systems. In other words, it is not what the family is doing wrong, but what it is doing right, in spite of the illness.

Four areas have been identified as important for families to accomplish. The mental health professional will appreciate the family's growth and development as the members gain experience and ability in these areas. (These areas are described in Figure 2-3.) The family has adaptational attributes that can be operationalized to cope with mental illness. The adaptational model provides a good framework for working with and understanding the family and can facilitate alliances between families and professionals. It is empowering and allows family members to actively acquire greater competency in coping with the mentally ill individual. In contrast, the pathology model is stigmatizing and alienating. Not surprisingly, many families have developed adaptations at several levels.

Two important aspects of adaptation are learning effective communication skills and creating a supportive environment. Both have usually been skewed due to the family members' responses to the symptoms of the illness. It is important to assess how the family has changed as a result of trying to cope with these symptoms. Often, one discovers a very guarded atmosphere where everyone fears they will upset the mentally ill individual. They may be rendered speechless and helpless by such fear. In other families, there is a great deal of disagreement as to what is wrong and how to deal with the ill person. One parent may think the other is being too lenient, while siblings may be jealous of so much attention being given to the mentally ill member. Arguing may result, throwing the household into a constant state of agitation and stress.

Cognitive Attributes
- Understanding of the illness and treatment as well as a solid knowledge of community resources.
- Understanding the prognosis and having realistic expectations.
- Being able to adapt to the demands of the illness.

Behavioral Attributes
- Communication skills including conflict resolution, problem solving, and assertiveness.
- Stress management and behavior management.

Emotional Attributes
- Maintaining a stable emotional climate and mature defenses within the family.
- Resolving the emotional burden of mental illness in the family.

Social Attributes
- Achieving a normal balance of activities for all family members.
- Use of support networks, both formal and informal, and friendships.
- Developing outside interests and activities.
- Collaboration with professionals.
- Becoming advocates in the community.

Figure 2-3. Competency Model

Much has been written about communication with mentally disabled people. One parent stated her guide as, "Say it in five words or less." This had gotten her by for the most part. Figure 2-4 suggests other ways in which families can learn to communicate more effectively. The suggestions are also helpful for health care professionals, particularly when the individual is in the acute stages of illness or the early stages of treatment. Knowing what to say in a difficult situation is critical to feeling competent about being in control and able to avoid an argument or crisis.

By helping the family members to see how the illness has caused changes in themselves in response to the symptoms, they can begin to learn new ways to cope. Establishing a supportive environment that is not overly stimulating will be important if the ill member is to live at home. This may not be possible, in which case the family will need to learn of other options, such as residential programs. Adapting may require being able to accept some of the symptoms, such as delusions, hallucinations, or poor motivation. For example, it is hard to watch someone struggle while hearing voices, but the family can learn ways to reduce the stimuli that tend to increase auditory hallucinations. Being able to have realistic expectations of the mentally ill member re-

It is often helpful to use the following guidelines when communicating to some-one with a mental illness.

1. Keep it simple — when confused or hearing voices, it is difficult to dis-criminate and understand what is being said. Also, if feeling depressed it takes a real effort to listen if the message is too complex.
2. Repeat if necessary — sometimes the message is not heard completely and needs repeating. Also asking to repeat it may help to know if the lis-tener really heard you.
3. Give only one message at a time. If you ask too many questions, or say too many things, it will further confuse the individual.
4. Speak slowly and calmly. How you deliver the message often determines how it is received.
5. Don't argue over delusions. Don't agree, either. Simply state you don't have the same view and change the subject.
6. Remember you are talking to someone who may have difficulty under-standing. Be patient and empathic. Don't talk down. You are speaking to another adult, not a child.
7. Speak with respect. Self esteem is important in getting cooperation and understanding. You can have a role in assuring improved self esteem gained from a satisfying communication that is respectful.
8. Be solution oriented, not problem oriented.
9. Know when to terminate the conversation and leave — or stay, and enjoy a quiet non-verbal communication with your loved one.

Figure 2-4. Effective Communication

garding family activities, family burdens, and changed family roles will be important to explore.

Much of this exploration will be directly related to how the ill individual responds to treatment. Do the family members understand the treatment and any possible limitations? Do they know the risks versus benefits of medica-tions? Are they aware that there is no cure and, for many, no return to their former life? Have they had enough experience with the illness to be able to predict causes and effects? This is very important if the family is to have some measure of control over the illness and be able to communicate to the pro-fessionals about what has happened in the past or may happen in the future.

The family members are the historians. They know by a look or a remark when something is not right and an individual is changing for the worse. They have been living with the illness and can be of critical importance in preventing a crisis. By listening to their alerts, mental health professionals can save pre-cious resources of time and money by responding in a timely manner to the individual's changing status.

A supportive environment is very important to the ill relative's recovery and continued stabilization. It is also critical for the caregiver. Sensitivity to the tension and stress on the family are important factors to consider when creating an environment that meets the needs of both. Ultimately, this may mean that the family cannot have the ill person live at home. However, if they do decide to have the ill member live with them, family caregivers can be taught to:

- keep things calm and quiet
- create a predictable schedule
- use words carefully
- support growth of confidence and self-esteem
- help the ill person come to terms with the illness
- come to terms with their own changed lives

THE PROFESSIONAL WORKING WITH FAMILIES

The exhaustion known to professionals as "burnout" is also likely to be felt by families and caretakers of people with persistent mental illness. The day-to-day demands and sacrifices may become too much of a burden. By helping families cope, develop realistic expectations, talk about their experiences privately or in a group, and deal with stigma, the professional can reduce the potential for burnout. The simple act of cooperating and sharing information includes rather than excludes the family. Developing trust with family members will establish a collaborative interaction that can improve the timeliness of interventions and reduce hospitalizations (Bernheim & Lehman, 1985).

The professional must develop empathy for the family caregiver. By understanding the burden that mental illness places on the family, the professional can offer sincere assistance for coping, thus helping the family to continue as the caregiver. One of the most important aspects of this process is establishing a balance between the ill person's needs and those of the other family members. As the latter gain education and experience in managing and coping with the symptoms and behaviors of the ill person, they will find more time to spend on themselves. It is important that they avoid becoming burned out or overstressed. Figure 2-5 provides guidelines for managing the inevitable increase in stress. The ability to find humor and have a life apart from the role of caregiver are important aspects of this process (Dearth, Labenski, Mott, & Pellegrini, 1986).

Family caregivers also need exercise, rest, regular and healthy meals, and time to socialize and play. Parents need time for intimacy, and everyone needs privacy. Paying attention to a family environment that provides for these needs will go a long way toward preventing burnout and reducing tension and stress.

The emotional response that the family members experience in adapting to their relative's illness needs to be recognized as normal. Providing encouragement to talk about their feelings and start taking care of themselves

Stress management classes are given all over the country, but families often do not realize the tremendous amount of stress they undergo on a day to day basis. Offering simple stress management exercises can greatly relieve them. The following list provides guidelines for managing the inevitable stress involved in being a caregiver.

1. Learn a simple breathing exercise that can be used whenever stressors increase.
2. Join a support group and attend one meeting a month for support and one meeting a month for education.
3. Identify a member or two from your support group that can be available when you need to "check in" with someone.
4. Offer to volunteer in your local organization. As you give, you learn that you are not alone and helping others often makes one feel better about oneself.
5. Find a place in your home or garden that can be your special retreat, even for a few minutes a day. Use it to remind yourself that you deserve a moment of peace away from the stress. If you can, visualize that place and the feelings of calm you have when you are there, at other times during the day when you cannot be physically present in your retreat area.
6. Get regular exercise, eat regular meals that are balanced and get plenty of rest. You need to take care of yourself before you can care for others.
7. Find your spiritual core. Somewhere, regardless of religion or culture, there is a place in all of us where we have our center of understanding and acceptance of ourselves. If you find this in church or temple, then maintain your connection to this support.
8. What other ways do you know that reduce your stress? Make a list and hang it where you can be reminded of them.

Figure 2-5. Stress Management Guidelines

is of primary importance. Through education they can gain a better understanding of mental illness, and through sharing experiences they can learn that they are not the only family with these problems and concerns. This will promote growth and compassion among the family members both toward their ill relative and toward each other.

ADVOCACY AND SUPPORT NETWORKING

Stigma has brought many individuals together in the fight for acceptance and self-esteem. Recently, a number of famous persons have been identified as having a mental illness and becoming successful in spite of their disabilities, including Abraham Lincoln, Ludwig van Beethoven, Patty Duke, Ernest Hemingway, Leo Tolstoy, and Tennessee Williams. Reducing stigma has helped to strengthen the determination among the mentally disabled to fight for better treatment, parity in benefits for other health problems, and rights as consumers through a grievance process.

A number of consumer, family, and community groups have arisen directly from the community mental health system. Many are actively engaged in changing the way treatment is provided, improving expedient access to care, developing housing and housing support programs, seeking increased funding, fighting for parity through legislation, advocating patient rights and equal entitlements under the Americans with Disabilities Act, the federal legislation that guaranteed equal civil rights to individuals with disabilities, and any number of issues and concerns that surface at the local and national level. Some of these organizations are listed in Figure 2-6.

Summary

The effects of mental illness reach far beyond the afflicted individual. They touch the family, friends, and caregivers as well. How the symptoms are managed depends to a great degree on the amount of information provided by the mental health professional. In addition, the cultural perspective will often

---

Each community may have different resources, but most will include a local chapter of one of these:

1. National Alliance for the Mentally Ill (NAMI)
   2101 Wilson Blvd. Suite 302
   Arlington, VA 22201
   (703) 524-7600

2. National Mental Health Association
   1021 Prince Street
   Alexandria, VA 23314-2971
   (703) 684-7722

3. National Depressive and Manic Depressive Association
   730 North Franklin, Suite 501
   Chicago, IL 60610
   (312) 642-0049

4. United Consumers (or other local name)
   (Check the local AMI or local telephone directory)

5. American Psychiatric Association (APA)
   1400 K Street, NW, Suite 1101
   Washington, DC 20005
   (202) 682-6000

Figure 2-6.   Organizations Arising from the Community Mental Health System

dictate the level of shame and stigma that must be overcome and how treatment will be provided.

The stress of coping with a persistent, serious mental illness can create challenging problems to be addressed by the treatment professionals. Including all support members in treatment has proven helpful, especially with the current general reduction in resources. Sometimes the genetic aspect of mental illness is evidenced in families, and more than one member has symptoms that are difficult to understand and accept. This may cause roles to change and communication to be strained and ineffective. Some of the emotions that must be dealt with are guilt, shame, fear, denial, grief, isolation, depression, and anger. Confidentiality laws complicate open discussion about the ill family member, and as a result, treatment plans must include methods to assure all members of the treatment team be included at times of crisis and in planning for intervention and prevention.

The family offers a resource to monitor changes in symptoms, provide history, support treatment goals, and assist with housing and the regular taking of medication. It also provides an important social network for the ill individual. Support groups such as AMI have promoted advocacy and education about mental illness. Education of both the family and the individual has improved understanding of the effects of the illness on both. Classes on stress management, understanding helpful responses to symptoms, improving socialization skills, and generally preventing burnout have allowed family members to return to fulfilling personal goals and achieving an improved quality of life.

Consumer groups have likewise provided a safe means to come forward for many individuals who have been too ashamed or afraid to admit they had a mental illness. As advocacy and support networks grow and as more and more famous personalities share their own perspectives of living with a mental illness, stigma will be reduced for both the individuals and the families. The caring professional who can adapt to working with the family as a resource and respect the mentally ill individual as potentially rehabilitatable, will come to appreciate the tremendous strengths and determination of those they serve.

The only true enemy is mental illness . . . not one another.

Review Questions

1. What are the effects of mental illness on the family?
2. How are family roles and rules changed by mental illness?
3. What are some points to remember for improving communications within the family?
4. Who are the members of a treatment team and what are their roles?
5. How can inclusion of the family enhance the treatment team?

Learning Activities

1. Imagine yourself in a situation where your relative is not thinking clearly and has disappeared. You don't even know if he or she is in a safe place. How would you feel and what might you do?
2. Compile a resource list of the following in your community: psychiatric emergency services; access point for nonemergency treatment; list of three dentists who take Medicaid; list of three physicians who take Medicaid; list of support groups for families of the mentally ill and individuals with a mental illness; list of housing sources for the psychiatrically disabled; list of disabled student programs for the psychiatrically disabled; and list of vocational programs for the psychiatrically disabled.
3. Locate and attend an AMI family support meeting (often called "Caring and Sharing"). Be sure to call first and request permission to attend the meeting, as admission to nonmembers varies from chapter to chapter.
4. Prepare and present an informational program about mental illness to a local club such as Rotary, Lions, or the chamber of commerce.
5. Contact your local library to create an informational bulletin board or other display with basic information on mental illness and the relevant community resources.
6. Ask AMI if you might visit one or two families to interview them regarding their experience with mental illness and present your findings in class.
7. Read one of the books listed in the suggested reading section and record your reaction to it.
8. Borrow one of the informational videos from your local AMI and record your reaction to it.

References

Bachrach, L. L. (1988). The homeless mentally ill. In W. W. Menninger & G. T. Hannah (Eds.), *The chronic mental patient II* (pp. 65–91). Washington, DC: American Psychiatric Press.

Bernheim, K., & Lehman, A. (1985). *Working with families of the mentally ill.* New York: W. W. Norton.

Bernheim, R., Lewine, R., & Beale, C. (1982). *The caring family: Living with chronic mental illness.* Chicago: Contemporary Books.

Dearth, N., Labenski, B., Mott, M. E., & Pellegrini, L. (1986). *Families helping families: Living with schizophrenia.* New York: W. W. Norton.

Hatfield, A., & Lefley, H. (1993). *Surviving mental illness: Stress, coping and adaptation.* New York: Guilford Press.

Marsh, D. (1993). *Families and mental illness: New directions in professional practice.* Westport, CT: Praeger.

Meinhardt, K. (1988). *Early symptoms recognition workshop.* Workshop presented to Santa Clara County Mental Health Department, San Jose, CA.

Talbot, J. A. (1988). The chronic adult mentally ill: What do we now know, and why aren't we implementing what we know? In W. W. Menninger & G. T. Hanna (Eds.), *The chronic mental patient II* (pp. 1–29). Washington, DC: American Psychiatric Press.

Woolis, R. (1992). *When someone you know has a mental illness: A handbook for family, friends, and caregivers.* New York: Tarcher/Perigee Books.

Suggested Reading

Andreasen, N. (1984). *The broken brain: The biological revolution in psychiatry.* New York: Harper & Row.

Cooney, C. (1986). *Don't blame the music.* New York: Putnam Books.

Duke, P., & Turan, K. (1987). *Call me Anna.* New York: Bantam Books.

Fieve, R. E. (1975). *Mood swing.* New York: Bantam Books.

Fuller Torrey, E. (1988). *Surviving schizophrenia: A family manual.* New York: Harper & Row.

Hyland, B. (1987). *The girl with the crazy brother.* Danbury, CT: Franklin Watts.

Isaac, R., & Armat, V. (1990). *Madness in the streets: How psychiatry and the law abandoned the mentally ill.* New York: Free Press.

Johnson, J. (1988). *Hidden victims: An eight-stage healing process for families and friends of the mentally ill.* New York: Doubleday.

Lefley, H., & Johnson, D. (1990). *Families as allies in treatment of the mentally ill: New directions for mental health professionals.* Washington, DC: American Psychiatric Press.

Papolos, D., & Papolos, J. (1987). *Overcoming depression.* New York: Harper & Row.

Sheehan, S. (1983). *Is there no place on earth for me?* New York: Random House.

Walsh, M. (1986). *Schizophrenia: Straight talk for families and friends.* New York: William Morrow.

Theory

CHAPTER 3

Psychological Models

Michael Allessandri, Ph.D.
Director and Research Assistant Professor
University of Miami, Florida

Jennifer T. Skinner, OTR
Special Education Department
San Francisco Unified School District

Key Terms

biopsychosocial focus
eclectic
paradigm

synthetic eclecticism
technical eclecticism

Chapter Outline

Introduction
Humanistic Model
    Development of the Model
    Applications in Occupational Therapy
Biological Model
    The Brain
    Causal Factors of Psychopathology
    Applications in Occupational Therapy
Psychodynamic Model
    Psychoanalytic Concepts
    Neo-Freudian Theories
    Applications in Occupational Therapy
Behavioral Model
    Classical Conditioning
    Operant Conditioning
    Modeling
    Applications in Occupational Therapy
Cognitive Model
    Expectations
    Appraisals
    Attributions
    Beliefs
    Applications in Occupational Therapy
Summary

Introduction

It is generally understood that a comprehensive understanding of a client, including relevant biological, psychological, and sociocultural factors, creates more effective and meaningful treatments. This greater understanding, including what is meaningful and motivating to them, is likely to enhance treatment compliance, thereby facilitating more positive outcomes. It is in this process of developing an understanding of the individual clients and their needs that an appreciation for psychological theory becomes critical. Nearly 100 psychological models have been identified (Harper, 1975). Among the more prominent of these are the humanistic, biological, psychodynamic, behavioral, and cognitive models. Each model, or **paradigm,** represents a unique set of basic assumptions about psychological disorder, including relevant etiological factors and appropriate treatment strategies. In order to familiarize the reader with these theoretical paradigms, the major concepts of each will be presented independently. Although presented separately, it is not our intention to convey that these models are necessarily incompatible. We believe strongly that in order to gain a comprehensive understanding of the client, an integration of concepts from the varied models is most useful. After all, no single model exists that is capable of explaining all psychopathology. An appreciation for all mediating influences on one's behaviors, thoughts, and emotions is essential. Attending to the complex array of biological, intrapsychic, and interpersonal factors that may be creating and/or maintaining psychological dysfunction allows for a comprehensive **biopsychosocial focus** understanding of the individual client. This, in turn, will foster the development of more individualized and effective treatment protocols.

Most contemporary therapists use an **eclectic** approach, employing ideas and techniques from a variety of psychological paradigms in order to understand and treat effectively a client's presenting problems (Davis & Adams, 1995). **Synthetic eclecticism** describes the integration of distinct theoretical principles, while **technical eclecticism** refers to the adoption of a variety of therapy strategies and techniques from multiple schools of thought. While eclectic approaches and attempts at theoretical integration have become quite popular, they have not always proven very successful (Patterson, 1989). Nonetheless, it seems reasonable to expect that practitioners who are eclectic in their orientation will have more tools available to them to treat the complex psychological disturbances they encounter.

HUMANISTIC MODEL

The humanistic model emphasizes the value, worth, and potential of the individual, with a focus on the integrity of the client–therapist relationship. This model of psychological functioning offers a philosophy and an approach to dealing with clients in psychological distress to which all practitioners, regardless of theoretical orientation, should attend. With its primary focus on broad dimensions of an individual's life experience, the humanistic model is generally more encompassing than the other paradigms, which attend to rather specific aspects of human functioning such as physiological processes, unconscious conflicts, learned behaviors, and cognitive processes. For example, humanism pays careful attention to the individual's concept of self as well as personal values. Because of their global perspective, humanistic theories are often seen as more than simply explanations of psychological adjustment and personality development. In fact, they are often viewed as philosophies of life (Davis & Adams, 1995).

Development of the Model

The basic tenets of humanistic psychology arose in the early twentieth century as an alternative to the two prominent theoretical models of the time: the psychodynamic and behavioral paradigms. Humanistic principles in psychology, however, were evident prior to the development of the more formal paradigm that emerged in response to the older theories of psychology. For example, early humanistic philosophies are evident in the work of G. Stanley Hall and William James, both of whom stressed the unique characteristics of human beings. In addition, the bridge between theoretical humanism and clinical practice was first seen in the early 1800s by Samuel Tuke, an English Quaker. Tuke developed a program, known appropriately as "moral treatment," stressing the humane treatment of the mentally ill. Prior to this time, clients with psychiatric illnesses were locked up in asylums, where they were provided with basic necessities (i.e., food, water, and shelter), but essentially removed from the community at large. Moral treatment encouraged active involvement in the care and upkeep of the asylum, as well as participation in selected self-care and leisure activities, which included woodworking, gardening, and sewing. Tuke found that engagement in daily tasks had a positive, reality-orienting effect on the psychiatric patients with whom he worked. Moral treatment, it seems, was quite consistent with the principles and practice of occupational therapy (Fidler & Fidler, 1963; Hopkins, 1988). Underlying Tuke's treatment principles lies the basis of a humanistic treatment approach: the ability to look beyond the psychiatric disease, unconscious conflicts, and environmental precursors of behavior and toward the inherent worth of each individual.

The popularity of humanistic approaches in clinical practice waxed and waned, but the theoretical principles continued to be expounded, especially in Europe, where humanistic principles were closely tied to existential philosophy. The sociocultural trends of the 1950s and 1960s contributed to the reemergence of humanistic principles and practices in psychology. In particular, the theories of Abraham Maslow and Carl Rogers helped humanism become the "third force" in psychology (Association for Humanistic Psychology, 1987), along with behaviorism and psychodynamic theory. Humanists stressed that behaviorism and psychodynamic theory were too reductionist, with the former focusing on environmental stimuli and resulting observable behavior and the latter focusing on human behavior as being primarily sexually driven (Reilly, 1962). Both Maslow (1968) and Rogers (1951) proposed more global and healthy perspectives of human functioning than these other paradigms, and both held as basic the belief that individuals were innately good and driven to achieve self-actualization (i.e., realize their potential as whole and self-contained beings).

Maslow defined a pyramidal hierarchy (shown in Figure 3-1) representing five levels of needs. The lower levels of the pyramid comprise "deficiency," or survival-based, needs (i.e., physiological needs, safety needs, the need to be loved, and the need to belong to a social group). As one moves up the hierarchy, needs become less survival driven and more focused on the components of happiness and personal success. Among these higher-level needs, or "meta-needs," is the need for esteem. Self-actualization, the point at which a person has realized fully his or her potential, lies at the peak of the pyramid.

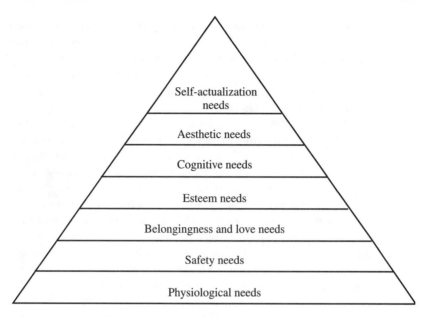

Figure 3-1. Maslow's Hierarchy of Needs

According to Maslow, a person is only able to concentrate on and meet higher-level needs after lower-level needs have been met (1968).

Carl Rogers was heavily influenced by Maslow's hierarchy of needs. He, too, felt the motivating drive of humans was to achieve a state of self-actualization. He believed that it is only through the process of trying to achieve self-actualization that an individual develops an increasingly differentiated self-concept. Reflecting on Maslow's need hierarchy, Rogers proposed that human beings have a basic need for positive regard, especially from parents and significant others in their lives. Rogers conceptualized positive regard as a freely provided and unconditional liking for another person as an individual, without demands or expectations on that person's behavior. When this regard is provided unconditionally to developing children, they will grow up in a better position to realize self-actualization. More often than not, however, children are not raised with unconditional positive regard. Instead, they are taught that positive regard is, in fact, conditional; that is, certain behaviors, thoughts, and emotions valued by the caregiver (typically the parent) are required in order to receive positive regard. What results is a set of conditions of worth, which impacts the child's subsequent behaviors. That is, in an effort to receive positive regard, the child begins to behave in a manner consistent with the conditions and expectations set forth by the caregiver rather than his or her own desires and needs. As a result, the child's need to self-actualize may be in direct competition with his or her need to receive positive regard from the caregiver. The adoption of the standards and values of others may inhibit self-actualization, especially if the standards are very restrictive. It is the discrepancy between one's experience (shaped by conditions of worth) and one's self-concept that creates psychological abnormality. In order to maintain the integrity of the self-concept, discrepant experiences are distorted and denied. The self-concept itself becomes distorted over time as it begins to internalize the conditions of worth set forth by others.

Rogers (1942, 1951, 1961) applied humanistic principles to create client-centered therapy, a nondirective therapeutic approach focused on helping individuals realize their potential by creating a safe, supportive environment to promote self-enhancement. Characteristics present in this nonjudgmental environment include empathy, unconditional positive regard, and genuineness (Davis & Adams, 1995). *Empathy* refers to experiencing the world from the client's perspective. This is accomplished through the use of active listening and reflecting techniques in which the therapist communicates an understanding and acceptance of the client. Genuineness involves responding to the client as a human and not just a therapist. It also requires that therapists stay in touch with their own feelings and be able to communicate them to the client in an effective, appropriate manner. Finally, an environment of unconditional positive regard should be created so that clients feel comfortable and secure when engaging in the change process. That is, clients should not feel judged in this environment; they should feel valued and accepted regardless of their thoughts, behaviors, and emotions.

Although notably more existential than humanistic, the beliefs of Victor Frankl (1967, 1972), a survivor of the Nazi concentration camps, represent another strong influence in this phenomenological domain. Frankl disagreed with Rogers and Maslow that the motivating drive toward fulfillment in life is self-actualization. Instead, he postulated that there was a basic drive toward meaning in life and, therefore, that psychiatric disturbances arose from an inability to find meaning in life. Frankl, along with other existentialists, asserted that there was an anxiety, shared by all humans, that resulted from the knowledge that death, or "nonbeing," is a known outcome of being. It was Frankl's belief that some people resolve this anxiety by finding meaning in their lives. *Meaning* represents different things to different people. It does not have to represent actions toward a specific goal, but it may represent the freedom to take responsibility for an attitude or belief, even if unspoken. Frankl argued that meaning could also be found through the ability to believe in one's inherent worthiness. Accordingly, a person could create meaning or purpose in life simply through the act of taking the responsibility to believe a certain way.

Applications in Occupational Therapy

Applications of the theories of Rogers, Maslow, and Frankl have been extended into the arena of occupational therapy practice through the integration of humanistic and existential principles into prominent occupational therapy models. Moreover, as noted by Mosey (1980), the philosophical basis of occupational therapy appears to be grounded in humanistic and existential principles. After all, inherent in the occupational therapy theory base is the belief that individuals find meaning through occupation (Fidler & Fidler, 1978). Occupational therapists are taught to see each client as an individual with unique qualities. This is reflected in the development of goals and treatment objectives, all of which are defined by the client. In today's managed care environment, insurance companies define which services are covered, thus dictating a structure within which goals must be chosen. However, occupational therapists can, and should, define treatment priorities within this structure according to client needs.

Humanistic principles reinforce the notion that no matter how well conceived the therapeutic protocol, the treatment outcome depends on both the client's capacities and his or her choice to utilize them (Yerxa, 1967). This basic concept highlights perhaps the most salient contribution of humanistic theory — the importance of the individual client in determining his or her own outcomes. Humanistic theories remind therapists that "man, through the use of his hands . . . can influence the state of his own health" (Reilly, 1962, p. 6). Approaching therapy with this dictum in mind encourages therapists to assume a more nondirective approach with the clients they treat. Taking such an approach with a client who has become disabled allows him or her to gain a better understanding of his or her own areas of interest and determine the extent to which his or her own cultural and spiritual identity will impact treatment priorities. Empowering a client to take an active role in the healing process may be the first step toward helping him or her to reestablish meaning in life and therefore the will to live. As Yerxa eloquently states, "I believe our broad purpose is to produce a reality-orienting influence upon the client's perceptions of his physical environment and self" (1967, p. 5).

In summary, the client-centered principles of the humanistic model are very useful in establishing rapport and trust between client and therapist. This is a significant predictor of treatment outcome in all disciplines, including occupational therapy. The practicing occupational therapist, therefore, would be well served by employing humanistic principles as part of the therapeutic process. Being nonjudgmental and genuine toward clients and understanding their perspective or frame of reference (i.e., providing empathy) may be critical to the change process. In general, therapists should make every effort to create a nonjudgmental environment in which the vulnerable client feels safe in expressing him- or herself and in learning new, and relearning old, skills.

BIOLOGICAL MODEL

The biological model of psychology has sought to understand the physiological mechanisms underlying behavior. This knowledge allows us to understand the behavior of clients from a biological or medical perspective. According to this model, symptoms of psychological disorder are caused by underlying biological factors. Included among these causal factors may be viral infections, neuroanatomical defects, biochemical (i.e., neurotransmitter and hormonal) imbalances, and genetic predispositions. Those who support a biological model for psychopathology typically approach psychological abnormality as medical researchers approach illness. Treatment generally follows a biological or medical perspective as well (e.g., the prescription of medication or electroconvulsive therapy). Thus, while other areas of psychology propose theories regarding the nature of thinking, learning, feeling, and perceiving, this branch attempts to reduce these processes to their simplest components in order to study the mechanisms that produce them.

Although biological factors were long considered as possible determinants of abnormal behavior, it was not convincingly demonstrated that psychological disorders had organic bases until syphilis was identified as the cause of a constellation of psychological symptoms, including delusions of grandeur as well as paralysis. From this key discovery, scientists began to speculate about the causal factors of other psychological disorders, stimulating revived interest in biological explanations of psychopathology. Biological psychologists view abnormal behavior as an illness caused by malfunctioning parts of the organism, primarily the brain (Gershon & Rieder, 1992). Therefore, a brief overview of brain structure and function is presented next.

The Brain

The brain is made up of billions of neurons and many more support cells, called glia. Groups of neurons form brain regions, such as the hindbrain, midbrain, and forebrain; further differentiation is noted within each region and is shown in Figure 3-2. For example, the hindbrain is comprised of the medulla, pons, cerebellum, and reticular activating system; it is connected to the spinal cord. The forebrain consists of the cerebrum (i.e., the two cerebral hemispheres), thalamus, and hypothalamus. The midbrain coordinates communication between the forebrain and hindbrain regions.

Within the forebrain, the cerebrum is further differentiated into the cerebral cortex, corpus callosum (which connects the two brain hemispheres), basal ganglia, and amygdala. The cerebral cortex has four distinct regions: the frontal, parietal, temporal, and occipital lobes, as is shown in Figure 3-3. The frontal lobe is located near the front of the brain and contains the motor cortex. The parietal lobe contains the somatosensory cortex. The temporal lobes are located on the sides of the brain and contain the auditory cortex, and the occipital lobe, at the back of the brain, contains the visual cortex. Finally, the limbic system is located at the base of the forebrain and includes portions of the thalamus, hypothalamus, and amygdala.

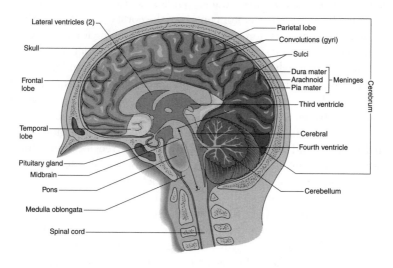

Figure 3-2. Structures of the Brain

Each of these brain regions and subregions is comprised of neurons responsible for specific brain functions. The medulla controls heart rate, respiration, and gastrointestinal function. The pons is involved in sleeping, waking, and dreaming; it is also a pathway for motor information traveling from the cerebral hemispheres to the cerebellum. The cerebellum receives and processes information from peripheral sensory structures (i.e., hair cells of the

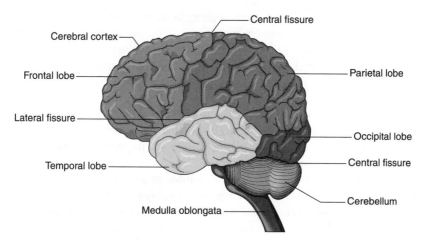

Figure 3-3. The Four Lobes of the Cerebral Cortex

inner ear, joint receptors, and muscle spindles). It also is responsible for processing feedback from the motor centers of the cortex (e.g., the coordination of head/eye movements; force and timing when reaching for an object, etc.). The reticular activating system screens incoming information and stimulates other brain regions whose pathways pass through the pons and medulla; it is thought to be primarily responsible for the mediation of states of arousal.

In the forebrain, the thalamus is important in processing and relaying information between other regions of the central nervous system and the cerebral cortex. Specifically, it directs incoming sensory information from the visual, auditory, and somatosensory systems to the correct locations within the cerebral cortex. The cerebral cortex is primarily responsible for sensory processing, motor control, and higher mental functions, such as learning, memory, planning, and judgment. The hypothalamus helps regulate body temperature, hunger/satiety, thirst, and the sex drive. It also controls the release of hormones by the pituitary and modulates feelings of pleasure and aggression. The amygdala is involved in the coordination of the autonomic nervous system and the endocrine system, as well as emotional states.

Similar to other brain regions, each of the lobes of the cerebral cortex has specific brain functions. The frontal lobe is involved in higher mental functions such as thinking and planning, as well as in the control of the body muscles. The parietal lobe processes information about pain, pressure, and body temperature. The temporal lobes are involved in memory, perception, and language processing, and the occipital lobe is responsible for visual processing.

Causal Factors of Psychopathology

Psychopathology can be caused by any number of physiological dysfunctions. Included among the possible physiological causes of psychopathology are infections, such as syphilis. Anatomical aberrations may also be present. That is the size or shape of certain brain regions may be abnormal, thereby creating abnormal behavior. For example, Huntington's disease, which presents with violent emotional outbursts, memory and other cognitive difficulties, delusions, suicidal thinking, and involuntary body movements, has been traced to a loss of neurons in the brain area called the basal ganglia.

However, infections and brain structure defects are not the only determinants of abnormal behavior. It may also be that neurons are not communicating effectively with one another due to improperly functioning neurotransmitter substances and systems. It is via the neurotransmitter substances that neurons transmit electrical impulses to other neurons; thus, these substances are critical in the transmission of information in the brain. Hormonal imbalances may also contribute to aberrant behavior. Neurotransmitter dysfunction and hormonal imbalances represent biochemical causal factors of psychopathology. In addition, genetic factors may also be operating in the manifestation of a psychological disorder.

Biochemical Factors.   Biochemical factors, including neurotransmitter dysfunction and hormonal imbalances, have been implicated as possible causal factors in many psychological disorders. Several of the neurotransmitter substances receiving particular attention in psychopathology research are serotonin, dopamine, gamma-aminobutyric acid (GABA), and norepinephrine. Each of these neurotransmitters has been found to be related to the symptom presentations of specific psychological disorders. To understand how neurotransmitter dysfunction can impact behavior first requires a good understanding of the structure of nerve cells and the mechanism of communication among these cells.

Neurons are comprised of several parts: the cell body, or soma; dendrites; and an axon (shown in Figure 3-4). Most neurons have one axon and numerous dendrites attached to the cell body. The cell body houses the basic cellular components (i.e., ribosomes, endoplasmic reticulum, mitochondria, and Golgi apparatus), which manufacture vital nutrients for the cell's survival. The cell body is also the manufacturing plant of neurotransmitters, the chemical messengers whose transport between cells forms the basis for cellular communication. The axon transports these chemical messengers to its distal end, where they are stored in vesicles until needed. The axon also serves to conduct an electrical signal from its proximal end (by the cell body) to its distal end (where the vesicles are stored). The dendrites are comparable to the antennae of a radio; they receive chemical messages from the axons of other

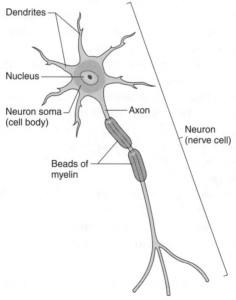

Figure 3-4.   The Neuron

cells. A neuron's axon does not form a direct connection with another neuron's dendrites. Rather, a small gap (approximately 20 billionths of a meter wide) separates them (Thompson, 1993). This space between two neurons is referred to as the synapse.

An electrical impulse is received by a neuron's dendrites (located at one end of a neuron) and then travels down its axon (a long fiber) to the axon's terminus, where it stimulates the release across the synapse of tiny packets of neurotransmitter substances in chemical form. These substances cross the synapse and bind to receptors (actually proteins) on the dendrites of the next neuron. Depending on the nature of the neurotransmitter substance, this binding either stimulates or inhibits the firing of the next neuron. In either case, neurotransmitter substances are essential to effective communication between the neurons.

Normally, the electrical current generated by the bonding of one neurotransmitter on a dendrite is not enough to excite a cell. However, if enough excitatory neurotransmitters bind to the dendrites of a cell in either a short time (temporal summation) or a small space (spatial summation), the cell will build a large electrical charge at the area where the cell body connects with its axon, called the axon hillock. If the axon hillock builds a large enough charge (normally −70 millivolts), gates on the membrane of the axon will open up and allow the charge to propagate down the axon.

A synapse has both a presynaptic and a postsynaptic terminal. The presynaptic terminal lies at the distal end of an axon and contains the vesicles that house the neurotransmitters. The postsynaptic terminal lies on the distal end of a dendrite and contains "locks" with shapes specific for the entry of certain neurotransmitter "keys." The electrical signal, upon reaching the distal end of the axon, causes a chain of reactions to take place as follows: Calcium ions are released, causing the vesicles (housing the neurotransmitters) to bind with the distal end of the axon and, in effect, opening a door through which the neurotransmitters escape from the vesicle within the axon and move into the open space of the synapse beyond. Once in the synapse, the neurotransmitter key is drawn towards the lock on the postsynaptic membrane (on the dendrites of the second cell). If the key fits the lock (in a chemical sense), the neurotransmitter will bind to the membrane and either excite or inhibit the next cell, depending on its function. At this point, the process begins again. This chain of events serves as the basis for communication between neurons.

Many different types of neurotransmitter substances have been discovered in the brain. It has also been discovered that different types of neurotransmitters serve different brain regions; that is, each neuron uses only certain kinds of neurotransmitters (Barondes, 1993). Neurotransmitter problems may include:

a. excessive or insufficient amounts of neurotransmitter substances in the synapse
b. too few receptor sites on the postsynaptic membrane

c.　the presence or absence of other chemicals that interfere with neural transmission

d.　the interrelationships between different neurotransmitter systems (environmental factors such as stress can also inhibit neural transmission)

Neurological studies have indicated that abnormalities in the activity of different neurotransmitters can cause different mental disorders. For example, generalized anxiety disorder has been linked to the insufficient activity of gamma-aminobutyric acid (GABA), an inhibitory neurotransmitter, in the brain (Braestrup, Schmiechen, Neef, Nielson, & Petersen, 1982). Individuals with this disorder may benefit from the use of anxiolytic drugs (e.g., Valium, Librium, Xanax), which facilitate GABA binding at the receptor site. Schizophrenia (most notably the "positive" symptoms such as hallucinations and delusions) has been linked to excessive dopamine activity (Angrist, Lee, & Gershon, 1974; Grilly, 1989; Wong et al., 1986). Antipsychotic medications (e.g., haloperidol, Mellaril, Thorazine) decrease levels of dopamine in the brain, thereby alleviating the positive symptoms. Depression has been linked to low activity of norepinephrine and serotonin (Schildkraut, 1965; Siever, Davis, & Gorman, 1991). Individuals suffering from depression may be relieved of their symptoms by taking antidepressant medication (e.g., Prozac, Paxil, Zoloft). These drugs work specifically to increase the levels of serotonin present in the synapse, thereby enhancing the likelihood it will bind to its receptors.

　　Increased understanding of the special regions of the brain, the mechanisms surrounding neural connectivity, and the functions of the neurotransmitters has certainly furthered our understanding of the biological basis of behavior. However, our knowledge of the physiological factors present in psychopathology is by no means complete. In an effort to develop a more comprehensive biological understanding of abnormal behavior, another biochemical system, the endocrine system, has become the subject of investigation. Unlike the neural connections, this system communicates by means of the circulatory system. The hypothalamus regulates endocrine system functioning in one of two ways: (1) by releasing hormones directly into the bloodstream, and (2) by emitting hormone release factors, which stimulate the anterior pituitary gland to release the appropriate hormone into the bloodstream. In both cases, hormones circulate throughout the body until they bind to target receptors. Similar to the lock-and-key mechanisms of neurotransmitters, the target receptors are selective for the particular hormones with which they bind.

　　One frequently studied hormone is adrenocorticotropin (ACTH). The target receptor site of ACTH is the adrenal gland. When ACTH binds to the adrenal gland, it causes steroid hormones to be released. One of these is cortisol, which serves to elevate blood sugar and increase metabolism. When a person is under significant stress, the hypothalamus stimulates the pituitary gland to secrete large amounts of cortisol. The increases in blood sugar, and thus in metabolism, are necessary for cells to sustain themselves in the midst of excessive activity. Physiological psychologists have determined that the energy expended in increasing metabolism and blood sugar levels lessens the energy available for other bodily functions (specifically, self-defense). Thus, the link between high levels of stress and a weakened immune system may lie in the excessive secretion of ACTH from the pituitary gland (Kalat, 1988).

Genetic Factors in Psychopathology.   Many theorists who follow the biological model believe that inherited vulnerabilities mediate psychological disorders. Certain personality traits, temperamental styles, and specific disorders may have a genetic component (Bouchard, Lykken, McGue, Segal, & Tellegen, 1990). In fact, researchers and clinicians have long noted that certain disorders tend to run in families. In an effort to study the genetic influence on psychopathology, researchers have utilized studies of twins, family pedigrees, adoptions, and risk. These research methodologies attempt to tease out the unique genetic contributions to psychopathology from the vast array of influential biological and environmental factors present. In many cases, a unique genetic contribution proves elusive to the investigator. In such cases, it appears likely that a combination of factors is essential to the manifestation of psychopathology. Thus, multiple genes — or, more likely, a genetic predisposition — coupled with psychological risk factors may be required for psychological disorders to manifest themselves. The theoretical model outlining this possibility is the diathesis-stress model. According to this model, diatheses (i.e., genetic or other biological predisposing factors) must be present along with psychological stressors in order for abnormal behavior to develop. This model has been used to explain the etiology of psychological disorders such as schizophrenia (Meehl, 1962), as well as the development of personality characteristics such as temperament (Plomin, DeFries, & McClearn, 1990).

Twins are frequently studied in the effort to learn more about the genetic influences on psychopathology. There are two types of twins, monozygotic (identical) and dizygotic (fraternal). While identical twins share all the same genes, fraternal twins have an average of only half their genes in common. Twin studies often help to tease out genetic contributions to psychology because twins are typically raised in the same environment, thus controlling external influences to a large degree. Research on several disorders, such as schizophrenia, autism, and bipolar disorder, has demonstrated that identical twins are more likely to share the same disorder than dizygotic twins. When both twins have a disorder, they are referred to as *concordant twins.* When only one twin has a disorder, they are *discordant.*

Family pedigree studies are designed to assess how many members of a given family have a specific disorder. The notion here is that if more members of a given family have a disorder than would be expected in the general population, there may be a genetic predisposition to the disorder that is being transmitted across the generations. For example, evidence from such studies has demonstrated that depression occurs at greater frequencies within families than in the general population (Bloom, Lazerson, & Hofstadter, 1985).

Adoption studies help to further delineate the roles of nature and nurture in the development of psychopathology. One type of adoption study is to compare adopted children to their adoptive and biological parents. Another, perhaps stronger, methodology is to study twins who have been adopted by different families and therefore reared apart. Studies such as these have demonstrated that numerous personality traits, such as IQ, alcohol and drug use, crime and conduct problems, depressiveness, danger seeking, and neuroticism are strongly related in identical twins and related, but to a much lesser degree, in fraternal twins (Bouchard et al., 1990; Bouchard & McGue, 1990; Waller, Kojetin, Bouchard, Lykken, & Tellegen, 1990).

Risk studies target the family members of identified patients to determine the frequency of an identical psychological disorder among them. Studies such as these help to clarify the relative risk of developing that psychological disorder. For example, it has been found that the risk of developing depression is greater for those family members whose biological relationship is closest to the identified patient (Gottesman, 1991).

Applications in Occupational Therapy

The biological model provides much useful information to the occupational therapist working with clients who have mental illness. An understanding of the biological basis of the disorder can guide clinicians in the formulation of appropriate treatment plans. For example, understanding the biological basis of schizophrenia allows a clinician to appreciate the importance of medication management in the treatment of symptoms. Thus, working with a patient to develop a medication routine or schedule may be a treatment priority. Furthermore, family members and caretakers may find some relief in understanding the biological basis of the disorder. Additionally, understanding that a disorder reflects overactivity in the limbic system and frontal lobe area of the brain may lead a clinician to develop theories of treatment focusing on the remediation of skills in the affected areas. For example, teaching appropriate social interaction skills and how to dress for a work environment may assist an individual with schizophrenia to acquire a job.

Understanding the biological basis of disorders such as attention deficit hyperactivity disorder (ADHD) or autism may allow the clinician to develop a teaching style that is appropriate for the particular child. For example, understanding that a child with ADHD may have an uninhibited reticular formation would allow a clinician to predict that this child will have difficulty focusing attention. When setting up to evaluate or treat this client, the clinician should prepare by modifying the environment. Modifications may include dimming bright fluorescent lights, choosing a confined work area with minimal distractions, selecting well-organized activities, and using a timer to allow the child to self-monitor the time left on a task. Knowing that attention requires a lot of energy for this child, periods of attentiveness should be handsomely rewarded.

In summary, the biological model may very well be the fastest growing perspective in psychology. Due to recent scientific advances such as magnetic resonance imaging (MRI), positron emission tomography (PET) scanning, and computerized axial tomography (CAT) scanning, scientists are now able to study the brain and its processes more closely. These technological breakthroughs, along with the tremendous advances in the use of pharmacological treatments to ameliorate psychological disorders, have enabled clinicians to develop a better understanding of the physiological mechanisms underlying aberrant behavior. The enhanced appreciation for the role of biology facilitates the work of all service providers, including occupational therapists, who work directly with clients with psychological disorders. Biological factors, however, are not the only determinants of psychological disturbance; psychological factors, such as unconscious conflicts, learning histories, and cognitive processes, may also be etiologically significant. The models described in the remainder of this chapter attempt to explain psychopathology in terms of these psychological factors.

PSYCHODYNAMIC MODEL

The psychodynamic model primarily focuses on the emotional and personality development of the individual and emphasizes early childhood experiences as formative. According to psychodynamic theorists, both normal and abnormal behaviors are largely determined by unconscious psychological forces and internal processes. It is the interaction among these forces that creates behavior, thoughts, and emotions. Abnormal behavior results when these dynamic forces come in conflict (intrapsychic conflict). Psychodynamic theorists assume a deterministic view of behavior. That is, all behavior can be seen as the product of forces beyond the immediate awareness and control of the individual. Although patterns of behavior are viewed as having their origins in early childhood, they may not emerge until adulthood.

The most prominent of the psychodynamic theories was developed by the Viennese neurologist Sigmund Freud in the early twentieth century. His interest in hypnosis as a form of treatment for hysterical illnesses (i.e., physical ailments with no apparent medical explanation) and his early work with the neurologist Jean Charcot and the physician Josef Breuer ultimately led to the formulation of his theory of psychoanalysis, which was the first truly psychological theory of normal and abnormal behavior. This theory postulates that unconscious factors are responsible, not only for hysterical illnesses, but for all psychological functioning, both normal and abnormal. Treatment involves the use of free association, hypnosis, dream analysis, and the interpretation of resistances and transference (i.e., the process by which the patient comes to attribute characteristics of important figures from childhood to the therapist) in order to help unconscious conflicts become conscious. Once available to consciousness, psychological conflicts can be worked through and resolved.

Psychoanalytic Concepts

Psychoanalytic theory represents a set of elaborate assumptions about human behavior that are quite complex and, due to their abstractness, often difficult to comprehend. Moreover, the theory has evolved throughout this century. Various therapists have expanded on the original theory, and it has been influenced by different cultural beliefs. Indeed, Freud expanded and changed his own ideas through his lifetime. In order to familiarize the reader with psychoanalytic theory, the following discussion is meant to be a cursory review of some of the key Freudian concepts, including structures of the mind, ego defense mechanisms, levels of consciousness, and psychosexual developmental stages (Comer, 1995; Freud, 1923/1976; Kaplan & Sadock, 1995). However, the intricacies and depth of Freud's theoretical notions cannot possibly be captured in such a review.

Structure of the Mind.   Freud believed that personality was comprised of three dynamic and interactive forces operating at the unconscious level. The terms used to describe these three forces are *id, ego,* and *superego;* they refer respectively to instinctual needs, rational thinking, and moral standards. It is the interaction among these three forces that shapes human behavior, thoughts, and emotions. In fact, psychoanalysts assert that what distinguishes abnormal and normal behavior is the manner in which psychic energy is distributed among these three "structures." If the id or the superego are too overpowering, it will render the ego ineffective and abnormal behavior will result.

The id, which is innate, represents an individual's instinctual needs, drives, and impulses. Freud believed that these instincts were primarily sexual in nature. The id, which was viewed by Freud to be the primary motivating force in personality, is most prominent in psychoanalytic theory. The id strives for immediate and constant gratification, thereby operating in accordance with the pleasure principle. The id operates without consideration of realistic constraints or regard for consequences. Two sources of id gratification have been described in psychoanalytic writings: direct or reflex activity and primary process thinking. An example of reflex activity is an infant seeking and receiving milk from the mother to satisfy hunger. A description of primary process thinking involves activating a memory or image of the desired object. For example, when a hungry child's mother is unavailable, the child may imagine her breast. As Comer (1995) notes in this example, such images are at least partially satisfying because the id is unable to distinguish between objective and subjective realities. *Wish fulfillment* is the Freudian term used to describe the gratification of id instincts by primary process thinking.

As we come to recognize that our environment will not meet every instinctual need, a separate force develops out of the id. This force, the ego, strives for gratification unconsciously but does so in accordance with the reality principle. The ego engages in secondary process thinking, which involves planning, reasoning, remembering, evaluating, and decision-making processes.

That is, the ego determines whether it is safe or dangerous to express an impulse by considering the factors present in reality. The ego experiences anxiety and/or guilt when the id presses to make its desires conscious or get them gratified.

In an effort to control unacceptable id impulses and reduce the anxiety and/or guilt they arouse, the ego develops unconscious coping responses, called ego defense mechanisms, to protect the self. Defense mechanisms are unconscious methods generated by the ego to protect itself from anxiety and guilt related to unacceptable id impulses. Examples of these mechanisms are repression, denial, fantasy, projection, displacement, rationalization, reaction formation, intellectualization (isolation), undoing, regression, identification, overcompensation, and sublimation (several of these are described in Table 3-1). The principal function of the ego, then, is to mediate the impulses of the id and also the moral and ethical value constraints posed by the superego (comprised of the conscience and the "ego ideal"). Psychological abnormality is thought to result when the ego is not mediating effectively, whereas psychological adjustment results when the ego is able to effectively regulate internal conflicts.

The superego develops from the ego during the phallic stage of psychosexual development. In interaction with our caregivers (typically parents), we learn that many of our id impulses are not acceptable and should not be expressed. Thus, parental values and judgments come to be unconsciously

Table 3-1. Ego Defense Mechanisms

Mechanism	Description
Repression	Preventing unacceptable impulses or desires from becoming conscious
Denial	A primitive or early defense mechanism by which a person disavows or refuses to acknowledge the external source of anxiety
Projection	Attributing personally unacceptable impulses or desires to the external world
Displacement	Shifting repressed desires and impulses from a dangerous object to one that is more safe and acceptable
Reaction Formation	Adopting behavior that is in direct opposition to one's unacceptable impulses or desires
Intellectualization	Repressing of the emotional components of one's experience, not the informational components
Regression	Retreating to an earlier, more immature developmental stage in response to anxiety
Identification	Adopting the values and feelings of a person who causes anxiety in an attempt to increase self-worth
Sublimation	Expressing sexual and aggressive impulses in a socially acceptable manner

introjected (incorporated), thereby becoming the standards against which we come to judge our own behaviors. The superego is comprised of two components, according to Freud: the conscience and the ego ideal. It is the conscience that reminds us that certain behaviors, thoughts, and emotions are acceptable or unacceptable. The ego ideal represents the person we are striving to become; it incorporates all the values and standards of our caregivers. It is important to remember that the superego is just as irrational as the id. It has no concern for reality and can be overly critical and controlling, generating feelings of guilt and worthlessness when standards are violated.

According to Freud, these personality forces are fueled by psychic energy. One critical component of this (finite supply of) psychic energy is sexual energy, which is present in the child long before adult sexuality develops. Prior to the development of mature sexual interests and expression, this sexual energy exists as libido according to Freudian theory. Early in life, libido is associated with pleasurable activities related to the gratification of biological needs; later in life, social and psychological needs become prominent. (This will be discussed further when the psychosexual developmental stages are presented in the next section.)

Levels of Consciousness. Freud (1923/1976) initially conceptualized that the human mind was comprised of three levels of consciousness: the unconscious, the preconscious, and the conscious. The intrapsychic conflicts he noted to be central to his theory of personality could occur at any of these varying levels of awareness. Relating these concepts to the structural model, the id is unconscious, while the ego and superego function at various levels of consciousness (shown in Figure 3-5). The unconscious contains elements, such as instincts or drives, that actively seek to become conscious but are typically prevented from doing so by psychic forces. That is, they may be viewed as unacceptable for expression by the ego (creating anxiety) or by the superego (creating guilt) and, therefore, prevented from being expressed consciously. A large portion of mental activity is unconscious, meaning that it occurs outside a person's normal awareness and is not readily accessible, according to this theory. In fact, psychoanalysts assert that most behaviors, thoughts, and emotions are unconsciously motivated. On the other hand, the preconscious level of the mind contains elements that can become conscious; this, however, requires efforts at retrieval on the part of the individual. Conscious material is that of which we are aware of at any given moment; thus, the contents change constantly. According to psychoanalysts, consciousness represents only a small part of actual mental life.

Developmental Stages. Freud believed that individuals pass through a series of psychosexual stages, each identified by a specific body region most sensitive to sexual stimulation and therefore most capable of gratifying id instincts (as described in Table 3-2). The satisfactory gratification of the impulses at one stage allows the individual to move to the next stage. Adjust-

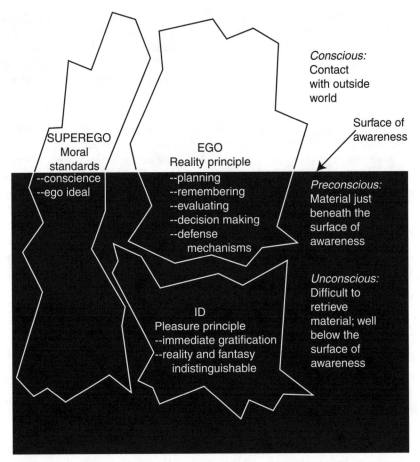

Figure 3-5. Levels of Consciousness and Related Structures of the Mind

ment problems are related to impulses that were ungratified or improperly gratified at earlier stages. Sometimes fixation — excessive attachment to someone or something that is appropriate to an earlier developmental level — may result. At other times, regression — a reversion to an earlier, more immature form of behavior, which is typically due to stress or internal conflict — may occur. The psychosexual stages are as follows: oral, anal, phallic, and genital. A fifth stage of development, the latency stage, occurs between the phallic and genital stages and represents a period when sexuality is repressed.

During the first psychosexual stage, called the oral stage, the maximum gratification of id impulses comes from sucking, feeding, biting, and other behaviors that center around the mouth or oral region, which represents an erogenous zone, or pleasure center. During the second year of life, pleasure shifts to the anal region as the primary source of gratification. The elimina-

Table 3-2.   Psychosexual Developmental Stages

Psychosexual Stage	Age Range	Source of Gratification
Oral	Birth–$1\frac{1}{2}$ years	Oral region (mouth, tongue)
Anal	$1\frac{1}{2}$–3 years	Anal region
Phallic	3–6 years	Genitalia
Latency	6–12 years	Sexual desires repressed
Genital	>12 years	Mature sexual relationships

tion and retention of feces become primary sources of libidinal satisfaction during this period of development.

Between the ages of three and five, children pass through the phallic stage, during which sexual gratification comes from manipulation of the genitalia. It is during the phallic stage that the superego develops in response to the Oedipus complex in boys and the Electra complex in girls. It is theorized that during these psychic conflicts, incestuous desire for opposite-gender parents is repressed and identification with same-gender parents occurs. Thus, boys begin to adopt aspects of their fathers' personalities, while girls adopt those of their mothers. It is through the process of internalizing parental standards, moral beliefs and values that the superego begins to develop.

Following the phallic stage, there is a much needed repression of sexual desires (referred to as the latency stage of psychosexual development) so that children can be primarily engaged in nonsexual learning and socialization experiences. This stage lasts roughly until the children are 12 years of age, the time when puberty generally has its onset. The genital stage is the final psychosexual stage. During this developmental period, Freud believed that sexual drives reappear and sexual gratification is achieved through mature sexual relationships. While earlier forms of sexual desire and expression are notably narcissistic (i.e., focused distinctly on self-gratification), this stage of development relates to an emerging and maturing interest in other people, who are no longer seen solely as objects of self-gratification but rather as unique and valuable in their own right. The defense mechanism of sublimation is likely to be evident during this stage of psychosexual development.

Neo-Freudian Theories

Freudian theory has been altered over the years by many theorists who believe strongly in the power of the unconscious and intrapsychic conflict but who disagree with other aspects of Freud's theory. The Neo-Freudians, as they have come to be called, placed less emphasis on the role of sexuality than did their predecessor. For example, Carl Jung developed analytical psychology, which combined Freudian and humanistic theories. Compared to Freud, he believed the unconscious to be more positive, creative, and spiritual, and he deemphasized the role of sexuality as a motivator of behavior. He also believed that in addition to the personal unconscious, there also exists a collective unconscious, which represents all the experiences of all people over the centuries.

Other theorists took exception to Freud's focus on psychosexual development and instead attended to psychosocial aspects of personality development. Alfred Adler, for example, believed that human beings were motivated more by social needs than sexual drives. According to Adler's theoretical notions, children's goals evolve from selfish to more social over the course of development. Harry Stack Sullivan similarly emphasized the importance of interpersonal relationships in personality development on the grounds that one's developing personality cannot be separated from one's social context. He also stressed that human beings have a basic need for security, as we live in a potentially hostile world. The concept of security and the importance of social relationships in achieving security were also addressed by Karen Horney, who believed that childhood relationships were most critical in determining security and adjustment later in life. The experience of anxiety, according to her theoretical notions, was due primarily to social (i.e., interpersonal) factors rather than factors that were biological or sexual. Finally, Erik Erikson conceptualized a life span theory of psychosocial development in which he emphasized the relationship between individuals and the social context in which they live their lives. Erikson also stressed the impact of this changing relationship on personality development from infancy through old age. Each of these stages is characterized by a specific developmental challenge, or crisis, whose resolution affects how the individual deals with subsequent stages.

Applications in Occupational Therapy

Gail S. Fidler has been credited as being the first occupational therapist to utilize a psychodynamic approach in treatment (Hopkins, 1988). She encouraged the study and use of projective techniques to guide the interpretation of nonverbal communication displayed by the patients within her activity groups (Fidler & Fidler, 1954). Fidler believed a person's relationships with objects in the environment to be integral to the development of the ego. Because occupational therapy used activities requiring patients to interact with both human and nonhuman objects, she felt it was a rich medium through which clients could reveal both feelings and needs and through which the therapist could ascertain unconscious conflicts and the strength of clients' ego defense mechanisms (Miller, Seig, Ludwig, Shortridge, & Van Deusen, 1988).

Anne Cronin Mosey was heavily influenced by Gail Fidler and also described psychiatric function from a psychodynamic frame of reference. She believed that "occupational therapy attempted to bring . . . unconscious content to consciousness and integrate it with conscious content" (Hopkins, 1988, p. 29). Since that time, other occupational therapists have written about the use of projective tests within the realm of occupational therapy but generally have cautioned that the interpretation of an activity in this way requires additional education and collaboration with psychologists and/or psychiatrists. Generally, such authors suggest that a therapist can learn about a client's self-esteem, the presence of underlying conflicts (i.e., control or expression of anger), the ability to relate to the therapist, and the use of ego defense mechanisms through such activities as making tile mosaics, drawings, clay sculpture, and magazine collages (Sheffer & Harlock, 1980).

In summary, psychodynamic theory has had a profound impact on Western culture. Its influence can be seen in our educational system, literature, the arts, and, of course, all the mental health professions. Although the theoretical concepts of Freud and his followers may be regarded as outdated and lacking in empirical validity, they are still in use today by many clinicians. In addition, even though psychodynamic principles may have had less impact on the practice of occupational therapy than the other paradigms, this does not negate the potential value they may have in practice. In particular, a knowledge of psychodynamic concepts can assist the occupational therapist in becoming sensitive to intrapsychic factors (e.g., psychological factors not immediately accessible to consciousness) and early childhood experiences impacting an individual client's functioning. An awareness of defense mechanisms and maladaptive coping mechanisms may also prove to be clinically useful for the occupational therapist. Moreover, a self-reflective, "analytical" way of thinking about the self as therapist stems from the psychoanalytical model. Assessing such factors may facilitate the therapy process as well as the development of more effective treatment plans for clients.

BEHAVIORAL MODEL

Behaviorism is the branch of psychology that studies the interaction of a person and her or his environment. Psychologists following the behavioral model stress the study of objective behavior and generally reject all schools of thought based on subjective reports of thoughts and feelings. Behaviorism is based on a mechanistic model of behavior that is reflective of the early thinking of René Descartes. Descartes described the difference between involuntary and voluntary behavior as a function of what initiated it; a stimulus from the external environment (involuntary) or a higher mental process (voluntary) (Nevin, 1973). Sir Charles Sherrington (1906) expanded this concept by describing the stimulus-and-response mechanisms of reflexes within the human nervous system. A classic example of a stimulus-response paradigm is the stretch reflex elicited by a tendon tap. A tap to the tendon of the quadriceps causes the quadriceps to shorten, resulting in knee extension (i.e., straightening of the knee). In this example, a tendon tap (the stimulus) elicits knee extension (the response).

According to behaviorists, all behavior, whether normal or abnormal, is learned. Furthermore, the learning of such behavior can occur in three distinct ways: through classical or respondent conditioning; operant or instrumental conditioning; or modeling.

Classical Conditioning

Psychologists became interested in the application of reflex properties to behavior through the work of Ivan Pavlov, a physiologist who separated and studied the difference between "inborn" behavior, such as the act of pulling one's hand away from a hot stove, and learned behavior, such as engaging in a withdrawal response after hearing someone scream "Fire!" (Schwartz & Reisberg, 1991). In studying the digestive processes in dogs, Pavlov observed that salivation was always elicited by placement of food in the dog's mouth. He termed the food an unconditioned stimulus (UCS), in that it always caused the same reaction (salivation). A UCS must be shown to produce reliably a desired response without prior training (Gormezano, Prokasy, & Thompson, 1987). He termed the salivation an unconditioned response (UCR), as it was always triggered by the taste of the food. Subsequently, Pavlov noticed that dogs salivated upon the sight of a person bringing the food to them. Pavlov then observed that ringing a bell on successive trials (a conditioned stimulus, or CS), in conjunction with presenting the animal with food (an unconditioned stimulus, or UCS) caused salivation (the UCR) to occur. After repeated pairings of the UCS with the CS, Pavlov found that he was able to elicit salivation using the CS in isolation. He now termed the appearance of salivation a conditioned response (CR) because the response was now elicited by the conditioned stimulus (bell) alone (i.e., without the presentation of the unconditioned stimulus). Over time, the conditioned stimulus fails to elicit the conditioned response if it continues to be presented without the unconditioned stimulus. This is referred to as extinction. This process of learning by temporal association is what behaviorists refer to as classical or respondent conditioning.

John B. Watson was strongly influenced by Pavlov's theories and rejected other psychological theories of his day as being too subjective. He felt that unobservable events (i.e., thought processes, perceptions of stimuli, and feelings and emotions) should not be a part of any scientific theory. Instead, Watson felt that stimuli and responses elicited by those stimuli should form the basis of scientific analysis. Watson is best known for applying Pavlov's theories of classical conditioning to human learning. In one study, Watson and Rayner (1920) "trained" a young boy to be frightened of a furry, white rabbit by presenting it in conjunction with a loud noise. Not only did the boy learn to associate the harmless rabbit with the fear response, he also generalized the response to other white, furry objects.

This study formed the basis for a technique developed by Joseph Wolpe (1958) to treat phobias, which is known as systematic desensitization. This technique focuses on the use of progressive muscle relaxation procedures and gradual exposure to feared stimuli at increasing levels of intensity in order to eliminate phobias. The basic premise is built on the concept of reciprocal inhibition, which simply states that one cannot feel anxious and relaxed at the same time. Thus, if you can create a state of relaxation and pair it with the presentation of a feared stimulus, the anxiety will ultimately be extinguished. This technique is often successful when used with clients who have specific phobias or who are afraid to engage in certain types of activities.

Operant Conditioning

Edward L. Thorndike studied the goal-directed behavior of cats attempting to escape from a box to obtain food (1898). The box was equipped with a lever that opened the door and allowed the cat to escape. Thorndike described the cat's initial attempts at escape as purely random movements that accidentally tripped the lever, allowing the cat to escape and obtain food. However, with increasing numbers of learning trials, the amount of time between placement in and escape from the box decreased. Thorndike also observed that the cat's behavior came closer and closer to the target behavior with each learning trial in that the cat used less random, unnecessary movements and more efficient, goal-directed ones. Thorndike concluded that when a response (i.e., pushing the lever) is followed by a positive event (i.e., escape and food), it is more likely to be repeated; conversely, if a response (i.e., random movement) is followed by a negative event (i.e., inability to escape and lack of food), it is likely to cease. This principle is known as the law of effect and serves as the basis for a type of learning known as operant or instrumental conditioning.

B. F. Skinner expanded Thorndike's theory by studying the behavior of hungry rats in a device known as the Skinner box, which contains both a lever and an empty food plate (1938). In his studies, lever pushing initially did not cause anything to happen. In this situation, the rats rarely pressed the lever. Subsequently, the lever was connected to a food container such that depression of the lever resulted in a few food pellets being delivered into the food plate. Skinner then observed that the incidence of lever pressing increased dramatically. He concluded that behavior followed by a positive consequence will result in an increase in that behavior. Skinner then hooked up a device that hit the rat's paw each time it attempted to press the lever. As predicted, the incidence of lever pressing decreased dramatically compared to the condition in which the rats were given food for reinforcement. Skinner thus concluded that behavior followed by a negative consequence (i.e., punishment) will result in a decrease in that behavior.

Skinner cited these and other studies to support his theory of operant conditioning, which states that behavior can be modified by its consequences. Operant and classical conditioning differ in that the behaviors elicited by operant conditioning are voluntary, while those elicited by classical conditioning are involuntary. Skinner then renamed the law of effect, now referring to the concept as the principle of reinforcement. He also asserted that reinforcement is the primary mechanism for learning and for explaining human behavior.

Skinner (1938, 1953) described the different types of reinforcement and punishment contingencies he used in operant conditioning trials. Positive and negative reinforcement both serve to increase the occurrence of target behaviors, while positive and negative punishment serve to decrease behaviors. Positive reinforcement can best be explained as rewarding a person or animal for a behavior after its occurrence. Rewards can be given in such forms as food, praise, hugs, or new clothes — anything qualifies as long as the person receiving the reward perceives it positively. Negative reinforcement also increases the likelihood of a behavior reoccurring, but it does so through the removal of an aversive stimulus. Positive punishment refers to the delivery of an aversive stimulus in response to a behavior. Spanking or yelling are examples of positive punishment. Negative punishment refers to the removal of a positive stimulus in response to a behavior. An example of negative punishment is taking food away from a brain-injured client who is purposefully spitting it out on the table. Taking away privileges (e.g., going for a walk, watching TV, earning an allowance or tokens) from a child for inappropriate behavior may be an effective negative punishment.

Edwin Guthrie conducted studies providing valuable insight into the importance of the time interval between the presentation of a stimulus and the subsequent presentation of a reward (1935). He found that if the reward is delayed following a correct response to a stimulus, the learner may attribute another response (made during the time delay) to reward acquisition. This principle is especially important when treating children or clients with cognitive deficits, for whom immediacy in delivering reinforcements is critical to promoting behavior change.

Reinforcement schedules describe differences in the elapsed time interval and rate with which behaviors are reinforced. Differences in schedules of reinforcement lead to different response sets. There are two general types of reinforcement schedules: continuous and intermittent. In continuous reinforcement, every occurrence of a target behavior is reinforced, while in intermittent reinforcement, some, but not all, instances of a behavior are reinforced. Intermittent reinforcement can be based on either the number of behaviors required for reinforcement (ratio schedules) or the amount of time that must elapse before a behavior is reinforced (interval schedules). Ratio and interval schedules can be either fixed (i.e., a set number of responses or elapsed time is required prior to the delivery of reinforcement) or variable (i.e., the number of responses and elapsed time required for reinforcement constantly changes). Response rates vary according to the reinforcement schedules used. The use of continuous reinforcement schedules is advised when teaching new behaviors, while intermittent reinforcement schedules are recommended for the maintenance of acquired skills (S. M. Deitz, 1985).

Skinner described different methods of teaching behaviors using principles of reinforcement. Shaping and chaining represent two such methods. Both can be used in clinical settings to teach more complex behaviors. Shaping involves reinforcing a person for closer and closer approximations of a target behavior. Initially, only a simple response is required. The criteria for reinforcement are then gradually made more stringent in an attempt to elicit more complex or refined target behaviors (Becker, 1985). This technique is widely used to teach verbal behavior (i.e., language), whereby closer and closer approximations of the required sound, word, or phrase are needed to obtain reinforcement. Clients with head injury, mental retardation, or autism often benefit from this form of teaching.

Chaining refers to a method of reinforcement involving the linking of component skills to teach a more complex behavior. This procedure involves reinforcing in a particular sequence simple behaviors that are already in the individual's repertoire in an effort to teach more complex skills (D. E. D. Deitz, 1985a). Chaining can be accomplished in either a forward or backward format. Forward chaining refers to the teaching of a task's subcomponents in the order in which they are to be performed so as to complete the task (D. E. D. Deitz, 1985b), while backward chaining teaches the subcomponent skills in reverse order. In this case, the final response is taught first, then the preceding response, and so on, until the first response in the sequence has been taught (Schreibman, 1985). A benefit of backward chaining is that the client produces the final product each time, which makes tasks more meaningful and less frustrating. Backward chaining generally appears to be the more effective of the two methods, although both are widely used clinically.

A final concept studied by Skinner was the extinction of behaviors. *Extinction* refers to the decline in rate of a target behavior and ultimate elimination of that behavior. Skinner found that he could eliminate (or extinguish) a response by removing the reinforcement that followed it; this is referred to as operant extinction (Poling, 1985). In laboratory studies, it has been demonstrated that animals initially continue to elicit behaviors following the removal of reinforcement, sometimes even at an increased rate, but that response rates decline and eventually fade with time. Skinner did note that some behaviors were more resistant to extinction than others, which had to do with the schedule of reinforcement used during the skill acquisition phase of learning. Specifically, behaviors that are reinforced more variably prove more resistant to extinction procedures, while those on a fixed schedule are extinguished more easily. Behaviors can also be eliminated using respondent extinction, in which unconditioned stimuli consistently fail to follow conditioned stimuli, thereby weakening the likelihood of the conditioned response reoccurring (Poling, 1985).

Modeling

In addition to the classical and operant conditioning explanations for the acquisition of behavior, Albert Bandura (1977) recognized that learning also occurred through observation and imitation of the behaviors of others. Bandura expanded Skinner's theory of operant conditioning by stating that persons can learn by observing the consequences that people receive for their behaviors. For example, if a child observes her sibling receive a piece of candy for making her bed, she may learn vicariously that making one's bed results in receiving treats. Consequently, she may be more likely to make her bed in the future. Bandura differs from Skinner in that he differentiates learning from the performance of learned behaviors. Bandura claims that although the child in this example may have learned that making one's bed results in reinforcement, she may nevertheless choose to not perform the task. This may be due, in part, to appraisals she makes about the relative value of the reinforcement to the task requirements. Thus, Bandura integrates cognitive components into his understanding of modeling and observational learning.

Bandura (1986) has cited four critical factors necessary for a behavior to be learned observationally and subsequently performed. First, in order for observational learning to occur, the learner must attend to the modeled behavior. Second, the learner must form and retain a mental image of the modeled behavior for later use. Third, the learner must reproduce the modeled behavior from the stored image. That is, he or she must take the stored mental image and convert it into overt behavior. Fourth, the observational learning process requires that the learner be sufficiently motivated to reproduce the modeled behavior. Bandura's understanding of behavior acquisition clearly reflects his appreciation for the mediating influence of cognitive processes in learning. Proponents of the cognitive model, in fact, assert that cognitive processes are primary in determining psychopathology.

Applications in Occupational Therapy

Behavioral principles are widely used in contemporary society (e.g., in the educational, legal, and employment systems) in an effort to promote productive and prosocial behaviors of individuals. Related procedures are also commonly used in the practice of psychology and related disciplines, such as occupational therapy. Behavioral systems are particularly used in programs for adolescents and milieu treatment. Additionally, some behavioral principles, such as reinforcement and reward, are commonly incorporated into day treatment models and long-term care facilities for people with mental illness.

Because behavioral strategies are relatively concrete and do not require complex verbal, cognitive, or psychosocial abilities, they can be used effectively with a variety of clinical populations (e.g., individuals with mental retardation, autism, or schizophrenia). Attending to a client's learning history, including reinforcement contingencies that influence behavior, can be very useful to the practicing occupational therapist when designing treatment protocols. In addition, using conditioning and modeling procedures in therapy certainly will facilitate more positive outcomes for clients (especially individuals with cognitive deficits, young children, and clients lacking sufficient internal motivation to comply with treatment).

COGNITIVE MODEL

Although interest in cognitive processes has a long history in experimental psychology, a clinical model of their etiological significance in psychopathology only began to emerge in response to traditional behavioral notions that rejected the mediating influence of mental processes on abnormal behavior. Proponents of the cognitive model, therefore, believe that behavior is influenced by factors other than observable environmental stimuli and the responses they elicit. These theorists argue strongly that what people think, believe, expect, remember, and attend to influences how they behave (O'Leary & Wilson, 1987). Specifically, dysfunctional cognitive processes are thought to produce psychological disorder. Furthermore, altering a person's cognitions (i.e., making them more functional and adaptive) can ameliorate psychological difficulties. Although the behaviorists, such as Skinner (1971), acknowledged that mental life existed, they denied the causal role of cognitions in behavior. Cognitive psychologists, on the other hand, view cognitions as primary causal agents in psychopathology, and therefore, as first-order treatment targets.

Cognitive psychologists take issue with the basic stimulus-response conditioning theories of behaviorists, which they find far too passive and simplistic. These theorists believe that the learner actively interprets novel information relative to previously acquired information, which they refer to as a schema (Neisser, 1976). Rescorla (1988) even conceptualizes classical conditioning as an active process by which individuals learn about relationships among events.

The application of cognitive psychology concepts and principles to the understanding and treatment of psychopathology is a relatively recent phenomenon and is becoming increasingly popular, especially when combined with behavioral approaches in what is referred to as cognitive-behavior therapy. The focus of related treatments generally is to alter cognitions and cognitive processes in order to facilitate behavioral and emotional changes. The general term for this treatment approach is *cognitive restructuring*. Several prominent professionals in the field have proposed cognitive theories of psychopathology that bear mentioning. Notable figures include Albert Bandura, Aaron Beck, and Albert Ellis. For the purposes of therapy, cognitive processes can be divided into those that are short term and those that are long term. Short-term processes, including expectations, appraisals, and attributions, are processes of which we either are or can become aware through practice. On the other hand, long-term processes, including beliefs, are generally not readily available to consciousness.

Expectations

Expectations refer to cognitions that anticipate future events. In his seminal work on modeling and observational learning, Albert Bandura assessed the impact of expectations on the performance of learned behaviors. Bandura demonstrated that individuals learn behavior, not only by receiving reinforcement directly for the expression of that behavior, but also by observing others receiving reinforcement for the same behavior. As a result of this evidence for vicarious learning, Bandura hypothesized that learning must involve expectations in addition to operant conditioning principles (Bandura, 1977, 1978; Bandura & Walters, 1959). According to Bandura's theory, two types of expectations are relevant to behavior change: an outcome expectation and an efficacy expectation. An outcome expectation is a person's belief that a given behavior will lead to a desired outcome, while an efficacy expectation is the person's belief that he or she can, in fact, perform the behavior necessary to produce the desired outcome. Both are critical to understanding the mechanisms underlying the acquisition and application of learned behavior. In fact, it has been shown that individuals may learn that a specific behavior will result in a desired outcome but, because they do not believe they have the capacity to perform the target behavior, it nonetheless fails to be produced. As a result, some desired outcomes do not occur (Bandura, 1977, 1978; Bandura & Adams, 1977).

Appraisals

Human beings are constantly evaluating events occurring in their everyday lives. Sometimes these appraisals are evident. Other times, these evaluative processes are not conscious, but rather automatic, most likely due to a lifetime of practice. In his cognitive explanations for psychopathology, Aaron Beck (1976) emphasizes automatic thoughts as causal agents of psychological disorder; in fact, he argues that emotion states are always preceded by related thought processes. In therapy, the individual is taught to slow down and become aware of relevant negative automatic thoughts so that they may then be restructured (Goldfried, Decenteceo, & Weinburg, 1974).

Beck is primarily interested in cognitive processes related to depression (Beck, 1967, 1976; Beck, Rush, Shaw, & Emery, 1979), but his theoretical concepts have also been successfully applied to other psychological conditions, including personality and anxiety disorders. Specifically, Beck noted that depressed individuals tend to distort their realities by engaging in dysfunctional thought processes. Beck's cognitive therapy of depression is primarily concerned with altering negative thoughts about one's self, the world, and the future and with correcting general misinterpretations of life events that individuals with depression typically possess. The pattern of negative thinking described by Beck is called the "cognitive triad," which refers to negative self-evaluation, a pessimistic view of the world, and a sense of hopelessness regarding future outcomes. These thoughts reflect the drawing of false conclusions by selectively attending to isolated aspects of a situation (selective abstraction), the exaggerating of the importance of negative events (magnification), and the generalizing of the significance of isolated events for one's life (overgeneralization). These pervasive negative thoughts represent primary treatment targets in Beck's cognitive therapy for depression. The goal of therapy, therefore, is to help the patient monitor and systematically refute illogical and negative self-statements.

Attributions

Attributions are an individual's beliefs about cause-and-effect relationships. For example, an individual might make internal or external attributions (Rotter, 1966), stable or unstable attributions (Weiner, 1974), or global or specific attributions (Abramson, Seligman, & Teasdale, 1978; Seligman, 1991); the specific array of attributions made determines differential behavioral outcomes. Internal attributions emphasize the causal role of intrapersonal variables, while external attributions focus on the role of the environment or other factors out of the individual's personal control. Stable attributions are those that are persistent over time, whereas unstable attributions are considered transient. Finally, global attributions emphasize the persistence of behavior across tasks, while specific attributions relate to one's understanding that a certain behavior is specific to a certain task. The goal of cognitive therapists is to alter the attributions that individuals make so that they become more rational and adaptive.

Beliefs

Albert Ellis (1962) argues that irrational beliefs, instilled in us over the course of our lives by parents and society, are at the root of psychological disorder. In addition to being maladaptive in and of themselves, these beliefs are also presumed to shape short-term, dysfunctional expectations, appraisals, and attributions. Specifically, maladaptive behaviors and emotions are due to false assumptions (e.g., illogical "shoulds" and "musts") that individuals make about their behavior and the world. As defined by Ellis, six such assumptions are as follows:

1. Adult human beings must be loved and approved by all significant others.
2. In order to be worthy, one should be competent, adequate, and successful in all possible respects.
3. It is catastrophic when things are not the way one would like them to be.

4. Unhappiness is externally caused, and one has little or no control over negative events.
5. Past history is the critical determinant of present behavior, and events that strongly affect one's life will continue to do so.
6. There is always a perfect solution to one's problems, and it is catastrophic if that ideal solution is not found (Ellis, 1962).

Ellis's rational emotive therapy (RET) actively confronts and challenges these assumptions or false beliefs and attempts to replace them with those that are more rational and, hence, more adaptive to an individual's functioning.

Applications in Occupational Therapy

The cognitive model of psychology is clearly among the more prominent of the contemporary theoretical paradigms. Its focus on cognitive processes that mediate behavior has proven to be a very rich area for empirical study. In addition, the inclusion of cognitive components in psychological assessment and intervention has resulted in more comprehensive and effective treatment outcomes for many clients. Psychology is certainly not the only discipline attending to the influential role of cognitions in the manifestation and amelioration of aberrant behaviors and emotions. Other service providers, including occupational therapists, also attend to cognitive processes in their assessment and treatment of clients. By attending to dysfunctional appraisals, expectancies, attributions, and beliefs, a therapist may be better able to facilitate and maintain behavioral and emotional changes in their clients. Research in the area of cognitive psychology has also enhanced our understanding of the importance of providing clients with meaningful tasks and therapeutic activities that are consistent with their level of cognitive functioning — factors that are critical across disciplines.

Summary

The broad psychological models discussed in this chapter contribute to occupational therapy's underlying philosophy and also contribute to the tools and strategies used in OT treatment. Occupational therapists integrate skills both in executing specific adjunctive activities and in developing a plan to increase their clients' independence and self-efficacy. The underlying belief of occupational therapy is that health is maintained through preserving and enhancing an individual's ability to carry out daily activities in the areas of work/education, self-care, and play/leisure. Since every client is unique, treatment plans must be personalized in order to assure that the goals of treatment are those that are most meaningful to the particular client. To understand clients' behavior, it is imperative that occupational therapists have a comprehensive understanding of the biological, intrapsychic, and interpersonal factors mediating that behavior. For example, it is essential to have an understanding of the clients' level of cognitive and perceptual functioning, their ability to process sensory input and produce motor output, their cultural belief system, personality factors that were present prior to injury or disease onset, and valued life roles. Only then can a therapist establish and carry out a treatment plan that is meaningful to the particular client. Psychological theory and research provides many of the tools necessary to develop effective treatment plans. Although the theoretical concepts presented here from the biological, psychodynamic, behavioral, cognitive, and humanistic models are distinct in their understanding and treatment of psychological disorders, they are not necessarily incompatible. In fact, the integration of concepts should provide the practicing clinician with a better understanding of the biopsychosocial factors influencing behaviors, thoughts, and emotions. Theoretical integration should also allow for the development of individualized treatment plans that are both more comprehensive and more effective.

Review Questions

1.–5. Identify the following key points for each of the psychological models presented in this chapter.
1. Humanistic model:
2. Biological model:
3. Psychodynamic model:
4. Behavioral model:
5. Cognitive Model:

       View of human beings

       Source of motivation

       Etiology of illness

       Cultural implications

       Implications for interdisciplinary treatment

       Implications for occupational therapy

6. Describe the benefits and disadvantages to using an eclectic approach to therapy.

Learning Activities

1. Choose one of the models presented in this chapter and prepare either a written or oral report explaining why you think the particular model is best suited for occupational therapy practice.
2. Choosing a different model, prepare a similiar report discussing the model's limitations in occupational therapy practice.
3. This textbook has many contibuting authors, each with different training and experiences with these psychological models. As you read the fol-

lowing chapters, try to identify the particular model that best matches each author's perspective.
4. Think about yourself and identify a daily life problem that you want help in resolving. Which model would be most helpful for a therapist to use with you?

References

Abramson, L. Y., Seligman, M. E. P., & Teasdale, J. (1978). Learned helplessness in humans: Critique and reformulation. *Journal of Abnormal Psychology, 87,* 49–74.

Angrist, B., Lee, H. K., & Gershon, S. (1974). The antagonism of amphetamine-induced symptomatology by a neuroleptic. *American Journal of Psychiatry, 131,* 817–819.

Association for Humanistic Psychology. (1987). *The meaning of humanistic psychology.* San Francisco, CA: Author.

Bandura, A. (1977). *Social learning theory.* Englewood Cliffs, NJ: Prentice-Hall.

Bandura, A. (1978). The self system in reciprocal determinism. *American Psychologist, 37,* 122–147.

Bandura, A. (1986). *Social foundations of thought and action: A social cognitive theory.* Englewood Cliffs, NJ: Prentice-Hall.

Bandura, A., & Adams, N. E. (1977). Analysis of self-efficacy theory of behavioral changes. *Cognitive Theory and Research, 1,* 287–310.

Bandura, A., & Walters, R. H. (1959). *Adolescent aggression.* New York: Ronald Press.

Barondes, S. H. (1993). *Molecules and mental illness.* New York: Scientific American.

Beck, A. T. (1967). *Depression: Clinical, experimental, and theoretical aspects.* New York: Harper & Row.

Beck, A.T. (1976). *Cognitive therapy and the emotional disorders.* New York: International Universities Press.

Beck, A. T., Rush, A. J., Shaw, B. F., & Emery, G. (1979). *Cognitive therapy of depression.* New York: Guilford Press.

Becker, R. E. (1985). Shaping. In A. S. Bellack & M. Hersen (Eds.), *Dictionary of behavior therapy techniques* (p. 205). New York: Pergamon Press.

Bloom, F. E., Lazerson, A., & Hofstadter, L. (1985). *Brain, mind, and behavior.* New York: Freeman.

Bouchard, T. J., Lykken, D. T., McGue, M., Segal, N. L., & Tellegen, A. (1990). Sources of human psychological differences: The Minnesota study of twins reared apart. *Science, 250,* 223–228.

Bouchard, T. J., & McGue, M. (1990). Genetic and rearing environmental influences on adult personality: An analysis of adopted twins reared apart. *Journal of Personality, 58,* 263–292.

Braestrup, C., Schmiechen, R., Neef, G., Nielson, M., & Petersen, E. N. (1982). Interactions of convulsive ligands with benzodiazepine receptors. *Science, 216,* 1241–1243.

Comer, R. (1995). *Abnormal psychology* (2nd ed.). New York: Freeman.

Davis, J. M., & Adams, H. E. (1995). Models. In L. A. Heiden & M. Hersen (Eds.), *Introduction to clinical psychology* (pp. 21–46). New York: Plenum Press.

Deitz, D. E. D. (1985a). Chaining. In A. S. Bellack & M. Hersen (Eds.), *Dictionary of behavior therapy techniques* (p. 53). New York: Pergamon Press.

Deitz, D. E. D. (1985b). Forward chaining. In A. S. Bellack & M. Hersen (Eds.), *Dictionary of behavior therapy techniques* (p. 131). New York: Pergamon Press.

Deitz, S. M. (1985). Schedules of reinforcement. In A. S. Bellack & M. Hersen (Eds.), *Dictionary of behavior therapy techniques* (p. 189). New York: Pergamon Press.

Ellis, A. (1962). *Reason and emotion in psychotherapy.* New York: Lyle Stuart.

Fidler, G. S., & Fidler, J. W. (1954). *Introduction to psychiatric occupational therapy.* New York: Macmillan.

Fidler, G. S., & Fidler, J. W. (1963). *Occupational therapy: A communication process in psychiatry.* New York: Macmillan.

Fidler, G. S., & Fidler, J. W. (1978). Doing and becoming: Purposeful action and self-actualization. *American Journal of Occupational Therapy, 32,* 305.

Frankl, V. E. (1967). *Psychotherapy and existential papers on logotherapy.* New York: Square Press.

Frankl, V. E. (1972). *The doctor and the soul.* New York: Alfred Knopf.

Freud, S. (1976). *The ego and the id.* In J. Strachey (Ed. & Trans.), *The complete psychological works* (Vol. 19). New York: Norton. (Original work published 1923)

Gershon, E. S., & Rieder, R. O. (1992). Major disorders of the brain. *Scientific American, 267,* 127–133.

Goldfried, M. R., Decenteceo, E. T., & Weinberg, L. (1974). Systematic rational restructuring as a self-control technique. *Behavior Therapy, 5,* 247–254.

Gormezano, I., Prokasy, W., & Thompson, R. (1987). *Classical conditioning* (3rd ed.). Hillsdale, NJ: Lawrence Erlbaum Associates.

Gottesman, I. I. (1991). *Schizoprenia genesis: The origins of madness.* New York: Freeman.

Grilly, D. M. (1989). *Drugs and human behavior.* Boston: Allyn & Bacon.

Guthrie, E. R. (1935). *The psychology of learning.* New York: Harper.

Harper, R. A. (1975). *The new psychotherapies.* Englewood Cliffs, NJ: Prentice-Hall.

Hopkins, H. L. (1988). An historical perspective on occupational therapy. In H. L. Hopkins & D. H. Smith (Eds.), *Willard and Spackman's occupational therapy* (7th ed., pp. 16–37). Philadelphia: Lippincott.

Kalat, J. (1988). *Biological psychology* (3rd ed.). Belmont, CA: Wadsworth Publishing Company.

Kaplan, H., and Sadock, B. (1995). *Comprehensive textbook of psychiatry* (6th ed.). Baltimore: Williams & Wilkins.

Maslow, A. H. (1968). *Toward a psychology of being*. New York: Van Nostrand-Reinhold.

Meehl, P. E. (1962). Schizotaxia, schizotypy, schizophrenia. *American Psychologist, 17,* 827–838.

Miller, R. , Seig, K., Ludwig, F., Shortridge, S., & Van Deusen, J. (1988). *Six perspectives on theory for the practice of occupational therapy.* Rockville, MD: Aspen.

Mosey, A. C. (1980). A model for occupational therapy. *Occupational Therapy in Mental Health, 1,* 11–31.

Neisser, U. (1976). *Cognition and reality*. San Francisco: Freeman.

Nevin, J. (1973). *The study of behavior: Learning, motivation, emotion, and instinct.* Reading, MA: Addison-Wesley Educational Publishers, Inc.

O'Leary, K. D., & Wilson, G. T. (1987). *Behavior therapy: Application and outcome.* Englewood Cliffs, NJ: Prentice-Hall.

Patterson, C. H. (1989). Eclecticism in psychotherapy: Is integration possible? *Psychotherapy, 26,* 157–161.

Plomin, R., DeFries, J. C., & McClearn, G. E. (1990). *Behavioral genetics* (2nd ed.). New York: Freeman.

Poling, A. (1985). Extinction. In A. S. Bellack & M. Hersen (Eds.), *Dictionary of behavior therapy techniques* (p. 124). New York: Pergamon Press.

Reilly, M. (1962). Occupational therapy can be one of the greatest ideas of twentieth century medicine. *American Journal of Occupational Therapy, 16,* 1–16.

Rescorla, R. A. (1988). Pavlovian conditioning: It's not what you think it is. *American Psychologist, 43,* 151–160.

Rogers, C. R. (1942). *Counseling and psychotherapy: Newer concepts in practice.* Boston: Houghton Mifflin.

Rogers, C. R. (1951). *Client-centered therapy: Its current practice, implications, and theory.* Boston, Houghton Mifflin.

Rogers, C. R. (1961). *On becoming a person: A therapist's view of psychotherapy.* Boston: Houghton Mifflin.

Rotter, J. B. (1966). Generalized expectancies for internal versus external control of reinforcement. *Psychological Monographs, 80*(1).

Schildkraut, J. J. (1965). The catecholamine hypothesis of affective disorders: A review of supporting evidence. *American Journal of Psychiatry, 122,* 509–522.

Schreibman, L. (1985). Backward chaining. In A. S. Bellack & M. Hersen (Eds.), *Dictionary of behavior therapy techniques* (p. 22). New York: Pergamon Press.

Schwartz, B., & Reisberg, D. (1991). *Learning and memory*. New York: W. W. Norton.

Seligman, M. E. P. (1991). *Learned optimism: The skill to conquer life's obstacles, large and small.* New York: Random House.

Sheffer, M., & Harlock, S. (1980). Tell us what your drawings say. *Occupational Therapy in Mental Health, 1,* 21–38.

Sherrington, C. S. (1906). *The integrative action of the nervous system.* New Haven, CT: Yale University Press.

Siever, L. J., Davis, K. L., & Gorman, L. K. (1991). Pathogenesis of mood disorders. In K. Davis, H. Klar, & J. T. Coyle (Eds.), *Foundations of psychiatry* (pp. 254–262). Philadelphia: W. B. Saunders.

Skinner, B.F. (1938). *The behavior of organisms: An experimental analysis.* New York: Appleton-Century-Crofts.

Skinner, B. F. (1953). *Science and human behavior.* New York: Macmillan.

Skinner, B. F. (1971). *Beyond freedom and dignity.* New York: Knopf.

Thompson, R. (1993). *The brain: A neuroscience primer.* New York: Freeman.

Thorndike, E. L. (1898). Animal intelligence: An experimental study of the associative processes in animals. *Psychological Review Monograph Supplement, 2*(8).

Waller, N., Kojetin, B., Bouchard, T., Lykken, D., & Tellegen, A. (1990). Genetic and environmental influences on religious interests, attitudes, and values. *Psychological Science, 1,* 138–142.

Watson, J. B., & Rayner, R. (1920). Conditioned emotional reactions. *Journal of Experimental Psychology, 3,* 1–4.

Weiner, B. (Ed.). (1974). *Achievement motivation and attribution theory.* Morristown, NJ: General Learning Press.

Wolpe, J. (1958). *Psychotherapy by reciprocal inhibition.* Stanford, CA: Stanford University Press.

Wong, D. F., Wagner, H. N., Jr., Tune, L. E., Dannals, R. F., Pearlson, G. D., Links, J. M., Wilson, A. A., Toung, J. K. T., Malat, J., Williams, J. A., O'-Tuama, L. A., Snyder, S. H., Kuhar, M. J., & Gjedde, A. (1986). Positron emission tomography reveals elevated D_2 dopamine receptors in drug naive schizophrenics. *Science, 234,* 1558–1562.

Yerxa, E. J. (1967). Authentic occupational therapy. *American Journal of Occupational Therapy, 21,* 1–9.

Suggested Reading

Diasio Serrett, K. (Ed.). (1985). *Philososophical and historical roots of occupational therapy.* New York: Haworth Press.

Ellis, A. (1973). *Humanistic psychotherapy: The rational-emotive approach.* New York: McGraw-Hill.

Frankl, V. (1978). *The unheard cry for meaning:Psychotherapy and humanism.* New York: Simon & Schuster.

Hopkins, H. (1988). Current basis for theory and philosophy of occupational therapy. In H. Hopkins & H. Smith (Eds.), *Willard and Spackman's occupational therapy* (7th ed., pp. 38–42). Philadelphia: Lippincott.

Shannon, P. (1977). The derailment of occupational therapy. *American Journal of Occupational Therapy, 31*(4), 229–234.

Yerxa, E. (1979). The philosophical base of occupational therapy. In *Occupational therapy — 2001*. Rockville, MD: American Occupational Therapy Association.

Occupational Therapy Models

Anne MacRae

Janet Falk-Kessler, Ed.D., OTR, FAOTA
Assistant Professor of Clinical Occupational Therapy
Associate Director of the Programs in Occupational Therapy,
Columbia University

Dorothy Julin, MA, OTR
Chief Occupational Therapist
Alameda County Medical Center, San Leandro, California

Rene Padilla, MS, OTR
Assistant Professor, Creighton University, Omaha, Nebraska

Sally Schultz, Ph.D., OTR
Coordinator of Graduate Studes
Associate Professor, Texas Women's University, Denton, Texas

Key Terms

dynamical systems theory
expectant treatment
general systems theory
in vivo
meta-models
occupational activity

occupational readiness
open systems theory
organizational abilities
relative mastery
task environment

Chapter Outline

Introduction

The basic psychological theories that underscore mental health treatment were outlined in the previous chapter. These broad-based belief systems are interdisciplinary in nature. Each specific discipline, including occupational therapy, uses one or more of these belief systems to forge its own professional expertise. In this chapter, a review of concepts specific to occupational therapy is presented. The authors of this chapter represent clinicians and educators who use these models and frames of reference in practice and teach clinical interpretations of them. It is not possible in the confines of this chapter to do justice to each model or concept. Readers are urged to use the primary sources listed in the reference and suggested reading sections for a complete discussion of the underlying theory. However, in order for the reader to understand how these models are used in practice, each author discusses a single case illustration from the perspective of a particular model.

The language of theory development includes such terms as *theory, model, frame of reference, approach,* and *paradigm.* While it could be argued that each concept is distinct, these terms are used in multiple fashions and no single set of definitions has appealed to all clinicians. Therefore, for the purposes of this chapter, the terminology that is used is consistent with the original sources and no further attempt is made at creating uniformity. However, we believe that a practice-based discipline such as occupational therapy benefits from a broad-based interpretation of the term *theory,* such as is presented by Lela Llorens: "Theory is not static, nor is it ever final. It merely represents the current state of knowledge on a given topic at a particular time. As more facts become available[,] . . . theory changes and improves" (1984, p. 9). Occupational therapy does not yet have a fully developed unifying "theory" on which to base its practice in mental health. Instead, several models, frames of reference, and theoretical concepts together form the basis for occupational therapy in mental health.

Occupational therapists practicing in mental health use a mixture of many different theories, models, concepts and techniques (Barris, 1984). For the purposes of this chapter, discussion is limited to commonly used and recently introduced models and concepts in occupational therapy mental health practice. They all differ in their level of theory development, expressed purpose, and applicability to different client populations, making them, metaphorically, a collection of "apples and oranges." Therefore, it is impossible to compare their relative value. The models of occupational performance and human occupation, as well as the occupational adaptation and the acquisitional frame of reference, are broad in scope and can be considered **meta-models,** whereas the theory of cognitive disability is restricted in its focus to a specific component of human functioning, namely, cognition.

OCCUPATIONAL PERFORMANCE MODEL

The concept of occupational performance pervades the theoretical thinking of the profession and is considered a basic premise of the field. However, the model is more than a single concept and instead is discussed in this chapter as a guide for practice.

The model of occupational performance was originally developed by the American Occupational Therapy Association (AOTA) as a guide for developing curricula for occupational therapy academic programs in the United States (AOTA, 1974). Pedretti developed the AOTA model further to form a frame of reference for the treatment of physical disabilities (1985), and Llorens (1991) contributed a developmental perspective to the model by describing occupational performance from infancy through extreme old age. Until recently, however, the potential use of this model for the treatment of psychosocial dysfunction had not been adequately explored.

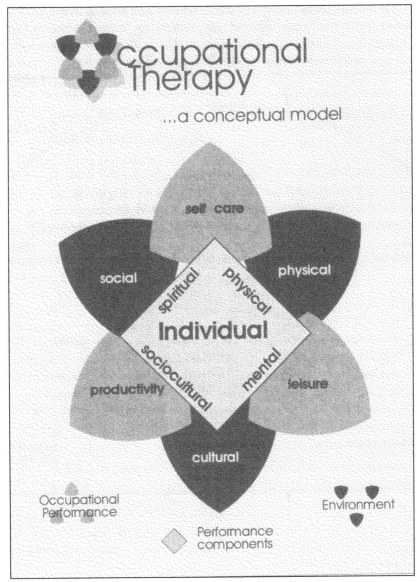

Figure 4-1. Interacting Elements of the Individual in a Revised Model of Occupational Performance

(From *Occupational Therapy Guidelines for Client-Centered Mental Health Practice* (CAOT, 1993).

The Canadian Association of Occupational Therapists (CAOT) developed their own version of the model of occupational performance in 1991. The revised model is shown in Figure 4-1. The model of occupational performance as articulated by CAOT was based on their *Occupational Therapy Guidelines for Client-Centered Mental Health Practice* (CAOT, 1993) and is, therefore, an ideal framework for this chapter. However, this presentation of this model is also substantially influenced by the AOTA version, and the discussion pertains to both versions.

The original model of occupational performance acknowledged the role of "life space influences," which included cultural background and the human and nonhuman environments. However, there was no built-in mechanism for applying this information, causing it to remain an evolving process for the profession. The third edition of the "Uniform Terminology for Occupational Therapy" (AOTA, 1994) describes environment as a performance context. This is consistent with the CAOT model, which depicts the social, physical, and cultural environments. As the discipline of occupational therapy becomes more culturally sensitive, increasing emphasis is being placed on examining all the occupational performance areas and components through the eyes of a culturally diverse "other."

Occupational Performance Areas

The occupational performance areas are divided into self-care, productivity, and leisure. If the model is viewed as representing the sum total of human activity, then these categories cannot be narrowly defined. The occupational performance areas also cannot be viewed as being mutually exclusive, as there is much overlap between self-care, productivity, and leisure. Actually, activities that do overlap by fulfilling more than one occupational performance area often are viewed as having more personal meaning for the individual and the potential of greater satisfaction. An example would be a professional athlete who exercises for leisure, work, and self-care. Another example is personal — being a professor is considered a work role, yet many people also consider reading, writing, research, and teaching to have leisure and self-care qualities. Academic activities can be relaxing and enjoyable, and they also provide a deep sense of personal fulfillment and satisfaction.

Depending on one's culture, diagnosis, and personal interests, an activity may be viewed by a client very differently than by the therapist. Care must be taken to understand how clients view their tasks of occupational performance, as that view must supersede the therapist's interpretation.

Self-Care Activities.   Self-care activities include the routine activity of daily living (ADL) such as grooming, hygiene, dressing, and feeding. However, especially in psychosocial practice, self-care implies much more. I believe that any activity in which an individual engages for the purpose of self-fulfillment can be considered "inner self-care." Doing yoga or other forms of spiritual meditation and exercise may be viewed as a "leisure" activity for many people, but this is more than leisure. It is personally and spiritually enhancing; therefore, it is essential self-care for both physical (body) and mental (mind) health, and should be honored by the clinician as such. Having respect for oneself is essential to mental health. By focusing on inner self-care, the clinician can facilitate healthy self-respect as well as personal growth.

Productivity.   The original model of occupational performance narrowly defined productivity as "work," but this had serious limitations. Western society typically views work as being synonymous with revenue-producing employment. While this is certainly included in the occupational performance model view of productivity, it is only one type of possible activity. The entire business of managing one's environment and maintaining one's position in a society involves productive activities. These may include managing a household, including tasks related to independent living such as housekeeping, money management, doing laundry, and cooking. Raising a family is also a productive activity, which requires not only independent living skills, but also requires mastering a complicated set of skills involving communication and relationship development. It is important for the clinician to understand the clients' view of a productive role. For example, a student therapist may tell a client that, based on her evaluation, there appears to be a deficit in work activity and that her treatment plan will focus on developing roles in this area. The client may look confused and respond rather curtly, "My job on this planet is to keep myself healthy and out of the hospital." For some people with serious mental illness, taking care of oneself is a full-time occupation, which goes beyond the usual scope of self-care and becomes a "work" role.

Leisure Activities.   As with the other two occupational performance areas, leisure pursuits are both individually and culturally defined. Occupational therapists have a rich background in many of the activities that are considered by Western society to be leisure pursuits. These include hobbies of all kinds, sports, games, music, arts, and crafts, as well as social and cultural celebrations. The value placed on involvement in leisure activities is highly variable with culture. Men in the United States, particularly those who are now elderly or approaching old age, have typically not valued many leisure pursuits, rather seeing them as frivolous, childlike, or feminine. Compared to his female counterpart, if a man from this society also loses his traditional work roles through disability or retirement, he may experience a greater sense of loss because he has fewer remaining perceived options for feeling productive. With such a client, the occupational therapist is in a difficult situation, which requires attempting to honor the values and beliefs of the client while also trying to facilitate the adoption of roles that will give the client an enhanced sense of usefulness.

Occupational Performance Components

"[Occupational performance components are] elements of human function that affect a person's ability to perform occupational tasks or performance skills" (Pedretti, 1985, p. 1). They also affect the intensity and meaning of the task experience for an individual. The occupational performance components are identified by CAOT (1993) as physical, mental, spiritual, and sociocultural, and by AOTA (1994) as sensorimotor, neuromusculoskeletal, motor, cognitive and cognitive integration, and psychological and psychosocial skills. The AOTA definitions are more specific and are helpful in determining the need for specific assessments. The point of having the performance areas broken down into components is to help the therapist pay attention to the complexity of any task and become able to pinpoint particular areas of strength and deficit.

The CAOT definitions are more general, but they are essentially the same except for the addition of the spiritual component. If the occupational performance components are meant to represent the totality of human function elements, then spirituality is an essential inclusion. In the past, spirituality was only associated with religious belief. When it was acknowledged at all, it was in the domain of life space or cultural influences. However, present attitudes about spirituality pervade every activity in which human beings may engage. Urbanowski and Vargo state, "Spirituality may be defined as the experience of meaning in everyday life" (1994, p. 89). A broad view of spirituality dictates an individual's relationship with the world at large, the meaning or purpose of life, and one's sense of ethics and values; it also determines one's beliefs regarding mortality, the afterlife, and the supernatural. While care should be taken to avoid either proselytizing one's own belief system or undermining the religious beliefs of the client, spirituality can be viewed as a large component of all human activity.

An underdeveloped section of the AOTA model of occupational performance involves the psychological and psychosocial components. AOTA (1994) defines these components as psychological, including values, interests, and self-concept; social, including role performance, social conduct, and interpersonal skills; and self-management, which includes coping skills, time management, and self-control. Implicit but not articulated in these descriptions is the importance of feelings and affect. Occupational therapists focus on the "doing" aspects of living, but in order to understand doing, one must explore thinking and feeling.

Evaluation and Intervention

The occupational performance model is not theory bound and does not have a set of prescribed evaluation tools, with the exception of the Canadian Occupational Performance Measure (COPM) (Law et al., 1994). The COPM measures a client's self-perception of occupational performance by using a semistructured interview. It can be administered at any time during treatment, but is best used as an outcome measure of the client's perception of performance and satisfaction, provided it is administered at the beginning of treatment and then readministered at the time of discharge.

The occupational performance model does not limit the use of any other forms of evaluation or theory-driven approaches. The strength of the model is that it does not limit the therapist's view of the client to one theoretical perspective. For example, a therapist who is heavily influenced by sensory integrative theory may easily identify strengths and deficits in the sensorimotor, neuromusculoskeletal, motor, and cognitive-integrative components, yet neglect functions of the psychological and psychosocial domain. Likewise, a clinician trained in cognitive disability theory may focus solely on the cognitive integration and cognitive components. Moreover, occupational therapists who react to the constraints placed on them by third-party reimbursers may overly emphasize the self-care area and neglect productivity and leisure. The use of this model requires that the clinician consider the broad picture first before zeroing in on any one area or component.

MODEL OF HUMAN OCCUPATION

The model of human occupation was introduced by Kielhofner and colleagues (Kielhofner, 1980a, 1980b; Kielhofner & Burke 1980; Kielhofner, Burke, & Igi, 1980) as an attempt to synthesize occupational behavior concepts into a practice and research model. The model evolved from earlier work on occupational behavior by Reilly (1962, 1969). One of the main themes of this tradition is that humans have a need for competence and achievement, and consequently for occupation. This achievement phenomenon begins in childhood play and is continued through adult work. It results in the development of interests, abilities, skills, and habits of competence, cooperation, and competence. The model of human occupation also draws on concepts from **general systems theory** (Berrien, 1968), **open systems theory** (von Bertalanffy, 1968), and **dynamical systems theory** (Haken, 1996) as a means of organizing seemingly disparate categories and levels of information. The model attempts to explain how occupation is motivated, organized, and performed by emphasizing the human system's spontaneous, purposeful, tension-seeking, and creative properties (Kielhofner, 1995).

The model describes occupational behavior as behaviors in which persons engage for most of their waking time and which include playful, restful, serious, and productive activities. These activities of work, play/leisure, and daily living are carried out by individuals in their own unique ways, based on their beliefs, preferences, the kinds of experiences they have had, the environments in which they live, and the specific cultural patterns they acquire over time (Kielhofner, 1995). The environment, then, is seen as intimately linked to the performance of occupation.

The human being maintains constant interaction with the environment, which provides input of many types (food, sensory stimulation, expectations of behavior, etc.). Humans use that input in many ways as well (food becomes energy; sensory stimulation is translated into touch, pain, temperature, and so on; words that were heard are interpreted, etc.). This usage is known as throughput. Part of the result of the process of input and throughput is that a behavior, called output, is produced. Finally, as a person performs the behavior, he or she experiences him- or herself doing the behavior and sees its results. This process, called feedback, becomes a new source of input into the system. The model of human occupation explains occupation as the cumulative expression of the entire circular process. To further explain the dynamic interaction between the person and the environment from which occupation arises, the model describes the external and internal environments of the human being as comprised by several subsystems.

The External Environment

According to the model of human occupation, the external environment offers opportunities for certain behaviors at the same time that it requires others. A restaurant, for example, offers a chef room to walk around, speak, cut up vegetables, cook at a stove, and so on. At the same time, the restaurant requires from the chef the behavior of actually preparing meals for the customers. If the chef does not meet that requirement, he or she will be fired. The actions of providing opportunity and requiring behavior are seen as forming a complementary relationship. The influence of this relationship comes from several sources in the environment, including the physical realm (such as objects and built or natural structures), the social realm (the tasks deemed appropriate and desirable and the social groups sanctioning the behavior), the settings in which occupation occurs (such as home, neighborhood, school or workplace, and gathering, recreation, and resource sites), and the overall culture (such as values, norms and customs) in which the person's life is unfolding.

It is difficult to make generalizations about the environmental circumstances of persons with psychosocial dysfunction. A lack of objects may lead to a person's failure to develop needed skills on which to build socially sanctioned habits and roles. An overabundance of objects, on the other hand, may cause overstimulation, which leads to the same consequence because the person will be unable to organize the environment sufficiently to develop skills selectively. A lack of acceptance of the individual's behavior or personal conditions by a respected social group may accentuate that individual's stress, leading to poor performance and an expectation of failure. Finally, social environments may be such that they actually expect or require maladaptive behavior, as in the street gangs.

The Internal Environment

The model of human occupation describes the internal environment of a person as also composed of a number of subsystems. These are the volition subsystem, which includes personal causation, values, and interests; the habituation subsystem, which includes habits and internalized roles; and the mind-brain-body performance subsystem, which includes musculoskeletal, neurological, and cardiopulmonary functions as well as symbolic images.

The Volition Subsystem. This subsystem is responsible for guiding the choices of occupations a person makes throughout the day. According to this model, choice of occupation is influenced by the outcome the person expects (dispositions) and the person's awareness of him- or herself as an active doer in the world (self-knowledge). Both these influences determine how a person anticipates, chooses, and experiences occupation.

In order to describe this process more specifically, the model of human occupation explains the volition subsystem as comprised of the areas of personal causation, values, and interests. Personal causation refers to the awareness people have over their abilities (knowledge of capacity) and their perception that they have control over their behavior (sense of efficacy). In other words, a person is more likely to engage in an occupation that he or she feels capable of doing. Values refer to the convictions people have that help them assign significance and/or standards of performance to the occupations they perform. Each person has a set of personal convictions that tells him or her how to view life and what matters in it. Out of these convictions arises a sense of obligation to do what one believes is good and/or right. Finally, interests are the dispositions to find pleasure, enjoyment, and satisfaction in certain occupations. Interests may also be understood as attractions people feel toward certain occupations and their preferences in the way of performing occupations.

All too often, people with mental illness perceive of themselves as helpless, inadequate, and under the control of external forces that they can do little to influence. This belief renders them dependent on others to identify their goals, structure their goal-directed behavior, and even communicate for them. If people do not believe they have a sufficient measure of control over their lives and environment, they are also not likely to believe that they have the type of skills needed to overcome those external forces. Expecting failure, these people are less likely to set goals and engage in meaningful occupations, instead becoming inactive and isolative. An extreme internal locus of control may also be part of a psychosocial dysfunction because people may not believe they have any limitations and consequently engage in activities that may harm them.

The Habituation Subsystem. In contrast to the volition subsystem, which has to do with conscious choice of occupation, the habituation subsystem has to do with the assumed and routine activity of daily life. These routine activities require very little deliberation because they are built on repetition. The habituation subsystem is comprised of habits and internalized roles. Habits have to do with the typical way in which one performs a particular occupation, how the performance of occupations is organized into a typical day or week, and the unique style the person puts into occupations, which gives a unique flavor to his or her performance.

While habits are typical ways of relating to occupations, internalized roles determine typical ways in which a person relates to other people. Roles are the identities and behaviors that people assume in the various social situations that comprise their lives. These roles have to do with the internal sense of what others expect a person to do and how they expect him or her to behave. In other words, roles have to do with a person's obligations and rights in various social contexts. According to the model of human occupation, of particular interest to the occupational therapy practitioner are the specific occupational behaviors that encompass a role, the style in which actions in the role occur, and the way in which a person's roles are prioritized or organized in relation to time.

Many people with psychosocial dysfunction have some disorganization in the habituation subsystem that limits their ability to fully enact roles. Role dysfunction may not only be a consequence of mental illness, it may be one of its causes as well. Role dysfunction may occur when people fail to internalize role expectations because of limited experience or a perceptual, motor, or cognitive deficit. Another cause for role dysfunction may be that people internalize dysfunctional roles to begin with, as in the case of children of abusive parents who lie to hide their parents' behavior because it is a family role expectation to protect the family; these children may grow up to be abusive because that was their experience of the parent role. Role dysfunction may also occur when there are too many roles and each demands effort and time at the expense of the others. Finally, the existence of too few roles may also be detrimental because the person lacks enough responsibility to structure time or because there simply is not sufficient social reinforcement to maintain a healthy activity level and degree of self-esteem.

The habit patterns of people with mental illness often gravitate toward being extremely rigid (as in the case of obsessive-compulsive disorders) or toward lacking any consistency from day to day (as with deeply depressed individuals or those with florid psychosis). Either extreme negatively impacts on roles because in the first case, habit completion becomes more important than the role itself, and in the second, there is no habit to support consistent role performance. The ideal number of roles required for a balanced lifestyle really depends on each person's abilities, interests, and personal circumstance.

The Mind-Brain-Body Performance Subsystem.   The final subsystem of the internal environment of the human being is the mind-brain-body performance subsystem. As its name implies, this subsystem represents the complex interplay between the musculoskeletal, neurological, perceptual, and cognitive abilities that is required to actually do an occupation or enact a behavior. It is through this subsystem that interaction with the environment occurs. A person perceives challenges and opportunities in the environment through the perceptual system and then processes this information in the brain, where it is interpreted and given meaning. According to the meaning ascribed to the perception, the brain plans an action, which is carried to the limbs where the muscles, joints, and so forth actually enact the action. Although the meaning of an occupation is ascribed by the volition subsystem and the habituation subsystem places it in social context, it is the performance subsystem that creates the actual actions related to the occupation. The complex interplay between mind, brain, and body that is inherent in the performance of any occupation occurs through the practice of specific skills, including motor skills, process skills, and communication-interaction skills. Table 4-1 is adapted from Kielhofner (1995) and provides a breakdown of each of these skill categories in order to help direct assessment and treatment.

Deficits in skills and their constituents have long been associated with psychosocial dysfunction. Debate exists as to whether psychopathology is due to organic causes (i.e., actual biologic disruptions in brain function) or environmental causes (i.e., poverty, limited opportunities for skills development, etc.). Because the human being is considered to be an open system, the most likely explanation is that psychopathology results from a combination of organic and environmental factors that influence each other and limit the person's ability to learn and acquire skills through exploration, imitation, and repetition.

The performance deficits of people with mental illness may be quite obvious or very subtle. For example, the cognitive and perceptual motor functioning of patients with borderline personality disorder often seem intact, and these people appear quite intelligent and talented. This outer appearance of functionality, however, masks impairments in process skills. When required to solve problems, people with this disorder are often unable to sequence tasks appropriately to meet a goal, have trouble anticipating consequences of their actions, may become rigid or impulsive, and may have difficulties concentrating. In contrast, deficits in the communication/interaction, process, and perceptual-motor skills of people with schizophrenia are usually more easily observed. They may be isolative and may show difficulties with motor coordination and with sequencing and completing self-care tasks.

Although deficits in skills may be the result of organic causes, they may also contribute to the worsening of the mental illness. For example, psychomotor retardation (difficult and slow movement) is often seen in depression, and, in turn, depression worsens when there is little movement. In addition, deficits in skills may be the consequence of the treatment of an illness. The side effects of many medications used in the management of mental illness include drowsiness, hyperactivity, muscle tightening, weakness, and sensory losses. Electroconvulsive therapy (ECT) may also affect memory and problem-solving abilities.

Table 4-1.   Performance Domains and Skills

Motor Domains and Skills

Posture:	stabilizes, aligns, positions
Mobility:	walks, reaches, bends
Coordination:	coordinates body parts, manipulates, flowing movement
Strength and Effort:	moves, transports, and lifts objects; calibrates force, speed, and movement
Energy:	endures, paces work

Process Domains and Skills

Energy:	paces, attends
Knowledge:	chooses tools and materials, uses and handles tools and materials appropriately, heeds directions, inquires for directions
Temporal Organization:	initiates, continues, sequences, terminates
Organization:	searches/locates, gathers, organizes, restores, navigates
Adaptation:	notices/responds, accommodates, adjusts, benefits

Communication/Interaction Domain, and Skills

Physicality:	gestures, gazes, approximates body appropriately, postures, contacts
Language:	articulates, speaks, focuses speech, emanates, modulates
Relations:	engages, relates, respects, collaborates
Information Exchange:	asks, expresses, shares, asserts

Social Interaction Domains and Skills

Acknowledging:	turns body/face toward others, looks at partner, confirms understanding, touches others appropriately
Sending:	greets, answers, questions, complies, encourages, extends, clarifies, sets limits, thanks
Timing:	times responses, speaks fluently, takes turns, times duration, completes
Coordinating:	approaches, places self at appropriate distance, assumes speaker's position, matches speaker's language, discloses, expresses emotion

Source: Adapted from Kielhofner (1995).

Evaluation and Intervention

A strength of the model of human occupation is the holistic view it provides of any dysfunction. Traditional health practice has often focused on one or two particular traits of a dysfunction and not looked at all the factors that contribute to it. The extent of the impact that dysfunction has in the person's life and environment is rarely fully explored (Kielhofner, 1995). This lack of understanding may be particularly detrimental to the person with mental illness.

The model of human occupation was designed for application to any person experiencing difficulties in performing occupation. According to the model, any traditional occupational therapy tool is valid for assessment and treatment. No one single assessment or treatment tool can completely address the complexity of a person. Some suggested evaluation tools include the Assessment of Communication and Interaction Skills (ACIS) (Salamy, Simon, & Kielhofner, 1993), the Assessment of Motor and Process Skills (AMPS) (Fisher, 1994), the Assessment of Occupational Functioning (OF) (Watts, Kielhofner, Bauer, Gregory, & Valentine, 1986), the Occupational Case Analysis Interview and Rating Scale (ACARUS) (Chaplain & Kielhofner, 1989), and the Occupational Performance History Interview (PHI) (Kielhofner, Henry, & Wakens, 1989). Interest and role checklists, activity configurations, manual muscle tests, range-of-motion tests, and cognitive tests are among the many other tools that can be used to evaluate each subsystem. Ultimately, data should be gathered regarding all subsystems of the person's internal and external environments. Once problems have been identified, steps for intervention are prioritized by keeping in mind that all subsystems are interdependent. Considering the current state of organization of the human system, occupational therapy treatment essentially is the provision of appropriate inputs into the system so that it may reorganize more adaptively as it produces occupation.

In summary, the model of human occupation serves to guide occupational therapy assessment in order to determine the areas of occupational dysfunction and plan intervention that addresses all problem levels. The model helps therapists integrate all subsystems into a holistic understanding of the strengths and deficits of the individual and the environment. Keeping in mind that all subsystems depend on each other to a certain degree, appropriate interventions are planned by the ways in which they will promote adaptive functioning in all areas described by the model, rather than in an isolated performance component. The model helps describe all the occupational dimensions of psychosocial dysfunction and integrates them into a whole. Based on the understanding of how function and dysfunction arose in the individual, intervention is elevated from the mere application of techniques to solve specific problems to the true art of therapy: lifelong adaptation.

OCCUPATIONAL ADAPTATION FRAME OF REFERENCE

Occupational adaptation (OA) is identified as a frame of reference in that it was designed to serve as an overarching guide to practice across populations and treatment settings (Schkade & Schultz, 1992, 1993; Schultz & Schkade, 1992). While many theories discuss the importance of both occupation and adaptation, this frame of reference is unique in that it proposes that these two concepts are not separate but in fact comprise an interactive phenomenon that explains the adaptation process experienced throughout the lifespan.

This brief discussion presents the distinguishing features of this frame of reference within mental health practice. The reader is referred to the reference and suggested reading sections for a more complete understanding.

Basic Principles

The practitioner who uses the occupational adaptation frame of reference is guided by a conceptual model that states the essential beliefs about the relationship between occupation and adaptation, the method of intervention, the outcome of therapy, and the roles played by the therapist and patient. This relationship is depicted in Figure 4-2. The fundamental tenets of this model, as articulated by Schkade and Schultz (1992), are as follows:

- Individuals respond to the demand for adaptation across the life span with varying degrees of adaptiveness.

- Adaptiveness is determined by individual uniqueness and the nature of interactions with the environment (occupation).

- The OA process describes the internal mechanism by which human beings experience the demand for adaptation, formulate a unique plan of adaptation, act upon their adaptation with an observable occupational response, evaluate the results, and integrate the effects into their adaptation repertoire.

- The demand for adaptation is embedded within the context of occupational environments (work, play, self-maintenance) and interwoven with the performance of occupational roles.

- The satisfying performance of occupational roles is a vital component of successful occupational functioning at each stage of life.

Evaluation and Intervention

Using this frame of reference, all therapy is directed toward improving the OA process (Schkade & Schultz, 1992). The plan for intervention is based on evaluating the individual's primary occupational roles and occupational environments, the degree of **relative mastery** in the performance of occupational roles, factors that may be interfering with relative mastery, and the occupational environments associated with primary occupational role.

The goal of therapy is to help patients gain increased relative mastery in their occupational roles. The focus on relative mastery, as opposed to functional independence, is a highly distinguishing feature of this theory. Therapists who practice from this approach place the role of evaluating occupational performance on the patient. Not only is the patient the primary contributor to developing the plan of intervention, he or she is also the primary evalua-

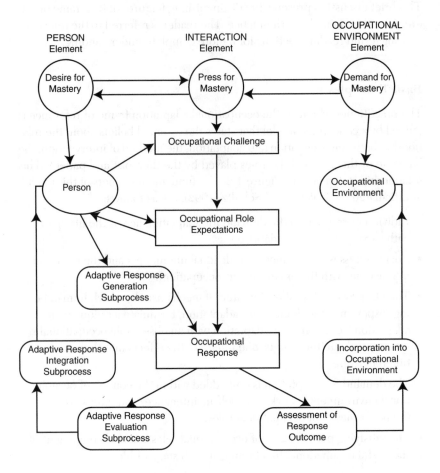

Figure 4-2. Schematic Representation of the Relationships among OT Constructs

Source: Schkade & Schultz (1992). Copyright 1992 by the American Occupational Therapy Association, Inc.

tor of its effectiveness. This approach ensures that the patient functions as the agent of change.

It is assumed that the ability to make the needed change is embedded within the patient's internal process of occupational adaptation. The role of the therapist is to create opportunities to intervene within the patient's internal occupational adaptation process. Such intervention is accomplished in two primary modes: **occupational readiness** and **occupational activity.** While readiness training affects the patient's personal systems (sensorimotor, cognitive, and psychosocial functioning), occupational activity is necessary to effect the occupational adaptation process.

The treatment plan is continually monitored to insure the desired effect on the OA process. This is accomplished by measuring improvement in the individual's perception of relative mastery in performing occupational roles, the spontaneous transfer of skills to novel situations, and the self-initiated adaptation of processes and techniques. To further elaborate on the use of the OA model in practice, "The Occupational Adaptation Guide to Practice" is shown in Figure 4-3.

Appendix
Occupational Adaptation Guide to Practice

Occupational Adaptation Data Gathering/Assessment
What are the patient's *occupational environments and roles?*
Which role is of primary concern to patient and family?
What occupational performance is expected in the primary *occupational environment* and *role?*
What are the *physical, social,* and *cultural* features of the primary *occupational environment* and *role?*
What is the patient's *sensorimotor, cognitive, and psychosocial* status?
What is the patient's level of *relative mastery* in the primary *occupational environment* and *role?*
What is facilitating or limiting *relative mastery* in the primary *occupational environment* and *role?*
Occupational Adaptation Programming
What combination of occupational readiness and occupational activity is needed to promote the patient's *occupational adaptation process?*
What help will the patient need to assess *occupational responses* and use the results to affect the *occupational adaptation process?*
What is the best method to engage the patient in the occupational adaptation program?
Evaluation of the Occupational Adaptation Process
How is the program affecting the patient's *occupational adaptation process?*

- Which *energy level* is used most often *(primary* or *secondary)?*

- What *adaptive response mode* is used most often *(preexisting, modified,* or *new)?*

- What is the most common *adaptive response behavior (primitive, transitional,* or *mature)?*
What outcomes does the patient show that reflect change in the *occupational adaptation process?*

- Self-initiated adaptations?

- Enhanced *relative mastery?*

- Generalization to novel activities?
What program changes are needed to provide maximum opportunity for *occupational adaptation* to occur?

Note: The italicized terms are constructs in the Occupational Adaptation Frame of Reference (Schkade & Schultz, 1992).

Figure 4-3. Occupational Adaptation Guide to Practice

Mental Health Application

Mental illness impairs people's ability to interact effectively with the environment. Symptoms such as depressed mood, anxiety, and psychosis cause individuals to disengage from meaningful occupation. Consequently, the ability to perform relevant occupational roles is severely affected. Even though symptoms may become managed through medication and support services, individuals with chronic mental illness oftentimes continue to deteriorate in their occupational functioning. This is explainable in that even though the symptoms may be resolved, the OA process may remain so impaired that it is not adaptive. Attempts to perform occupational roles fail due to impaired internal adaptive processes, and the individual continues to disengage from meaningful occupation. This prevents him or her from having the very experiences necessary to improve adaptiveness and thereby gain increased satisfaction (relative mastery) from performing occupational roles.

In contrast to traditional psychiatric approaches (with their emphasis on behavior modification, psychodynamics, and medication management), OA intervention is focused on increasing the individual's wherewithal to experience satisfaction in the performance of occupational roles. This is seen not as a by-product of intervention, but as the direct focus of intervention. In contrast with psychosocial rehabilitation, which emphasizes skill building (Anthony, 1992), OA places primary importance on the individual's internal adaptation process and on identifying avenues to improve that process. The measurement of improvement is, therefore, not based on the acquisition of functional skills but rather on the improvement of adaptiveness aimed at increasing the individual's experience of relative mastery.

Even though the majority of individuals with severe mental illness are inundated with skills training, most appear to lack the ability to generalize learning from one setting to another. This is typically attributed to the mental illness. However, an OA approach hypothesizes that the block to such generalization is not addressed in most therapy programs. I routinely observed this phenomenon in my role as a consultant to a forensic psychiatric hospital where all programming was based on skill acquisition. Once the program was restructured using principles of OA, the staff reported a demonstrable difference in the patients, who became more interested, more attentive, and more interactive during the group sessions.

The primary change in programming was a shift from what the staff thought the patients needed to learn to asking the patients what they wanted to learn. This shift reflects the necessity of engaging the patients in occupations that they find meaningful to ensure that the program is expected to be therapeutic.

The second most significant change in restructuring the program was teaching the staff how to promote the patient's adaptiveness. Without exception, the staff resisted this approach. They wanted to "show and tell" patients how to do their work. Practice based on OA demands that the therapist have a different approach. The therapist's role is to provide the opportunity — the "just-right challenge"—that will demand, **in vivo,** an adaptive response from the patient. It is only when patients tap into their adaptive processes that the therapist can observe the nature of that process and identify ways to help them break through dysadaptive modes. These elements cannot be talked about; they must be experienced through occupational activity. The challenge for therapists being trained in this approach is to allow patients to make mistakes, to struggle, and to create individual adaptations.

Within the context of meaningful occupation, the therapist will, of course, provide essential occupational readiness, such as time management training; budgeting, assertiveness and job skills; and techniques associated with the activity. These, however, are provided as a precursor to occupational activity wherein the individual is engaged in a form of actual "doing" that has personal meaning relevant to occupational roles. For the majority of individuals with serious mental illness, their greatest occupational environment deficit lies in the lack of work. Traditional psychiatric occupational therapy seems to have been focused on leisure-time pursuits. Leisure or play is conceptualized in the OA frame of reference as restorative for work because without meaningful work, leisure has no relevance. In my experience as a consultant for numerous psychiatric programs, three key elements are missing within intervention: the development of occupational roles, meaningful occupation, and the opportunity to increase adaptiveness. It is these elements that the OA frame of reference addresses in the mentally ill population.

ACQUISITIONAL FRAME OF REFERENCE

The use of an acquisitional frame of reference allows the occupational therapist to provide a pragmatic approach to assessment and treatment that is consistent with historical beliefs yet ideally suited to the current and future trends in mental health care. Treatment approaches that were initially organized into acquisitional frames of reference (Mosey, 1970) share a belief that functional behavior is rooted in, or a reflection of, one's interaction with one's current and/or expected environment; that areas of human functioning are not interrelated but rather are specific entities that can be focused on as independent arenas for treatment; that skills and abilities can be viewed on a continuum (e.g., simple to complex) rather than from a developmental perspective or hierarchy; and that inadequate learning, interaction, and/or improper environmental responses can contribute to an inadequate repertoire of functional skills. The components and relationships of the acquisitional frame of reference are depicted in Figure 4-4. As distinguished from many other models of treatment where one's behavior may be symptomatic of some underlying problem or conflict, acquisitional models assume that one's behavior *is* the area of function or dysfunction and therefore should be targeted directly in treatment. The fundamental goal when using an acquisitional frame of reference is to enable the individual to acquire those behaviors appropri-

ROLE ACQUISITION:
An Acquisitional Frame of Reference

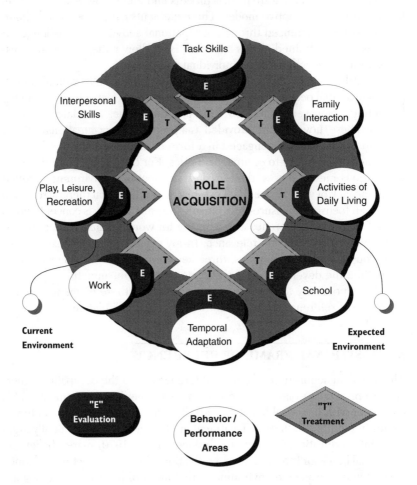

Figure 4-4.   Role Acquisition: An Acquisitional Frame of Reference

ate for his or her present and anticipated circumstances and expected environment (Mosey, 1986).

Basic Principles

Historically, the philosophy that guided occupational therapists working with psychiatric patients was based on the assumption that the way one organized one's daily routine was a reflection of one's behavior and personality. Moreover, in order to be able to function appropriately in a variety of roles (specifically work and self-care), individuals needed to *acquire* specific skills and abilities related to those roles (Gibson, 1993; Mosey, 1986). Activities that would facilitate **organizational abilities** along with promoting adequate social interaction were the primary tools of intervention. Contemporary acquisitional models are rooted in these same principles, but have evolved toward a comprehensive approach to assessment and treatment that allows for the application of specific theories in treatment dedicated to promoting functional skills. For example, if Mr. Smith has schizophrenia and is expected to live independently in his community, then a therapist using an acquisitional frame of reference needs to identify what tasks Mr. Smith will be expected to carry out each day and whether he has the appropriate skills and abilities to carry out those tasks. If, for example, Mr. Smith is planning to apply for a part-time job, the therapist must determine if he can fill out a job application, properly groom and present himself, respond appropriately to interview questions, organize his routine in order to carry out his responsibilities, and so on. Treatment for Mr. Smith in this particular area would include having him actually fill out a job application and come properly dressed and groomed for a simulated job interview. Acquisitionally based treatment focuses on those activities that one anticipates or actually carries out within all environments; it attends to the inherent and learned skills and behaviors necessary to carry out those activities.

Evaluation and Intervention

While environmental and personal attributes appear to be the overriding framework for establishing goals in treatment, assessment and intervention are actually guided by specific theories that enable the individual to learn the skills and abilities necessary to meet functional goals. Frames of references that fall under the acquisitional umbrella are those related to learning theories, such as behavioral approaches, and those that focus on socialization and its role in all facets of daily life, as exemplified by the Role Acquisition Frame of Reference (Mosey, 1986). Role acquisition in particular identifies, not only which roles one needs to assume, but which task and interpersonal skills are needed in order to carry out these roles. All these approaches allow the therapist to identify, not only what needs to be acquired, but how the individual can best acquire the necessary skills. How one learns within a reinforcing environment is as important to acquisitional models as what is to be learned.

Function and dysfunction are reflected through the display of adaptive or maladaptive behaviors within domains of concern, such as work or home management, and assessment is directed at the individual's current functional status rather than on past experiences or causal factors. More specifically, assessment is made of the individual's skills and behaviors that are appropriate to the current and expected environments, of meaningful motivators for the individual, and of the actual living and working environment. Postulates regarding change reflect the notion that appropriate and adaptive skills and behaviors can be learned through a reinforcing environment and that learning can be done through the context of social roles (Mosey, 1986). Though much is discovered from the careful use of, and observation in, the actual activities that one needs to carry out in one's expected environment, as well as through one's roles, specific assessment tools such as the Comprehensive Occupational Therapy Evaluation scale (COTE) (Brayman, Kirby, Misenheimer, & Short, 1976), and the Bay Area Functional Performance Evaluation (BaFPE) (Bloomer & Williams, 1987) can provide a systematic way of identifying, organizing, and assessing task and interpersonal skills, while an activities configuration such as the Activities Health Assessment (Cynkin & Robinson, 1990) can help identify daily patterns and habits that are adaptive or maladaptive. Readers are encouraged to consult the suggested reading section at the conclusion of this chapter for further details of how to use this frame of reference as well as its theoretical underpinnings.

Trends in Health Care

Current and future trends in mental health care are focused on restoring and maintaining functional skills. Since acquisitional models approach assessment and treatment from a pragmatic perspective, the client, family members, other health professionals, and third-party payers all must be able to understand the relevance and significance of occupational therapy interventions. Using this particular model helps to establish a strong partnership between all the stakeholders involved in an individual's care.

It is particularly important when working within interdisciplinary teams to be able to actively collaborate with other professionals. Therefore, the conceptual model, or frame of reference, used by occupational therapists should be congruous with other treatment approaches yet specific to occupational therapy, so that the field's unique contribution is retained. The acquisitional frame of reference is especially compatible in this way with some of the more recent trends in treating people with mental disorders. One example of this is the improved relationship between acquisitional models and psychiatric rehabilitation.

Psychiatric rehabilitation is a treatment approach aimed at enabling clients with mental disorders to accomplish those activities that are related to the roles of their choice. It does this by targeting individuals' skill levels and environmental supports (Anthony, 1992). A primary goal within the psychiatric rehabilitation model is to enable individuals to live as independently as possible. This treatment approach clearly articulates as one of its aims the restoration of abilities that can allow individuals to assume social and instrumental roles (Bridges, Huxley, & Oliver, 1994). From a historical perspective, the principles of occupational therapy contributed to the foundation of psychiatric rehabilitation (Munich & Lang, 1993). From a treatment perspective, the thrust at using realistic environments to address functional status demonstrates the parallel framework between psychiatric rehabilitation and acquisitional models, and therefore the compatibility. The added and significant role that acquisitional frames of reference play when used in conjunction with the psychiatric rehabilitation model is to articulate how to appropriately assess and treat functional status.

Given the variety of treatment contexts in which occupational therapists work, it is important to note that acquisitional frames of reference are particularly well suited for a range of settings. These include the following:

- treatment environments that have time constraints, such as acute care settings, in which the assessment and monitoring of skills and behaviors are of primary concern

- community mental health settings where treatment needs to be focused on enabling individuals to be independent and community living skills are a primary area of emphasis

- private practice settings in which attention to discrete functional domains may be the primary purpose of referral

- community settings, such as homeless shelters, where intervention needs to be focused specifically on the management of activities of daily living, and in managed care environments where individuals receive occupational therapy services for specific conditions and outcome measures are emphasized. In such environments, where capitation mechanisms may dictate reimbursement, acquisitional approaches tend to target specific outcomes so directly that the change process is facilitated.

In summary, using acquisitional frames of reference allows the therapist to focus immediately on those skills and behaviors needed by the individual in order to promote adequate function in all life circumstances.

THEORY OF COGNITIVE DISABILITY

Cognitive disability is a "restriction in sensorimotor actions originating in the physical or chemical structures of the brain [and] producing observable and assessable limitations in routine task behavior" (Allen & Allen, 1987, p. 185). Cognitive disability theory is, then, biologic in orientation. It states that such a disruption in brain function causes limitations in a person's ability to complete routine tasks such as work and daily living activities.

The Allen Cognitive Level assessment and associated treatment theory were developed and first published in 1985 (Allen, 1985). It divided cognitive disabilities into six levels of function, with level one indicating the lowest level of task ability (unable to complete any task) and level six indicating normal task activity. Table 4-2 describes patient function at each of the cognitive levels.

Cognitive disability theory is important to occupational therapists because it assists in determining a patient's ability to carry out tasks. Just as a physical

Table 4-2. Cognitive Levels of Patient Function

Cognitive Level	Sensory Processing of Information	Capacity for New Learning	Task Abilities	Length of Time Person Can Attend to Tasks
1	Internal/ Reflexive Cues	0	Automatic actions	Few seconds Reactive only for basic bodily function, intake, elimination.
2	Proprioceptive Cues	0	Postural actions May follow demonstrated body movements	5-10 minutes
3	Tactile Cues	0	Manual actions One step tasks Goals set by therapist Repetitive manual tasks	Up to 30-40 minutes
4	Visual Cues	Rote learning	Goal-directed for familiar tasks Must see all aspects of task	Approx. 45 minutes
5	Related Cues	Trial and error learning Inductive reasoning	Exploratory actions Learning new ways of doing tasks	Can carry over tasks for several days
6	Symbolic Cues	Deductive reasoning	Planned actions	Unlimited

limitation may alter the ability to do a task, a cognitive limitation will change task ability as well.

Philosophy of Practice and the OT Role

The underlying philosophy of occupational therapists is that we treat patients to make them more independent in the area of self-care, work, and leisure.

We work to restore normal abilities first — but what happens when the person has a residual disability that prevents "normal" functioning? Occupational therapists may then change or "adapt" a task so that it can be done at the individual's functional level. For example, in a physical rehabilitation setting, an occupational therapist may suggest adding hand controls to a car for a person with paraplegia. Often in mental health practice, occupational therapists have focused on changing the person rather than adapting the environment. We are teachers of skills, but we must also assess the level of a person's ability to learn new skills. There is a body of literature focusing on cognitive disabilities that addresses these issues by discussing ways of grouping psychiatric patients according to functional abilities and altering tasks based on a patient's capacity to function (Allen, 1985; Denton, 1987; Kaplan, 1988).

The occupational therapists' role when applying cognitive disabilities theory is that the focus is more on changing the task rather than changing the person. The clinician determines what the individual's cognitive ability will enable him or her to do and then adjusts the **task environment** in which the task is done and structures the task to eliminate problems the person cannot cognitively solve. Assessing a patient's level of function and attempting to predict how well he or she will eventually be able to care for him- or herself provides valuable information for the entire treatment team when determining discharge plans and appropriate aftercare needs.

Applicability of Theory

Persons with psychiatric diagnoses often have cognitive disabilities; however, in all areas of OT practice it is the person's cognitive abilities that we must determine. Many other diagnoses, such as cerebrovascular accidents (CVA or "stroke") and brain damage, may also lead to cognitive dysfunction and impact task ability (Allen, Earhart, & Blue, 1992).

It has been noted that during the acute phase of a psychiatric illness, and particularly with psychosis, a person's cognitive level of function may drop. This diminished function is not diagnosis specific but rather is related to the acuity of the disease. During the acute phase of a psychiatric illness, individuals may be hospitalized but are typically not confined to bed. They are generally up and about throughout the day. Such patients may exhibit decreased or heightened energy levels. There is often a desire to be engaged in activities but decreased ability to think about how to do so. According to Claudia Allen (1985), individuals with certain psychiatric diagnoses (e.g., affective disorders) will see an increase in cognitive function as the acuity of the disease diminishes, while other psychiatric disorders appear to have residual cognitive disabilities that will stabilize at less than normal function in the chronic phase of the illness. In every case, however, occupational therapy can serve both phases of the illness. During the acute phase it can support the current level of function and provide **expectant treatment** while waiting for the disabling symptoms to subside, and during the chronic phase it can provide supportive treatment. This includes intervention with the patient, family, and caregivers and providing vocational programs that structure the environment, eliminate elements of the task demands that cannot be performed, and implement longer-term rote learning for desired task completion.

Evaluation and Intervention

The Allen's Cognitive Level (ACL) evaluation consists of the verbal and demonstrated instruction of three lacing stitches: the running stitch, the whip stitch, and the single cordovan stitch. The patient is asked to complete each of these stitches in sequence, and a determination of the cognitive level is based on the ability to follow these instructions and complete the task (refer to Allen et al., 1992, for the complete instructions on how to conduct this evaluation). There are an additional 24 standardized craft projects compiled in the Allen Diagnostic Module (ADM), which were designed to help verify the ACL scores and to provide for more patient choice in activity (Allen & Reyner, 1996)

In addition to the ACL assessment, I suggest conducting a structured interview with the patient that addresses the areas of living situation, education, work history, leisure pursuits, and social support networks. This provides a history of how well he or she has functioned in the past and, when combined with the results of the ACL, it allows the therapist to predict future abilities.

The Routine Task Inventory (Allen et al., 1992) is also suggested when planning long-term rehabilitation. This inventory gives detailed information on the patient's ability in self-care, major life roles, and social roles.

Once the evaluation is completed (this includes a determination of the patient's current cognitive level of function and information on the prior level), the therapist can begin to plan appropriate treatment. Is this illness acute, with a drop in a previously higher cognitive function? Treatment in this case will be expectant. That is, the therapist will provide activities that the patient is willing to do and watch for a spontaneous remission of symptoms. The documentation of observations of change in the person's ability to do tasks is an objective record of the changes in the severity of an acute illness. In planning supportive treatment, the therapist relies on task analysis and on changing the task or the task environment so the patient can experience successful task achievement within his or her cognitive range of function. An example of altering the task environment is the elimination of distracting sounds or excess visual stimulation so a person may more easily concentrate. Many persons with manic-depressive illness complain of losing concentration when there is background music or noises and often have increased sensitivity to light. Such individuals may wish to wear sunglasses while completing a task. For other diagnoses, such as schizophrenia, other affective disorders, and personality disorders, the therapist also determines how tasks can be changed to support the current level of function. For example, a patient assessed at cognitive level four needs to have all elements of a task clearly visible and within an arm's-length range of vision. Therefore, all materials to be used should be placed in front of the patient and no further away than the person can reach while positioned at a work station (table, countertop, etc.). There should be a finished sample that the patient may examine while working, thus supporting his or her ability to succeed in the task.

Palliative treatment also involves changing tasks to fit the cognitive function. In general, therapists wish to alleviate the pain and distress of psychiatric symptoms. For example, it often is very distressing to a patient when he or she feels unable to perform a task. A potential patient reaction is to become angry, frustrated, and/or defensive; some may blame others for their inability to complete a task or may become anxious or agitated (Allen, 1985). If the therapist knows the patient's cognitive level of function, the task can be altered (e.g., having all elements of the task readily visible or showing the patient how to do something rather than "telling" them how) to enable him or her to succeed and thus experience mastery.

Treatment Settings

Acute Care Hospital.   Psychiatric patients are admitted to acute care hospitals when their symptoms are so severe that they have become dangerous to themselves or to others. Self-endangerment ranges from thoughts or behaviors of suicide or self-harm to an inability to care for one's basic needs of food, clothing, and shelter. Danger to others may be the result of an inability to control anger and aggressive behaviors brought on by delusional thinking or of failing to understand the effects of one's actions on people. These behaviors can be linked to diminished cognitive function. The loss of ability to figure out how to do tasks contributes to a person's inability to care for him- or herself or for others. A graphic example is a mother who was admitted for endangering her infant child by scalding him in a tub of hot water. Her perception was that she must bathe him in this way before taking him to church. A religious preoccupation dictated that the child must be clean in the presence of God. At cognitive level four, unseen properties are not understood, and in this case there is a great likelihood that the patient did not comprehend that a water temperature that she could tolerate was beyond the tolerance of an infant's body. This woman needed hospitalization so that she could be protected from carrying out such behaviors until medication could be administered that would impact her cognitive dysfunction. In this way, occupational therapists can apply task analysis for the acutely ill person to allow appropriate interaction with the environment.

Outpatient Settings.   Many patients attending outpatient programs such as day treatment, individual counseling, sheltered workshops, and vocational rehabilitation have a chronic cognitive disability. The therapist with knowledge of a patient's cognitive level can, through task analysis, structure activities and provide the repetition of needed skills to promote the rote learning of new tasks such as using public transportation or setting up a workstation.

Home and Work.   There is also the opportunity within this framework to intervene with the family or board and care home operators and with vocational rehabilitation programs to teach ways to set up tasks for people with chronic cognitive disabilities.

Summary

In summary, this discussion of cognitive disability theory and application has briefly outlined the sensorimotor capabilities of persons functioning at Allen Cognitive levels one through six. A major consideration for occupational therapy practice is the assessment and treatment of an essentially biologic limitation of cognitive functioning that impacts patients' ability to complete tasks in the areas of self-care, education, work, and leisure. Occupational therapists have the capacity through observation of a patient's task performance (e.g., the ACL test) to determine the level of a patient's functional abilities and to provide graded task opportunities and appropriate task environments that will support and enhance successful task completion and promote greater psychosocial independence.

CASE STUDY APPLICATION

The focus of this chapter is on the clinical application of models, theories, and frames of reference. In order to more clearly understand the similarities and differences between the five approaches presented, all the chapter authors developed a response to the following case illustration, each using a different theoretical perspective. In Tables 4-3 through 4-7 on pages 130–136 they discuss goals and treatment for this case according to the specific models.

CASE ILLUSTRATION: LAVON

LaVon is a 38-year-old woman who has been attending a day treatment program based on the clubhouse model with a vocational focus for the past five years. Since the start of her attendance at this program she has not been hospitalized. However, in the past, she attended other programs, including partial hospitalization and day treatment. She has also had multiple acute hospitalizations. LaVon had her first psychotic episode when she was 17 years old, at which time she was placed on Thorazine. She has had several hospitalizations since that time as well as repeated medication changes. Within the last five years she developed moderate tardive dyskinesia, for which she was prescribed Cogentin. Her current medications include Clozaril, which she is tolerating well.

At this time, LaVon does not experience psychotic symptoms, although in the past she experienced auditory hallucinations and delusions that she was being followed. She is, at times, guarded and hypervigilant. LaVon met her current husband three years ago in this program. They live in an assisted independent living apartment. Other than her husband, LaVon has no close friends or family, although she participates in group activities in the program.

LaVon completed high school as an average student. She has held some jobs for short periods of time (3 to 6 months), working as a dishwasher, cleaning person, and clerical assistant. She was fired from her last three jobs after becoming belligerent after she thought her boss was unfair or other employees were following her. Currently, she is in a vocational training program working on a supervised janitorial work crew four hours per week. She often comes to the clubhouse looking somewhat disheveled. She states that this is because she does not like water and her husband does not do the laundry. When asked about her leisure activities, she states that she watches television with her husband and goes regularly to a coffee shop near her house.

Summary

Theoretical concepts and approaches are the necessary starting point for effective occupational therapy intervention, but simple knowledge of these approaches is insufficient. In addition, occupational therapists must accurately apply these frameworks in their clinical practice. The choice of approach is based on many factors, including academic training, clinical exposure, institutional policy, and personal preference. However, the most important factor in the choice of approach should be the clinical needs of the client. Some occupational therapists choose to develop an eclectic approach to practice, based on several models and theories. An eclectic approach may at times best meet the needs of clients or patients, but therapists should understand the specific borrowed elements of the approaches before attempting to create their own framework for practice. A haphazard application of theoretical elements can create confusion and be difficult to articulate.

Although a single, unifying theory base does not exist in occupational therapy, several **meta-models** and specific intervention theories have been developed. Theory is not static, so it can be expected that the approaches discussed here will change; some will be further developed, and others may be discarded. Furthermore, additional theories and frames of reference are also being developed. Among them are McCormack's Mindbody Model (1994) and Fidler's Life-Style Performance Model (1996). Both these models add to the body of knowledge in occupational therapy and provide mechanisms for addressing the complexities and nuances of occupational therapy. It remains to be seen how they will be used in mental health clinical practice.

Table 4-3. Goals of Treatment Using the Occupational Performance Model

OP Areas	Goals of Treatment
Productivity	Stable employment (identified by client through the COPM)
Self-Care	Improved personal care demonstrated by consistent clean hair and clothes (identified by the therapist through observation)
Leisure	Not a priority in this treatment plan. I would encourage LaVon to continue with clubhouse program for ongoing exposure to a variety of leisure opportunities.

Components	
Physical	Further evaluate potential functional deficits secondary to tardive dyskinesia. Assist client in developing coping strategies for managing symptoms.
Mental	Cognitive strategies, psychoeducational instruction, and practice in anger management, reality-testing techniques, and coping skills
Spiritual	An integral part of all treatment is to help the client identify activities that have personal meaning and the capacity for self-fulfillment.
Sociocultural	Encourage continued participation in social groups (i.e., the clubhouse). Practice social skills in groups. Identify culture through expressive activities.

Note: All intervention can, directly or indirectly, affect the client's main goal of stable employment and therefore can be presented to her with that focus.

Table 4-4. Treatment Considerations Using the Model of Human Occupation

Volition	
Personal Causation	Identify intact skills to serve as source of competence; identify past successes that can serve as encouragement of effectiveness of skills; structure successful participation in increasingly complex activities that require independent decision making; provide feedback and encourage analysis of skills
Values	Set very short-term, concrete, and visibly achievable goals. Break down long-term goals into shorter, more achievable sequences. Activities chosen should be relevant to her married, worker, and homemaker roles.
Interests	Provide opportunities and encourage the exploration of new and realistic interests. Explore community resources for the continued pursuit of new interests.
Habituation	
Roles	Increasingly give her responsibility for planning activities with husband. Utilize groups for the graded development of skills for workers within a social content. Explore opportunities in the community for participation in other roles. Role-play various roles and discuss expectations in order to promote the internalization of expectations.
Habits	Set clear expectations of habits and routines during participation in OT program. Grade opportunities in order to have her practice skills within the framework of roles. Balance daily schedule with ADL, work, and leisure tasks.
Mind-Brain-Body Performance	
Skills	Develop skills and an awareness of body and motor abilities through activities that require large movements, sports, and so on. Provide training and allow the practice of specific skills and problem-solving steps in a variety of contexts. Provide specific training in social and communication skills incorporating methods for obtaining feedback (i.e., video-tape, group discussion, etc.).
Environment	The treatment environment should encourage increased responsibility in making choices, managing the self, setting goals, and so forth. Expectations for participation in treatment should be made clear. Sanctions for inappropriate behavior should also be maintained. Transitions from structured programs to community life should be supported by the use of community resources. LaVon should be encouraged in the observance of cultural and social traditions that match her background. This will increase her sense of social ties and reinforce her attention to social cues regarding her behavior.

Table 4-5. Application of the Occupational Adaptation Model

Data Gathering and Assessment	Discuss occupational roles and assess LaVon's perception of how she performs these roles. LaVon should then identify the primary role and relevant occupational environment for focus in therapy. The therapist and client should identify the array of factors that limit relative mastery in an occupational role. (In this case, an assumption is made that LaVon wants to return to work.)
OA Programming	While the client may be in need of specific person-system interventions, the OA therapist places these deficits as secondary to what is viewed as LaVon's greatest impairment, an impoverished ability to adapt. Impacting the internal adaptation processes (particularly the adaptive response mechanism)—namely, the reaction LaVon experiences that *precedes* the observable dysfunctional behaviors—is the focus of therapy. All programming is designed to determine the "blocks" within her processes and improve her occupational adaptation processes so that LaVon can experience greater mastery as a long-term worker. Therapy would consist of two parts.
PART I—Occupational Readiness	The therapist involves LaVon in learning the skills necessary to experience increased mastery in the worker role. This may involve: °work relations training and conflict resolution techniques °work habits, work appearance, and medication management °handling insensitive remarks from others °knowledge about her psychiatric diagnosis and its effect on everyday experiences °knowledge of human adaption and OA theory, as relevant
PART II—Occupational Activity	This part of the intervention emphasizes LaVon's adaptive processes. The therapist engages LaVon in occupation-based activities that provide an opportunity to learn modes of adaption and, more importantly, that give her in

(continues)

Table 4-5. Application of the Occupational Adaptation Model (continued)

PART II—Occupational Activity (continued)	vivo experiences that demand her to adapt to the task at hand. The client must be given naturalistic experiences that foster the generalization of adaptive approaches learned in one setting to similar, yet slightly different, tasks. As LaVon begins to learn new ways of responding to different situations, the therapy will facilitate generalization through carefully directing the client into and through therapeutic activities that promote adaptiveness.
OA evaluation	The effect of occupational readiness and occupational activities is the therapist's primary measure of therapeutic effectiveness; the acquisition of performance skills and independence provides supplemental measures. Changes are based on whether the program is facilitating positive change in the client's internal adaptive processes. Such changes are observable and include self-initiated adaptions, enhanced relative mastery, and generalization to new tasks. Determining the client's assessment of relative mastery is vital in making programming decisions.

Table 4-6. Application of the Acquisitional Frame of Reference

Assessment of Current Status

History and Observation	LaVon's roles include: wife, resident of an assisted living apartment, member of a day treatment program, and possible worker. She also has some degree of motor impairment. We also know that she has deficits in task (e.g., task initiation) and interpersonal (e.g., social interaction) skills, and within specific domains; ADL (unkempt appearance), work (unable to sustain employment), and family/friends (social network is limited to treatment and residential settings). It is likely that she has impaired time management skills as well.
	LaVon does have strengths, as indicated by her marriage of three years, her ability to live somewhat independently, her ability to gain employment, and her ability to recognize motoric symptoms.
The COTE Scale	This tool is useful in monitoring changes in levels of task skills on a daily basis. Within the task skills continuum, for example, posture, physical strength and endurance, gross and fine motor coordination, rate of performance, and the use of tools and materials may all be affected by LaVon's motor impairment. This would influence her performance in the various domains, such as her ability to carry out her activities of daily living (hygiene, meal preparation, etc.).
An Activities Health Assessment	This should be carried out so that LaVon's ability to establish and organize her routine can be examined. It is also important to identify what activities would be interesting and motivating for LaVon and and to determine how to place them within a nonthreatening social context. These assessment components are vital to the establishment of an activity-based treatment program that targets the relevant skills and behaviors

(continues)

Table 4-6. Application of the Acquisitional Frame of Reference (continued)

Ongoing Assessment and Treatment

Simulated and Practice Activities	Each of the skill areas should be assessed within the contexts of LaVon's expected roles. For example, if, in her role in the assisted living residence, she is expected to prepare a simple meal for herself and her husband, one needs to determine if she can plan out a simple menu and prepare it. How might her skill deficits, such as her difficulty in task initiation and her motoric impairments, affect her performance? This is assessed by actually having LaVon plan and prepare a meal. Other activities within each of the domains need to be similarly constructed so that the range of task and interpersonal skills can be addressed within their contexts. Activities chosen in treatment need to reflect those activities engaged in within the environment, those that are of interest to LaVon, those that involve partnerships or other means for interpersonal interaction, and those in which learning theories can be applied. If LaVon does have difficulty with meal preparation, placing her in a thematic-based cooking group would be appropriate for teaching her the initial skills within a social context. This should be reinforced, if possible, by promoting meal preparation activities in her residential setting. Her deficits in hygiene and appearance can be addressed in an appropriate thematic group as well.

Table 4-7. Evaluation and Treatment Based on Cognitive
            Disability Theory

Evaluation

Functional History Interview	Self-Care: Disheveled appearance and soiled clothing for past 5 years.
	Living Situation: Lives with husband, dependent on him for her laundry.
	Work History: Menial labor, poor attendance, 3–6 mos. job longevity.
	Social/Leisure: Poor task initiation and socialization, no friends or family, guarded and hypervigilant
ACL Test	Completed running stitch and whip stitch, corrected a twist error by pulling out lacing—Cognitive Level 4.3/4.4

Treatment

Self-Care	Grooming: Establish daily grooming routine to promote rote learning. Use full-length and hand-held mirrors. Demonstrate the use of mirrors to check the front and back of the body when dressing and combing hair. Post list of grooming tasks near mirror (wash, brush teeth, comb hair, check clothing, etc.)
Living Situation	Encourage LaVon to participate with her husband in the laundry activity. Structure clothes washing by having all needed supplies (soap, bleach, softener) clearly visible and in the same location at all times. Clear, printed instructions for loading, turning on machines, unloading laundry, and use of the dryer should be mounted in clear view and there should be repeated demonstrations of the steps. Show LaVon how far to turn each faucet to achieve the appropriate mix of hot and cold water (temperature is an unseen property).
Vocational	The therapist will interact with the job coach to assure that work materials are in plain sight within 3–4 feet, cleaning routines are focused in 4-foot areas, routine sequences of activities are posted at workstations, and procedures to be followed are demonstrated.
Social/Leisure	If LaVon wishes to continue her day treatment program, structure task materials for craft projects within arm's reach and have a finished sample for comparison. The therapist should demonstrate unknown steps and assist the patient to rotate her work in order to achieve accurate completion of the task.

Acknowledgment

Anne MacRae authored the section on occupational performance, Janet Falk-Kessler authored the section on the acquisitional frame of reference, Dorothy Julin authored the cognitive disabilities section, Rene Padilla authored the model of human occupation section, and Sally Schultz authored the occupational adaptation section.

Review Questions

1. In what way is the occupational therapist's role changed by applying each of the approaches discussed in this chapter? How does the use of these approaches explain the role of occupational therapy?
2. What are the major theoretical differences in each of the approaches presented?
3. What are the theoretical commonalities?
4. Which approach would you use for LaVon (featured in the case illustration)? Why did you choose this approach?
5. How does each approach influence the evaluation process?

Learning Activities

1. Practice the evaluations referred to in this chapter and discuss why they are pertinent to the particular model.
2. Based on any of the case illustrations in this book, develop an evaluation and treatment plan using each of the approaches discussed in this chapter.
3. View the C. Allen and Earhart videotape, *Why Therapists Use Crafts* (available through S&S Worldwide, P.O. Box 513, Colchester, CT 06415-0513).

References

Allen, C. (1985). *Occupational therapy for psychiatric diseases: Measurement and management of cognitive disabilities.* Boston: Little, Brown.

Allen, C., & Allen, R. (1987). Cognitive disabilities: Measuring the social consequences of mental disorders. *Journal of Clinical Psychiatry, 48,* 185–191.

Allen, C., Earhart, C., & Blue, T. (1992). *Occupational therapy treatment goals for the physically and cognitively disabled.* Rockville, MD: American Occupational Therapy Association.

Allen, C., & Reyner, A. (1996). *How to start using the Allen Diagnostic Module.* Colchester, CT: S & S Worldwide.

American Occupational Therapy Association (AOTA). (1974). *A curriculum guide for occupational therapy educators.* Rockville, MD: American Occupational Therapy Association.

American Occupational Therapy Association (AOTA). (1994). Uniform terminology for occupational therapy (3rd ed.). *American Journal of Occupational Therapy, 48* (11), 1047–1054.

Anthony, W. (1992, Fall). Psychiatric rehabilitation: Key issues and future policy. *Health Affairs,* 164–177.

Barris, R. (1984). Toward an image of one's own: Sources of variation in the role of occupational therapists in psychosocial practice. *Occupational Therapy Journal of Research, 4,* 3–23.

Berrien, F. K. (1968). *General and social systems.* New Brunswick, NJ: Rutgers University Press.

Bloomer, J., & Williams, S. (1987). *The Bay Area Functional Performance Evaluation (BaFPE): Task oriented assessment and social interaction scale manual.* Palo Alto, CA: Consulting Psychologists Press.

Brayman, S. J., Kirby, T. F., Misenheimer, A. M., & Short, M. J. (1976). Comprehensive occupational therapy evaluation scale. *American Journal of Occupational Therapy, 30*(2), 94–100.

Bridges, K., Huxley, P., & Oliver, J. (1994). Psychiatric rehabilitation: Redefined for the 1990's. *International Journal of Social Psychiatry 40*(1), 1–16.

Canadian Association of Occupational Therapists (CAOT). (1993). *Occupational therapy guidelines for client-centered mental health practice.* Ottawa, Canada: Minister of Supply and Services.

Chaplain, K., & Kielhofner, G. (1989). *Occupational Case Analysis Interview and Rating Scale.* Thorofare, NJ: Slack.

Cynkin, S., & Robinson, A. (1990). *Occupational therapy and activities health: Toward health through activities.* Boston: Little, Brown & Co.

Denton, P. (1987). *Psychiatric occupational therapy: A workbook of practical skills.* Boston: Little, Brown & Co.

Fidler, G. (1996). Life-style performance: From profile to conceptual model. *American Journal of Occupational Therapy, 50*(2), 139–147.

Fisher, A. (1994). *Assessment of Motor and Process Skills* (version 8.0). Unpublished test manual. Colorado State University, Department of Occupational Therapy, Fort Collins, CO.

Gibson, D. (1993). The evolution of occupational therapy. In H. Hopkins & H. Smith (Eds.), *Willard and Spackman's occupational therapy* (8th ed., 535–542). Philadelphia: Lippincott.

Haken, H. (1996). *Principles of brain functioning: A synergetic approach to brain activity, behavior and cognition.* Berlin, NY: Springer.

Kaplan, K. (1988). *Directive group therapy.* Thorofare, NJ: Slack.

Kielhofner, G. (1980a). A model of human occupation: Part 2. Ontogenesis from the perspective of temporal adaptation. *American Journal of Occupational Therapy, 34*(6), 657–663.

Kielhofner, G. (1980b). A model of human occupation: Part 3. Benign and vicious cycles. *American Journal of Occupational Therapy, 43*(7), 731–737.

Kielhofner, G. (1995). A model of human occupation: Theory and application (2nd ed.). Baltimore, MD: Williams & Wilkins.

Kielhofner, G., & Burke, J. P. (1980). A model of human occupation: Part 1. Conceptual framework and content. *American Journal of Occupational Therapy, 34*(5), 572–581.

Kielhofner, G., Burke, J. P., & Igi, C. H. (1980). A model of human occupation: Part 4. Assessment and intervention. *American Journal of Occupational Therapy, 35*(7), 777–780.

Kielhofner, G., Henry, A., & Wakens, D. (1989). *A user's guide to the Occupational Performance History Interview.* Rockville, MD: American Occupational Therapy Association.

Law, M., Baptiste, S., Carswell, A., McColl, M. A., Polatajko, H., & Pollock, N. (1994). *Canadian occupational performance measure.* Toronto: CAOT Publications.

Llorens, L. (1984). Theoretical conceptualizations of occupational therapy: 1960–1982. *Occupational Therapy in Mental Health, 4*(2), 1–14.

Llorens, L. (1991). Performance tasks and roles throughout the life span. In C. Christiansen & C. Baum (Eds.), *Occupational therapy: Overcoming human performance deficits* (pp. 45–66). Thorofare, NJ: Slack.

McCormack, G. (1994). Holism revisited: Toward a mindbody model for occupational therapy. *Physical Disabilities Special Interest Section Newsletter.* (American Occupational Therapy Association, Rockville, MD), pp. 2–4.

Mosey, A. C. (1970). *Three frames of reference for mental health.* Thorofare, NJ: Slack.

Mosey, A. C. (1986). *Psychosocial components of occupational therapy.* New York: Raven Press.

Munich, R., & Lang, E. (1993). The boundaries of psychiatric rehabilitation. *Hospital and community psychiatry, 44*(7), 661–665.

Pedretti, L. W. (1985). *Occupational therapy practice skills for physical dysfunction.* St. Louis: C. V. Mosby Co.

Reilly, M. (1962). Occupational therapy can be one of the great ideas of 20th century medicine. *American Journal of Occupational Therapy, 16,* 1–9.

Reilly, M. (1969). The education process. *American Journal of Occupational Therapy, 23*(3), 299–307.

Salamy, M., Simon, S., and Kielhofner, G. (1993). *The assessment of communication and interaction skills* (Research version). University of Illinois at Chicago, Department of Occupational Therapy.

Schkade, J. K., & Schultz, S. (1992). Occupational adaptation: Toward a holistic approach for contemporary practice: Part I. *American Journal of Occupational Therapy, 46,* 829–838.

Schkade, J. K., & Schultz, S. (1993). Occupational adaptation: An integrative frame of reference. In H. Hopkins & H. Smith (Eds.), *Willard and Spackman's occupational therapy* (8th ed., pp. 87–91). Philadelphia: Lippincott.

Schultz, S., & Schkade, J. K. (1992). Occupational adaptation: Toward a holistic approach for contemporary practice: Part II. *American Journal of Occupational Therapy, 46,* 917–916.

Urbanowski, R., & Vargo, J. (1994). Spirituality, daily practice, and the occupational performance model. *Canadian Journal of Occupational Therapy, 61*(2), 88–94.

vonBertalanffy, L. (1968). General systems theory — A critical review. In W. Buckley (Ed.), *Modern systems research for the behavioral scientist* (pp. 11–30). Chicago: Aldin.

Watts, J., Kielhofner, G., Bauer, D., Gregory, M., & Valentine, D. (1986). The Assessment of Occupational Functioning: A screening tool for use in long-term care. *American Journal of Occupational Therapy, 40,* 231–240.

Suggested Reading

Barris, R., Kielhofner, G., & Watts, J. (1988). *Occupational therapy in psychosocial practice.* Thorofare, NJ: Slack.

Bruce, M., & Borg, B. (1993). *Pyschosocial occupational therapy: Frames of reference for interventions.* Thorofare, NJ: Slack.

Florey, L. (1969). Intrinsic motivation: The dynamics of occupational therapy theory. *American Journal of Occupational Therapy, 23*(3), 319–322.

Stein, F. (1983). A current review of the behavioral frame of reference and its application to occupational therapy. *Occupational Therapy in Mental Health, 2*(4), 35–62.

Christiansen, C., & Baum, C. (1991). *Occupational therapy: Overcoming human performance deficits.* Thorofare, NJ: Slack.

Fidler, G., & Fidler, J. (1978). Doing and becoming: Purposeful action and self-actualization. *American Journal of Occupational Therapy, 32,* 305–310.

Hopkins, H. (1988). Current basis for the theory and philosophy of occupational therapy. In H. Hopkins & H. Smith (Eds.), *Willard and Spackman's occupational therapy* (7th ed., pp. 38–42). Philadelphia: Lippincott.

Hopkins, H., & Tiffany, E. (1988). Occupational therapy — Base in activity. In H. Hopkins & H. Smith (Eds.), *Willard and Spackman's occupational therapy* (7th ed., pp. 93–101). Philadelphia: Lippincott.

Yerxa, E. (1979). The philosophical base of occupational therapy. In *Occupational therapy — 2001.* Rockville, MD: American Occupational Therapy Association, 26–30.

Diagnosis and Dysfunction

Psychopathology and the Diagnostic Process

Anne MacRae

Key Terms

diagnosis

DSM

dysfunction

psychopathology

symptom

Chapter Outline

Introduction
Psychopathology
    Thought
    Language
    Perception
    Affect
    Orientation
    Memory
    Sensorimotor
Diagnosis
    Overview of the *Diagnostic and Statistical Manual of Mental Disorders*
        (DSM)
    Theory and the DSM
    The Role of Occupational Therapy
Summary

Introduction

The purpose of this chapter is to provide a brief overview of psychopathology and diagnosis. It is not intended to replace or represent the more extensive knowledge found in abnormal psychology courses or textbooks. Indeed, several of the authoritative psychiatric and psychological texts are sources for this chapter (American Psychiatric Association, 1994; Comer, 1995; Gelder, Gath, & Mayou, 1989; Hales, Udofsky, & Talbott, 1994; Kaplan, Sadock, & Grebb, 1994; Heiden & Hersen, 1995; Maxmen & Ward, 1995; Templer, Spencer, & Hartlage, 1994). Rather than simply restating the information from these sources, there is an emphasis in this chapter on OT clinical application, and specifically on the functional implications of psychopathology and diagnosis.

The terminology used in mental health settings can often be confusing, especially since the terms are often misused by the general public. It is important to be as specific as possible and to be clear as to whether a phenomenon is a **symptom, dysfunction,** or **diagnosis,** even though there is often much overlap. In other words, an individual may experience a particular symptom that is typical of a specific disorder but still not meet the criteria for that diagnosis. Moreover, neither the symptom nor the diagnosis will give the clinician a true indication about the level or type of dysfunction. It is a common error to assume that some diagnoses automatically imply a greater level of dysfunction, when actually, "[P]sychiatric diagnosis does not always predict functional performance" (Bonder, 1991/1995, p. xxi). The following case illustrations compare brief psychiatric histories of three people in order to show the differences between symptoms, diagnosis, and dysfunction.

CASE ILLUSTRATIONS

Ms. Jones complains of feeling bored and depressed (symptoms). She has alienated all of her friends and is now isolated from social contact (dysfunction). Ms. Jones also meets the criteria for borderline personality disorder (diagnosis).

Mr. Nguyen has recently been fired from his job for reportedly "slipshod" work (dysfunction). His doctor has been treating him for dysthymia (diagnosis) for several years, but lately Mr. Nguyen has been feeling more lethargic and melancholic (symptoms).

Mrs. Garcia is hospitalized for an episode of major depression (diagnosis). She expresses feelings of hopelessness and suicidal ideation (symptoms) and is disinterested in performing basic self-care tasks such as caring for personal hygiene (dysfunction).

PSYCHOPATHOLOGY

Symptoms of mental illness may present in a wide variety of combinations, and there are various schemas for organizing the information. The following is one example of a categorical organization of **psychopathology** and descriptions of common symptoms within each category.

Thought

Thought includes what are considered to be the higher intellectual functions of abstraction, reasoning, judgment, and analysis. The most common deficits seen in this area are concrete thinking and an inability to recognize or correct errors (which may be due to increased impulsivity). Concrete thinking includes thought processes focused on immediate experiences and specific objects or events as well as an inability to think metaphorically or abstractly.

A specific form of psychopathology involving the content of thought is delusions, which are deep-seated beliefs not based in reality. The presentation of factual proof will not typically change such beliefs. There are many types of delusions, including delusions of grandeur as well as self-deprecating and paranoid delusions. These are typically not an exaggeration of real experiences, but rather an essentially inaccurate, though powerful, belief. For example, an individual with a delusion of grandeur may believe he or she has supernatural powers, is a famous historical figure, or has an important secret mission to accomplish. Some delusions are relatively harmless with little associated dysfunction, while others leave an individual extremely incapacitated in daily living activities, or, as sometimes is the case with paranoid delusions, make him or her a danger to him- or herself or to others.

Another form of disordered thought is obsession, which is a specific and repetitive thought that is typically unwanted and cannot be eliminated by reason. Obsessions are often found in conjunction with compulsions, whereby a person attempts to extinguish the obsession by acting upon it. Although obsessive-compulsive disorder (OCD) is a diagnosis, it is possible to have either or both symptoms without meeting the criteria for OCD or any other diagnosis. Again, the level of associated dysfunction is quite variable.

Language

Speech disturbances are often considered to be part of thought disorder, but they are so common in severe mental illness that it is easier to study them as a separate category. Some people who experience these symptoms seem oblivious to the oddity of their speech, but other people find it exhausting to engage in casual conversation and may avoid it whenever possible. Occupational therapists must be knowledgeable of these symptoms in order to appreciate the effort clients may be expending in conversation and also to understand the meaning of their communication. Table 5-1 provides examples of some of the abnormal speech patterns that can occur with severe mental illness.

Perception

Perception is the ability to attain information via the senses and then process and interpret the stimuli. It is well documented that people with persistent mental illness (particularly schizophrenia) commonly experience hallucinations and illusions, but it is also true that there is a higher than average incidence of other perceptual disturbances in this population (Blakeney, Strickland, & Wilkinson, 1983). These include distorted time and spatial awareness, poor visual perception, poor body scheme, and astereognosis, which is an inability to identify common objects by touch.

Hallucinations.   Hallucinations are perceptual images experienced as sensations but not based on actual stimulation from the external environment. Hallucinations can involve any of the senses: visual (seeing images), auditory (hearing voices or sounds), tactile (feeling sensations on the skin surface), gustatory (taste), olfactory (smell), and somatic (feeling sensations within the body). There have been many attempts to correlate kinds of hallucination with an actual diagnosis, but care must be taken not to oversimplify the relationship between symptom and diagnosis. For example, there are many theories regarding damage to the brain and the presence of visual and tactile hallucinations, yet there are also many exceptions. Nevertheless, there are some significant patterns regarding kinds of hallucinations and diagnosis. For example, visual or olfactory hallucinations may precede grand mal seizures. Tactile hallucinations are often experienced during alcohol or drug withdrawal, and gustatory hallucinations may indicate brain trauma.

Hallucinations seem very real to the person experiencing them and can cause dysfunction in several ways. The relationship between the manifesta-

Table 5-1. Abnormal Speech Patterns Associated with Mental Illness

Term	Description	Example
Concreteness	Extremely literal verbal responses due to concrete thinking patterns. The speaker does not recognize the nuances of language, including abstractions or metaphors	"Reading can open a whole new world." *Response:* "And then the lava flows out of the cracks."
Loosening of Associations	Ideas shift from one subject to another that is completely unrelated. The speaker does not show any awareness that the topics are unconnected	"What is your name?" *Response:* "A rose by any other name. . . . I wish I could get out of here. . . . Jigsaw puzzles are fun."
Perseveration	Repetition of the same word, phrase, or idea. Also, an inability to shift from one task to another.	"What do you want to do today?" *Response:* "Today is Tuesday, I always do wash on Tuesday, always on Tuesday it's wash."
Circumstantiality and Tangentiality	The person digresses, giving unnecessary, irrelevant information. When speech is circumstantial there is difficulty getting to the point of the conversation, yet in the person's mind, the answers are related. In tangential speech the person starts answering a question but then rapidly digresses.	"When were you in the hospital?" *Circumstantial response:* "I went to this great concert last summer after I visited my aunt." *Tangential response:* "In the fall . . . the leaves were so beautiful. . . . They were like my paintings. . . . My art is my soul."
Echolalia	Repetition (echo) of the words and phrases of others. This speech is repetitive and persistent.	"What is your name?" *Response:* "What is your name? Your name, your name."
Clanging	The sound or rhyme of the words takes precedence over the meaning or content of the replies.	"What is your occupation?" *Response:* "I used to be a lawyer, now a liar, lollipops, licenses, and licorice."
Neologism	An invented word that may closely resemble an existing word or may be known only to the individual.	"Why were you admitted to the hospital?" *Response:* "It come from too much normiation, a sort of infesteration of some sort. I was being institized."

Table 5-2. Model of Functional Deficits Associated with Hallucinations

Classification		*Observable Behavior*
Class 0	Insufficient information	None identifiable
Class I	No hallucinations	None
Class II	Intermittent hallucinations with minimal or no functional deficits	Phenomena reported upon questioning or in appropriate settings. Individual may appear withdrawn
Class III	Intermittent or persistent hallucinations with functional deficits related to the content of the phenomena	Evidence of poor self-esteem such as frequent self-deprecating remarks, poor posture, lack of social interaction, and poor motivation
Class IV	Intermittent or persistent hallucinations with functional deficits directly related to the intrusiveness of the phenomena	Inappropriate behavior while apparently responding to internal stimuli. Inappropriate affect such as giggling not related to the outside environment. Conversations with the self. Poor attention to the task on hand but can be redirected to task and surroundings
Class V	Intermittent or persistent hallucinations with functional deficits related to *both* content and intrusiveness of the phenomena	See classes III and IV
Class VI	Persistent hallucinations with profound functional deficits. Generally acute	Inability to appropriately respond to the external environment.

Source: From MacRae (1997).

tion of hallucinations and specific dysfunctions is described in the model of functional deficits (MacRae, 1997) and shown in Table 5-2.

The model of functional deficits is a framework for examining the phenomenon of hallucinations from an occupational therapy perspective. In this model, various types of dysfunction are correlated to specific manifestations of hallucinations. For example, when the dominant feature of the hallucinations is the *content* (such as what the voices are saying), typically there is evidence of poor self-esteem and observations may include frequent self-deprecating remarks, poor posture, lack of social interaction, and poor motivation. However, when the dominant feature of the hallucinations is the *intrusiveness* of the phenomenon, dysfunctions will more likely include inappropriate behavior while apparently responding to internal stimuli. Observations might include behaviors such as giggling for no apparent reason, conversations with the self, and poor attention to tasks.

Illusions.   A milder form of perceptual distortion is an illusion, in which the outside object causing the stimuli is real but the person misinterprets the object (for example, a lamppost may be mistaken for a robot). Like hallucinations, illusions may involve any of the senses, but auditory and visual illusions are most common.

Affect

Affect refers to the observable behavior representing one's emotions, but (as shown in Figure 5-1, which depicts classical drama masks) it is not always possible to know what someone is feeling. It is also sometimes difficult to determine a pathological affect because there are normal fluctuations in everyone's emotional state. The demonstration of emotions is partially dictated by culture, so awareness of and sensitivity to a person's background are essen-

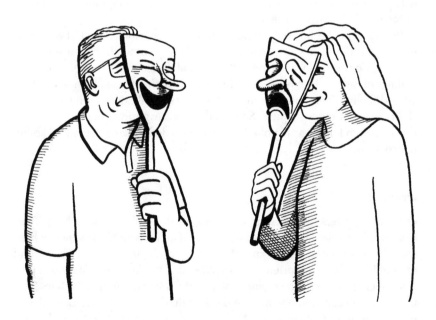

Figure 5-1.   Affect Is an Observable Behavior Representing Emotion

tial. Disturbances of affect can be a direct result of a mental illness or a neurological disorder such as cerebrovascular accident (CVA). Changes in affect can also be drug induced. *Flat affect* refers to a lack of observable emotion. Other emotional states, such as anxiety or hostility, may be considered pathologic if the emotional state is either inappropriate or out of proportion to the environmental stimuli.

Depression.   Depression is one of the most common affective symptoms. It may be seen with many psychiatric diagnoses, including not only major depression and dysthymia but also schizophrenia, the dementias, and personality disorders. Mania is a condition in which the individual responds in an eager, exuberant, and even joyful manner, regardless of the environmental reality. Although mania is considered a disordered affect, the dysfunction resulting from the manic state is usually caused by the associated features of poor judgment and impulsivity. Therefore, mania might best be described as a syndrome consisting of affect, thought, and motor dysfunctions.

Lability.   Lability is a state of unstable emotions, which may present in many different ways. For example, one individual may swing rapidly between laughter and tears, while another person may cry uncontrollably yet may be unable to identify a reason for the tears. Paying particular attention to the individual's previous level of emotional display and cultural background is necessary to accurately identify a true lability.

Because *affect* refers only to the observable behavior associated with feelings, it is difficult to categorize or even identify some altered or impaired feelings. For example, a person with a mental illness may experience intense feelings of rage and yet have no visible signs of such intense feelings. Another altered feeling state common in mental illness is anhedonia, which is an inability to experience pleasure. Some individuals experience a milder form of this symptom known as hypohedonia, which is defined as a decreased ability to experience pleasure.

Orientation

Orientation refers to a person's awareness of time, place, and person. Typically, the first orientation to be lost is time. The individual may know where and who he or she is, yet not know the date, month, or even year. The second orientation to be lost is orientation to place, and the last is orientation to person, which includes the recognition of both the self and significant others. This pattern is so predictable that a standard method of charting has been developed to represent orientation. O (orientation) × 3 means that the individual is oriented to time, place, and person; O × 2 means orientation is to place and person only; and O × 1 means that the person is oriented only to person. If orientation was lost in a different order than that of time, place, and person,

Table 5-3. Orientation to Time, Place, and Person

Description	Clinical Interpretation	Charting
Mrs. Wong states that she is in Hong Kong in 1948 when she is actually in present-day San Francisco. She recognizes her children and can report her own name.	Mrs. Wong is not oriented to place or time; she is oriented to person.	O x 1
Mr. Geary recognizes all of his family members, as well as his doctor. He is aware that he is presently hospitalized in his hometown but frequently is unclear about the day and month and occasionally does not know the year.	Mr. Geary is clearly oriented to person and place; however, his time disorientation fluctuates in severity.	O x 2
Ms. Tenaka was administered a mental status exam during which she was able to accurately report her name, her presence in the psychiatric emergency room, and the correct date.	Ms. Tenaka is fully oriented to time, place, and person.	O x 3

this must be explicitly stated. Table 5-3 provides examples of this form of documentation.

Memory

The most common categorization of memory is the simple division into short term and long term. However, memory is quite complex and further categorization is helpful to determine specific functional deficits associated with its loss. Table 5-4 describes one classification system of types of memory and their clinical significance. A knowledge of these specific types of memory will help the clinician identify an individual's assets as well as deficits and plan treatment accordingly. For example, procedural memory is often retained when declarative memory is not. By designing a treatment plan that allows desired responses to become automatic, the therapist can help patients become more functional.

Another example of clinical significance is the identification of prospective memory, which is important for independent living. Examples of prospective memory include remembering to pay bills, go to the doctor, and turn off the stove.

People who have severe memory deficits, as is found with dementia of the Alzheimer's type or substance-induced persisting amnestic disorder, often engage in confabulation. Confabulation is the unknowing fabrication of events

Table 5-4. Types of Memory

Type	Description	Example
Procedural memory	An automatic sequence of behavior such as conditioned responses	Despite significant deterioration of her mental status, Mrs. Makiba remembers to retrieve the newspaper from the porch and make a pot of coffee by 8 A.M. as she has done every day for years.
Declarative memory	Memory specific to consciously learned facts such as school subjects.	Mr. Alvarado is diagnosed with schizophrenia. He has a history of failure in jobs and has been unable to pass classes at the community college due to poor attendance. Nevertheless, he is able to recall much of the material from the lectures he was able to attend and he is quite knowledgeable about current events.
Semantic memory	The knowledge of the meaning of words and the ability to classify information or ideas.	Mr. Hackett lives in a supervised residential care home, where he is considered to be quite proficient at solitary crossword puzzles.
Episodic memory	The knowledge of personal experiences	Mrs. Yen spends three mornings a week meeting at the cultural center, where she enjoys sharing stories and reminiscing with her friends.
Prospective memory	The capacity to remember to carry out actions in the future. In essence, "to remember to remember"	After a home evaluation, the occupational therapist concluded that Ms. Cohen can live independently. She has been able to keep all her appointments and safely operates a stove in the kitchen.

to fill in the gaps of true memory. It is not intentional lying, as the person is not aware that he or she is doing so. It is also not delusional, as the person will not be particularly invested in, or attached to, the confabulated statements.

Sensorimotor

Observable changes in the activity level of a person with a mental illness are sometimes assumed to be a consequence of psychotropic medications. The fourth edition of the **DSM** includes new classifications of drug-induced movement disorders to assist the clinician in identifying specific neurological patterns associated with high levels of psychotropic medication (APA, 1994). While drugs can have such effects, it is also common to experience increased or decreased activity levels due directly to a mental illness. It is not always possible to predict when, or if, a motor symptom will accompany a mental illness or what form the motor response will take. For example, one person with depression may appear lethargic while another person is quite agitated and yet a third person with depression shows little or no change in motor response.

Specific motor symptoms may also be related to the severity of the mental disorder. Catatonia, which is rigidity or immobility, would most likely be observed during an acute and severe psychotic episode rather than as a persistent state. Other possible symptoms involving motor function are stereotypy, the repetition of apparently senseless actions; tics, involving muscular spasms or twitching; and compulsions, which are repetitive, irrational behaviors acted out in response to an overwhelming urge.

A variety of sensorimotor symptoms may be found in mental illnesses with an organic basis. These include abnormal muscle tone, abnormal gait, and apraxia, which is an inability to plan and coordinate complex motor actions. Sensory-integrative dysfunctions, including decreased pain and temperature sensation, may also be present. These deficits are often subtle and may go unrecognized.

DIAGNOSIS

The determination of a clinical diagnosis in psychiatry is, at best, an inexact process based on both deductive and inductive reasoning. One view of this process is that it is a constructive way of ordering knowledge about a person's dysfunction in order to better understand the mental illness. However, diagnoses are also viewed by some as a destructive force that serves only to inappropriately label and dehumanize individuals. There are inherent dangers in labeling, and it is the clinician's responsibility not to make assumptions about an individual's behavior or abilities based on diagnosis alone. On the other hand, a structured diagnostic process attempts to make psychiatric terminology more uniform, which is important because of the stigma attached to mental illness. The implications of these disorders at a societal level are great, which means that the careless use of volatile terms must be avoided, regardless of the purpose of diagnosis. Indeed, the occupational therapist can play an important role in educating the public about the myths of mental illness and the misuse of clinical terminology. For example, calling someone "a schizophrenic "implies that the individual's main identifying feature is an illness, which is simplistic and dehumanizing. It is both more appropriate and more accurate to identify the individual as a "person with schizophrenia." Figure 5-2 suggests other ways to use labels intelligently and sensitively.

LANGUAGE

Mental illnesses are frequently the subject of news stories, or of dramatic films or television programs. The National Alliance for the Mentally Ill offers the following guidelines for use of medical and slang terms about mental illnesses:

- words like "crazy," "nuts," "wacko," "sicko," "psycho," "lunatic," "demented" and "loony" are offensive

- terms like "insane" are inappropriate except when used in a specific medical or legal context (e.g., the term "criminally insane" in a courtroom scene)

- referring to a "mentally ill person" or a "person with a severe mental illness" is preferable to "the mentally ill," which depersonalizes—highlighting the illness, not the person

- terms like "schizophrenia" and "manic depressive illness" have very specific meanings and apply only to certain groups of ill people; such scientific labels need to be checked carefully for accuracy; they should **not** be used to refer to "schizophrenic weather" or other uses unrelated to the illnesses themselves

■ ■ ■ ■ ■ ■ ■

For more information, contact the National Alliance for the Mentally Ill, a self-help organization providing mutual support, public education, research and advocacy for people with serious mental illnesses:

> Public Relations Department
> National Alliance for the Mentally Ill
> 2101 Wilson Boulevard, Suite 302
> Arlington, VA 22201
> 703/524-7600

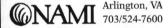

ABOUT MENTAL ILLNESS

Figure 5-2. Language about Mental Illness

Another criticism of the diagnostic process is the lack of precise data on psychiatric illness. It is rare that measurable or visible objective data such as X-rays and blood tests, as are used in physical diagnosis, can be used in psychiatry." Much of the controversy stems from a lack of accurate measurements to validate the diagnosis, thereby allowing for differences of opinion of a highly subjective nature" (Mathis, 1992, p. 253).

Still another significant concern about diagnosis is cultural bias. "In a world in which ethnic and cultural pluralism is daily becoming more politically salient, it is striking that North American professional constructs of person-ality and psychopathology are mostly culture bound" (Lewis-Fernandez & Kleinman, 1994, p. 67), with, specifically, a white, male, Judeo-Christian ori-entation. The awareness of this limitation is increasing, but it remains essen-tial that clinicians be aware of the inherent ethnocentrism found in the current diagnostic system. "A clinician who is unfamiliar with the nuances of an indi-vidual's cultural frame of reference may incorrectly judge as psychopathol-ogy those normal variations in behavior, belief, or experience that are particular to the individual's culture" (APA, 1994, p. xxiv).

Given these limitations, why are diagnoses used at all? Despite legitimate controversy, the diagnostic process helps facilitate interdisciplinary commu-nication and fosters research, both of which are essential for high-quality men-tal health care. It is hoped that as research continues, the process of diagnosing will become increasingly objective, culturally sensitive, and accurate.

Overview of the Diagnostic and Statistical Manual of Mental Disorders (DSM)

The concept of multiaxial diagnosis had been discussed in the European psy-chiatric literature since the 1940s. Nevertheless, it is a relatively new idea in American psychiatry and has only had practical application since the publi-cation in 1980 of the third edition of the American Psychiatric Association's *Diagnostic and Statistical Manual of Mental Disorders* (DSM-III). This multi-axial system provides a comprehensive view of an individual's mental health, with each axis addressing a different domain. This system minimizes the like-lihood that pertinent information will be overlooked in interdisciplinary treat-ment planning. An overview of the multiaxial assessment process according to DSM-IV is provided in Table 5-5.

Study of the DSM is a significant part of the academic curricula of mental health professionals. Unfortunately, it is sometimes difficult for students to keep in mind that the information being presented is not clear-cut, concrete, or complete. It is important to critically analyze the data and be aware of its limitations. As stated in the DSM-IV, "The specific diagnostic criteria included in DSM-IV are meant to serve as guidelines to be informed by clinical judg-ment and are not meant to be used in a cookbook fashion" (APA, 1994, p. xxiii). Furthermore, the process of evaluation and treatment planning is far more comprehensive than can be covered in a manual such as the DSM, and each particular discipline has something unique and specific to offer. It is impor-tant to be familiar with the information in the DSM; however, it should not be assumed that this knowledge is all that is required for practice, as it barely constitutes a beginning.

Table 5-5. An Overview of the DSM-IV Axes

Axes	Description	Comments
Axis I	Clinical Disorders; Other conditions that may be a focus of clinical attention	Reason for referral or principle diagnosis is listed first if multiple diagnoses are present
Axis II	Personality Disorders, Mental Retardation	May also be used to record maladaptive personality features and defense mechanisms
Axis III	General Medical Conditions	Condition is related to the mental disorder and is consistent with the International Classification of Diseases (ICD)
Axis IV	Psychosocial and Environmental Problems	If the problem is the primary focus of treatment it is also recorded on Axis I under "Other conditions that may be a focus of clinical attention"
Axis V	Global Assessment of Functioning	Impairment in functioning due to physical or environmental limitations is not considered

Source: Reprinted with permission from the Diagnostic and Statistical Manual of Mental Disorders, Fourth Edition (APA, 1994). Copyright 1994, American Psychiatric Association.

Theory and the DSM

Although the APA stated that the DSM is atheoretical, theories pervade both our conscious and unconscious thought, so it may not be possible to eliminate theoretical bias. However, the association did make a serious attempt to avoid defining disorders based on the beliefs of a particular school of thought. This is a valuable unifying concept for all the professions involved in mental health because of the diversity of beliefs that are found in practice, particularly regarding the etiology of mental illness. Rather than defining disorders based on an individual theory, such as behaviorism or psychoanalytic thought, the multiaxial system uses what is known as a biopsychosocial approach to assessment. This model is an attempt to be holistic by providing a wide range of information without necessarily referring to the etiology of the disorder or defining it according to one theoretical belief. Figure 5-3 illustrates the communication difficulties encountered when theoretic beliefs are the sole basis of diagnosis. While various theories have significance for treatment, diagnosis becomes problematic when clinicians base their diagnosis solely on theoretical premises.

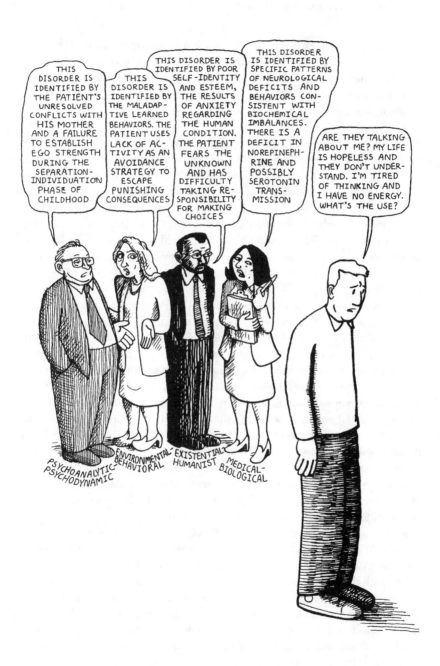

Figure 5-3. Problems with Theoretically Based Communication

The Role of Occupational Therapy

Occupational therapists work within a system in which diagnosis is important, but their view of disorder differs from that of other mental health professionals. The difference revolves around the importance of function in everyday activities, the causes of dysfunction, goals of treatment, and methods for intervening (Bonder, 1995, p. 17).

Occupational therapists are not responsible for determining diagnosis; however, in settings where an interdisciplinary approach is utilized, they often contribute to the diagnostic process by providing the team with specific information from evaluations. A knowledge of the first three axes is essential for effective communication with the team, but from an occupational therapists' perspective, a more valuable focus is on axes IV and V. Occupational therapy intervention is based on the assessment of an individual's unique assets and deficits, and diagnosis on Axis I and Axis II alone cannot provide this information. An attempt is made in the DSM to denote the severity of some disorders; however, this is not always indicative of the individuals' functional level.

Axis IV is used to report the psychosocial and environmental problems in an individual's life. The problem groups used with this axis include problems with the primary support group and those related to the social environment; educational, occupational, housing, and economic problems; problems with access to health care services and those related to interaction with the legal system and crime; and other psychosocial and environmental problems (APA, 1994). Occupational therapists often uncover relevant information for this axis during an initial assessment and use the data in the development of the treatment plan. Axis IV is used to specify all problems that are deemed relevant to the individual's diagnosis and treatment. This is a significant improvement from the Axis IV rating scale in the DSM III because it documents specific, concrete problems, whereas the former scale rated a problem's severity based on an assessment of an "average" person's response to the same stressor without consideration of the role of multiple stressors.

Axis V is the Global Assessment of Functioning (GAF) scale. The purpose of the GAF (reproduced in Figure 5-4) is to assess a person's overall levels of psychological, social, and occupational functioning. Clearly, this is very much in line with the evaluation process of occupational therapy, where assessment is based on task performance in work, leisure, and self-care activities and the motor, sensory, emotional, cognitive, and social components of those tasks. Axis V measures are somewhat reliable and valid; however, they are not widely used (Goldman, Skodol, & Lave, 1992). Occupational therapists should have a major role in the determination and increased implementation of this scale.

The DSM-IV has proposed several additional scales for more specific tracking of an individual's functioning. These include the Social and Occupational Functioning Assessment Scale (SOFAS), the Global Assessment of Relational

Global Assessment of Functioning (GAF) Scale

Consider psychological, social, and occupational functioning on a hypothetical continuum of mental health or illness. Do not include impairment in functioning due to physical (or environmental) limitations.

Code *(Note: Use intermediate codes when appropriate, e.g., 45, 68, 2.)*

100 | 91	Superior functioning in a wide range of activities, life's problems never seem to get out of hand, is sought out by others because of his or her many positive qualities. No symptoms.
90 | 81	Absent or minimal symptoms (e.g., mild anxiety before an exam), good functioning in all areas, interested and involved in a wide range of activities, socially effective, generally satisfied with life, no more than everyday problems or concerns (e.g., an occasional argument with family members).
80 | 71	If symptoms are present, they are transient and expectable reactions to psychosocial stressors (e.g., difficulty concentrating after family argument); no more than slight impairment in social, occupational, or school functioning (e.g., temporarily falling behind in schoolwork)
70 | 61	Some mild symptoms (e.g., depressed mood and mild insomnia) OR some difficulty in social, occupational, or school functioning (e.g., occasional truancy, or theft within the household), but generally functioning pretty well, has some meaningful interpersonal relationships.
60 | 51	Moderate symptoms (e.g., flat affect and circumstantial speech, occasional panic attacks) OR moderate difficulty in social, occupational, or school functioning (e.g., few friends, conflicts with peers or co-workers).
50 | 41	Serious symptoms (e.g., suicidal ideation, severe obsessional rituals, frequent shoplifting) OR any serious impairment in social, occupational, or school functioning (e.g., no friends, unable to keep a job).
40 | 31	Some impairment in reality testing or communication (e.g., speech is at times illogical, obscure, or irrelevant) OR major impairment in several areas, such as work or school, family relations, judgment, thinking or mood (e.g., depressed man avoids friends, neglects family, and is unable to work; child frequently beats up younger children, is defiant at home, and is failing at school).
30 | 21	Behavior is considerably influenced by delusions or hallucinations OR serious impairment in communication or judgment (e.g., sometimes incoherent, acts grossly inappropriately, suicidal preoccupation) OR inability to function in almost all areas (e.g., stays in bed all day; no job, home or friends).
20 | 11	Some danger of hurting self or others (e.g., suicide attempts without clear expectation of death; frequently violent; manic excitement) OR gross impairment in communication (e.g., largely incoherent or mute).
10 | 1	Persistent danger of severely hurting self or others (e.g., recurrent violence) OR persistent inability to maintain minimal personal hygiene OR serious suicidal act with clear expectation of death.
0	Inadequate information.

Figure 5-4. The Global Assessment of Functioning (GAF) Scale

Functioning (GARF), and the Defensive Functioning Scale. As these are newly introduced scales in the DSM, their usefulness in clinical practice is yet to be shown. However, in some settings they would be ideal data collection tools for research conducted by many disciplines, including occupational therapists. The case illustrations of Cathy and David illustrate the use of the axis system in diagnosis. As you are reading, look for the pertinent information that led to the information on the axes.

CASE ILLUSTRATION: CATHY — APPLICATION OF THE DSM

Cathy is a 33-year-old woman who was referred to the day treatment center with the goals of increasing structure in her life, improving social skills, and enhancing her poor self-image. Despite having a Master's degree, she has never held a job for more than a couple of months and has been unemployed for the last three years. She presently receives disability payments and lives alone in an apartment. However, she is angry at her landlord so she stopped paying the rent. He, in turn, is threatening to evict her. Cathy freely admits that it is hard for her to "pay bills and stuff," stating, "I'm just not that organized a person." She frequently spends her entire monthly check on the day it is cashed and then resorts to "borrowing" money from her sister and neighbors.

Cathy has a history of getting quite enthusiastic about a particular therapist for a short while and then "firing" him or her. She has dropped out of several mental health programs in the past. Cathy has had several hospitalizations for attempted suicide. Her suicidal threats and attempts are usually very dramatic (i.e., slashing her wrists or threatening to jump out of a building) and often coincide with the perceived "failure" of the most recently fired therapist. Recently, she has become quite attached to the occupational therapist at the day treatment center and states, "She is the only one who really understands me."

AXIS I   V71.09 — No diagnosis on Axis I

AXIS II   301.83 Borderline Personality Disorder

AXIS III   None

AXIS IV   Occupational problems — unemployment; housing problems — discord with landlord

AXIS V   60 (current)

CASE ILLUSTRATION: DAVID — APPLICATION OF THE DSM

David is a 14-year-old boy who was brought to the emergency psychiatric service after it took three police officers to subdue his vicious physical attack, in which he used a baseball bat on another youth. It was originally thought that David might be on the street drug PCP, but his blood levels proved negative and he became quite calm and somewhat aloof during the hospital admission process. Formal charges against David are pending.

David is presently undergoing evaluation on the adolescent psychiatric unit. Reports from the school and family reveal a history of aggressive behaviors at school since third grade, but with a recent increase in frequency. David has been involved in several physical fights with classmates over the past two semesters and was reported for two incidents of vandalism. He also is frequently truant from school. David says he has no "real friends," and he shows no remorse for his acts of violence. His academic record shows substantially below-average reading ability, although he maintains a passing grade in math and workshop classes. His mother reports that she cannot control him and that, in order to provide basic care for David and his four sisters, she must work two jobs, one as a housekeeper and the other on a night shift at a local factory. Six months ago, David's father was convicted of assault and robbery and is presently serving a five-year sentence in the state penitentiary.

AXIS I	312.8 — Conduct Disorder, Childhood-Onset Type, Severe; 315.00 Reading Disorder (Provisional)
AXIS II	V71.09 — Deferred on Axis II
AXIS III	None
AXIS IV	Problems with primary support — father incarcerated, mother unable to provide discipline; educational problems — below-average academic performance, discord with teachers and classmates; problems related to interaction with legal system/crime — recent arrest
AXIS V	50 (current)

Summary

This chapter provides a brief overview of the terminology commonly used in mental health settings. Much of the terminology related to mental health care is misunderstood or misused. Consequently, clinicians practicing in the field need to be as specific and clear as possible in professional discussions and documentation. Furthermore, clinicians can be role models for the sensitive use of terminology and advocates for educating the public about mental health.

Occupational therapists primarily focus their practice on the alleviation of dysfunction, but a thorough understanding of symptoms and diagnoses is essential for all clinicians working in mental health. People with mental illness present with a range of symptoms and dysfunctions of varying frequency and severity, and it is not possible within this chapter to do justice to all presentations. However, forthcoming chapters on specific disorders provide more in-depth discussions of commonly seen diagnoses, dysfunctions, and symptoms.

Review Questions

1. How are symptoms related to diagnosis?
2. What is the relationship between thought and language in relation to psychopathology?
3. How would you justify the use of the DSM for diagnosis?
4. What argument would you offer against use of the DSM?
5. How does occupational therapy differ from the other mental health professions in regard to diagnosis?

Learning Activities

1. Organize groups of two to six people. Write each of the following terms on an index card.
   Catatonia
   Compulsion
   Lability
   Mania
   Perseveration
   Disorientation
   Confabulation
   Each group member should choose a card and take a turn play-acting the disorder, while the other members attempt to identify it. Give feedback to each performer regarding your perception of the accuracy of the representation.
2. Create a "memory log." Spend a block of time, such as a whole morning or afternoon, writing down your activities and recording the type of memory you needed to use to complete that activity (refer to Table 5-4 for definitions). How would your life be different if you had a deficit in each type of memory?
3. Review magazines and television commercials and programs. How many instances of insensitivity about mental illness do you find?
4. Conduct an analysis of your own current level of stress and functioning. How would you presently rate yourself using Axes IV and V?

References

American Psychiatric Association (APA). (1994). *Diagnostic and statistical manual of mental disorders, Fourth Edition.* Washington, DC: Author.

Blakeney, A., Strickland, L. R., & Wilkinson, J. (1983). Exploring sensory integrative dysfunction in process schizophrenia. *American Journal of Occupational Therapy, 37*(6), 399–407.

Bonder, B. (1995). *Psychopathology and function* (2nd ed.). Thorofare, NJ: Slack. (First edition published 1991)

Comer, R. (1995). *Abnormal psychology* (2nd ed.). New York: Freeman.

Gelder, M., Gath, D., & Mayou, R. (1989). *Oxford textbook of psychiatry* (2nd ed.). New York: Oxford University Press.

Goldman, H., Skodol, A., & Lave, T. (1992). Revising Axis V for DSM-IV: A review of measures of social functioning. *American Journal of Psychiatry, 149*(9), 1148–1156.

Hales, R. E., Udofsky, S. C., & Talbott, J. A. (Eds.). (1994). *Textbook of psychiatry* (2nd ed.). Washington, DC: American Psychiatric Press.

Heiden, L. A., & Hersen, M. (Eds.). (1995). *Introduction to clinical psychology.* New York: Plenum Press.

Kaplan, H., Sadock, B., & Grebb, J. (1994). *Kaplan and Sadock's synopsis of psychiatry* (7th ed.). Baltimore, MD: Williams & Wilkins.

Lewis-Fernandez, R., & Kleinman, A. (1994). Culture, personality, and psychopathology. *Journal of Abnormal Psychology, 1*, 67–71.

MacRae, A. (1997). The model of functional deficits associated with hallucinations. *American Journal of Occupational Therapy, 51*, 57–63.

Mathis, J. (1992). Psychiatric diagnosis: A continuing controversy. *Journal of Medicine and Philosophy, 17*, 253–261.

Maxmen, J., & Ward, N. (1995). *Essential psychopathology and its treatment* (2nd ed.). New York: W. W. Norton.

Templer, D., Spencer, D., & Hartlage, L. (1994). *Biosocial psychopathology: Epidemiological perspectives.* New York: Springer.

Suggested Reading

Many new terms have been introduced in this chapter that will also be used in other chapters. Therefore, it is strongly recommended that students have at least one medical dictionary to study clinical terminology. Suggested sources include the most recent editions of the following:

Dorland's medical dictionary. Philadelphia: Saunders.

Miller, B., & Keane, C. *Encyclopedia and dictionary of medicine, nursing, and allied health.* Philadelphia: Saunders.

Taber's cyclopedic medical dictionary. Philadelphia: F. A. Davis.

Disorders of Children and Adolescents

William L. Lambert, OTR
Occupational Therapist
First Hospital, Wyoming Valley
Wilkes Barre, Pennsylvania

Barbara Jo Rodriques, OTR
Lead Occupational Therapist
Dominican Santa Cruz Hospital
Santa Cruz, California

Key Terms

acting out	latency age
consistency	mentor
crack babies	parallel task group
dynamic	structure
ego strength	tic
identified patient (ip)	time-out

Chapter Outline

Introduction

This chapter presents an overview of occupational therapy practice with children and adolescents who are emotionally disturbed. Basic concepts used in providing occupational therapy to children and adolescents with mental illness are described. Occupational therapy programming is discussed based on our experience and on successful interventions used in other settings (Hoffman, 1982; Llorens & Rubin, 1967). Treatment, intervention groups with examples of group protocols, and activities appropriate for this population are presented.

It is often hard for individuals outside child psychiatry to fathom the need to treat children and adolescents for mental disorders. Nonetheless, such treatment has occurred for some time. Indeed, the primary site for the treatment of mental illnesses in general has traditionally been the hospital, whether a small inpatient unit or a large state institution. Residential treatment facilities traditionally have provided long-term treatment for children and adolescents.

DSM-IV DIAGNOSES

The *Diagnostic and Statistical Manual of Mental Disorders, Fourth Edition* (DSM-IV, APA,1994) lists disorders usually first diagnosed in infancy, childhood, or adolescence. Many of these disorders, such as mental retardation and

Tourette's disorder, can continue to cause problems during adulthood. Many disorders that are discussed in other chapters of this volume, such as schizophrenia and major depression, may also first be encountered in childhood and adolescence (Morrison, 1995). Figure 6-1 summarizes DSM-IV disorders beginning in infancy, childhood, or adolescence.

Limitations of Intellectual Functioning
    Mental Retardation. Beginning before the age of 18, these individuals have low intelligence that causes them to need special help in coping with life. The criteria for this diagnosis are an IQ of less than 70 as determined by an individual test and impaired ability to adapt to the demands of normal life. The individual may have difficulty in communicating, caring for self, living at home, relating to others, using community resources, academic functioning, working, using free time and in maintaining health and safety. Individuals may exhibit behavioral problems, such as, aggression, dependency, impulsivity, self-injury and poor frustration tolerance. This disorder is coded on Axis II and is assigned a code number according to its severity: Mild, Moderate, Severe, Profound or Unspecified. About 1% of the population has Mental Retardation. 80% have mild mental retardation IQ of 50-70 and males outnumber females by about three to two.
    Borderline Intellectual Functioning. This is a V-code (not a diagnosis, but the presenting problem) used for persons in the IQ range of 71-84, without the problems in coping with life associated with mental retardation.

Learning Disorders. This diagnosis indicates substantially more difficulty than normal in learning specific academic skills. The diagnosis must be made on the basis of a standardized individual test. These are coded on axis I.
    Reading Disorder. Reading skills develop far more slowly than those of peers.
    Mathematics Disorder. Skills are markedly less than expected for person's age.
    Disorder of Written Expression. Writing skills are slow to develop.
    Learning Disorder Not Otherwise Specified. This can be used for other categories, such as spelling, that do not meet the criteria above.
    Academic Problem. A V code (not a diagnosis but the presenting problem) used when scholastic problems are the focus of treatment.

Motor Skills Disorder
    Developmental Coordination Disorder. The person is slow to develop motor coordination as shown by dropping things, general clumsiness, poor handwriting , poor sports abilty or delays in achieving developmental milestones, such as sitting, crawling or walking, and is not necessarily mentally retarded. The incoordination is not due to a general medical condition and substantially impedes daily living and academic achievement. This is coded on Axis I.

Communication Disorders. These disorders are measured by standardized tests that are given individually and they substantially interfere with social and educational life.
    Expressive Language Disorder. Patients may have small vocabularies or trouble producing grammatically correct sentences.
    Mixed Receptive-Expressive Language Disorder. A person has the problems listed above but with problems understanding words or sentences.
    Phonological Disorder. Speech develops slowly for the person's age or dialect.
(continues)

Figure 6-1.   Disorders Beginning in Infancy, Childhood, or Adolescence

Stuttering. Frequent disruption in the normal fluency of speech. All of the above disorders are coded on Axis I.

Pervasive Developmental Disorders

Children fail to develop normally in a number of areas including the ability to interact socially, to communicate verbally and non-verbally, and to use their imaginations. These are coded on Axis I. These conditions may continue to affect adults, but they will rarely be the focus of evaluation of an adult.

Autistic Disorder. The child has impaired social interactions and communications and develops stereotyped behaviors and interests before age three.

Rett's Disorder. After six months of apparently normal development, the child has abnormal development as shown by slow head growth, delayed language, poorly coordinated gait , loss of purposeful hand movements and of social engagement.

Childhood Disintegrative Disorder. Following two years of normal development the child loses acquired skills.

Asperger's Disorder. Similar to autistic disorder, except children with this disorder do not have delayed or impaired language.

Pervasive Developmental Disorder Not Otherwise Specified. Used for conditions such as atypical autism.

Attention-Deficit and Disruptive Behavior Disorders

Attention-Deficit/Hyperactivity Disorder (ADHD). A common condition in which children are hyperactive, impulsive or inattentive or all three. Symptoms typically begin before the child goes to school, but it is usually diagnosed around age nine. Developmental milestones may occur early. They usually have trouble sitting quietly and cannot focus in school. They tend to be impulsive and say things that may hurt others' feelings, so they may be unpopular. They may be so unhappy that they may also fit criteria for Dysthymic Disorder.

Attention-Deficit/Hyperactivity Disorder Not Otherwise Specified. Used for symptoms of hyperactivity, impulsivity or inattention that do not meet the criteria for ADHD.

Conduct Disorder. The individual violates rules, age approriate norms or the rights of others, evidenced by aggression against people or animals, property destruction, lying or theft, or seriously violating rules. The symptoms cause impairment in job, school, or social life. Childhood onset type is coded if at least one problem occurs before age 10. Adolescent onset is coded if there are not problems before 10. Severity, such as mild, moderate or severe, is also coded. This is a common precursor to Antisocial Personality Disorder.

Oppositional Defiant Disorder. Multiple examples of negativistic behavior, such as losing temper, arguing with adults, defying rules, doing things to deliberately annoy others, blaming others for own mistakes, being angry and resentful or being spiteful or vindictive, persist for at least six months. The symptoms cause much distress or impairment in work, school or social life.

Child or Adolescent Antisocial Behavior. This is a V-code (not a diagnosis but a presenting problem) where antisocial behavior occurs but cannot be ascribed to a mental disorder.

Disruptive Behavior Disorder Not Otherwise Specified. This is used for disturbances of conduct or oppositional behaviors that do not meet the criteria for Conduct or Oppositional Defiant Disorder.

Feeding and Eating Disorders of Infancy or Early Childhood

Pica. The child eats material that is not food.

(continues)

Figure 6-1.   (continued)

Rumination Disorder. There is persistent regurgitation and chewing of food already eaten.

Feeding Disorders of Infancy or Early Childhood. A child's failure to eat enough leads to weight loss or a failure to gain weight.

Tic Disorders

Tourette's Disorder. Multiple vocal and motor *tics* (any stereotyped movement or vocalization that is sudden, nonrhythmic, rapid, and repeated) occur frequently throughout the day. It usually occurs at age seven or at least by early teens. It lasts throughout life, with periods of remission, and reduction in severity when one is mature.

Chronic Motor or Vocal Tic Disorder. A patient has either motor or vocal tics, but not both.

Transient Tic Disorder. Tics occur for no longer than one year.

Tic Disorder Not Otherwise Specified. This is for tics that do not meet the above criteria.

Elimination Disorders.

Encopresis. At the age of four years or later, the child repeatedly passes feces into clothing or onto the floor.

Enuresis. At the age of five years or later, there is repeated voiding of urine into bedding or clothing (it can be voluntary or involuntary).

Other Disorders of Infancy, Childhood or Adolescence

Separation Anxiety Disorder. The child becomes anxious when separated from parent or home.

Selective Mutism. The child elects not to talk.

Reactive Attachment Disorder of Infancy or Early Childhood. Beginning before age five, the child does not relate appropriately to others.

Stereotypic Movement Disorder. Patients repeatedly rock, bang their heads, bite themselves or pick at their own skin or body orifices.

Parent-Child Relational Problems. A V code (not a mental disorder, but a presenting problem) used when a parent and child have problems getting along.

Sibling Relational Problems. A V code used for difficulties between siblings.

Problems Related to Abuse or Neglect. A V code used to cover difficulties that arise from neglect or from physical or sexual abuse.

Disorders of Infancy, Childhood, or Adolescence Not Otherwise Specified. A catchall category for mental disorders that begin in early life and do not meet the criteria for any other disorder described above.

Figure 6-1. (continued)

Children seen by occupational therapists in solely mental health settings commonly have diagnoses of conduct, oppositional defiant, or separation anxiety disorders. Other disorders described in the DSM-IV, such as mental retardation and pervasive developmental disorders and attention deficit/hyperactivity disorders may commonly be seen by occupational therapists in school, after-school and private clinics, or general hospitals that are not specifically designated as mental health settings. This chapter will focus on the disorders that are typically seen in settings designated specifically for the treatment of mental illness.

The presenting problems encountered by occupational therapists treating children with emotional problems are varied. Some may be specified by the V-codes listed in Figure 6-1. Other "typical" psychosocial stresses may include the parents' divorce; verbal, physical, and/or sexual abuse; other traumatic events, such as the death of a sibling, parent, or grandparent; and socio-economic conditions that may be coded according to axis V of the DSM-IV. The child may respond to traumatic events by withdrawal, aggressive or atypical behavior, or regression to behavior expected from a younger child. Sometimes the child is confronted by a physical condition such as diabetes, which may limit the child's ability to play and eat what others are eating or require an unusually strict adherence to a medication and blood-monitoring situation (see Chapter 7 for further information regarding psychosocial factors in physical illness). The child may find the illness overwhelming and consequently start **acting out** at home or become noncompliant with the treatment of the illness in an attempt to exert control.

In other cases a dysfunctional family situation may have led to treatment. Parents sometimes lack the parenting skills required for rearing a normally developing child. In such circumstances, it may be a lack of parental supervision, an inability to set and enforce limits and rules, or the failure to distinguish and differentiate the needs of the parent from the needs of the child. In other situations, parents have placed expectations on children that the latter find overwhelming, such as a parental need to see a child excel in academics or athletics. Sociological factors, such as poverty, violence, and crime, may constitute a stressful environment, resulting in depression or anxiety and leading to a need for treatment. Whatever the antecedents that lead to a child receiving professional treatment, the primary reasons are similar to any psychiatric intervention situation. These factors include the following:

- danger of presenting harm to oneself or others
- a breakdown in role functioning, namely, appropriate behavior as a sibling, student, playmate, son, or daughter
- a decrease in obedience to, or compliance with, authority figures
- social withdrawal
- increase in aggression or other unacceptable or inappropriate acting-out behaviors, such as fighting, truancy, criminal activities such as theft or vandalism, fire setting, and violence directed toward pets or other animals

Other factors that contribute to emotional problems in children include fetal alcohol syndrome and fetal alcohol effects, which sometimes impair a child's ability to learn from experience or impair the usual responses to medical interventions. The offspring of mothers who used or abused drugs during pregnancy, **crack babies** may display a wide range of often unpredictable developmental deficits.

Regardless of the unique circumstances that are part of a child's particular situation, the onset of the illness varies with each child, based on diagnosis, level of disability, and equality-of-life factors such as income level, access to health care, and stability of the family situation. Children's emotional problems and the consequences of interpersonal and social impairments become more visible once they reach the age where they can be observed by others at day care, preschool, or the school system setting. At this time difficulties tend to become more evident and families often seek professional, clinical help. Problems may become evident in childhood and continue into adolescence. Alternately, difficulties may first be identified during adolescence, which is a period of great change and, therefore, vulnerability. In fact, some researchers (Gilligan, 1979, 1991; Gilligan, Lyons, & Hammer, 1990) believe that adolescence is a particularly difficult time for females due to their extreme vulnerability to social and psychological pressure.

The period of adolescence is a time in which there is a great deal of transition, learning, and growth. Changes are occurring physically, emotionally, and socially as the adolescent moves from childhood to adulthood. The advent of adolescence presents special challenges for the child with a mental disorder. As teenagers move through this period, they begin to assume new roles with increasing independence from the adults in their lives. This transition to adulthood requires an expanding repertoire of cognitive, intellectual, social, language, and motor skills, which are essential for adult living. This is typically a gradual process in which the adolescent rapidly moves in and out of new and old roles. These changing roles sometimes make it difficult for parents and clinicians to know how to treat individuals, either as children or as adults. On the one hand, adolescents need to be provided with opportunities to learn how to assume responsibilities independently. On the other hand, they must learn to comply with expectations, provided they are not too demanding, restrictive, or permissive. Work and life roles must be experienced so that behaviors can be developed for self-identification and emotional independence. These tasks become more complex in modern society, in which there are few rituals or religious ceremonies that indicate the rite of passage from childhood to adulthood. Unlike the ritual ordeals of primitive societies, which presented youths with challenges that enabled them to prove themselves as adults and join their society, modern-day behaviors that could be considered substitutes for rituals, such as substance use or sexual behavior at an earlier age with more than one partner, are maladaptive and threaten physical and mental health. Moreover, the period of adolescence has been lengthened by lowering the age of entrance and raising the exit age. For example, 10- and 11-year-old girls are encouraged to wear makeup, adolescent clothes, and teenage jewelry and to present themselves as "sexy," while 22- to 24-year-olds may still be living at home and have trouble participating in the economy as self-supporting, independent adults (Newton, 1995). There may also be identity confusion; for example, a person aged 18 or older is able to vote, own property, and participate in military actions, although banks may refuse to loan money to adolescents aged 18 to 20 for financing a car or housing. Therefore, this time period can be filled with fear, anxiety, and ambivalence, making change extremely difficult for the emerging adolescent. The teenager may sometimes want to be both a responsible adult who makes autonomous decisions and a child who surrenders responsibility to adults. Though adolescents may mistakenly believe they have acquired the maturation and skills necessary for adult responsibility, at the same time they may feel out of control of changes taking place in their own bodies.

As a result of psychological and social ambivalence, adolescent behavior may seem precipitous or ill timed. Hence, this is a common time for eating and conduct disorders to appear, as well as anxiety and mood disorders. Although typically, this period is described as a tumultuous period for all teens, some researchers (e.g., Block et al., 1981; Offer & Schonert-Reichl, 1992) suggest that tumult is not necessarily the norm. The idea that normal adolescence consists of rebellion, stress, conflict, and trouble is particularly noted in the biological and psychodynamic theories (Papalia & Olds, 1992; Sigelman & Shaffer, 1995). While this is a popular framework for clinicians working with adolescents, researchers have identified adolescent personalities that do not show the otherwise pathological or disturbed behavior that is considered normal in adolescence (Block et al., 1981). In fact, three paths of development from childhood to adulthood have been described (Offer & Sabshin, 1984). The first path is one of a smooth, consistent transition with little conflict. The second is a "surgent growth," including spurt periods characterized by minor conflicts and difficulty. A third path is marked by "tumultuous growth," involving behaviors and problems considered "normal" by many developmental theorists. Adolescents from this third path of growth often come from crisis-oriented families with some evidence of pathology, yet it is they who have been mistaken for the norm. Additionally, those who study temperament (e.g., Chess & Thomas, 1984; Thomas & Chess, 1986) find that if a child's temperament "fits" within his or her developmental trajectory, he or she may go through adolescence in a relatively nontroubled manner. These findings suggest that disturbance and conflict are pathological rather than normal for this period.

There are many normal developmental tasks for the healthy, growing adolescent, including:

- accept physical changes in the body, such as changing voice and size, hair growth, maturing genitals and other body parts, menstruation, acne, and perspiration
- establish more adult relationships with others
- develop masculine and feminine roles
- develop a sense of sexuality
- develop **ego strength**
- establish a personal philosophy and unique values and attitudes

These developments will influence life in all occupational performance areas and components, including family, school, work, church, and peer group activities. Adolescents are generally anxious to try out "adult" roles. They often require consistent direction, guidance, structure, and limits provided by others (parents, teachers, treatment staff) for help in taking on roles that are congruent with developing maturity.

HELPFUL CONCEPTS FOR TREATING CHILDREN AND ADOLESCENTS

Because children and adolescents are developing a self-identity and learning how to behave in their social world, concepts such as structure and consistency, interpretation, time-out, limit setting, avoidance of power struggles, modeling, and a consistent team approach are important to keep in mind when working with children and teenagers. Although these concepts are used when working with adults, who presumably have developed some sense of identity and social norms, they are particularly important for the time period when individuals are learning who they are and how to act in the world.

Structure and Consistency

Two fundamental principles guiding treatment in pediatric and adolescent psychiatric occupational therapy are **structure** and **consistency**. For individuals with poor impulse control, attention deficits, hyperactivity, or poor response to limits and rules, increasing the amount of structure can improve their response to activity interventions, help them learn how to modulate their own emotions, and assist them in learning appropriate role behavior. The environment itself is used to provide cues to appropriate behavior similar to those used in milieu therapy or therapeutic communities.

Structure can be verbal, such as the tactic of redirection, or physical and tangible, depending on the specific activity or equipment used. Activities can begin with the imposition of verbal structure, such as directions and limits or rules regarding the activity. For example, the group leader or therapists may say: "Today in group we are going to share the toys in the playroom. There can be no hitting. If anyone hits someone else, he or she will have to leave the group." This introduction provides an idea or standard that can be referred to throughout the group session to provide consistency. For children, a poster that lists the rules of the group or activity provides an additional reference point that can be used to remind them of the structure (see Figure 6-2). For adolescents, a brief discussion of what the rules mean for each participant or periodic reminders from the therapist will serve to reinforce the structure, and an age-appropriate graphic form of reminder is also handy. Depending on the type of group, teenagers might elect their own rule keeper for each session or time period.

Occupational Therapy Group Rules
  1. Have Fun
  2. Share
  3. Listen to Staff
  4. Clean Up

Figure 6-2.   Rules Poster

When conducting groups it is important to ensure that the group begin and end at the designated times and follow the established routine as much as possible. Naturally, a variety of unpredictable and unavoidable circumstances can interfere with the daily course of programming. For example, a therapist may be sick or on vacation, or special events, such as holiday parties, may take temporary precedence over scheduled programming. In such cases it is important to inform patients of changes in the established consistency. This practice can prevent the eruption of acting-out behavior from a patient who may otherwise feel unable to trust the adults and the therapeutic environment responsible for his or her care. A clinical example of this phenomenon can be seen in the case of a child, Joanie, who was not made aware of the impending absence of the therapist who normally ran her group.

CASE ILLUSTRATION: JOANIE

When Joanie, 8, arrived in the therapy room, she learned that the group had been changed from an art group to a play group, which caused her to cry, kick, and scream. When an interpretation was made that the child appeared very upset, she blurted out: "I wanted to have art! I have to paint my project so I can give it to my mother!"

Discussion

Had she been informed of the change beforehand, the incident might have been averted and, instead, Joanie might have (1) been able to calmly present her disappointment and concerns, (2) been provided with options for completing her project, and (3) thereby learned how to acceptably express her internal feelings and thoughts.

A point that may be implicitly understood by occupational therapists is that another way to provide structure is through activities themselves. "The child's developmental progression is facilitated by play, games and activities, integral functions of a child's daily life" (Abramson, 1982, p. 61). An example is making a tile mosaic project in a **parallel task group**. Structure is provided:

• when each patient has his or her own project, which encourages work in a specific spot and focuses attention on a personal project

- when an example or sample is provided that may be followed to enhance redirection to task
- when the instructions are clear (e.g., "put tiles in the tray like this."). This encourages following the stated direction
- when steps are graded according to therapy goals (e.g., "pick up each tile and glue it in place.").

Children and adolescents enjoy the structure of individual activities, which can serve as a means of exploring their abilities and skills and possibly learning about their strengths and limitations.

> Puppetry, doll play, and drawing provide a technique for dramatizing and externalizing intrapsychic issues. For the older latency-age child, board games may become catalysts for communication and interpersonal relationships. . . . At all times, play, games and activities are active experiences, and their focus on productivity and participation offer intrinsic satisfaction for the child: To cultivate those skills necessary to fulfill life roles. (Abramson, 1982, p. 61)

Although there are common considerations when choosing an activity for any person, for a child or adolescent it is particularly important to be mindful of dangerous parts such as sharp edges, toxic chemicals, or toxic paints or parts that can be ingested, such as small wheels found on a toy car for toddlers. Another consideration is whether there are any parts that could be used in a suicide attempt, such as when knives are being used in a cooking group. In general, in planning activities for children or adolescents it should be constantly considered whether:

- the activity chosen is age appropriate
- the activity is broken down into steps that the child can understand
- the steps are age appropriate for a child to carry out independently
- the therapist wishes the child to carry out independently or by asking for assistance.

For example, if an activity should involve a child sustaining attention to a task, perhaps a tile mosaic project involving the selection of a number of small tiles placed in a trivet is the activity of choice. If improving self-esteem is a consideration, an easy-to-do, foolproof activity such as painting a sun catcher or lacing a small coin purse may do. Where individual play skills are lacking, perhaps the creation and assembly of a toy car that the child can use independently or in conjunction with other children is the activity of choice. In any case, the activity should facilitate developmentally appropriate skills and be fun and intrinsically motivating for the child or adolescent.

Interpretation

Interpretation of, or putting words to, behavior is a therapeutic technique that provides a child or adolescent with an avenue to express feelings with words, which is more often appropriate than other means such as aggression or acting out. This is often an effective way of de-escalating a child or adolescent who is displaying behavioral problems that result from an inability to use words for self-expression. In the example of Joanie, interpretation involved the therapist identifying to the child in a clear and supportive manner what she observed. Joanie could then better express the behavior's cause (whether the change in routine, a reminder of a **dynamic** within her family, or a feeling she could not identify). The identification of these issues by using interpretation clarifies the situation at hand and teaches a more adaptive coping strategy: the use of words to express feelings and reach acceptable solutions to problems. Activities can be used to provide opportunities to externalize intrapsychic issues or facilitate communication. Once issues have been externalized or communicated, interpretation helps children and adolescents to understand, learn, cope, and adapt emotionally (Abramson, Hoffman, & Johns, 1979).

Time-Out

Time-out is an intervention technique that results in behavioral changes and increases the children's and adolescents' understanding of their role in a situation. If a child is asked to take time-out for kicking a peer while fighting over a toy, he will learn that aggression leads to the loss of the chance to play. Time-out also provides an opportunity for the adult to teach the child how to share. Thus, the child becomes better able to perceive the situation and learn from it. Similarly, if an adolescent is removed from group for aggression or breaking the rules, she will become better able to think about the situation and learn from it. Time-out is the process of removing a young person from a problematic situation to a specific area away from the group and, at the same time, allowing him or her to think about the behavior that led to removal from the group.

The length of time-out should vary with the individual's age and mental capacities. For example, when a child has provoked a fight with a peer, he will be removed to a time-out chair, a "think about it" area, or another room, where he will be requested to remain for a specified amount of time. Depending on his age, he may be asked to remain in time-out until he can count to 10 or until a minute goes by on a timer. After a time-out has been completed, it is important to critically analyze the incident. The patient and staff should meet briefly to discuss the behavior that led to the time-out, evaluate whether the intervention was useful for the client, and develop a plan of action that will be utilized in future situations. A plan of action may involve identifying with the client alternative coping strategies (such as a self-assigned time-out) or the use of assertive responses (such as letting a staff person know when he or she is feeling frustrated or agreeing on a "code word" to indicate the need for a behavior change). This process should be kept as brief as possible so that acting-out behavior is not reinforced. When used properly, a time-out can be efficacious in changing maladaptive behavior to that which is more socially appropriate. Time-out should not be conceived of as a punishment, nor should the individual taking a time-out think of it in this way. It is important to present the time-out as a way to learn new behavior so that a positive learning experience may occur.

Limit setting

Limit setting involves informing others what is permissible and what is unacceptable; it lets individuals know "how far they can go." Setting limits is especially important for children and adolescents because they need, and look for, limits, which eventually become internalized as a set of rules that guide socially accepted behavior. The teaching of behavior such as learning to respect the property of others and not taking what doesn't belong to them begins when children are told, in effect, "Thou shalt not steal" (whether this occurs at home, school, or in a religious setting), and the rule is enforced by the parent. When consistent enforcement of the rule or limit occurs, appropriate behavior will be learned or thus becomes a part of that person's internal code of values, morals or conscience. Children and adolescents are protected by rules or limits, such as saying that they may play in the yard but not in the street, they must be home before a certain hour, or they should not drive recklessly. This not only teaches safety and prevents harm, it also shows children and adolescents that their welfare is the concern of the parent or other adult. Limits that are thus enforced clarify the relationship between the parent (or other adult) and child and teach appropriate role behavior. Limits should be friendly but firm, and short and impersonal. Limits can be put in the context of the group rules, as when the occupational therapist says: "We must share the toys," or, "The house rules say that fighting over what program to watch on TV leads to an early bedtime for everyone." Although setting limits may be interpreted as punishment, if done in a protective and supportive way, it will foster more mature behavior. Naturally, the amount of limit setting depends on the needs of the child and the comfort level of the therapist (Abramson et al., 1979).

Since adolescents are more cognitively advanced and bigger than children, setting limits for them can be more complex. When setting limits during treatment it is particularly important to consider why you are asking that a particular limit be maintained. Is this a safety consideration, a limit necessary for maintaining a therapeutic environment, an attempt to stop a behavior that is disruptive and irritating? If the behavior is compromising safety in a serious way, limits must be placed immediately and follow-through must occur prior to any further incident. Interventions and policy set forth by the facility must be initiated to eliminate any further compromise of safety or risk to the patient or others.

If the behavior is one that destroys the therapeutic environment, such as name calling or sexual comments, the clinician may make some choices regarding the appropriate intervention and consequences for behavior. He or she will base the intervention on the program rules or policy, which may include imposing a time-out or exclusion from the next group or activity, or there may be the opportunity to choose a response to this behavior based on his or her rapport with the adolescent, interventions that have worked in the past, and the group's developmental level. The therapist may choose to ignore behavior but at the same time utilize the opportunity by asking peers in the group to comment, thereby encouraging assertive responses to this intrusive behavior; alternately, the therapist may set the limit immediately.

Some useful methods in setting limits that have stood the test of time can be taken from the popular assertiveness movement of the 1970s. They include the "broken record" technique and the "rule of five" (Alberti & Emmons, 1978; Jakubowski & Lange, 1978; Smith, 1975). The broken record method involves a repetition of a limit or direction until the desired response results. Slight variations can be allowed in this method to address a child or an adolescent and reassure them that the therapist is listening. However, he or she also continues repeating the main directive. The "rule of five" is particularly useful when the child or adolescent is not able to reason due to developmental age or to escalating behavior and the loss of impulse control with the potential for continued escalation. The directive statement to the patient is to have no more than five words in it, with no more than five letters in each word. The goal at this point is to "keep it simple." The statement is made directive in an effort to establish control immediately and is often utilized in escalating situations.

Imposing consistent limits and consequences aids children and adolescents in understanding that they will not be harmed by each other's behavior; rather, they will be helped to maintain self-control and will learn to modulate feelings and emotions approriate to various situations and contexts.

Avoiding Power Struggles.   Because of their particular developmental tasks and ambivalence, power struggles are more likely to occur with teens. The following is an example of a situation that threatens to create a standoff between therapist and client. However, the therapist's nondefensive behavior avoids a power struggle.

CASE ILLUSTRATION: AVOIDING A POWER STRUGGLE

Therapist talking to a 15-year-old male: "If you're going to come into crafts group, you have to make something."

Adolescent: "All you have is girl stuff."

Therapist: "We have plenty of other crafts for you to try. If you don't want to make something, you can leave."

Adolescent, becoming angry: "I can be here! That's a stupid rule, my parents are paying for this stupid group and you can't make me leave."

Therapist, after thinking about it: "You know, you're right, it is a stupid rule. You're welcome to stay as long as you're not disruptive. Does that sound reasonable?"

Adolescent, looking smug and smiling: "Yeah."

Therapist: "Let me know if you'd like a deck of cards or something."

Discussion

The therapist avoided a potential conflict by recognizing his rigid behavior and response and genuinely acknowledging his mistake. Providing children and adolescents with a choice of activities within a group setting is beneficial for many reasons. In most treatment settings, much power and control have been stripped away from patients, who are no longer in their own environment and are now more restricted. A person may be in the treatment setting as a consequence of an action in which he or she was not able to maintain control and thus may feel a great deal of remorse and guilt, which may not be expressed openly. The therapist's task is to help the individual regain self-confidence and improve the ability to modulate his or her emotions and regulate his or her own behavior.

Therapeutic Use of Self

The therapeutic use of self entails the development of an individual style that works with patients in a specific way to promote change and growth and help to provide a corrective emotional experience. This is a difficult concept, or "art," to describe. "The art of occupational therapy involves captivating the child through toys, objects, and games or through the therapist's own actions so that the child becomes involved in the therapeutic process. This art is almost intangible" (Kramer & Hinojasa, 1993, p. 443). An occupational therapist responds to a child in a therapeutic manner, conveying appreciation of the child's uniqueness, kindness, love, and understanding; guiding the child through each step of occupational therapy intervention; and encouraging him or her to accomplish the task that has been chosen to meet the treatment goal. Each therapist will develop a unique and personal style or therapeutic personality for working with patients. The therapeutic use of self requires providing a new response to an old situation, which enables the patient in turn to respond in a new manner that is both adaptive and appropriate.

CASE ILLUSTRATION: KAY — THE THERAPEUTIC USE OF SELF

Kay, a patient on a children's unit, was a young woman with impulsive behavior who could not sustain her interest or complete tasks as assigned. During a cooking group, the occupational therapist assigned her the job of chopping vegetables to be put in a salad. However, Kay did not stay with her task, and, moments later, she was in another part of the room engaging in an activity that had been assigned to another child. The young occupational therapist, in a raised voice, told Kay, "You are not where you belong," and asked what was her task. Kay said, "I'm supposed to be chopping vegetables." The therapist said, "You are driving me crazy," to which she responded, "You sound just like my mother: she always says that." At that point, the therapist realized he was not being therapeutic and was indeed responding to Kay in the same manner in which adults had always responded to her. Therefore he acknowledged that fact, apologized for sounding impatient, and redirected Kay to the task at hand (as he should have done previously).

Discussion

As demonstrated by the therapist in this case, the therapeutic use of self involves responding to patients in a way that will guide them onto a new path through developing behaviors that are appropriate and socially acceptable. This involves responding to patients in a different manner than nontherapeutic individuals in past situations.

Children and adolescents in a psychosocial setting may have experienced emotional, physical, and sexual abuse or neglect. A child or teenager may experience many emotions surrounding abuse and neglect yet be unaware of them or unable to express them directly. Sometimes emotions may be displaced toward a therapist, particularly if he or she is trusted not to retaliate or withdraw. For teens, this displacement behavior may be especially apparent because a major task of adolescence is to establish a separate identity, apart from adults and authority figures. It is important for therapists to maintain the therapeutic role, understand the young person, and respond in ways that indicate an understanding nature and a wish to understand the individual client. Therapists may help clients find other ways of coping by providing alternative reponses to those given previously by hurtful adults, providing opportunities to express emotions that assist in modulating their responses, putting words to feelings and providing age-appropriate opportunities to explore and master the self and the environment.

More often than with other age groups, and particularly in periods when young people experience in their environment numerous threats such as drugs, violence, and gangs, working with teens necessitates that one's beliefs be set aside and an understanding, empathic attitude be adopted. For example, young teens may become pregnant and find themselves alone in deciding whether to terminate the pregnancy, choose adoption, or raise the child. As a therapist, even though your beliefs and values may dictate the decision you would make for yourself, it is ethically and morally correct to assume a neutral attitude and assist clients to come to their own conclusions. Children and teenagers may be involved in addiction to drugs or alcohol, violence, or self-mutilation. Moral judgments must be suspended to permit teenagers to reflect and think about their lives in a context of support and allow therapists to provide the best possible treatment based on the needs of the client. As a therapist, one way of suspending judgments and providing treatment driven by an understanding of the clients' needs is to know your own thoughts, feelings, values, and biases and to acknowledge and accept the emotions and thoughts evoked by working with children and teenagers. You will then be able to provide respect, empathy, genuineness, sensitivity, and warmth to adolescents who may not have hitherto received enough of these responses. A single factor that has been described (Carrillo, 1992) as making the difference for an adolescent from a troubled environment with low socioeconomic levels between becoming a troubled or healthy adult in terms of mental health, substance use, and criminal behavior is the presence of a "caring" adult to provide support, responsibility, and advocacy for the young person. Such support and advocacy can be natural roles for an occupational therapist working with adolescents.

Team Approach

The team concept is particularly essential in providing services for the child or adolescent because their life roles are as family members. Other family members should be consulted and included on the team whenever possible. Developmental life roles also are demonstrated to children and adolescents by other professionals such as teachers and education specialists, and other therapists, such as psychologists, speech therapists, psychiatrists or pediatricians, and activity and sports leaders, such as coaches and community activity leaders. Others who participate in a child or adolescent's life should be regularly consulted. (Naturally, consultation will be with permission of the client or the responsible parent whenever possible.) Contemporary descriptions of the role of occupational therapy show that more than just sensorimotor or neuromuscular skills are being addressed for the child and adolescent population. "They [occupational therapists] are [also] beginning to develop assessment and treatment strategies that provide valuable information to the interdisciplinary clinical team and that are based on theory unique to occupational therapy" (Sholle-Martin & Alessi, 1990, p. 873).

Medications

Even though some medications, such as Ritalin Hydrochloride, have received controversial media attention, a variety of other medications are judiciously used in the treatment of children and adolescents. Medication is often needed to assist the patient in gaining control over his or her behavior or stabilizing symptoms so that patients may more readily participate in therapy. Medication is often selected only after all members of the team have been consulted or the patient has been observed in various settings. The occupational therapist can contribute observations of the client in various life roles or occupational settings.

While medication is often needed to assist the patient (and a psychiatrist is ultimately responsible for prescribing medications), it is important for the occupational therapist and other team members to carefully monitor the medicated client's behaviors and status. The occupational therapist works closely with the individual, and may be the first to observe emerging side effects or changes in behavior. It is particularly important to monitor medications closely in young people because psychoactive medication sometimes interacts with the neurochemistry of the synapses and may interfere with development of new neuron networks and neurologically based competencies (Newton, 1995). Therefore, cognitive and behavioral approaches are usually attempted before a consideration of pharmacology.

CHILD AND ADOLESCENT SETTINGS AND PROGRAMS

When considering a program, the need is to always provide the least restrictive environment for the patient. The best program will provide the most normalized and balanced program, always with the goal of needing no further intervention. Children and adolescent programs may be based on a habilitative rather than a rehabilitative approach. Habilitation involves addressing skills and behaviors that were previously unlearned and undeveloped. This is opposed to the rehabilitative approach used with adults, which focuses on the retrieval of skills patients already have or had prior to their current illness (Lambert, Moffitt, & Rose, 1989).

The role of the registered occupational therapist has been described broadly in the literature. Kent described the OTR working with children with psychosocial dysfunction as a developmental therapist with an assessment role of evaluating functioning level in skills and interests (cited in Sholle-Martin & Alessi, 1990). The OTR's role with children has been described as based on social learning, behavioral, psychoanalytic, systems analysis, and developmental models, as well as the occupational therapy theories of Mary Reilly. Evaluation emphasizes play history, temperament, family dynamics and patterns of behavior, and treatment modalities include play, behavioral management, sensorimotor integration, values clarification, and activity groups (Reilly, Kielhofner, Ayres, Nelson, Llorens, & Rubin, cited in Sholle-Martin & Alessi, 1990). According to Lambert & Moffitt, OTRs also implement parent-child activity groups to improve parents' ability to interact with their children (cited in Sholle-Martin and Alessi, 1990).

Inpatient hospitalization, long-term residential treatment, outpatient settings, community-based programs, partial hospitalization programs, and school-based settings may all offer opportunities for the therapist. Anywhere there are children and adolescents there is a possible treatment setting in which their psychosocial needs may be met. Newer developments within the school system and in partial hospitalization programs are discussed here.

School-based Programs

School districts are required to meet the special needs of their students in cases where a student's performance in the classroom is affected. Depending on the county and the particular office of education, there may be opportunities for the occupational therapist interested in working to meet the school-aged clients' psychosocial needs. Some counties are meeting the psychosocial needs of so-called severely emotionally disturbed (SED) students through programs offered on public school campuses. Such programs typically provide services through a special education teacher, psychiatrist, and social worker as well as teacher's aides and assistants who work with the clinical staff. Occupational therapists are included in some of these programs and may provide services including assessment, treatment, home programs, school programs, and consultation. In the school-based setting, the goal is to increase the student's function in the special education classroom with the long-term goal of participation in a regular classroom. All treatment goals should indicate progress toward this end. The occupational therapist is able to view students holistically, look at their performance in the classroom, and provide the necessary services for skill development and improved classroom success.

Partial Hospitalization

Partial hospitalization programs are sometimes referred to as day treatment programs. They are another alternative designed to prevent children and adolescents from entering or staying in an inpatient hospitalization setting. These programs also provide a useful service of transitioning the patient from an inpatient to an outpatient setting. Typically, these programs are affiliated with a psychiatric unit or residential program in the community. The clients will attend a program during typical school hours and will receive treatment groups or therapy more intensively than if they were outpatients. The student may attend a program like this to avoid hospitalization or to make necessary adjustments to medication under a supervised setting. As with the school-based program and most treatment programs, the goal is to improve the clients' functioning to the degree to which they can be placed in a less intensive environment. The adolescent in this type of program, however, may not be attending school, may be in need of transitioning back into the school system, or may require assistance in becoming emancipated and therefore need life skills training.

IMPLEMENTING A CHILDREN'S PROGRAM

When developing a program of occupational therapy, it is important to assess the needs of the patients, demands of the service delivery system, and structure of the program. For example, if developmental motor lags are an area of concern, sensorimotor groups may be planned. Where play skills are lacking, play groups and opportunities to develop age-appropriate play skills are of prime importance. If children in the treatment setting have difficulty expressing their thoughts and feelings appropriately, programming should address these needs (Lambert et al., 1989; Lambert & Moffitt, 1988).

The second critical step is to look at the service delivery system itself. In acute care settings there is relatively little time to provide treatment before discharge looms. Often it is the role of occupational therapy and the team to begin treatment with the idea that it will be continued outside the hospital setting at school, in a partial hospitalization setting, or in an outpatient office. In a longer term setting, treatment may be carried out entirely in one place, although because of the recent changes in health care delivery, there may not be an extended period of time to bring about change. In terms of planning occupational therapy for an existing program, it is important to understand how therapy fits into the current program in terms of philosophy and program needs. This makes an understanding of theory important and flexibility imperative. The therapist must assume a systems approach, involving an awareness of the current program, the service delivery system, and the clients' needs.

In addition to occupational therapy assessments based in specific frames of reference, groups and activities are determined by the developmental needs of individual children. For example, a child may be 12 years old chronologically but function at a 3- or 4-year-old level, with a limited ability to express feelings in words and impaired cognitive skills secondary to a diagnosis of pervasive developmental disorder or mental retardation. Such a child may be placed in a play group that meets the needs of his or her developmental, age-appropriate level. The child's play and social behavior can be observed at the same time he or she is provided with opportunities for developmentally appropriate play activities. When a child is observed to be playing successfully at a developmentally appropriate level, he or she may then be moved up from a play group to a skills group to learn further personal and social skills (Lambert et al., 1989).

Evaluation and Assessment

General areas of assessment concern the occupational performance areas of self-care and play. Play can be evaluated by observing a child at play and obtaining a play history concerning what toys and games the child chooses. The occupational performance components to be assessed are primarily sensorimotor, cognitive, psychological, and social. Formal evaluations such as the Test of Visual Motor Skills (TVMS), the Good-Enough-Harris Draw-A-Person test, or the Erhhardt Developmental Prehension Assessment (EDPA) may further evaluate adaptive motor skills and coordination as well as a basic assessment of achievement on expected developmental milestones (cited in Asher, 1996). A useful tool for a quick assessment of the other components is the Kinetic Self-Image Test (Abramson, 1982b), was developed as part of the Initial Play Interview at Mount Sinai Hospital in New York. In this test, the child is asked to draw a picture of him- or herself doing something. Besides data regarding sensorimotor and cognitive components, valuable information such as interests, relationships, and self-concept can be determined.

CASE ILLUSTRATION: JOSH — KINETIC SELF-IMAGE

Josh, a newly admitted boy, drew a picture of "me, my mom and Dad going for ice cream." Although the boy was 11 years old, he provided basically stick figures and a poorly drawn house. During the evaluation, Josh kept looking at the clock, and he also asked to go to the bathroom several times. When asked if he had an appointment or was waiting or looking for someone, he said, "I have a family session at 3 o'clock." However, when asked if he was leaving group to see if his parents had arrived, he angrily denied it.

Discussion

This simple assessment can be helpful in determining mental age and motor coordination, what the child is thinking about, and the quality of family or personal functioning and relationships.

Evaluation and Treatment

Play is often referred to as the work of the child; it is generally defined as the way children learn basic skills and resolve intrapersonal and interpersonal conflicts.

> From a child's play we can gain understanding of how he sees and construes the world[;] . . . play refers to a young child's activities characterized by freedom from all but personally imposed rules, . . . by fantasy involvement and by the absence of any goals outside of the activity itself. (Bettelheim, 1987, p. 15)

It is helpful to distinguish play from games because the latter are a predominant occupation of older children and adolescents. Games are usually competitive, and they have agreed-upon rules that are imposed externally. Games require that the activity be pursued in a prescribed manner, without one's personal fantasy, and there is often a goal, such as winning, outside the activity (Bettelheim, 1987). With the basic acceptance of the importance of play (and later, games) as treatment, and also with the recognition of play as the predominant occupation of childhood, it is the primary occupation used in pediatrics and the primary activity used in pediatric groups (Abramson et al., 1989; Hoffman, 1982; Jack, 1987; Lambert, 1988; Sholle-Martin & Alessi, 1990). In fact, "play therapy has become the main avenue for helping young children with their emotional difficulties" (Bettelheim, 1987, p. 15).

Play is also the primary mode of evaluating children, which is done through specific assessments and interviews and by ongoing observation. There are various ways to initially evaluate and continue to observe play. Some useful categories to think about while observing play are (C. Grandison, personal communication, January 28, 1997):

- developmental or stage of play, such as solitary, exploratory, parallel, project, or cooperative (Hoffman, 1982). A 2-year-old can be expected to engage mostly in parallel play, whereas a 10-year-old can be expected to cooperate with other children in play.
- entrance to play; for example, does a child hesitate to play or quickly bolt toward the toys?
- initiation toward play; that is, (1) does a child intiate play independently or wait for someone to start with, and (2) is the same pattern consistent throughout play?
- energy level: what is the level of energy of the child at play and does it change within or over sessions? Is it the same with or without structure? Is it the same with a parent present?
- body movement and use of space; that is, does the child know where others are? Does he or she define a small area or fill up every space? Does the child use furniture?
- emotional tone; that is, what is the emotional tenor to the play (e.g., is it angry or sad?) and does it remain the same over time?
- materials: what materials does the child gravitate toward and how are they used?
- symbolic nature of play, for example, does the child use objects and play symbolically? What are the themes of play, and are they consistent throughout?

An ongoing, regularly scheduled play group also provides information as to the child's current developmental level of play as reflected in the choice of toys, games, and peers while engaged in play.

There are various play scales (Asher, 1996), play classifications (Florey, 1968), and histories that include other observations and categories. The Knox Play Scale (Reilly, 1974) uses categories of space and material management, imitation, and type of participation. A play observation that we ourselves use looks at toys chosen, time of participation, quality of interaction with the toy, language, and social qualities to play. There is an emphasis on the play's developmental level (e.g., solitary, exploratory, parallel, etc.) and theme (such as aggressive, destructive, nurturing, etc.). A Parent-Teacher Play Questionnaire (Scutta & Schaaf, 1989) elicits information from others concerning a child's favorite toy, choices of toys, playmates, preferred locations for play, and any changes in the past week.

Groups.   Play group is a nondirective group that occurs in the occupational therapy playroom. On an acute inpatient unit such a play group has been particularly efficacious for early **latency age** children. "[It] is a valuable diagnostic tool as well as a developmentally appropriate way for the children to interact with their peers and to deal with potentially stressful situations" (Abramson et al., 1979, p. 391). The group's protocol is illustrated in Figure 6-3.

The room includes toys, water and sand play areas, dress-up clothes for fantasy play, and a table and chairs. It serves to encourage the development of play skills, which in turn facilitates the development of social skills. The play group also has the goal of providing an arena whereby children may resolve conflicts

NAME OF GROUP: Occupational Therapy Play Group

DESCRIPTION:Play is an important part of a child's development. Children learn, express themselves, and develop interpersonal interaction skills through play. Through play, children are able to express inner feelings and conflicts in a non-threatening way. This group's primary goal is to evaluate skills and provide an adequate environment where the children's dynamics, developmental level of play and socialization skills can be observed and practiced.

THERAPIST NAME: William Lambert, OTR/L

TITLE: Occupational Therapist

GOALS:

1.)Provide a stimulating environment where the children will be motivated to play.
2.)Encourage peer interaction through play.
3.)Provide insightful interpretations related to the play when appropriate.
4.)Allow the children to work through dynamic issues through the play.
5.)Encourage the highest developmental level of play and interpersonal interaction possible.

ENTRANCE CRITERIA:

1.)Group members are selected by the OTR according to their developmental levels of play.
2.)Five children is an optimal number of group members.
3.)Patient has appropriate level of privileges.
4.)Patient has been medically cleared by physician.

GROUP RULES:

1.)Have fun
2.)Share
3.)Listen to staff
4.)Clean up

FORMAT:

   Group meets two times per week for 45 minutes with two leaders: the OT and a member of the nursing staff.

EXIT CRITERIA:

1.)Change in level of privileges.
2.)Change in developmental status.
3.)Discharge from the hospital.

Figure 6-3.   Play Group Protocol

and issues that led to their current problems and dysfunction. For example, two children may use dolls to express anger at parents who abused them. They may also recreate arguments or scenes they observed in the home. For example, by using toy sharks, a child may safely and appropriately show anger or jealousy toward a sibling or peer by "eating" him or her during water play or "burying" him or her in the sandbox. A game like Sorry™ helps increase frustration tolerance, and a game like Twister™ develops not only laterality but also the ability to be close to others appropriately and respect body space. Beanbag toss games are an appropriate outlet for anger and aggression and also provide the opportunity to engage in turn taking and mild competition.

There are countless ways in which play can help children learn new skills and accomplish treatment goals. For example, it is better to ask children to try to clean up the entire playroom before you can count to 10 than it is to just command them to clean up the playroom because "it's time to end group." Turning an activity into a game or play, as in this example, is often more effective than other approaches. It is also congruent with the philosophy of occupational therapy and the general approach of using play as a treatment modality. The active experiences of play and the focus on productivity and participation offer intrinsic satisfaction for a child's needs. Aside from conflict resolution, play also offers children the additional ability to work on treatment goals of improving impulse control, developing cognitive skills, mastering the environment, and developing age-appropriate social interactions. Through the mastery of tasks, latency-aged children will be able to benefit from the successful interaction with objects and people in occupational therapy group and gain mastery over themselves in the process.

Creative task groups also serve as highly effective interventions with latency-aged children. The use of tiles to make mosaics, wood projects such as creating a bookshelf or making a toy car, painting sun catchers, or participating in seasonal activities such as carving a pumpkin or baking Christmas cookies offer children rewarding experiences. In addition, the experiences teach appropriate interactions and cognitive skills, such as the ability to follow directions, increase attention span and concentration, and complete tasks, and comments made about the projects often provide a valuable additional perspective on a child's emotions and concerns. Copper tooling is a highly successful creative task project. Children frequently ask, "Can I do more than one?" or after successful completion of the project, they will ask, "Can we do copper tooling projects again?" When I ask them why they liked the project, they often reply, "Because it's fun to do — because it's easy to make." Indeed, the steps of copper tooling are easy to grade according to the therapeutic purposes of the group.

Of course, it is important to take precautions such as removing the solution as soon as all group members have used it and conducting the group in a well-ventilated area. In general, copper tooling is one of the most successful activities that I've used with emotionally disturbed children. Cries of "Can I make more than one?" generally attest to its value to the children who participate in the project.

Most often, creative tasks are provided as part of a parallel task group. This structure provides opportunities to develop appropriate interpersonal interactions on a limited basis, share through the use of supplies that are common to the group activity, and develop impulse control by waiting to follow the steps and to see the project through to completion.

Group goals may include learning how to follow simple, step-by-step verbal directions; sharing materials and space; interacting without being intrusive; sustaining an increasing attention span; and developing impulse control. Other information that can be gained even through the use of a simple craft project includes who the gift or project is to be given to, and, therefore, who is important in the child's life.

A skills development group is provided for older children who have adequate play and social skills and need to improve problem-solving, coping, and communication skills. See the group's protocol in Figure 6-4. Group topics and discussion focus on common problems and situations that children face as well as the specific problem areas that led to treatment.

While a variety of activities can be used in the skills development group, including crafts, therapeutic board games are usually used. "Stress Strategies" is a game used to develop coping skills, and "The Talking, Feeling and Doing Game" (Lambert et al., 1989) facilitates the expression of thoughts and feelings. Both are examples of games that are effective in meeting treatment goals. Because they use a board game format, children are usually willing to participate and an appropriate amount of structure is provided. Children are often happy to have an outlet for their unexpressed feelings and thoughts and view the game as a safe and nonthreatening means of personal expression.

CASE ILLUSTRATION: THE TALKING, FEELING, AND DOING GAME

Seven children aged 8 to 12 years old are playing the game with the occupational therapist, a member of the nursing staff, and an OT student. Sam rolls the dice, lands on a yellow space, and selects a "feeling" card, which reads: "Name three things that could cause a person to be angry." He pauses and then says, "Being told to shut up, being hit, and being lied to." Dave lands on a white space and selects a "talking" card, which reads, "What kind of work does your father do? What do you think about that kind of job?" Dave answers, "He fixes trucks," although he does not mention that his father is in prison. "I'm going to race motorcycles when I grow up," he says when asked what he thinks of his father's job. Christine rolls the dice and also lands on a white space. Her card asks, "What is the best thing you can say about your family?" She replies, "They bring me candy and lots of things." John lands on a red space and picks a "doing" card, which reads, "Skip across the room and then return to your seat." He says, "I'm not doing that," but he agrees to take another card. This one asks him to pretend that he is having an argument with someone and to tell

NAME OF GROUP: Occupational Therapy Skill Development Group

DESCRIPTION: A developmental task group for children who have developed basic play and social skills and need to acquire skills in cognition, interpersonal interactions and self-expression.

THERAPIST NAME: William Lambert, OTR/L

TITLE: Occupational Therapist

GOALS:
1.) To improve cognitive skills such as:
    a.) problem-solving
    b.) organization of thoughts
    c.) ability to follow directions
2.) To improve interpersonal interaction skills and facilitate sharing cooperation.
3.) To improve ability to express thoughts and feelings appropriately.

ENTRANCE CRITERIA:
1.) Group members are selected by the OTR according to developmental need.
2.) Patient should be on appropriate level of privilege to attend groups.
3.) Patient is medically cleared by physician.
4.) Five to seven children is the optimal number of group members.

GROUP RULES:
1.) Have fun
2.) Share
3.) Listen to staff
4.) Clean up

FORMAT:
    Group meets two times per week for 45 minutes with two leaders: the OT and a member of the nursing staff. Activities will be planned to develop specific skills through the use of games and creative tasks.

EXIT CRITERIA:
1.) Change in level of privileges
2.) Discharge from hospital

Figure 6-4.   Skills Development Group Protocol

---

the group what it is about. "I'm arguing with Melissa. She won't share," John replies. The therapist then rolls and lands on a "feeling" space. His card reads, "When was the last time you cried?" He says, "I cried when my dad died." Then he talks about how crying is helpful in expressing feelings of sadness. Linda and Rhonda, the other adults in group, reinforce what the therapist has said. This helps the children talk about their feelings and express them appropriately.

Discussion

This game promotes, through talking, the expression of what is on children's minds. The game facilitates the expression of feelings, promotes the discussion of personal problems, and can explore family dynamics without threat and in a manner that matches the children's emotional age. It is important to have a good working knowledge of the children to effectively lead a game such as this.

The parent-child activity group (Lambert, 1989) involves engaging the parents of the emotionally disturbed child in an activity with the child. It is held weekly in the occupational therapy room, where families usually work on an arts and crafts activity together with the goal of completing it in one session. This group improves the parent-child interaction by engaging them together in a pleasurable, successful activity, something that may not otherwise be possible due to the child's illness. The therapist provides encouragement and support and models appropriate caregiver behavior such as setting limits on inappropriate actions and giving praise for desirable ones. He assists parents in differentiating between behavior that is maladaptive and behavior that is typical for the child's developmental level. Beyond providing occupational therapy for families and their disturbed children, the OTR is able to provide the treatment team with information about family interactive patterns, the child's response to therapy with the parents, and how well the parents are implementing what they are being taught about how to interact with their child. The parent-child activity has expanded the scope of occupational therapy in the hospital setting to areas traditionally reserved for individual and family therapists. By providing information on how the child acts and what he or she does in the group, occupational therapy has enhanced the team's ability to see the child and family more globally and respond with more integrated treatment for both.

INTERVENTION WITH ADOLESCENTS

Just as for children, the family is important to the adolescent. Although the teenager may be establishing a self-identity that is autonomous from the family, it is still a pertinent shaper of values and interests and represents the primary foundation from which the adolescent can build an individual identity. Just as play is the overall occupation of childhood and individual play activities are formative, the overall occupation of adolescence is to form an identity that includes work as well as play or leisure, toward which vocational and leisure activities are formative. Along with the family, the peer group assumes a role as a pertinent shaper of values and interests. Therefore, when working with an adolescent client, the treatment process must include his or her peers. Since the essential developmental process occurring for this age group is establishing independence and an autonomous identity (which is sometimes interpreted as being different from the family), the adolescent often relies heavily on peers. In a treatment setting, the treatment milieu is a powerful tool because it allows the group to assume responsibility and empowers individuals in the group to make decisions for the good of the whole. An example of utilizing the milieu as a treatment tool is to have the adolescent group define the rules for the program, with the help of staff guidance that is nondidactic and instead asks the group members to reflect on the process and think for themselves. The OTR is included as a member of the milieu and also can duplicate the process in occupational therapy. For example, the group can make decisions such as what modalities will be used for the week, where the group will go on the weekly outing, or what will be made in cooking group.

Because the family is the primary foundation from which the individual can build self-identity, parental and family factors are essential to consider. There may be demands by parents for the adolescent to take on a role of independence before he or she is developmentally able or to become a caretaker of his or her siblings, which may disproportionately interfere with the developmental tasks of the period. Conversely, a parent may inadvertently keep the adolescent in a dependent role and may reinforce childish behaviors. Either of these situations may result in a disruption to the normal developmental tasks for the adolescent, leading to frustration at the least, at worst, acting-out behaviors. For example, the adolescent may sever all communication and set out to prove he or she is independent. Parents and teens may conflict when, in fact, what the child needs are differing degrees of security, limits, and responsibilities appropriate to different situations. Conflicts with parents often occur around social life, such as customs or family traditions, home responsibilities, school and grades, social values and morals, use of the telephone or family car, and family rules. To learn social values and appropriate behavior in society, parents must maintain consistent behavior during their offsprings' childhood and adolescence while at the same time providing a flexible, caring, communicative environment that expresses love, trust, and a respect for privacy. Thus, the task of adolescence is also a challenge for parents.

When a child or adolescent enters the mental health system as "the patient," the family and the individual should be helped to realize that the family is a system in itself; that is, each family member affects, and is affected by, each other. The family member in the hospital may become the **identified patient (ip)**, but the family may have to acknowledge how the family as a whole, or family system, fits into the creation and solution of problems that may be expressed by the identified patient. Therefore, the family should be informed, included, and involved as much as possible in treatment. As with children, occupational therapy for adolescents can involve the family, particularly when focusing on activities that may be shared by a family as a group.

There are ever-increasing numbers of blended and nontraditional families in the United States. The traditional family may no longer be constituted of a biological mother and father with biological siblings. Children and adolescents may be adopted and raised by extended families, grandparents, relatives, stepparents, or family friends. Whoever the child or adolescent considers to be "family" may be permitted to join in treatment, as is often the case in the parent-child activity group (Lambert, 1990).

Because of the adolescent tasks of establishing independent self-identity and learning about vocational and leisure interests and values, having a **mentor** may become important during this developmental time. Therefore, it is particularly important that the therapeutic staff be aware of the symbolic nature that their relationship and interactions may have for guiding adolescents in their quest for establishing independent values and interests in occupational areas and their components.

Activities

For adolescents as well as younger children, care must be taken to choose modalities appropriate for the client's developmental age. Games are generally appropriate for older children, as they are for adolescents, due to their externally imposed parameters and rules and to the opportunity for competition and achieving a goal other than the game itself. Those modalities and games that offer ease of adaptation and opportunities for creativity are useful due to the varied developmental age ranges possible in a group of teenagers. Because the peer group is so important, success-oriented activities that provide a sense of mastery and self-confidence are key tools to increase the adolescent's willingness to participate.

Generally, the more opportunity there is for the group participants to be a part of the decision making, the more sense of cooperation will be developed and the more smoothly the group will progress. In fact, an ongoing theme in therapy with adolescents is helping the client move cognitively and behaviorally from a style of decision making and coping that is guided only by outside pressure to a style that becomes internally self-initiated and is based on integrated and flexible thinking and social norms and mores (Newton, 1995). Therefore, therapy should encourage the adolescent to move from an emotion-focused problem-solving style, which can be more impulsive and rigid, to a more mature, flexible, thoughtful, and reflective style.

Some theorists, such as Kohlberg (cited in Cole, 1993; Sigelman & Shaffer, 1995), suggest three levels and six stages of moral development, any of which may be found to operate in adolescents. They state that motivation to move to the next level is created by experiences that contradict former beliefs and bring into question one's own reasoning. Occupational therapists can encourage growth in moral reasoning by exposing group members to reasoning at a higher level and by encouraging role taking and role reversal (Bruce & Borg, 1993). Developmental learning can be accomplished through introducing moral dilemmas for discussion and problem solving (Cole, 1993) or, in other words, utilizing concepts of values clarification (Simon, Howe, & Kirschenbaum, 1995). By using the occupational therapy knowledge base of activity analysis, occupational therapists can assist teenagers to develop this cognitive learning process. Table 6-1 lists some developmental goals, modalities, and specific activities for treating adolescents that are grounded in these ideas.

Specific activities often meet more than one developmental goal and utilize more than one occupational performance component. For example, it is impossible to work on social skills without considering cognitive abilities, self-esteem, and communication skills. Activities improve skills in more than one area. For example, meal preparation may be utilized for training and assess-

Table 6-1. Developmental Goals, Modalities, and Activities for Adolescents

Occupational Performance Areas

Self-Care		Play/Leisure	Work/Education (Productivity)

Components

Motor	Cognitive	Social	Psychological

Goals

Motor	Cognitive	Social	Psychological
• develop self-identity, uniqueness • develop healthy body image and acceptance of physical self	• concentration • attention • sequencing • decision making • problem solving • critical thinking • representing	• learn appropriate social forms, rules, identity, communication • relating to, connection with, and getting along with others	• develop self-identity, uniqueness • develop healthy body image and acceptance of physical self

• recognizing, acknowledging, and expressing emotion/affect

• learning and understanding others' points of view

• managing frustration, stress, and time
• developing vocational skills and interests
• developing avocational skills and interests

Activities

| • budgeting
 • meal preparation
 • household
 • daily life activities | • career search
 • getting and maintaining a job (calling/ applying and interviewing
 • volunteerism | • games and hobbies
 • sporting and cultural events
 • organized altruism
 • parties
 • crafts
 • peer teaching | • journal writings
 • lifeline
 • biography
 • values clarification |

Structure

| team and partner tasks | role-plays | outings graded tasks | discussion structured "workbook" exercises |

ment in the areas of cognition (following a recipe), socialization (using a group format), and independent living (practicing safety in the kitchen).

Team building.   One activity that is extremely useful in working with adolescents (particularly when developing social and relational skills, cognitive reasoning, and self-awareness) is team building, which includes experiential activities, such as a ropes course (Voight, 1988), or Outward Bound program (Godfrey, 1980). While these programs vary, the basic premise is to have the group find itself faced with what seems to be an impossible task initially and then successfully mobilize as a team to accomplish the presented tasks. The tasks are conquered throughout one or more days while the participants face increasing fears that demand increasingly complex problem solving and teamwork. This modality is excellent in developing a young group of peers into a team whose members support and care for each other and recognize the value of cooperation. The experience enhances individual strengths and weaknesses, develops leadership roles, and encourages creative, group problem solving. The key to the utilization of team building involves activity analysis and facilitator training. The therapist must have the training required for this specific program and for working with this specific age and population. Many elements of the challenging tasks may need to be adapted to meet the needs of the group, which means that activity analysis is essential.

CASE ILLUSTRATION: TEAM BUILDING

A sample of a simplified task element is stated as follows: "There is a huge spider that lives underground. It has built this web in front of you and your group must get to the other side of it." The group is standing in front of a six-foot-square "spider web" made from ropes and elastic cords with holes of various size and shape; the number of holes must equal or exceed the number in the group. "There is no way to go under or around this web, and once someone goes through one hole in the web, no one else can go through that hole. In addition, if the web is touched, the spider will come out of the ground and eat the group." This is obviously not a true situation, and therefore humor and fun can be brought into the task.

Discussion

As the group works to solve this situation, the facilitator listens, allowing the group to process the new information and progress together. A key element for the facilitator of such groups is knowing how to let the group work on its own but also knowing at what point to intervene so that the group does not become totally frustrated. With training in facilitation, occupational therapists can use their knowledge of activity analysis and grading activities to utilize team building as a rich and developmentally corrective experience for adolescents.

Creative expression.   The creative modalities are useful for the adolescent who is attempting to establish an understanding of the changing emotions and thoughts that often prevail at this stage. Creative expression activities may be verbal or nonverbal and may include art, crafts, movement, dance, music, song writing, singing, poetry, writing, or keeping a journal or diary. Due to the expressive nature of these modalities, an adolescent may initially be uncomfortable or shy in sharing with the group. One useful method of encouraging sharing is to begin with dyadic interaction, in which you ask the adolescent to choose at least one person in the group with whom to share his or her work. This method also shows respect for the individual's desire for privacy. Consider establishing the trust, safety, and security of the group by including discussions about confidentiality and reassurance that "what is shared with the group stays within the group." This is a time to facilitate the process of individuals in a group establishing their own rules and standards for their group. Teaching, modeling mutual respect, and giving assurance that work will not be "analyzed" for hidden meaning and that creative talent will not be judged are useful means in establishing an environment of creative sharing.

An example of a creative expression activity with a focus is the "Lifeline." One variation of this activity is to ask the group to: "Indicate your life on this piece of paper — you can use symbols, words, or drawings. Include events that are important to you or things that you remember as you were growing up and also things that you would like to happen or that may occur in your future." Have supplies available and offer encouragement that "there is no right or wrong way to complete this task."

Figure 6-5 shows an example of a lifeline created by an adolescent female diagnosed with a severe eating disorder. Of note initially is the extreme creativity and the obvious amount of work that went into this task. The themes are family: both brother and mother are mentioned, as are pets, ballet, and the stresses of moving, braces, illnesses, and accidents. In a 50-minute treatment session, the individual learns about and integrates various aspects of herself and the group members learn, and hopefully understand, a great deal about each other.

The therapist may be tempted to analyze the artwork; however, this may interfere with what the patient is telling us about her work and herself. It is essential to allow the patient to explain the meaning of her work and answer any questions the therapist or others may have about the drawing (Remocker & Storch, 1979; Simon et al., 1995; Korb-Khalsa, Azok, & Leutenberg, 1990, 1991, 1994, 1995).

Summary and Current Trends

There are various diagnoses and presenting problems of children and adolescents that include DSM-IV disorders such as depression and eating disorders (APA, 1994), in addition to disorders first diagnosed in infancy, childhood, and adolescence. Environmental psychosocial stresses, such as family dys-

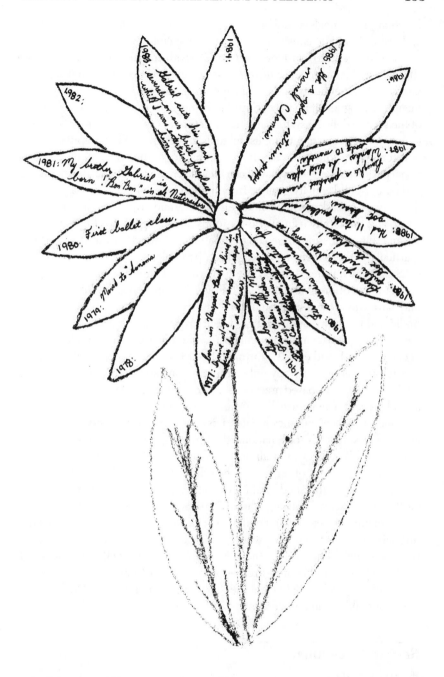

Figure 6-5: Lifeline

function, abuse, neglect, violence, and poverty, as well as developmental stages and tasks, should be considered when treating children and adolescents.

Useful concepts to consider when working with children and adolescents are structure and consistency, interpretation of behavior, time-out, limit setting, a personal therapeutic style, the team approach, and medications. When implementing a program, it is vital to consider the needs of the patients, the demands of the service delivery system and the structure of the current or planned program. Various assessments are useful tools for occupational therapists.

Intervention for children is based primarily on the concept and occupational performance area of play; it can include creative task, skill development, and parent-child activity groups. Intervention for adolescents is based on the developmental task of establishing self-identity and involves issues of the peer group and the family using various groups, including groups for team building and self-expression, based on occupational performance and components (particularly those focusing on cognitive, psychological and social skills).

"Sicker and quicker" has become an often-used phrase when describing the trend toward offering less time for therapy for children and adolescents who may have the most severe emotional problems. As managed care replaces traditional insurance and reimbursement programs, time frames for therapy are becoming shorter and inpatient hospitalizations are being curtailed in favor of community-based care. Unfortunately, cost containment may also limit access to occupational therapy unless therapists make the transition from hospital- to community-based practice. Since, due to their age and status, children and adolescents cannot usually be effective self-advocates (especially in a "bottom line"–driven economic climate), it is important for therapists to advocate appropriate services — occupational therapy included — for children and adolescents. Unfortunately, not all hospitals and localities currently offer occupational therapy and other mental health services to children who require them. Addressing the needs of this population may include an increased focus on the public school setting, where OT continues to be a strong presence. Children and adolescents in need of occupational therapy for emotional disturbances can be found everywhere: in the hospital, the school, at day care, and in your neighborhood (Forness, Florey, & Greene, 1993). Therapists will, most likely, need to become stronger advocates for their patients, as well as their profession, in order to meet the need for community mental health treatment for children and adolescents.

Review Questions

1. What do the terms "acting out" and "setting limits" mean? Why are they important in working with children and adolescents?
2. What are the most likely diagnoses of children and adolescents that you may encounter in a mental health setting?

3. What or who constitutes the system or environment of a child or adolescent that must be considered in treatment?
4. Why are expressive and team-building groups important for adolescents?
5. What is the underlying base of treatment for children and why is it so important?

Learning Activities

1. Visit day care centers, preschools, and grade schools to observe children in this age group. Not only may you have the opportunity to view symptoms of dysfunction such as hyperactivity or aggression, you can become familiar with typical behavior.
2. Fill out a play history for yourself by following any assessment listed in Asher (1996) or mentioned here. Was play driven by your own internal rules and fantasy? When do you remember starting to play games? How was playing games different than solitary play?
3. Can you see yourself as a therapist with adolescents? Would you be willing to listen to and agree with an adolescent who has challenged your authority and "the rules"?
4. Think back to when you were a teenager. How did you like to be spoken to? Who were the people you admired, respected, or wanted to be like? What was your favorite activity? How did you spend most of your time? What did you care most about? How did it feel when adults complained about "the youth of today"?
5. Electronic media bring information to individuals from all over the world in an instant. This cultural innovation seems to appeal greatly to young people and means that children and teens may spend more time in solitary pursuit on a computer, but, paradoxically, have more opportunities to connect with many people. How can the Internet and World Wide Web be used in the treatment of children and adolescents?

References

Abramson, R. M. (1982a). Therapeutic activities for the hospitalized child. In L. Hoffman (Ed.), *The evaluation and care of severely disturbed children* (pp. 61–69). New York: SP Medical & Scientific Books.

Abramson, R. M. (1982b). Developmental and Diagnostic Assessment. In L. Hoffmann (Ed.), *The evaluation and care of severely disturbed children* (pp. 37–44). New York: SP Medical & Scientific Books.

Abramson, R. M., Hoffman, L., & Johns, C. A. (1979). Play group psychotherapy for early latency-age children on an in-patient psychiatric unit. *International Journal of Group Psychotherapy, 29*, 383–392.

Alberti, R., & Emmons, M. (1995). *Your perfect right* (7th ed.). San Luis Obispo, CA: Impact.

American Psychiatric Association (APA). (1994). *Diagnostic and statistical manual of mental disorders* (4th ed.). Washington, DC: APA.

Asher, I. E. (1996). *Occupational therapy evaluation tools: An annotated index* (2nd ed.). Bethesda, MD: American Occupational Therapy Association.

Bettelheim, B. (1987, March). The importance of play. *Atlantic Monthly*, 35–46.

Block, B. M., Arney, K., Campbell, D. J., Kiser, L. T., Lefkovitz, D. M., & Speer, S. K. (1991). American Association for Partial Hospitalization, Child and Adolescent Special Interest Group: Standards for child and adolescent partial hospitalization programs. *International Journal of Partial Hospitalization, 7*(1), 13–21.

Bruce, M., & Borg, B. (1993). *Psychosocial occupational therapy: Frames of reference for intervention* (2d edition). Thorofare, NJ: Slack.

Chess, S., & Thomas, A. (1984). *Origins and evolution of behavior disorders: From infancy to early adult life.* New York: Brunner/Mazel.

Dryfoos, J. G. (1992). Adolescents at risk. A summary of work in the field: Programs and policies. In D. Rogers & E. Ginzberg (Eds.), *Cornell University Medical College Seventh Conference on Health Policy* (pp. 128–141). Boulder, CO: Westview Press.

Florey, L. L. (1968). *A developmental classification of play.* Unpublished master's thesis, University of Southern California, Los Angeles.

Forness, S., Florey, L., & Green, S. (1993). *Hidden in plain sight: Children with behavior disorder in school systems.* Paper presented at the 73rd annual conference of the American Occupational Therapy Association, Seattle, WA.

Gilligan, C. (1979). Woman's place in man's life cycle. *Harvard Educational Review, 49,* 431–446.

Gilligan, C. (Ed.). (1991). *Women, girls and psychotherapy: Reframing resistance.* New York: Haworth Press.

Gilligan, C., Lyons, N. P., & Hammer, T. J. (Eds.). (1990). *Making connections: The relational worlds of adolescent girls at Emma Willard School.* Cambridge, MA: Harvard University Press.

Godfrey, B. (1980). *Outward bound: Schools of the possible.* New York: Doubleday.

Hoffman, L. (1982) *The evaluation and care of severely disturbed children.* New York: SP Medical & Scientific Books.

Jakubowski, P., & Lange, A. (1978). *The assertive option: Your rights and responsibilities.* Champaign, IL: Research Press.

Kaplan, H., & Sadock, B. (1995). *Comprehensive textbook of psychiatry* (6th ed.). Baltimore: Williams & Wilkins .

Korb-Khalsa, K. L., Azok, S. D., & Leutenberg, E. A. (1990). *Life management skills I.* Beachwood, OH: Wellness Reproductions.

Korb-Khalsa, K. L., Azok, S. D., & Leutenberg, E. A. (1991). *Life management skills II.* Beachwood, OH: Wellness Reproductions.

Korb-Khalsa, K. L., Azok, S. D., & Leutenberg, E. A. (1994). *Life management skills III.* Beachwood, OH: Wellness Reproductions.

Korb-Khalsa, K. L., Azok, S. D., & Leutenberg, E. A. (1995). *S E A L S + plus/self-esteem and life skills.* Beachwood, OH: Wellness Reproductions.

Kramer, P., & Hinojosa, J. (1993). *Frames of reference for pediatric occupational therapy.* Baltimore: Williams & Wilkins.

Lambert, W. (1990). *Parent-child activity: Assessment and treatment of families.* Paper presented at the Pennsylvania Occupational Therapy Association Annual Conference, Philadelphia, PA.

Lambert, W., & Moffitt, R. (1988). *A collaborative approach to developmental group in child psychiatry.* Paper presented at the Pennsylvania Occupational Therapy Association Annual Conference, State College, PA

Lambert, W., Moffitt, R., & Rose, J. (1989). *Therapeutic use of toys and games in child psychiatry.* Paper presented at the Pennsylvania Occupational Therapy Association Annual Conference, Hershey, PA.

Llorens, L., & Rubin, E. (1967). *Developing ego functions in disturbed children: Occupational therapy in milieu.* Detroit: Wayne State University Press.

Morrison, J. (1995). *DSM-IV made easy: The clinician's guide to diagnosis.* New York: Guilford.

Newton, M. (1995). *Adolescence: Guiding youth through the perilous ordeal.* New York: Norton.

Offer, D., & Schonert-Reichl, K. (1992). Debunking the myths of adolescence: Findings from recent research. *Journal of the American Academy of Child and Adolescent Psychiatry, 31,* 1003–1013.

Papalia, D. E., & Olds, S. W. (1992). *Human development .* New York: McGraw-Hill.

Reilly, M. (Ed.). (1974). *Play as exploratory learning.* Beverly Hills, CA: Sage.

Remocker, A. J., & Storch, E. T. (1979). *Action speaks louder: A handbook of nonverbal group techniques.* New York: Churchill-Livingstone.

Scutta, C., & Schaaf, R. C. (1989, October). *A Time for Play?* Paper presented at the Pennsylvania Occupational Therapy Association Annual Conference, Hershey, PA.

Sholle-Martin, S., & Alessi, N. E. (1990). Formulating a role for occupational therapy in child psychiatry: A clinical application. *American Journal of Occupational Therapy, 44*(10), 871–882.

Sigelman, C. K., & Shaffer, D. R. (1995). *Life-span human development* (2nd ed.). Pacific Grove, CA: Brooks/Cole.

Simon, S. B., Howe, L. W., & Kirschenbaum, H. (1995). *Values clarification: a handbook of practical strategies for teachers and students* (Rev. ed.) New York: Warner Books.

Smith, M. J. (1975). *When I say no I feel guilty.* New York: Dial.

Thomas, A., & Chess, S. (1986). The New York longitudinal study: From infancy to early adult life. In R. Plomin & J. Dunn (Eds.), *The study of temperament: Changes, continuities, and challenges.* Hillsdale, NJ: Erlbaum.

Voight, A. (1988). The use of ropes courses as a treatment for emotionally disturbed adolescents in hospitals. *Therapeutic Recreation Journal, 12*(2), 57–64.

SUGGESTED READING

Banus, B. S., Kent, C. A., Norton, Y., Sukiennicki, D. R., & Becker, M. L. (1982). *The developmental therapist* (2nd ed.). Thorofare, NJ: Slack.

Berger, K. S. (1994). *The developing person through the lifespan* (3rd ed.). New York: Worth.

Bingham, M., Edmondson, J., & Stryker, S. (1983). *Choices: A teen women's journal for self-awareness and personal planning.* Santa Barbara, CA:Advocacy Press.

Blake, J. (1990). *Risky times: How to be AIDS-smart and stay healthy: A guide for teenagers.* New York: Workman. (Spanish version published in 1993)

Byrne, K. (1987). *A parents' guide to anorexia and bulimia.* New York: Henry Holt.

Freud, Anna. (1967). *The ego and the mechanisms of defense.* New York: International Universities Press.

Gil, E. (1983). *Outgrowing the pain: A book for and about adults abused as children.* New York: Dell.

Hall, Calvin S. (1982). *A primer of Freudian psychology.* New York: Harper & Row.

Heron, A. (Ed.). (1994) *Twenty writings by gay and lesbian youth.* Boston: Alyson Publications.

Hunter, M. (1990). *Abused boys: The neglected victims of sexual abuse.* New York: Ballantine Books.

Levy, B. (1993). *In love and in danger: A teen's guide to breaking free of abusive relationships.* Seattle: Seal Press.

McCoy, K., & Wibbelsman, C. (1992). *The new teenage body book.* New York: BodyPress/Perigee.

New Games Foundation. (1976). *The New Games Book.* Garden City, NY: Doubleday.

Outward Bound, USA. (1981). *Learning through experience in adventure based education.* New York: Morrow.

Pratt, P., & Allen, A. (1989). *Occupational therapy for children* (2nd ed.). Baltimore: Mosby.

Stein, M. B., Hyde, K. L., & Monopolis, S. J. (1991). Child and family outreach services as an adjunct to child and adolescent mental health treatment. *International Journal of Partial Hospitalization, 7*(1) 69–75.

Steiner, H. (1995). *Treating adolescents.* San Francisco: Jossey-Bass.

Vogler, R., & Bartz, W. (1992). *Teenagers and alcohol.* Philadelphia: Charles Press.

The Psychosocial Issues of Physical Illness and Disability

Alice Kibele, MS, OTR
Assistant Professor, San Jose State University

Rene Padilla

Gordon U. Burton, PhD, OTR
Professor, San Jose State University

Key Terms

accommodation
acute hospitalization
adaptive response
autonomy

dual diagnosis
individuation
roles

Chapter Outline

Introduction
Psychiatric Diagnosis with Physical Disability
The Psychosocial Needs of Children with Physical Disabilities
    Psychosocial Development
    Impact of Altered Development on Psychosocial Functioning
    Occupational Therapy Intervention
Psychosocial Issues in Acute Medical Hospitalizations
    Disruption of Routines and Habits
    Fear
    Intervention in Acute Settings
Psychosocial Issues of Chronic Disability
    Loss
    Hope
    Acceptance and Love
Summary

Introduction

This chapter explores the occupational therapist's role in addressing the psychosocial needs of people of all ages with physical dysfunctions. In some cases there may be evidence of a distinct mental illness concurrent with the physical disorder but even in the absence of a diagnosable condition, there are significant psychological issues related to physical illness and disability.

PSYCHIATRIC DIAGNOSIS WITH PHYSICAL DISABILITY

Occupational therapists consistently encounter patients with **dual diagnosis** in a myriad of settings, including general, psychiatric, and rehabilitation hospitals as well as schools and community-based treatment settings. Occupational therapists are trained to address all areas of human performance, but this is often not recognized either by patients, health care administrators, third-party reimbursers, or sometimes even the therapists themselves. For example, an occupational therapist working in a very busy outpatient rehabilitation clinic may feel pressured by real or perceived constraints to simply "fix" the patient's physical damage. However, if the time is not taken to address the patients' emotional issues, progress in rehabilitation may be very slow or even nonexistent.

Mental illness may precede a physical disorder, occur simultaneously, or develop following physical illness. The following illustrations are examples of each of these scenarios.

CASE ILLUSTRATION: MR. HARRISON

Mr. Harrison has a long history of bipolar disorder with repeated hospitalizations for both manic and depressive episodes. He is currently in intensive care following a suicide attempt, in which he jumped out of a fifth-story window. His fall was partially broken by electrical wires, resulting in burns over 30 percent of his body. He also sustained multiple fractures of the lower extremities and left hip. At the present time, it is not clear what long-term deficits he may have, but he states that it doesn't matter because he does not plan on living. Although Mr. Harrison is on a medical unit, the occupational therapist from the psychiatric unit was consulted to help prepare him for rehabilitation. The occupational therapist knew the patient from previous psychiatric admissions and used their preexisting therapeutic relationship to help Mr. Harrison focus on expressive activities, values clarification, and personal goal setting.

Discussion

In this case Mr. Harrison's mental illness preceded his physical illness and was most likely a factor in his suicide attempt and later physical problems. His mental illness also continues to influence his recovery.

CASE ILLUSTRATION: MR. LAURETO

Mr. Laureto is in an intensive care unit (ICU) because significant paralysis caused by his Guillain-Barré syndrome prohibits independent breathing. His only means of communication is blinking his eyes to answer yes (two blinks) and no (one blink). Through a series of interviews with yes/no answers, the occupational therapist determined that Mr. Laureto was experiencing intense and frightening hallucinations, possibly due to the sensory deprivation brought about by the sudden paralysis. The consulting psychiatrist concluded that Mr. Laureto was suffering from what the DSM-IV (APA, 1994) terms a "psychotic disorder due to a general medical condition." The occupational therapist arranged with the ICU nursing staff to provide multiple reality-orienting cues close to Mr. Laureto's bed. These included a radio, a large poster with a schedule of baseball games for his favorite team, photographs of his family, a clock, and a calendar.

Discussion

In this case, the mental illness was a result of Mr. Laureto's physical condition. Once that was determined, interventions were implemented to alleviate the mental condition.

CASE ILLUSTRATION: MS. SHAKIR

Ms. Shakir sustained a cervical spinal cord injury in an automobile accident, resulting in quadriplegia. She successfully completed the rehabilitation program. The occupational therapist noted on the discharge plan that Ms. Shakir appeared to be well adjusted to her disability and had reached her optimum level of function with the use of necessary adaptive equipment. Upon returning home, however, Ms. Shakir found functioning in the community to be quite a bit more difficult than she experienced in the hospital. She became withdrawn, often staying in bed all day and refusing to see friends. Her home attendant noted that she was not eating regularly and often refused personal care. It was recommended that Ms. Shakir begin seeing a psychotherapist for depressive symptoms. She was also prescribed a tricyclic antidepressant and referred to a day treatment program that was wheelchair accessible.

Discussion

In the case of Ms. Shakir, a mental illness—depression—developed, not as a result of her physical injury or even a disability, but because of her underestimation of what she needed in her own environment. Once she had been diagnosed and treated and had received further help for community living in day treatment, her symptoms abated.

The interrelations of psychiatric and physical disabilities with people's functioning have been examined, but an in-depth understanding of all aspects of this dual diagnosis is lacking. This may be due to the dynamic interchange between mind, body, and functional activities. It is known that when a client has a dual diagnosis, a speedy recovery of the physical illness may be impeded and compliance after discharge may be decreased (Fulop, 1991).

Depression in the physical disability setting is a very common second diagnosis, which increases with age and poor health (Caine & King, 1993). Depression tends to increase as function decreases. In a study by Morris, Raphael, Samuels, and Molloy (1992), older age was found to be related to major depression when there was a personal or family history of affective or anxiety disorders, and depression was found by Ames (1993) to relate to, and increase in, physical disabilities.

Drug abuse can be both a cause and a result of a physical disability. For example, painful medical conditions may lead to prolonged alcohol and narcotic abuse. Conditions such as hepatitis and HIV infection can also be caused by intravenous drug use. Woosley (1991) suggests that alcohol used by a patient as a coping strategy can severely limit success in rehabilitation. Therefore, a history of drug use or signs that substances are being used as a coping strategy should always be ruled out by the health care team.

THE PSYCHOSOCIAL NEEDS OF CHILDREN
WITH PHYSICAL DISABILITIES

Occupational therapists must be aware of the child's development in all areas, and of the **roles** played by the child within the context of family, peers, the culture, and its institutions. Readers are encouraged to review the primary psychosocial and cognitive tasks identified by theorists such as Freud, Erikson, and Piaget. The Papalia and Olds (1995) text on human development is a particularly thorough description of developmental theorists. In this chapter, discussion is limited to a brief overview of psychosocial development at various stages of childhood and adolescence, a discussion of the effects of altered development on psychosocial functioning, and the nature of occupational therapy intervention.

Psychosocial Development

Treatment of the child implies the involvement of the entire family. The treatment team, including occupational therapists, develops an Individualized Family Service Plan (IFSP) that identifies the strengths and needs of the family and as a basis for determining effective intervention strategies (Hanft, 1989). In the United States, this process is mandated by federal law governing the provision of special education services for children from birth to three years of age. The most effective occupational therapy goals are those that are aligned with family and cultural expectations regarding the developing infant, child, and adolescent. The child may be part of a traditional, blended, multigenerational, or single-parent family. As they grow from infancy, children assume responsibility within the family and gain additional roles in the wider circle of the community in which they live.

The infant's role in the family is appropriately defined by dependence but is by no means a passive one. The healthy infant and primary caregiver (or caregivers) bond; they establish a pattern of give-and-take in an exchange of mutual admiration that creates the foundation for a lifetime of emotional, as well as physical, strength. The unfolding personality of the healthy infant born into a psychologically healthy family reflects adjustment, on the part of the family and the infant, to each other's expectations and demands (Brazelton, 1990).

During the years of early childhood, the child's role is characterized by a passion for **autonomy**, which alternates with clinging dependency. Vigilance regarding children's safety and well-being must be balanced with opportunities for them to expand the boundaries of experience and develop a sense of self as separate from the parent. In the years that follow, steadily increasing demands on children include developing the ability to contain their physical energy for extended periods of time, listen and absorb quantities of new information, and display evidence that they have retained and interpreted the new knowledge. Parental and sociocultural expectations for school-aged children are incorporated into play experiences as they interpret, in settings of their own making, the variety of roles they may assume in adulthood.

During middle childhood, play, school, and the primary family arena provide opportunities for the development of ethical and meaningful interactions with others. The child develops the cognitive capacity for considering increasingly complex issues. However, the (still largely egocentric) school-aged child primarily sees the world from the perspective of an evolving sense of self and through the lens of the family, without regard for his or her emotional health or the degree of "fit" within culture and society.

During adolescence, increasing demands are made on the individual for responsible and independent decision making in the realms of self-care, school and work, and leisure pursuits. Some adolescents experience premature parenthood, thus aborting, delaying, or altering their own process of **individuation**. In school, work, and meaningful relationships, they begin to experience the pressures and challenges of the adult world.

The need to belong—to be unlike those adults whose values they reject— is a recurring theme of adolescence, as is the sense of invulnerability in the face of physical and psychological danger. Risk-taking behavior is a hallmark of the adolescent, who, while in effect examining in a new way the two-year-old's issues of autonomy versus dependence, may literally fight to establish him- or herself as separate from the family of origin. Such risk can run the gamut from experimentation with clothing and hair to unprotected sexual exploration and leisure pursuits deemed dangerous by adults.

Those without a history of strong family interaction and those who reject the family may seek involvement in peer groups or gangs to establish a sense of congruence and belonging. Adolescents experience conflicting sexual tension, both hormonal and societal. Unprotected and promiscuous sexual behavior exposes adolescents to the risks of unplanned pregnancy and sexually transmitted disease, which can inexorably alter the course of their future or even threaten their lives. The pressure to conform to traditional gender roles and sexual orientation can be particularly difficult for adolescents who identify themselves as gay or lesbian, further contributing to a sense of isolation from the norm (Hersch, 1991). Even for adolescents whose primary family has supported their healthy psychological development, ambivalence, uncertainty, and questioning of society's prevalent norms are characteristic of the movement toward adulthood and autonomy.

Impact of Altered Development on Psychosocial Function

There are potentially serious psychosocial implications for children who are born prematurely or with congenital disorders, as well as for those who acquire a disability through trauma or acute or chronic illness.

Prematurity. As ever-younger premature infants are saved as a result of advances in neonatal technology, increasing numbers of parents must raise a newborn who is different from the one anticipated and deal with the loss of the idealized child whose birth they had anticipated. There is a high risk of parental alienation as the parent views the neonate in the complex and technical world of the intensive care unit, where privacy and peace are scarce and explanations by medical personnel may be difficult to understand.

The nervous system of the premature and medically unstable infant is not prepared for the world outside the mother's womb. Such infants commonly react to handling, feeding, and other components of the normal parental role with a behavioral display of nervous system immaturity. Behaviors may include tremors, failure to make eye contact, and the inability to stabilize respiration, heart rate, and other automatic functions. If an infant's evidently negative response to handling produces in the parent a sense of incompetence, frustration, and fear, that response cycle can interrupt the formation of the bond between infant and primary caregiver that is a foundation for childhood and adult mental health.

Infants born to mothers who have abused alcohol or other substances during pregnancy may face the dual challenges of an immature, unstable, or damaged nervous system and an emotionally or literally absent parent. Following hospital discharge to the home or a foster placement, infants identified as being at risk for developmental disability become candidates for occupational therapy services and are placed in community-based and school district–funded infant and preschool intervention programs.

Congenital disabilities and birth trauma. Children who sustained birth trauma with oxygen insufficiency or were born prematurely may be diagnosed with cerebral palsy, a term used to describe a wide variety of abnormalities in motor function and associated developmental skills deficits. Mental retardation may be present, but it is not a component of the diagnosis. This group and children with other congenital abnormalities, including spina bifida and arthrogryposis, are at risk for psychosocial difficulties beyond those related to problems in infant/caregiver attachment. Such children, whose movement patterns are altered, miss many developmentally appropriate opportunities to explore and engage the environment, their peers, and others. As they grow and find many of their needs met by parents, teachers, and other caregivers, children with such disabilities often miss opportunities to delay gratification, discover cause-and-effect relationships, negotiate their needs with others, assume age-appropriate responsibilities, and experience the consequences of their own actions.

Acquired disability and acute illness. Serious pediatric illnesses include meningitis, encephalitis, some tumors of the nervous system, and Guillain-Barré disease. Accidents, the current leading cause of death in children, may also contribute to long-term disability in those who survive. For families of many of these children, guilt regarding the illness or accident compounds the grief and loss regarding the child whose functional skills have changed. In children who retain memory of their former level of function and were old enough to have demonstrated their emerging skills and personality, grief, rage, denial, and/or confusion may complicate the rehabilitation process. Loss of function in familiar roles and occupational tasks can compound weakness, fatigue, and other effects of illness, further contributing to initial disorientation and poor motivation.

Chronic illness.   Acquired disabilities and a deterioration in function are associated as well with certain chronic illnesses, such as cystic fibrosis, asthma, juvenile diabetes, sickle cell disease, significant seizure disorders, and juvenile arthritis. Children and adolescents with such disorders must often alter their occupational roles and performance in self-care, school, and leisure pursuits to accommodate complicated and life-sustaining treatment regimens. Pain may be a part of the daily life experience, while necessary medications can produce unpleasant side effects, including drowsiness, sun sensitivity, and changes in appetite. An altered physical appearance, dependence on the parents for self-care assistance, or the need to use assistive devices challenge the emerging sense of self and may influence the child's ability to make and sustain meaningful friendships. Engaging in independent and age-appropriate role exploration through play and adolescent work experience can be impossible for some of these children.

CASE ILLUSTRATION: CHRISTINA

Christina is a 12 1/2-year-old-girl with juvenile arthritis, which was first diagnosed when she was 24 months of age. She has been hospitalized seven times during the course of her disease and takes daily medication for pain and joint swelling and to minimize destruction of her joints. The arthritis affects her neck, shoulders, jaw, left elbow, and both wrists. Most of her fingers now show noticeable changes, and her grasp is weak and inefficient.

Christina has trouble completing writing assignments and occasionally, when her pain and fatigue are greatest, she receives home schooling. She complains that missing school makes her feel isolated from her friends, as does her limited ability to walk. She lacks complete movement in her hips, knees, and ankles and will likely need hip and knee replacements once the bone growth in her legs is complete. During periods when her disease "flares," walking is limited to short distances.

Now that she is entering puberty, Christina is especially sensitive to her appearance. She notes that at the middle school she attends, children she does not know make cruel comments about the way she walks and moves. She is concerned that boys do not seem to like her, and she refuses to attend school dances. Her concern with her appearance also leads to her refusal to wear her protective hand splints during school.

Christina's pain is worse when she awakens in the morning, which slows her progress in getting ready for school. She often needs assistance from her mother with bathing, hair washing, and dressing, just at a developmental stage when most girls her age want complete privacy for self-care.

Discussion

Because of her chronic disability and her age, a time when many developmental changes take place, Christina's occupational roles and performance in self-care, school, and leisure pursuits were affected by having to accommodate complicated and life-sustaining treatment regimens.

Occupational Therapy Intervention

The occupational therapist who honors and responds to all areas of the child's development, as well as the family's unique cultural perspective and needs, will provide the most meaningful and effective intervention. Successful occupational therapy intervention considers the child's developmental level, occupational roles, and the psychosocial impact of prematurity, disability, and illness. Table 7-1 outlines common barriers for children and families and gives suggestions for occupational therapy intervention.

For all members of the treatment team, including the occupational therapist, children are most often meaningfully engaged through play. To the untrained observer, it may be difficult or impossible to identify by discipline the professional working with the child. Collaboration with other team members may be interpreted as duplication by those unfamiliar with the specific role of each member of the treatment team. In each treatment setting, the unique role as occupational therapists is to challenge the child's **adaptive response** toward functional independence through engagement in meaningful activity in the realms of self-care, play and school readiness, school, or prevocational tasks (Llorens, 1970). According to Clark (1993), the role of the occupational therapist can be likened to that of a coach for individuals with disabilities, who, like star athletes, must identify and practice those skills necessary to achieve success.

Therapist as interpreter and guide.   The occupational therapist's most critical role is facilitating an understanding of the child's signals that indicate pleasure and overstimulation. This is especially crucial in the neonatal intensive care unit, where, in addition to addressing the infant's medical and developmental needs, the occupational therapist works with bedside nursing staff and parents to improve the environment and position the infant to mimic the intrauterine state, which is most appropriate for the child's immature

Table 7-1. Barriers to Successful Pediatric Psychosocial Adaptation

Condition	Common Barriers or Difficulties for the Child and/or Parents	Suggested Occupational Therapy Intervention Strategies
Prematurity	• Infant's appearance, medical status, and developmental level are inconsistent with parents' expectations. • Infant's immature nervous system results in inability to respond normally to sensory stimuli, thus interrupting the early sensorimotor learning cycle. Infant at risk for developmental delay or disability. • Infant's medical status and technology of intensive care nursery may limit handling and thus prevent or interrupt formation of the parent-infant bond. Barriers may produce in the parents feelings of incompetency, frustration, fear, and anger, often directed at medical staff.	• Acknowledge parents' emotional reactions; educate them regarding infant's immaturity and its impact on development. • Help parents read infant's state of arousal and readiness for socialization; facilitate parent-infant bonding by helping parents see their child's individual personality and potential to develop despite a difficult start. • Work with bedside nursing staff and parents to provide privacy during parents' visits; modify environment and infant's position to accommodate immature nervous system. • As needed, intervene to improve specific skills. With parents, design alternate strategies to promote attachment.
Congenital Disabilities and Birth Trauma	• Sensory, motor, and cognitive deficits may limit the infant's ability to appropriately explore and respond to the environment. • Child's ongoing care needs may consume most of the parents' time, limiting the quiet playtime together that is necessary to build a healthy relationship	• Model for the parents intervention with the child that focuses on child's strengths, individual personality, and potential for growth toward individuation. • Acknowledge parents' feelings about child (may include fear, anger, depression, denial, hopelessness).

(continues)

Table 7-1. Barriers to Successful Pediatric Psychosocial Adaptation (continued)

Condition	Common Barriers or Difficulties for the Child and/or Parents	Suggested Occupational Therapy Intervention Strategies
Congenital Disabilities and Birth Trauma (continued)	and a role for the child within the family. • Provision of care by the parents limits child's experience of cause and effect, normal delay in having needs met, negotiation of needs with others, and consequences of own action.	• With parents, design strategies that build components of OT treatment into everyday care routine; help parents conserve energy to allow time for quiet play and bonding with the child. • Help parents provide for the child the appropriate developmental challenges to enable adaptation. • Design with the parents play experiences that adapt normal childhood activities.
Acquired Disability and Acute Illness	• Parents and caregivers (as well as the child) may experience guilt, grief, rage, and a profound sense of loss associated with changes in child's functional skills or threat of death. • Rapid change may be associated with nervous system healing, ongoing disease process, and medical treatment, further contributing to anxiety, agitation, and emotional lability in the child and family. • Disruption of the entire family unit, including siblings, is common. • Loss of function in familiar roles and tasks may exacerbate	• Build choice, no matter how minor, into each treatment session; allow the child time to process the challenge you have provided before expecting a response. • Provide developmentally appropriate treatment methods and materials. Address the child with respect and use language that is appropriate to his or her developmental level. • Plan for and acknowledge the child's verbal and nonverbal emotional expression. • Provide for appropriate privacy. Limit all unnecessary stimulation during treatment; as

(continues)

Table 7-1. Barriers to Successful Pediatric Psychosocial Adaptation (continued)

Condition	Common Barriers or Difficulties for the Child and/or Parents	Suggested Occupational Therapy Intervention Strategies
Acquired Disability and Acute Illness (continued)	weakness, fatigue, passivity, regression, depression, or other effects of acute illness.	needed, help nursing staff similarly limit stimulation on the medical or rehabilitation unit. • Involve the entire family unit in treatment to the extent possible; encourage family celebration with small rituals that duplicate life in their home. • Model for parents appropriate challenges and limit-setting if child is emotionally regressed.
Chronic Illness	• Progressive deterioration or exacerbations and remissions, requiring ongoing adjustment. • Pain & recurrent hospitalizations may result in regression and a sense of isolation; this requires further adaptation by the child and family and contributes to a sense of losing control. • Occupational roles and performance may need to be altered to accommodate pain, fatigue, and complicated and disruptive treatment regimens. • Necessary medication and medical treatment may produce side effects that delay or	• For the infant and toddler, the presence of a parent during painful or emotionally threatening procedures is the single most important factor in promoting the child's emotional health and cooperation. • Dolls, toys, and simulation materials allow the expression of fear and misconceptions. • Allow the infant or young child to maintain the necessary physical and emotional comfort zones before proceeding; work initially through the parents, if necessary. • With cooperation, and within the cultural guidelines of the family, use a token

(continues)

Table 7-1. Barriers to Successful Pediatric Psychosocial Adaptation (continued)

Condition	Common Barriers or Difficulties for the Child and/or Parents	Suggested Occupational Therapy Intervention Strategies
Chronic Illness (continued)	disrupt development and impact self-concept and self-esteem. • Altered physical appearance, dependence on parents for assistance, and the need to use assistive devices can challenge the emerging sense of self, particularly in middle childhood or adolescence.	system to reward adaptation and gains in skill. • Older children and adolescents benefit from education about the disease process and knowledge of the consequences of noncompliance with care routines. • Participation in, and increasing responsibility for, therapy and other care routines improves compliance and contributes to necessary individuation. • Assertiveness, self-advocacy, and emotional coping strategies are necessary survival skills for those with chronic illness. The use of group treatment, role-playing, and journal keeping are all appropriate methods. • Provide parent education about family celebrations, developmentally appropriate challenges, and effective limit setting.

nervous system. Guidelines may be given to nursing staff and parents to minimize overstimulation in the brightly lit, mechanized hospital setting.

Therapist as resource.   Parents and other caregivers frequently need help in understanding how to incorporate the often-complex care needs of the growing infant, child, and adolescent into their daily lives. The occupational therapist can help with environmental modifications and suggest adaptations to care routines that support psychosocial development and motor, sensory, cognitive, self-care, and play skills. The most meaningful interventions for parents are those that help them adapt normal childhood activities and play experiences for their child.

Accordingly, one critical task for the therapist is to help the family build components of treatment into the normal, daily routines of child care. For example, promotion of the complete upper and lower extremity range of motion can be incorporated into a diaper change. Using such strategies, the parent can make the treatment most meaningful. The caregiver can thus build on the relationship with the child rather than perform an isolated "duty," which the child must endure.

Therapist as role model.   The acceptance of the child as a unique and lovable individual is a vital first step toward that child's healthy emotional development. With support from the occupational therapist and other care providers, parents and families are more likely to accept the child's disability and provide an atmosphere in which therapy needs are balanced with everyday life and activity.

A crucial and early role for the occupational therapist is to build for the family an image of the infant and preschooler as an older child, adolescent, and, then, adult, when he or she will function at the most independent level. Picturing their child's future can help parents maintain hope. With such an early picture of the individual that their infant may become, families can put into perspective the relative importance of early therapy intervention. They can then be better prepared for the inevitable cessation of therapy services when they are no longer needed. At that point, the child may have achieved all appropriate goals or the family may now be capable of successfully instituting a home program addressing any remaining goals. With assistance, families can view the end of therapy services as a rite of passage and transition of their child to the next stage of life, rather than evidence of a failure of the system or the family unit to do enough to effect a cure.

The therapist can model for caregivers those behaviors that incorporate appropriate limit setting and expectations for developmentally appropriate behavior. Parents of children with disabilities often fail to establish for their disabled child many of the important behavioral expectations that are provided to children without physical and cognitive disabilities. Providing opportunities to experience behavioral consequences and assume responsibilities for meaningful chores that they are capable of completing provides all children, with and without disabilities, the same opportunities to learn and prepare for adult life, where they may function to the limit of their capabilities.

PSYCHOSOCIAL ISSUES IN ACUTE MEDICAL HOSPITALIZATIONS

Webster's Seventh New Collegiate Dictionary (1976) defines the term *acute* as an adjective that describes an event of sudden onset that has a sharp rise and short course and that seriously demands urgent attention. Webster further lists the words *critical* and *crucial* as synonymous with *acute*. These terms draw for us a picture of intensity of emotion and the need for immediate action, with a dimension of suspense and uncertainty of outcome. By this definition, the term certainly captures the experience of many individuals who require **acute hospitalization**.

The reasons for hospitalization in an acute medical care setting are as varied as the individuals who require the service. For many individuals, this type of hospitalization is ridden with anxiety and fear, while for others it is simply a passing inconvenience or an event full of expectation. To make sure that occupational therapy services are relevant, it is important that we understand the perception our clients have of both their personal health situation concerning hospitalization and their beliefs and expectations of what an acute hospitalization involves.

Hospitalization in an acute medical setting is usually necessary for persons who have suffered a sudden threat to their health, whose physical condition has deteriorated to the point of being life threatening, or whose condition requires an intervention that may itself be life threatening. Common reasons for hospitalization include sudden heart attacks, cerebrovascular accidents (CVA, commonly called strokes), and injuries sustained in an automobile collision or other type of accident. People may also be hospitalized to undergo planned interventions to correct, limit, or prevent deterioration in their health, as in the case of joint replacements, tumor removals, aneurysm clippings, coronary bypass surgery, radiation treatment, rehydration, and antibiotic treatment. Finally, there is also a group of persons for whom hospitalization is necessary because their health has deteriorated to such an extent that they require a period of receiving comfort measures, such as pain management, until death occurs. No matter the reason for hospitalization, however, acute hospitalization is associated with some type of physical disability that, in most cases, creates a disturbance in the neurological and/or musculoskeletal constituents of occupational skills (Kielhofner et al., 1985). These disturbances may be temporary, as in the decrease in endurance and strength that results from maintaining bed rest for a prolonged time, or long term, as in hemiplegia resulting from a stroke or cognitive impairments resulting from head injuries. In either case, however, the afflicted person's occupational behavior will be interrupted, limited, or jeopardized.

Disruption of Routines and Habits

Because daily routines and habits are built on a person's ability to physically perform them, they may become disorganized or be eliminated, modified, or delegated to others. In addition to not being able to complete the usual personal routines, the patient may have to learn new routines associated with the illness or the hospital environment. For example, a person may be dealing with the loss of ability to walk because of a lower extremity amputation. Besides now having to take extra time and expend extra energy to walk with crutches or propel a wheelchair, he or she must also incorporate routines of stump care and skin protection into his or her daily habits. This pattern of decreasing normal routines and replacing them almost immediately with new ones is not necessarily related only to the person's illness. It may also be due simply to the fact of seclusion in a hospital, which precludes the possibility of continuing with work, home activities, and leisure pursuits. Residence in the hospital requires adapting to different sleep, meal, medication, and treatment schedules. For some people, hospitalization may mean a significant decrease in the amount of usual daily activity, while for others, it may mean a significant increase. In either case, hospitalization requires a significant adjustment in a person's daily routine at a time when there may be decreased physical or cognitive abilities available with which to do so.

An added dimension of limitation imposed upon the individual during hospitalization has to do with its effects on his or her accustomed **roles**. Hospitalization not only has an impact on the individual's habits and daily routines, it also has an influence on the social context within which he or she is used to performing occupational behavior. During hospitalization, worker and homemaker roles must be completely put aside, at least temporarily. Other factors, such as the need for protective isolation or a hospital's restrictive visiting hours, may constrain social contact, thus hampering parenting or friendship roles. In the same way that habits and daily routines may be lost while others are being learned or adapted, the person's role repertoire undergoes a transformation. Because the management of the medical condition is often the focus of attention during hospitalization, the person may be in danger of placing him- or herself—or being placed there by others—in a "sick" or "invalid" role. This role is characterized by the patient's passive dependence on others to meet his or her needs and by social interactions centered on the person's illness or inability, whether real or only perceived, to perform other important roles. When a person loses a role, he or she may also lose the identity that the role had provided. Decreased self-esteem may result when the person takes on roles believed to be less important, productive, or socially acceptable. Role disbalance occurs when a person is unable to perform in a sufficient number of roles to maintain a sense of identity, purpose, and structure in everyday life.

At its best, hospitalization is fraught with changes for the patient: in physical capacities, in habits and routines, in environment, and in self-esteem.

Acute hospitalization is also associated in most people's minds with a high level of risk and uncertainty about the outcomes of intervention. Having to absorb information and sign numerous consent forms outlining the risks and potential side effects of treatment adds to the overwhelming sense of inability to process emotionally or fully understand what is happening to them. The sense of engulfment, coupled with the reduction in function that the person is already experiencing due to the medical condition, ultimately contradicts his or her view of the self as competent and erodes the belief that he or she possesses the necessary skills to overcome the illness and feel satisfaction in life. Physical limitations, both short and long term, may present the patient with a contradiction between the current limitations and personal or cultural values regarding what he or she ought to be able to do.

Fear

During hospitalization, fear frequently becomes a background feature of every moment because the person has no confidence in his or her ability to control events within his or her body or in the foreign hospital environment. It is not rare for patients to refuse therapy or other interventions designed to help them because they fear that any action may worsen their condition. Under the circumstances of hospitalization, it is very difficult for a person to maintain a sense of goals in life toward which to strive because the present focus is simple survival.

Depending on the person's cultural and social experience, he or she may anticipate rejection from others and avoid social contact. The concept of hospitalization itself may hold a negative meaning in the person's culture, representing death, infection, weakness, disability, misery, or pain. In these cases, the person will struggle with fear about the future and consequent dependence on others for medical help and with conscious or unconscious negative feelings about the symbolic meaning of the place where they are getting their needs met. If the hospital's routines and the patient's medical needs preclude cultural practices that the patient and family view as important during times of illness, the sense of alienation from oneself, one's significant relationships, and one's culture will be compounded.

CASE ILLUSTRATION: MR. BEHJATI

Mr. Behjati, a recent emigrant from Iran, was hospitalized for severe chest pain. While his condition was being evaluated, he was confined to bed and visiting was curtailed. Mr. Behjati is a devout Muslim and is concerned about his ability to engage in his five-times-daily prayers. He is also without his artifacts for the prayer ritual. His fear and anger are compounded by the absence of his family, who would traditionally speak for him in a crisis situation. Although he considers Western medicine to be effective and powerful, he does not understand why he is not getting aggressive treatment, nor does he think to relay any of his concerns to the health care providers. The physician noted that the patient seemed highly anxious and restless but he assumed this to be related to a cardiac condition.

Discussion

The recognition of Mr. Behjati's cultural and social mores could relieve his anxiety and restlessness and perhaps prevent misdiagnosis.

The fear of physical pain, disability, or death invariably is magnified through this temporary or permanent need to modify or disregard one's own values, and a sense of hopelessness and helplessness may be engendered. This process is depicted in Figure 7-1.

Intervention in Acute Settings

By the time patients in an acute medical setting are referred to occupational therapy for evaluation and treatment, they have usually already experienced a disturbance in their physical or cognitive capacities and are well on their way along a continuum of increasing fear. Occupational therapy intervention, then, cannot be limited to the simple prescription of exercises or adapted self-care routines but rather must consider several additional domains.

First, the therapist must have a thorough understanding of the medical condition of the patient and its real or potential functional implications. Because fear of the unknown may be immobilizing the patient, the therapist must help him or her understand the reality of the diagnosis and clarify any misconceptions about it. It is also essential for the therapist to clearly acknowledge to the patient which of the uncertainties being faced are real. The initial priority of occupational therapy intervention is to strategize practical ways to cope with uncertainty and fear and to demonstrate the power of occupation over one's emotional and physical well-being. Useful interventions include the use of expressive media, visualization exercises, progressive muscle relaxation, and active listening. (These techniques are elaborated in Chapter 12, "Anxiety Disorders.")

Once the patient's fears have been clarified, the second priority for occupational therapy is to understand the personal and cultural values he or she holds. If the patient is to sufficiently overcome the fear of the future and engage in occupation, he or she must have a sense of purpose or goal toward which to work. If, in fact, the outcome of hospitalization is uncertain or highly likely to end in death, the occupational therapist should empathically help the patient to accomplish tasks to help him or her die more peacefully and with a greater sense of completion. Interventions may include structured crafts projects for the patient to use as a farewell gift and graded self-care activities, energy conservation techniques, and communication skills training in order for the person to better focus on significant social relationships.

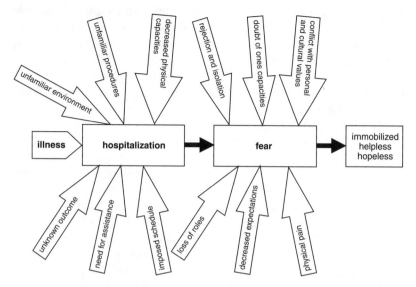

Figure 7-1.   Hospitalization Leading to Fear and Hopelessness

If the outcome of hospitalization is not likely to be life threatening, then occupational therapy should focus on the temporary or chronic limitations the patient will experience. To do so, the therapist must understand the roles the patient occupies and the environments in which they are enacted. This knowledge will assist in prioritizing skill training and guide the patient in the process of learning, reclaiming, modifying, delegating, or discontinuing roles. A supported exploration of the reality of the patient's fears of social rejection is an integral part of this process, and many patients will need to learn skills to cope with rejection when and if it occurs.

Acute medical hospitalization is fraught with fear for most patients. A knowledge of a variety of medical conditions and the precautions and functional limitations associated with them complements the occupational therapists' understanding of the performance dimensions that underlie the tasks of living. The occupational therapy intervention is focused, first, on overcoming fear and, second, on finding meaning in the experience of hospitalization through goal setting, activity, role modification, and values exploration. Occupational therapy offers each patient the opportunity to integrate all dimensions of function and often is the source of wholism in a reductionistic medical environment.

PSYCHOSOCIAL ISSUES OF CHRONIC DISABILITY

Human beings are in a constant state of change, adaptation, and adjustment to life, cognition, and the environment (Cairns & Baker, 1993). The normal physical changes of aging, such as those affecting body weight and hair color, are gradual and therefore easier to accommodate. This is the same process as **accommodation** to a chronic disability. After the original shock of the diagnosis of a long-term disabling condition or the inevitable adaptation to a congenital disability, the person will be in a position to start the process of adjustment to a chronic disability. This process requires constant accommodation and adaptation just like what the "nondisabled" population must go through on a daily basis. Factors that increase adaptability are shown in Figure 7-2.

Adaptation and adjustment to disability are not really any different than adjustment to other aspects of life change. This may seem obvious, but the biases of society and the health care system separate health care professionals from people with disabilities, which may result in alienation and a process of dehumanization of people with disabilities.

In all aspects of life, individuals compensate for a lack of physical prowess by empowering themselves with additional information or abilities. With a chronic disability, an individual must create new structures or more effectively use existing ones in order to keep gaining empowerment and knowledge of how to deal with the disability, overcome problems, and adapt. This is true not only for the individual with a chronic disability but for his or her significant others as well.

Loss

When people undergo a major loss in life, such as the loss of a loved one or special property (like a house), each person deals with it individually. Usually, a person first goes into shock (feeling overwhelmed); then he or she may start focusing on the problem as if it were all that there was in the world; and finally, he or she will, hopefully, put the loss into perspective and move on. Individuals with disabilities tend to go through the same process (Braithwaite, 1990). After a while it is hoped that the client will reach a point at which the focus is not on the disability and the client has started instead to anticipate future life tasks. This is not easy in cases where everyone the person encounters serves as a reminder of the loss. In the case of people with an obvious disability, the stares and comments of people around them may serve to remind them of their loss on a constant basis. Even if the disability is not obvious, the person may be continually reminded of the loss by being regularly confronted with the loss of skills or facility in doing simple tasks. In the face of these constant reminders, it takes additional time to grieve the loss and put it into perspective, since the perspective is continually changing and the loss is constantly being seen in new ways. Flagg-Williams stated that people "grow and change, experiencing different emotional patterns over time" (1991, p. 244). There appears to be an acculturation process that takes place, and the therapist may play a role in this process (Burton & Volpe, 1993). The first step may be to help the client and the family change their possible view of the patient's role

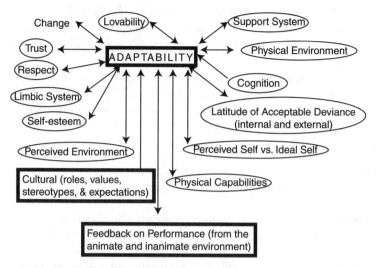

Figure 7-2. Elements That Increase Adaptability

from a sick role to a disabled role. This may not sound important, but if the disabled person remains in a sick roles, he or she may wait to get better and may feel the need to be cared for rather than take charge of his or her personal affairs in a responsible manner. The family may need help in changing their perceptions so as to help the client facilitate this role change.

Hope

The concept of hope needs to be addressed with a person with a disability throughout his or her lifetime, and also with the significant others who surround him or her. Hope keeps us moving forward through life. Some people get through life hoping that things will get better. Maybe they will win the lottery, their "big break" will come, or their children will have a better life. Since the client is no different than the rest of the population, hope is clearly important. Beliefs that may be perceived as full of denial, unrealistic, or delusional by a member of the health care team may in fact be helpful to the client or the family. Care must be taken not to inadvertently destroy their hope. The impact on the client that the occupational therapist makes in the acute stage of rehabilitation may later affect the long-term adaptation of the client and the family in ways that the therapist may not even think about.

CASE ILLUSTRATION: MR. BROWN

Mr. Brown suffered a cerebrovascular accident (CVA), or stroke, which could benefit from treatment in a rehabilitation center. While residing as an inpatient on the rehabilitation service, Mr. Brown and his family were told by his occupational therapist that "there is a one year window of opportunity to gain spontaneous return, and the most positive change will be seen within one year after the stroke." Mr. Brown and his family interpreted her comments to mean that within a year of discharge he would gain all the return that he would ever get.

At the one year anniversary of his stroke, Mr. Brown told his wife that he had looked at his present level of functioning and decided that he could not live with it. Without hope of further improvement, he contemplated suicide 12 months after his initial hospitalization.

Discussion

In Mr. Brown's case, an early statement by the occupational therapist was interpreted in such a way that it precluded hope.

The very concept of chronic disability highlights the fact that improvement does not always mean a return to normal levels of function. The therapist should strive to find a vocabulary that will communicate clearly to the client and family. This information will be client specific and may need to be changed over time as the client changes.

Acceptance and Love

There exists a very strong need for all individuals to feel accepted, part of a group, loved, and respected. Depending on how well we feel we have accomplished these tasks, we will tend to have high self-esteem and feel that we are lovable. The problem with having a disability is that it brings with it unique restrictions. For example, the disabled person may feel that he or she is not as lovable or as approachable as other people since equipment or societal restrictions may get in the way. As one person with a disability stated, "It is hard to be hugged if you are in a metal wheelchair with a computer on the lapboard and a hard, cold brace keeping you secure." The restrictions that physically stop the disabled person from expressing loving needs and the societal restrictions that dictate who is a lovable and worthy member of society create barriers that may prevent the disabled person from feeling valuable and worthy.

Beyond just providing the disabled person with physical aid in the area of physical adaptation, there is a need to provide structures in the community that foster hope, a feeling of need, worthiness, productivity, and purposefulness. Without these supports, the person with a disability may feel overwhelmed and believe that to hope for a better life, maturational development, adjustment, and growth is unrealistic. At a certain point there may be no visible hope of ever gaining reinforcement from life, and the person may feel that there may be nothing positive to look forward to. Society must find ways to allow for the support of people with disabilities so that they can feel that they can continue with the developmental aspects of life despite their impairments. The need for respite care for the caretaker is starting to be realized (Dell Orto, 1990; Ell & Northern, 1990; Kaitz, 1993; Schulz, 1994; Schwartzberg, 1994), but for people with a disability there has been little recognition of the need to provide an opportunity to have positive interactions with others and allow them to hope that adaptation can be positive and that there is reason to keep adapting and growing as individuals. The conditions that allow for adaptation and change are culturally specific as to the role of the person who is disabled or aging. This role can be used to help the individual grow and develop, or it can be used to damage the client. If a person with a disability is not forced to spend every bit of energy on physical function, he or she may be able to change, adapt, mature, and grow in other developmental aspects of life. By being freed from the need to focus on physical activities of daily living (ADL), the person may find time and energy to work on other developmental tasks that need to be accomplished. The therapist may be remiss if the focus is placed only on physical independence since physical abilities are not always reflective of the maturational hurdles that the person may be attempting to accomplish in life.

A statement that is often made by the elderly as they continue to age is that they are interested in quality, and not quantity, in later life. It is felt that this is not just a rationalization to deal with the body slowing down but the reflection of a maturational process that demonstrates an appreciation and a willingness to enjoy life by not rushing through it. When working with people with a disability, this same concept can be nurtured and developed as one aspect of a meaningful activity of daily living. In many cases clients have communicated that the acquired disability allowed them to become what they really wanted to become in their lives. Until they became disabled, they had had no compelling reason to focus on what was important, but now they had found a need to do so and feel that they are better off as a result. The use of the disability to create a higher quality of life for the individual is often overlooked (Fine, 1991). Although none of us would ask to become disabled in order to reap the possible benefits, disability can be a positive stimulus for change if the client is encouraged to perceive it in this way.

CASE ILLUSTRATION:
THE POSITIVE ASPECTS OF DISABILITY

Because of her arthritis, Mrs. Anderson could not keep up with her children and her spouse when they were hiking. She needed constant rest stops, and she felt that she was impeding the natural movement and development of the family. The occupational therapist helped her analyze the situation. As a result of OT intervention, what had looked like a negative situation to her was now viewed as a more positive situation and the outings were adapted. The rest stops were used to look up information about the area, to help her children learn about the plants and animals around them, and to permit the discussion of ecology and the natural flow of life. It could be perceived that Mrs. Anderson's disability allowed her children and her spouse to learn how to "stop and smell the roses" and thus enjoy the quality of life rather than spending all their time running through it. The disability in this case allowed them to enjoy a quality of interaction that they may not have had otherwise.

Discussion

The occupational therapy intervention did not include adaptive or assistive devices, but rather—and most important—it faciliated Mrs. Anderson's ability to "reframe" what could be viewed as negative into a positive experience for herself and her family.

Summary

The psychosocial component of illnesses and disabilities must be addressed in all occupational therapy treatment plans, regardless of the treatment setting. This chapter described the phenomenon of dual diagnosis, whereby a distinct psychiatric condition is related to a physical disorder, and discussed the role of the occupational therapist in such cases. In addition, a major portion of the chapter discussed the general psychosocial issues found with physical disabilities of all ages, even in cases where distinct psychiatric diagnoses do not exist. Occupational therapists are in a unique position on health care teams to assess and treat psychosocial issues regardless of diagnosis.

Occupational therapists are justifiably proud of their generalist background. By training, they are prepared to identify and treat functional deficits related to both physical and mental disorders. However, in clinical practice it is possible to lose some skills because not all may be used in a particular work setting. A conscientious therapist acknowledges personal limitations and knows when to ask for help. The use as consultants of occupational therapists who are experienced in mental health settings can be of great benefit to both staff and patients. However, regardless of whether the needs for OT are addressed by one therapist or a primary therapist plus consultants, it is only when all areas of occupational performance are acknowledged that the needs of each patient can be thoroughly addressed and the richness and depth of the profession of occupational therapy can be demonstrated.

Review Questions

1. Identify key occupational roles at each developmental level: infancy, early childhood, middle childhood, and adolescence.
2. Using material from Table 7-1, identify the likely barriers to age-appropriate psychosocial development and specific treatment strategies for the support of adaptation based on the following case study:

CASE STUDY: DIONDRA

Diondra is an 18-month-old female transferred to the rehabilitation unit at the children's hospital where you work. She sustained a head injury and fractures to her ribs, pelvis, left leg and arm in an automobile accident. She was an unrestrained passenger in a car driven by her grandfather, who was also seriously injured in the accident. Prior to the accident she lived with her mother, two older brothers, and her grandparents. Her parents are divorced. Her father lives out of the area and is not involved.

Diondra was unconscious for 10 days following the accident and in intensive care for an additional week. Now, 2 months following injury, her casts have been removed and she is medically stable. She has not regained any language, however, and she frequently appears agitated and confused, although she clearly recognizes and responds to her family. Her use of the right side of her body is limited, and she has poor balance in sitting although her head control is good. You will work with her on improving her balance, eye-hand coordination, and fine motor skills in order to achieve appropriate movement, play, and social behaviors. In addition, as her occupational therapist you will work on feeding.

3. Think about the disability that you most fear. Based on the information in this chapter, discuss how this disability would limit the activities you now enjoy performing and what daily routines or habits you would have to change or give up. What new routines would you have to learn in order to cope with the disability?
4. Name five ways that the principles discussed in this chapter relate to your life.

Learning Activities

1. Locate a hospital, educational setting, day program, or overnight camp in your area that provides services for children with disabilities. Volunteer your time with children who live with a physical disability on a daily basis.
2. Imagine that you have been hospitalized and told that your condition is likely to result in death within a few weeks. On a sheet of paper list the names of three or four people who are very important to you. After completing the list, next to each name write briefly why that person is significant to you (the reason may include that the person has been supportive, always makes you smile, has helped you through a particularly difficult time, etc.). Once you have noted the significance of each person, think of an object you could make or buy or an activity you could do with that person that would symbolize the uniqueness and special meaning of your relationship. As a last step, reflect on why you have not done that activity together or given that person the gift you thought of. Why have you

held back? What would happen if you did do these things? Would this help make you "ready to die"?

3. Write down the five best adjectives to describe your personal experiences with hospitals or the medical establishment. Did you feel safe or uncomfortable in your early experiences with health care? Write a short essay on what you could do as an occupational therapist to improve the experience for a patient/client. If possible, share this essay with an individual who is in a patient/client role and ask for feedback.

Acknowledgment

Alice Kibele is the author of the section on the issues of children and adolescents, Rene Padilla addresses specific issues in acute medical hospitalizations, and Gordon U. Burton discusses the psychosocial issues related to chronic disability.

References

American Psychiatric Association (APA) (1994). Diagnostic and statistical manual of mental disorders (4 ed.). Washington, D.C.: APA.

Ames, D. (1993). Depressive disorders among elderly people in long-term institutional care. *Australian-New Zealand Journal of Psychiatry, 27*(3), 379–391.

Braithwaite, D. O. (1990). From majority to minority: An analysis of cultural change from able-bodied to disabled. *International Journal of Intercultural Relations, 14*, 465–483.

Brazelton, T. B. (1990). *The earliest relationship.* Reading, MA: Addison-Wesley.

Burton, L., & Volpe, B. (1993). Sex differences in the emotional status of traumatically brain-injured patients. *Journal of Neurologic Rehabilitation, 2*, 151-157.

Caine, E. D. L., & King, D. A. (1993). Reconsidering depression in the elderly. *American Journal Geriatric Psychiatry, 1*, 4–20.

Cairns, D., & Baker, J. (1993). Adjustment to spinal cord injury: A review of coping styles contributing to the process. *Journal of Rehabilitation, 4*, 30–33.

Clark, F. (1993). Occupation embedded in a real life: Interweaving occupational science and occupational therapy. 1993 Eleanor Clarke Slagle lecture. *American Journal of Occupational Therapy, 47*, 1067–1078.

Dell Orto, A. E. (1990). Respite care: A vehicle for hope, the buffer against desperation. In P. W. Power, A. E. Dell Orto, & M. B. Gibbons (Eds.), *Family interventions throughout chronic illness and disability* (pp. 265–284). N.Y.: Springer.

Ell, K., & Northern, H. (1990). *Families and health care: Psychosocial practice.* New York: Aldin de Gruyter.

Fine, S. B. (1991). Resilience and human adaptability: Who rises above adversity? 1990 Eleanor Clark Slagle Lecture. *American Journal of Occupational Therapy, 45,* 493–503.

Flagg-Williams, J. B. (1991). Perspectives on working with parents of handicapped children. *Psychology in the Schools, 28,* 238–246.

Fulop, G. S., & Strain, J. J. (1991). Diagnosis and treatment of psychiatric disorders in medically ill patients. *Hospital and Community Psychiatry, 42,* 389–400.

Hanft, B. (1989, June). Providing family-centered occupational therapy services. *Sensory Integration Specialty Interest Section Newsletter, 12*(2), 1–3.

Hersch, P. (1991). Secret lives. *The Family Therapy Networker, 15*(1), 37–43.

Kaitz, S. (1993, May/June). Strategies to prevent caregiver fatigue. *Headlines,* 18–19.

Kielhofner, G., Shepherd, J., Stabenbow, C., Bledsoe, N., Furst, G., Green, J., Herlong, B., McLellan, C., & Owens, J. (1985). Physical disabilities. In G. Kielhofner (Ed.), *A model of human occupation: Theory and application* (pp. 170–247). Baltimore, MD: Williams & Wilkins.

Llorens, L. (1970). Facilitating growth and development: The promise of occupational therapy. *American Journal of Occupational Therapy, 24*(2) 93–101.

Morris, P. L. R., Raphael, B., Samuels, J., & Molloy, P. (1992). The relationship between risk factors for affective disorder and poststroke depression in hospitalized stroke patients. *Australian-New Zealand Journal of Psychiatry, 26* (2), 208–217.

Papalia, D. E., & Olds, S. W. (1995). *Human development* (3rd ed.). New York: McGraw-Hill.

Schulz, C. H. (1994). Helping factors in a peer-developed support group for persons with a head injury: Part 2. Survivor interview perspective. *American Journal of Occupational Therapy, 48* (4), 305–309.

Schwartzberg, S. L. (1994). Helping factors in a peer-developed support group for persons with a head injury: Part 1. Participant observer perspective. *American Journal of Occupational Therapy, 48* (4), 297–304.

Webster's Seventh New Collegiate Dictionary. (1976). Springfield, MA: G. & C. Merriam Co.

Woosley, E. (1991). Psycho-social aspects of substance abuse among the physically disabled. *American Archives of Rehabilitation Therapy, 29,* 1–4.

Suggested Reading

Atwood, M. J. (1985). Occupational therapy intervention for the adolescent with juvenile rheumatoid arthritis. *Occupational Therapy in Health Care, 2*(3), 344–348.

Baxter, C. (1989). Investigating stigma as stress in social interactions of parents. *Journal of Mental Deficiency Research, 33*(6), 446–455.

Belgrave, F. Z. (1991). Psychosocial prediction of adjustment to disability in African Americans. *Journal of Rehabilitation, 57,* 37–40.

Bowlby, John. (1982). *Attachment.* New York: Basic Books.

Bray, G. (1987). Family adaptation to chronic illness. In B. Caplan (Ed.), *Rehabilitation psychology desk reference.* Rockville, MD: Aspen.

Bukowski, W. M., & Hoza, B. (1989). Popularity and friendship: Issues in theory, measurement, and outcomes. In T. Berndt & G. Ladd (Eds.), *Contributions of peer relationships to children's development* (pp. 15–45). New York: Wiley.

Bullard, D. J., & Knight, S. E. (1981). *Sexuality and physical disability.* St. Louis: C. V. Mosby.

Christiansen, C. (1991). Performance deficits as sources of stress: Coping theory and occupational therapy. In C. Christiansen & C. Baum, (Eds.) *Occupational therapy: Overcoming human performance deficits* (pp. 69–96). Thorofare, NJ: Slack.

Harper, D. (1991). Paradigms for investigating rehabilitation and adaptation to childhood disability and chronic illness. *Journal of Pediatric Psychology, 16*(5), 533–542.

Kennedy, G. J. K., Kelman, H. R., & Thomas, C. (1990). The emergence of depressive symptoms in late life: The importance of declining health and increasing disability. *Journal of Community Health, 15,* 93–104.

Kibele, A., & Flint, S. (1990). The challenge of pediatric pain: The role of occupational therapy in multidisciplinary management. *Occupational Therapy Practice, 1*(3), 39–46.

Lilliston, B. A. (1985). Psychosocial responses to traumatic physical disability. *Social Work in Health Care, 10*(4), 1–13.

Lyness, J. M., Caine, E. D., Conwell, Y., King, D. A., & Cox, C. (1993). Depressive symptoms, medical illness, and functional status in depressed psychiatric inpatients. *American Journal of Psychiatry, 150*(6), 910–915.

Mahler, M., Pine, F., & Bergman, A. (1975). *The psychological birth of the human infant: Symbiosis and individuation.* New York: Basic Books.

Marinelli, R. P., & Dell Orto, A. E. (1984). *The psychological & social impact of physical disability* (2nd ed.). New York: Springer.

Pulaski, M. A. (1971). *Understanding Piaget.* New York: Harper & Row.

Stern, D. J. (1985). *The interpersonal world of the infant: A view from psychoanalysis and developmental psychology.* New York: Basic Books.

Versluys, H. P. (1989). Psychosocial accommodation to physical disability. In A. Trombley (Ed.), *Occupational therapy for physical dysfunction* (3rd ed., pp. 13–27). Baltimore: Williams & Wilkins.

Substance Abuse and Occupational Therapy

Kate Riley, MEd., MFCC
Chemical Dependency Counselor
Kaiser Permanente, San Francisco

Ruth Ramsey, MS, OTR
Director and Chair of Occupational Therapy
Dominican College of San Rafael, California

Elizabeth Cara

Key Terms

codependency
cross-dependency
defense
dual diagnosis
enabling
preferred defense structure

recovery
sobriety
substance abuse
substance addiction/dependence
twelve step groups

Chapter Outline

Introduction

One of America's leading health and social problems is the abuse of addictive substances, specifically drugs and alcohol. In the late 1800s, during the Industrial Revolution, the medical profession began to recognize the effects of alcohol abuse on factory workers and on pregnant women and their unborn children. Malnutrition, brain damage, liver disease, fetal alcohol syndrome, and child abuse were linked to the habitual abuse of alcohol. This concern eventually led to the Prohibition movement and resulted in passage of the 18th Amendment (1920-1933), which prohibited the manufacture, sale, or transportation of alcohol. The Prohibition movement failed and the law was ultimately repealed, in part because it did not distinguish social use from abuse (Royce, 1981).

Since Prohibition, substances other than alcohol have been identified and targeted as contributing to significant social problems. For example, there was a rise in the use of heroin and marijuana during the "jazz age" of the 1920s and 1930s. In the 1960s and 1970s, some members of the "hippie counter-culture" experimented with psychedelic, mind-altering drugs such as lysergic acid diethylamide (LSD) and mescaline. Cocaine—a stimulant drug that enables people to work long hours without fatigue—became popular during the achievement-oriented decade of the 1980s, and in the 1990s synthetically manufactured drugs such as ice (a long lasting methamphetamine) and ecstasy (a euphoria-inducing hallucinogen) achieved notoriety within the drug-using subculture.

The effects of **substance abuse** are widespread. According to the National Institute on Alcohol Abuse and Alcoholism, alcohol is involved in more than half of all child abuse cases, rapes, traffic deaths, felonies, fire fatalities, and homicides and a third of all suicides. Conservative estimates indicate that the problem of alcoholism and drug addiction exists in 4 to 13 percent of the population (Blume, Neider, Suemnick, & Westermeyer, 1991; Royce, 1981), with those affected coming from every economic, educational, and age level and from every race and gender. Furthermore, each substance abuser directly affects at least four to six other individuals, whether a spouse, children, parents, employer, employee, or innocent victim of an accident or crime (Royce, 1981).

In the workplace, substance abuse has a major impact on job performance, productivity, and profit. Substance abuse has been estimated to cost U.S. industries over $1,000 billion a year (Inaba & Cohen, 1993). Comparing substance abusers to nonabusers in the work arena, substance abusers are late 3 to 14 times more frequently, absent 5 to 7 times more often, have lower actual work output, and are more likely to be involved in grievance procedures. Medical costs for substance-abusing employees are much higher than for other employees since the former experience 3 to 4 times more on-the-job accidents, use 3 times more sick leave, and file 5 times more workmen's compensation claims (Inaba & Cohen, 1993).

Alcoholism is the third leading cause of death by disease in the United States, and 20 to 40 percent of all hospital beds are filled by people whose illnesses are alcohol related (NIAAA, 1978). Alcohol and drug use directly and indirectly contributes to the development of health problems such as hepatitis, heart disease, cerebrovascular accidents, high blood pressure, and diabetes. People with psychiatric disorders become increasingly dysfunctional when abusing alcohol and drugs, since these substances directly affect brain chemistry. **Substance addiction/dependence** greatly increases the likelihood of premature death in all illnesses and injuries.

Substance abuse plays a major role in accidents resulting in head, hand, and spinal cord injury and in other impairments typically requiring rehabilitation services. All too often, the substance abuse is left untreated in these individuals, who, tragically, frequently reinjure themselves or further endanger their health by continuing to abuse substances after their injuries.

The tremendous increase in awareness regarding the scope and severity of alcohol and drug abuse in the last 20 years has spurred increased scientific study of effective approaches to substance abuse treatment (Morgenstern & Leeds, 1993; Wallace, 1992). No longer focusing on the treatment of specific substances, chemical dependency treatment is now a generic or umbrella term that represents a marriage between the alcoholism and drug treatment fields (Wallace, 1992).

Regardless of the area of specialization, occupational therapists need to be well informed about the problems of substance abuse and methods of chemical dependency treatment. As rehabilitation professionals, occupational therapists can assess functional deficits contributing to, and resulting from, the illness of chemical dependency. This chapter is intended to provide an overview of basic information about alcoholism and other chemical dependencies. A definition and description of chemical dependency and types of addictive substances will be provided, and current treatment philosophies and models will be described. Occupational therapy interventions for treating people with primary chemical dependency or **dual diagnosis** problems will be outlined, along with a description of the optimal treatment focus for each stage of chemical dependency recovery.

DEFINITIONS—ABUSE, DEPENDENCE, AND ADDICTION

The *Diagnostic and Statistical Manual of Mental Disorders, Fourth Edition* (DSM-IV) (APA, 1994) makes a clear distinction between abuse and dependence:

Abuse

Drug and alcohol abuse is defined as use that has been harmful or is potentially harmful to the extent that the substance use negatively affects one or more important areas of the user's life for at least one month. There is continued use of the substance despite awareness that it is causing a problem or making an existing problem worse. There also may be repeated use in situations where it is known to be physically hazardous. The substance use is excessive and harmful but has not yet reached the dependence state.

Addiction and Dependence

Substance dependence is commonly referred to as drug addiction, and often the terms are used interchangeably. The diagnosis of alcohol or substance dependence is more severe than that of substance abuse. Substance dependency is the chronic, excessive use of a substance that is harmful to the individual. Addiction is characterized by physical tolerance, psychological dependency, deterioration in overall functioning, and a marked loss of control over the frequency and amounts of the substance used.

DSM-IV Diagnostic Criteria

The American Psychiatric Association (APA) lists diagnostic criteria for psychoactive substance dependence in DSM-IV (see Table 8-1). The APA requires at least three of the following nine characteristics to be present for diagnosis:

Persons with chemical dependency use substances in ways that disrupt their lives and cause harm. In the majority of substance-abusing people who present for treatment, the addiction is progressive (is becoming worse over time) and is characterized by a loss of control. The individual has often tried unsuccessfully to quit or cut down. The ability to limit or predict the amount, frequency, and duration of substance use has been lost, while the consequences of the addiction increase in frequency and severity over time.

The popularity and variety of drugs that are abused by people in our society are influenced by many factors, including cost, availability, ease of manufacturing and distributing, and potency. Table 8-2 lists types and varieties of addictive substances.

Table 8-1. Diagnostic Criteria for Substance Abuse

1. The substance is often taken in larger amounts of over a longer period of time than intended.
2. There exists a persistent desire or there have been one or more unsuccessful efforts to cut down or control substance use.
3. A great deal of time is spent in activities necessary to get the substance, in taking the substance, or in recovering from its effects.
4. There occur frequent intoxication or withdrawal symptoms at times when the person is expected to fulfill major role obligations at work, school, or home, or when substance use is physically hazardous.
5. Important social, occupational, or recreational activities are given up or reduced because of substance use.
6. There occurs continued substance use despite the user's knowledge of having a persistent or recurrent social, psychological, or physical problem that is caused or exacerbated by the use (e.g., the person continues using despite family arguments about heroin, cocaine-induced depression, or an ulcer that is made worse by drinking).
7. There is marked tolerance involving the need for continually increasing amounts of the substance (i.e., at least a 50 percent increase) in order to achieve intoxication or the desired effect and a markedly diminished effect with continued use of the same amount.
8. There are characteristic withdrawal symptoms.°
9. The substance is taken to relieve or avoid withdrawal symptoms.°

To meet the criteria for substance abuse, some symptoms of the disturbance must persist for at least one month or have occurred repeatedly over a longer period of time.

°May not apply to cannabis, hallucinogens, or phencyclidine (PCP).

Table 8-2. Types and Varieties of Addictive Substances

Alcohol	Historically has been, and remains, the most widely abused substance. Alcoholic beverages come in various strengths or "proofs." Wine is typically around 13 proof (or 6% alcohol); vodka , whiskey and other hard liquors range from 60 to 100 proof (or 30 to 50% alcohol). Many of the new wine coolers and malt beers are extra strong and are especially designed to create quick intoxication.
	Regardless of what form alcohol comes in, the body metabolizes it in the liver at the rate of one ounce an hour. A person becomes intoxicated if he or she consumes alcohol faster than the body can process it. People are considered intoxicated if they have a blood alcohol level above .08%. Chronic alcohol abuse causes damage to every organ in the body, especially the liver, heart, and brain. Withdrawal symptoms include tremors, hallucinations, sweating, seizures, and diarrhea.
Hallucinogens	In the 1960s hallucinogenic drugs such as LSD, mescaline, and psilocybin ("magic mushrooms") were introduced to American youth culture. Hallucinogens have recently again risen in popularity among 13–30-year-old substance users. "Designer" psychedelics such as MDMA, MDA, and MDM (methylenedioxymethamphetamine, also referred to as Ecstasy, X, and Adam) are synthetically manufactured drugs that cause stimulatory experiences and mild distortions of perception. These hallucinogenic amphetamines are said to calm the user and increase empathy with others.
	PCP, once a tranquilizer for animals, is now illegal to manufacture. PCP removes inhibitions and deadens pain, and its users can develop superhuman strength and lose any memory of their behavior while under the influence of the drug. There are many adverse reactions to moderate doses of PCP, including muteness, rigid robotic attitude, disorientation, paranoia, and seizures.
	Hallucinogenic drugs are used to alter reality by inducing an overwhelming sensory experience. Frightening and dangerous psychotic episodes can occur with experimental or chronic use of hallucinogenic drugs because they distort brain-sensory perception in unpredictable ways.
Cannabis	Marijuana is widely used and is frequently part of polysubstance dependency (chronic use of more than three drugs). Scientific cultivation techniques for growing marijuana plants have dramatically increased the potency of marijuana in the last decade (Inaba & Cohen, 1993). It is not uncommon to lace (adulterate) marijuana joints with crack cocaine, heroin or PCP. The most common route of ingestion is by smoking. Short-term effects of marijuana include talkativeness, increased appetite, a distorted sense of time and space, introspection, and impaired intellectual performance. Chronic smokers report serious paranoid ideation and feelings of depersonalization.
Cocaine	A stimulant grown from coca plants and distilled into white powder, which is inhaled through a straw into the nose or injected with a syringe, producing an intense sensation of pleasure lasting 20

(continues)

Table 8-2. Types and Varieties of Addictive Substances (cont'd.)

	minutes to $1^{1}/_{2}$ hours. Crack is cocaine that is crystallized into small yellowish rocks, which are smoked by the user to produce rapid and extreme euphoric sensation lasting 4 to 30 minutes. Frequent users of cocaine become paranoid and delusional. Addiction and psychosocial deterioration can occur very rapidly as the drug produces very intense cravings for continued use. The high is followed by intense depression with irritability and a need for sleep. Cocaine use causes muscular damage to the heart and weakens blood capillaries thereby increasing the likelihood of heart attacks and strokes.
Amphetamines and Other Stimulants	Methamphetamines are manufactured from chemicals and can be injected into the body, smoked in a pipe, joint, or cigarette; dissolved into a beverage such as coffee; or taken in pill form. Amphetamines are manufactured in illegal laboratories or gotten legally or illegally from doctors and pharmaceutical companies. Street names for different types of amphetamines include crank, shabu, ice, glass, meth, speed, crystal, and cross tops. Ritalin Hydrochloride and Dexedrine are examples of prescription stimulants that have the potential for abuse. The effects of amphetamines last 4 to 8 hours.
	The heavy use of stimulants causes the individual to become very jittery, malnourished, sleep deprived, extremely impulsive, and sometimes paranoid and delusional. Amphetamine or cocaine psychosis can last for several weeks. In some cases, users with persistent symptoms of delusions and paranoia may require hospitalization and medication to provide safety and stabilization until they withdraw ("come down") from the drug.
Narcotics	Narcotics are pain killers, which cause sedation, euphoria, impaired intellectual functioning, and impaired coordination. Narcotic drugs include heroin, codeine, opium, morphine, and Percodan, Demerol, and Darvon (trade names of narcotics prescribed for pain relief). Heroin has had a resurgence in popularity and it is now being smoked as well as used intravenously.
	During the early phases of narcotic abuse, the drug produces a feeling of euphoria and pleasure. However, as the user becomes habituated, *tolerance* develops and the pleasurable feelings diminish. The habitual narcotic users must continue taking the drug to ward off withdrawal symptoms such as painful muscle cramping, fever, chills, and diarrhea. These withdrawal symptoms can last 5 to 14 days. Methadone, a synthetic opiate, is sometimes prescribed for heroin detoxification or for the medical-social maintenance of the opiate-addicted person who has been unsuccessful achieving opiate abstinence. Naltrexone, a medication that blocks the effect of opiates, is used to prevent relapse on heroin and other narcotics. Naltrexone is being experimentally used to decrease the cravings and severity of alcohol and cocaine relapse (Inaba & Cohen, 1993).

(continues)

Table 8-2.	Types and Varieties of Addictive Substances (cont'd.)
Tranquilizers/ Benzodiazepines	Minor tranquilizers such as Valium, Librium, Xanax, Tranxene, Klonopin, and Ativan are widely used, and abused, prescription drugs. These drugs are prescribed for anxiety, irritability, insomnia, restlessness, and tension. Physical addiction to benzodiazepines can occur after two to three weeks of daily use. Detoxification should be medically supervised, as seizures and other serious medical complications can occur.

CAUSES OF ADDICTION

Despite many years of extensive research there is no one single widely accepted theory about what causes addiction. One of the major difficulties blocking a unified theory is the immense variety in the patterns of addiction and types of people who become chemically dependent. There has been acceptance of the idea that there are multiple pathways to addiction and many types of addiction (White, 1991). The origins of addictions are attributable to biological, psychological, and sociocultural factors (Schuckit & Hagland, 1978).

Biopsychosocial

Addiction is seen as a biopsychosocial disease affecting many important life areas, including family life, vocational performance, self-care abilities, physical and emotional health, social relationships, and financial well-being. The biopsychosocial approach emphasizes the contribution of biological, psychological, cognitive/behavioral, and social/cultural factors in the prevalence, development, and course of addictions (Wallace, 1992). It also is a useful theoretical framework for prevention, intervention, and treatment efforts, and especially for relapse prevention (Blume et al., 1991).

Biological and genetic components.   In the past 20 years scientists have come closer to validating the long-suspected link between biological and genetic factors and addiction (Deitrich, 1993). Pharmacological evidence indicates that the brain's opiate receptor system plays an important role in the maintenance of alcoholism (Friehlich & Li, 1993). Some studies, including studies of heredity in twins and generational transmission in families, suggest that genetic factors are more important than social factors in the development of addiction (Goldman, 1993; Goodwin, 1991; Schuckitt & Hagland, 1978). Laboratory researchers have begun establishing specific neurochemical factors in biological-based susceptibility. They speculate that the predisposition to addiction stems from differences in brain chemistry (Davies & Walsch, 1970; Myers, 1978; Wallace, 1992).

Psychological components.   In addition to biological factors, there are distinct psychological components that are thought to play an important role in initiating and then maintaining addiction (Brown, 1985; Gomberg, 1991; Zweben, 1992). Theorists have long debated the chicken-and-egg dilemma of whether the individual becomes addicted as a result of preexisting psychological conflicts or the psychological and emotional deterioration is a consequence of the addiction process itself? Low self-esteem, anxiety, depression, paranoia, emotional numbness, and poor handling of frustration may be outcomes rather than causes of chemical dependency.

Substance abuse does affect the brain chemistry and leads directly to symptoms that mimic psychiatric problems (Inaba & Cohen, 1993). Health care professionals must remember that psychopathology observed in substance users or newly abstinent individuals may be due to the disrupting effect of psychoactive substances on the brain (Pires, 1989; Zweben, 1992).

Sociocultural components.   Addiction is also significantly influenced by sociocultural factors (Tarter, 1983). The prevalence and patterns of addiction seem to be influenced by social conditions such as economic impoverishment, sociocultural oppression, and cultural norms that dictate the availability of drugs and alcohol and behavioral expectations for their use (White, 1991). Ethnicity has long been cited as a factor in the variance of addiction (Wallace, 1992); however, it is difficult to tease apart biological from cultural factors in ethnic group variations. It is important to note that while sociocultural factors may help to explain patterns and rates of addiction across different groups, they do not explain individual differences in consumption and addiction within a family or even within a culture.

Recently, theories on the etiology of addiction have proposed an interaction between psychodynamic factors and environmental stressors. For example, the stress-coping theory sees substance abuse as a habitual, maladaptive attempt to cope with stress and strain (Brehm, Khantzain, & Dodes, 1993). Severely traumatized individuals, such as combat survivors, rape victims, and victims of childhood abuse, attempt to use drugs and alcohol to induce dissociative states and ward off painful memories (Herman, 1992). The social ostracism experienced by homosexual individuals has been thought to be a factor in the higher incidence of alcoholism found in gay and lesbian populations.

Dual Diagnosis

Patients who have coexisting major mental illness and substance abuse disorders are referred to as having a dual diagnosis. According to a 1990 National Institute of Mental Health survey, 53 percent of drug abusers and 37 percent of alcohol abusers had at least one serious psychiatric problem in addition to their substance abuse problem (Zweben, 1992).

Alcohol and drugs are psychoactive substances, that is, they affect brain function, including sensory processing and cognition. The use and abuse of psychoactive substances can both cause and mask psychopathology. In individuals with dual diagnoses, some psychopathology may abate when the individual abstains from the abused substances. Psychiatric symptoms that persist usually require specific treatment and medication. The psychiatric disorders that most frequently co-occur with substance abuse are major depression, anxiety disorders, manic depressive illness, and personality disorders (Zweben, 1992).

While psychological factors are only posited to contribute to the development of addiction, they definitely play an important role in the maintenance of addiction through a process known as denial. Denial is a **defense**, a psychological process of distorted thinking and impaired reality testing, which maintains addiction. (This cognitive process is discussed in the section on denial and the defense system.)

Addiction and HIV

Intravenous drug abusers and other chemically dependent people are at high risk for contracting and transmitting HIV disease. Many become HIV positive because they have shared needles; traces of infected blood from an HIV positive person are transmitted when the drug user injects him- or herself with a contaminated needle. Addicted individuals may exchange sex for drugs or money to buy drugs. Alcohol and drugs impair judgment and reduce inhibitions, so many people under their influence also forget or ignore safe sex guidelines for the prevention of HIV.

TREATMENT APPROACHES

The many different approaches to treating substance abuse reflect theoretical beliefs about the causes of addiction and dominant social attitudes toward addicted and chemically dependent people. Social attitudes toward addiction have vacillated considerably throughout history, with hotly debated and widely divergent solutions being proposed (Keller, 1991). These solutions range from rehabilitation and decriminalization to imprisonment and the mandatory sentencing of drug users and sellers.

Cognitive-Behavioral Model

The cognitive-behavioral approach reflects the belief that addiction is largely a learned behavior, which therefore can be unlearned. The primary goals of behaviorally based treatments are the elimination of the behavioral habits and cognitive patterns of distorted thinking that maintain drug use (Zimberg, Wallace, & Blume, 1985).

Identifying behavioral consequences.   Cognitive-behaviorists first attempt to identify the potentially rewarding aspects of drugs and alcohol, which may motivate someone to continue using despite negative consequences. Some of the potential rewards include increased comfort in social situations, drug-induced feelings of pleasure, an illusory sense of personal power, and the cultural association of alcohol and drug use with increased status and sexual desirability.

A variety of cognitive behavioral approaches are used to enable the substance user to examine false beliefs about the benefits of substance use and then to focus on the negative consequences that have resulted, or could result, from the drug or alcohol use. Approaches could include homework assignments to list harmful consequences, sharing with group members personal examples of painful experiences with substances, interviewing family members about the effects of the drug and alcohol use on the family, and role-playing the sober self and the addicted self.

Identifying behavioral warning signs.   The individual identifies behavioral cues that represent warning signs leading to a relapse, or return to substance use.

**CASE ILLUSTRATION: ALAN—
PREVENTING RELAPSE BY IDENTIFYING BEHAVIORS**

Alan, in his third attempt at recovery, learned through the use of a written homework assignment that he displayed a specific sequence of behaviors before every relapse. When on this "slippery slope," Alan would feel bored with the Alcoholics Anonymous (AA) groups, become argumentative and critical, isolate himself at home, take the phone off the hook, and then begin to feel he could handle "a little" alcohol.)

Discussion

When Alan was assisted by an OTR to identify behaviors such as boredom with the AA groups, isolation, and criticism, he became acutely aware of exactly which behaviors could precipitate relapse.

Restructuring the environment.   Strategies in behaviorally based treatment include restructuring the living environment to reduce physical and emotional factors in the sequence leading to use.

CASE ILLUSTRATION: SHANTELLE— RESTRUCTURING THE ENVIRONMENT

Early in treatment, Shantelle was instructed to remove all drugs and alcohol from her apartment. She was told to take an alternative route home to avoid passing the area of her drug connection and to cut up her ATM card until she was able to successfully cope with her drug cravings.

Discussion

Shantelle restructured her environment to prevent any possibility of reconnecting with drugs or alcohol or with her previous addictive behaviors.

Aversion.   Some programs utilize aversion techniques that pair substance use with a mild, but unpleasant, electrical sting or with medications such as Antabuse, which, when taken with alcohol, causes vomiting, nausea, and stomach spasms. The goal is to change the pattern from one of inducing pleasure to one of inducing physical and/or emotional pain and then associating that with the substance use.

Rewarding abstinence.   Remaining abstinent is reinforced in many ways, including verbal encouragement, peer approval, and awarding medallions recognizing the length of time since the substance was last used. Attending twelve step meetings, finding substitute activities, and practicing nonhabitual responses also reinforces abstinence-based attitudes and behaviors (Zimberg et al., 1985).

Cognitive therapy.   In cognitive therapy, patients are taught to examine the connection between thoughts, feelings, and actions. They are taught to identify typical patterns of thinking that lead to substance use and shown how to change these patterns to promote **recovery**.

Psychodynamic/Psychoanalytic Model

This treatment approach emphasizes underlying psychological conflicts that maintain the individual's destructive relationship to substances. The focus of psychodynamic treatment is on internal, unconscious conflicts resulting from early family patterns. Early psychoanalytic theories emphasized the regressive nature of drug taking and the user's intense need for oral gratification (Rothchild, 1992). Current psychodynamic theories speculate that addictions result from unfulfilled dependency needs, which the individual attempts to soothe with alcohol or drugs. The substance use becomes a substitute for mature psychological functioning in individuals with deficits in the ability to handle and regulate feelings and maintain healthy self-esteem (Brehm et al., 1993).

Individual psychodynamic psychotherapy as an early intervention with alcohol and drug addiction is generally less effective than cognitive-behavioral approaches. Newly recovering people are vulnerable to becoming confused by a variety of feelings as conflicts or early traumas are explored because these feelings are often experienced as physiological states. For example, anger may be experienced as physical tension and sadness as physical pain (Morgenstern & Leeds, 1993). Intense cravings for drugs and alcohol will be experienced as the person looks for a way to soothe these painful feelings or states.

A toxic brain physiologically influenced by chemicals can neither absorb nor remember insights achieved in psychotherapy. This is true for both the active substance user and the newly recovering individual. Therefore, a supportive, directive approach has been found the most helpful to the newly recovering person, with psychodynamic approaches introduced as the individual strengthens and stabilizes in later **sobriety** (Rothschild, 1992).

Disease Model

The disease model, a medical approach, is one of the most widely used and accepted models of addiction and strongly influences many of the treatment approaches utilized by hospitals and clinics (Zimberg et al., 1985). According to this theory, the individual is born with a susceptibility to addiction because of biological and neurological deficiencies. Willpower, personality characteristics, and environmental factors are deemphasized.

From 1939 to 1960, Dr. E. M. Jelling conducted the first large-scale scientific study of alcoholism, from which he developed the disease model. Jelling proposed that alcoholism is not a single disease, but rather a disorder of at least five distinct types, some of which have a progressive, deteriorating course (Blume et al., 1991). The biological abnormality theory and subsequent approach to treatment known as the disease model was applied to explain uncontrolled compulsive drinking by the founders of Alcoholics Anonymous (Alcoholics Anonymous, 1955). Jellinik's disease model has also been successfully adapted to describe the course and progression of other addictions.

The acceptance of the concept of substance abuse as a disease has required continuing public education and reinforcement because the use of illegal "street" drugs such as cocaine, heroin, and marijuana and chronic "drunkenness" are often viewed with moralistic disapproval as failures of will. Within the disease model, addiction is viewed as a chronic, progressive, incurable, but treatable, disease. Throughout treatment the individual is encouraged to adopt the label of "recovering alcoholic/addict." The dangers of **cross-dependency** are emphasized, and complete abstinence is seen as the only viable goal. Medically supervised detoxification is indicated in cases where there has been prolonged intoxication or the person has a history of severe withdrawal symptoms, a history of seizure disorders, or suicidal ideation.

The medical model seeks to reinforce the importance of lifelong abstinence by encouraging the patient to attend counseling and **twelve step groups.** These support groups are frequently used as adjunctive interventions and are philosophically interwoven into many social and medical model treatment programs. Alcoholics Anonymous (AA) was founded in the 1930s by Bill Wilson and Dr. Bob Smith, two alcoholics who discovered that they could maintain their sobriety by helping other alcoholics. AA is often referred to as the most effective and widely utilized treatment for addictions (Royce, 1981). It is now an international self-help fellowship which offers support to all people who want to quit drinking.

Narcotics Anonymous, Cocaine Anonymous, and other anonymous support groups are structured on the AA model and utilize its "Twelve Steps and Twelve Traditions" (see Table 8-3) as the basis of their recovery program. The fellowship and principles offered at meetings encourage individuals to remain sober by taking life "one day at a time" and to work toward spiritual development and character change.

Codependency.   The process of addiction also impacts the people who live with, work with, care for, and depend on the substance-dependent person. Often, addiction treatment centers have programs that treat the family members for the dysfunctional way of relating referred to as **codependency**.

Codependency refers to a set of unhealthy characteristics that are adopted by many family members and other people close to, and affected by, a substance abuser. Being in a long-term relationship with an actively substance-addicted individual often results in extremely low self-esteem, many stress-related illnesses, chronic anger, and depression. As the substance abuse worsens, family members and concerned people may attempt to control the addict's addiction (e.g., by nagging, threatening, pouring out liquor, or spending money so there is less for drugs); they may also attempt to lessen the negative impact by compensating for the addict (e.g., taking over household chores or child care or managing finances), as well as making excuses (e.g., for the intoxicated behavior, absences from work, or mood swings). This behavior is referred to as **enabling**. While attempting to be helpful, the codependent person is actually enabling the addict to continue using by shielding him or her from the harmful effects of the addiction. Chemical dependency treatment programs attempt to intervene in the dysfunctional family system by altering the way family members deal with conflict, communication patterns, interpersonal needs, and domestic responsibilities.

TREATMENT ISSUES

There are some treatment issues that are experienced by the whole treatment team. Each member of the team should be aware of, and ready to resolve, such issues, whether individually or in the group.

Table 8-3. The Twelve Steps of Alcoholics Anonymous

Step One: We admitted that we were powerless over alcohol—that our lives had become unmanageable.

Step Two: Came to believe that a power greater than ourselves could restore us to sanity.

Step Three: Made a decision to turn our will and our lives over to the care of God as we understand him.

Step Four: Made a searching and fearless moral inventory of ourselves.

Step Five: Admitted to God, to ourselves, and to another human being the exact nature of our wrongs.

Step Six: Were entirely ready to have God remove all these defects of character.

Step Seven: Humbly asked God to remove all our shortcomings.

Step Eight: Made a list of all persons we had harmed, and became willing to make amends to them all.

Step Nine: Made direct amends to such people where ever possible, except when to do so would injure them or others.

Step Ten: Continued to take personal inventory and when we were wrong promptly admitted it.

Step Eleven: Sought through prayer and meditation to improve our conscious contact with God as we understood him, praying only for the knowledge of his will for us and the power to carry that out.

Step Twelve: Having had a spiritual awakening as the result of these steps, we tried to carry this message to alcoholics and to practice these principles in all our affairs.

Source: Alcoholics Anonymous (1955).

Denial and the Defense System in Addiction

The denial system consists of all the attitudes, behaviors, and beliefs that serve to maintain the addictive process (Zimberg et al., 1985). In the initial stages of treatment, the substance-dependent individual's denial system needs to be identified and emphatically challenged. Defensive communication styles, such as minimizing and rationalizing, and maladaptive interpersonal coping mechanisms that maintain the addiction need to be unlearned. Frequently a direct, sometimes confrontational, approach is necessary to help patients overcome their minimization, rationalization, and denial (see Table 8-4).

CASE ILLUSTRATION: JULIE (MINIMIZING AND RATIONALIZING) AND STAN (DENIAL)

Julie was induced to come for treatment by her employer after a coworker reported her for smelling of alcohol at work. Julie believed that she had conquered her previous cocaine addiction because she has been able to limit her use to weekends, and she felt in control of her drinking because she drank at

Table 8-4. Commonly Occurring Defenses in Addiction

1. Minimization—attempting to downplay the negative impact of the behavior—"I only drink after work and on weekends. . . . It's only been a problem for the last few years."

2. Rationalization—attempting to create a "rational" explanation for the drug use (which usually makes no sense)—"Alcohol helps me be more creative. . . . Pot is an organic natural weed, not a drug like heroin. . . . I need to do a few lines of cocaine to keep up with the kids and the housework."

3. Blame—holding others responsible for your choices and actions—"The pressure at work is so intense that I need a few drinks to relax. . . . My son is fat and lazy, and I drink because I can't stand seeing what he is doing to himself."

4. Denial—disregarding the obvious truth of a situation—"I was not that drunk. . . . The reason I have four DUI citations is that the police in this town are out to get me."

---

a local tavern in the company of friends instead of alone at home as she had in years past. Julie felt that she had been unjustly "caught" just when she actually had it "all under control."

Stan denied using any substance other than alcohol. He explained his urine test, which came back positive for cocaine, as follows: "Someone must have snuck it [the cocaine] into the vodka I was drinking." He disappeared from treatment immediately after being asked to provide another urine sample.

Discussion

Both Julie and Stan displayed active denial even after admitting they had substance abuse problems. Julie did respond to the treatment process and later recognized her minimizing and rationalizing defenses. Stan returned after several days' absence but was unable to be honest about his addictions. He took himself out of the program after a few weeks.

In order to address the addictive person's denial system, recovery programs place heavy emphasis on individual responsibility for behavior, attitude change, and an acceptance of responsibility for the past.

Enabling by the Staff and Codependency

Health care professionals sometimes unknowingly support a patient's addictive process, including denial. This can occur when the health care provider is insecure or unsure about how to best set limits on inappropriate behavior without offending the patient. This unwitting support of the addiction is also called enabling. Examples of a therapist's enabling behaviors include not confronting a patient when there is a concern about relapse, allowing the patient to blame others for his problems, bending the rules for the patient, and keeping secrets for him or her. For example, Julie, an OTR in an outpatient program, had overheard a patient, Don, bragging to the other patients at lunch about using marijuana over the weekend. Julie incorrectly hesitated to tell other staff because she felt she had been "eavesdropping" on a private conversation.

Setting limits on unacceptable behavior is an important staff function, with which every team member needs to be comfortable. This is especially important for patients who are in active denial of their addiction problem and are resistant to the treatment process. Such patients are adept at finding the "weak link" in the chain of treatment providers and may unconsciously attempt to sabotage their recovery through manipulative behavior. Treatment team members can thus become drawn into the patients' unhealthy ways of relating.

Many individuals with an early onset of addictions have failed to move through the normal emotional developmental milestones (Brown, 1985). Remaining emotionally immature, they may act very similarly to adolescents, with behavior that is rebellious, temperamental, demanding, and sometimes dishonest. For these individuals, learning how to be responsible, accountable, mature, and independent adults is a process that occurs gradually in recovery, sometimes taking 3 to 10 years (Royce, 1981).

CASE ILLUSTRATION: BILL—
IMMATURE BEHAVIOR IN TREATMENT

Bill is a 32-year-old businessman in treatment for cocaine and alcohol addiction. He is socially gregarious and frequently flirtatious with the staff and female patients. He has a strong sense of entitlement and devalues the occupational therapy cooking group. On several occasions during his treatment, Bill slipped out of the group and into a nearby vacant office to make personal phone calls. When confronted by the OTR about his absence from the activity, Bill attempted to be flirtatious and evasive, saying, "Oh, sweetie, I didn't know you cared so much about me," while placing his arms around the therapist and asking loudly in front of the rest of the patients: "Are you feeling better now that I am back? I promise to make it up to you; here, let me get the rest of these people organized." Bill abruptly walked off and busily participated in the remaining activities. When approached individually, Bill dismissively said: "My business calls are more important than your class on cooking burgers. I always eat out anyway." He was quite angry when he was further confronted about his dishonesty and disrespectful behavior of sneaking into a private office. Bill proceeded to create a snide nickname for the OTR and engage in subtly hostile adolescent teasing whenever he was in her groups.

Discussion

Overlooking inappropriate behaviors can impede, hinder, and even damage the therapeutic process. The occupational therapist in this case should monitor her own actions and attitudes, taking care not to react to defensive hostility and rejection from the patient. Supervision and team meetings can help the staff develop skills and gain comfort in setting firm and therapeutic bounds for working with chemically dependent patients. In this example, the occupational therapist met with the patient, reviewed the goals of the group, clearly stated the behavioral expectations, and also outlined the consequences of noncompliance. She suggested that the patient use individual or group psychotherapy to explore his resistance to treatment, devaluing of the staff, and indirect communication style.

OCCUPATIONAL THERAPY CONTEXT OF TREATMENT

The occupational therapist treats the chemically dependent patient as a member of a treatment team whose composition will vary somewhat depending on the treatment setting. In a hospital, the team is led by a physician (usually an internist, psychiatrist, or addiction medicine specialist), who supervises medical aspects of the treatment, often with the assistance of a nurse. Other team members may include a social worker or counselor, who provides family treatment, individual therapy, case management, and group treatment; a chaplain, who can be available to address spiritual concerns of the patient; and a dietitian for individual nutrition concerns. In a nonmedical setting, the team will probably be smaller and may be led by a clinical supervisor such as a psychologist, social worker, or physician, with counselors trained in chemical dependency and recovery (Nace, 1993).

It is always important for the occupational therapist to have direct and frequent communication with all members of the team. This usually happens in treatment planning or case conferences, where the specifics of the case, including discharge planning, are discussed. The occupational therapist contributes by reporting the results of functional assessments, observations of patient progress toward identified goals, and recommendations for discharge planning.

The use and abuse of substances in our society is so widespread that all occupational therapists are likely to encounter dependent or addicted individuals in the course of their professional careers. Whether in a skilled nursing facility, general hospital, pediatric clinic, day treatment, or partial hospitalization program, occupational therapists must be alert to the possibility that substance abuse is, or will be, an issue in treatment.

Functional Deficits and Domains of Concern

In considering the functional deficits of individuals with substance dependency diagnoses, it is useful to review occupational therapy's domains of concern as delineated in the AOTA *Uniform Terminology for Occupational Therapy, Third Edition* (AOTA, 1994) (see Table 8-5). Individuals with substance abuse problems can have deficits in all three domains of concern. Deficits in sensorimotor, cognitive, and psychosocial performance components affect all performance areas of work, leisure, and self-care. The temporal and environmental aspects of addiction must also be recognized and considered. General interventions are necessary and more suitable at different times in the process of treatment.

Performance Areas

Functional impairments can be seen primarily in the leisure and work performance areas.

Leisure. Functional impairments in the chemically dependent population often are evident initially in leisure areas, becoming quite pronounced as the individual gives up valued pursuits to devote more time to the acquisition and use of the addictive substance. For example, an alcoholic may drop out of the softball team to spend more time at the bar; a cocaine addict may neglect family outings to make a connection with a drug dealer.

Work. The social and economic value of work often strongly motivates addicted individuals to continue working until the progression of the disease interferes. However, physiological and psychological effects of addiction often result in decreased concentration, poor judgment, poor problem-solving skills, increased absenteeism, and poor time management. Therefore, addicted individuals may be required by employers or the legal system to seek treatment or face losing their jobs.

Table 8-5.   Occupational Therapy Domains of Concern

Performance areas: broad categories of human activity that are typically part of daily life, including activities of daily living, work and other productive activities, and play or leisure

Performance components: fundamental human abilities that are required for successful engagement in performance areas and include the sensorimotor, cognitive, psychosocial, and psychological

Performance contexts: situations or factors that influence an individual's engagement in desired performance areas

---

Performance Components

There is ample evidence that prolonged substance abuse affects many performance components.

Sensorimotor and perceptual-motor.   Significant impairments in sensorimotor and perceptual-motor function (defined as the ability to interpret sensory information and manipulate the self and objects) sometimes occur with prolonged abuse, especially of alcohol. Losses in tactile perception, figure-ground perception, visual-spatial functions, and fine motor coordination have been recorded in alcoholics (Van Deusen, 1989), with the greatest impairments evident in the area of visual-spatial function. Improvements have been noted with prolonged recovery; however, some losses may be irreversible and need to be compensated for.

Cognition.   Neurocognitive deficits have been demonstrated in as many as 75 percent of persons entering alcohol treatment (Butters & Cermak, 1980). Many areas are affected, especially memory, attention span, concept formation, problem solving, and learning. Although some of these areas show recovery after two to three weeks of sobriety, in other areas there may be a permanent loss of function. Areas of loss can include abstract reasoning, nonverbal problem solving, short-term memory, and perceptual-motor integration.

Psychosocial and psychological.   Many psychosocial skills are affected by substance abuse, including values, self-image, interpersonal and role-related skills, and self-management skills such as time management and coping (Mann & Talty, 1991; Moyers, 1991; Stoffel, Cusatis, Seitz, & Jones, 1992).

As the individual's substance abuse increases, his or her actions may be in conflict with deeply held values, such as honesty and responsibility. For example, Marsha, a home health aide, addicted to narcotics and benzodiazepines, began diverting drugs from her patients when she could no longer get them from her doctor.

Self-image and self-esteem suffer as the individual experiences losing control of his or her behavior. Poor interpersonal skills including dishonesty regarding the drug use, argumentative communication patterns, difficulties resolving conflicts, and avoidance and withdrawal may be present. For example, after entering treatment, Rick admitted that he would often pick a fight with his wife so he could justify his need to "cool off" with several drinks at the bar.

Poor stress management and coping skills can contribute to both initial drug use and increased usage levels. Drugs and alcohol tend to be used, to the exclusion of other coping skills, to enable individuals to tolerate unpleasant situations and difficult emotions. The expression of emotions in general is difficult for people with chemical dependency (Royce, 1981). Emotions that are perceived as intolerable, such as sadness, fear, anger, and loneliness, can

be anesthetized with substances, effectively also "numbing out" the individual's ability to experience joy, happiness, and excitement. Many chemically dependent people do not know how to moderate the expression of anger before
it turns into rage or leads to rejection by others. The negative consequences
of these deficits can be job loss, marital separation, loss of child custody, and
the alienation of prior support networks, such as friends and family.

Performance Contexts

Consideration must be given to the context of the substance abuse, and especially the developmental, cultural, and social aspects. For example, does the
patient drink or use alone or with others? Does he or she go to bars as a way
to meet people? Is there adolescent peer pressure to try the latest drug? Is a
lonely widow or widower self-medicating grief? What are the cultural norms
of the patient regarding substance abuse? Most important, how will the positive values of the patient's sociocultural community be strengthened through
treatment and the recovery process? These are critical factors that will guide
the treatment planning and implementation process and serve to either foster success or impede progress. For example, it is not sufficient to simply tell
the patient not to drink if, in the community to which he or she belongs, most
socializing occurs in the bars.

TREATMENT PLANNING

Occupational therapy and other rehabilitation services bring a functional perspective to the treatment of substance abuse that is often lacking in cognitively
based treatment programs. Because of the toxic action of chemicals on the
brain, chemically dependent individuals may not be able to function as well
as they appear to be, and they may experience significant cognitive limitations,
especially in early recovery.

Assessment

Occupational therapy assessment provides information regarding strengths
and weakness in the performance of culturally relevant roles and aids in developing an occupational therapy diagnosis, that is, in understanding and analyzing the patient's occupational behavior and needs.

Occupational therapy assessment of the chemically dependent patient
should consider the biological, psychological, and social impairments that have
resulted from the substance abuse. Assessment and specific occupational therapy evaluations should consider all performance areas, components, and contexts, but the process may be modified or condensed if time constraints exist.

Goals

The overall goal of the occupational therapist working with people who are chemically dependent is to support the development of a functional, recovery-oriented, abstinence-based lifestyle. As part of a multidisciplinary team, the therapist must make sure that the identified goals are relevant to the level of treatment, overall direction of treatment, and, most important, the patient's own priorities (Moyers, 1988).

Goals should always be set in consultation with the patient but with some caution about achievability. Unrealistic expectations for performance can lead to frustration, a sense of failure, and lower self-esteem for the patient and therapist.

CASE ILLUSTRATION: TANYA—EARLY RECOVERY

Tanya, who had only a few months' sobriety after 10 years of alcohol abuse and social isolation, wanted to attend her niece's wedding. Even though she had developed a relapse prevention plan for the event, Tanya underestimated both the degree of emotional stress inherent in the event and her vulnerable self-esteem. She stayed sober during the wedding and reception but then became depressed and drank all weekend. When she returned to her treatment program, she worked with the OTR to develop a specific behavioral plan for similar future events. She reexamined her choices and came to understand that a better course would have been to go to the ceremony but skip the reception.

Discussion

Tanya realized that she had been unrealistic about her goals, and although she did feel a sense of failure, she felt hopeful that in the future she would understand what the OTR meant when she mentioned goal "achievability."

Intervention

A useful model (Moyers, 1992b) for establishing goals and interventions conceptualizes phases of the recovery process that correspond to the levels of treatment (see Table 8-6).

First level, or phase, of treatment.   The **preferred defense structure** (PDS) of the patient at this level of treatment is the need to externalize locus of control. This means that in order to maintain sobriety, the patient accepts the need for treatment and allows the treatment team to provide the necessary support and structure. Counseling is generally directive and supportive. The patient may be going through a medically supervised detoxification process lasting from a few days to a few weeks. Occupational therapy treatment focuses on normalizing routines of daily living, organizing temporal be-

Table 8-6. Stage of Recovery/Levels of Treatment

Treatment level	One	Two	Three
Preferred Defense Structure	Need to externalize locus of control, accept help	Develop internal locus of control, be responsible for behavior	Develop insight into origins of behavior
Patient goals	Maintain early sobriety, accept need for treatment, stabilize daily routines	Develop healthy coping strategies, develop capacity for cooperative social interactions	Return to work/productive roles, grieve losses, maintain ongoing recovery plan
OT Treatment Focus	Normalize ADL routines, provide structure to increase temporal organization, begin to regain cognitive-perceptual abilities, increase self-esteem	Communication skills, stress management, problem solving, leisure interests, clarify values and interests	Return to work, self-awareness, self-expression, promote healthy family interactions, conflict resolution
OT Treatment Modalities	Fitness/body awareness, structured task groups, daily life management, meal preparation, structured leisure activities	Assertive communication, stress management, relaxation training, interest checklists, sports activities, community outings	Prevocational training, expressive therapy, psychoeducational topic groups (i.e., grief work, family issues)
Group Types	Parallel, project, thematic	Egocentric-cooperative, thematic	Cooperative, mature, task, instrumental

Source: Adapted from Moyers (1992). Group structure is based on that developed by Mosey (1970, 1981).
Note: The preferred defense structure (PDS) of the patient distinguishes the phases of the recovery process. The PDS changes over time and signifies progress in treatment. Levels of treatment correspond to stages of recovery.

haviors into routines and patterns, and beginning to regain cognitive and perceptual motor abilities.

Second level, or phase, of treatment. The PDS is the need to develop an internal locus of control and learn to be responsible for one's behavior. In accepting responsibility for behavior, the patient focuses on developing healthy coping strategies to replace unhealthy ones. These include learning to express emotions assertively, seek help when needed, and use relaxation techniques to control tension. The newly recovering person at this stage of treatment benefits from activities that promote cooperative social interaction, such as cooking, structured socialization, and community outings. Stress management and relaxation-training techniques could also be included at this level.

Therapy in this early stage is behaviorally and cognitively focused. For example, many times substance-addicted individuals have difficulty assertively saying no to invitations to drink or use. Role-playing and group activities focused on learning and practicing refusal skills can be quite beneficial. Cognitive therapy approaches can help the patient deal with persistent, obsessive thoughts of drug use and relapse.

Starting or increasing a regular fitness routine can help manage stress, develop healthy body awareness, and promote increased sensorimotor functioning. Persons recovering from chemical dependency often have a strong interest in sports and physical activities (Stoffel et al., 1992) and may appreciate opportunities to rebuild fitness levels while engaging in meaningful activities.

Third level, or phase, of treatment.   The PDS is the need to develop insight into the origins and consequences of addictive behavior. Patients often become depressed and ashamed as they realize much they have lost control of their lives and have hurt others because of their addiction. There is a need to grieve the losses created by the addictive behavior, such as the loss of a job, relationships, financial stability, or health. Patients also need to say good-bye to the addictive substances, their own addictive behaviors, and their substance-user identities and must learn new ways to live in the world. Educational topics can include the grief cycle and process. Activities that increase self-awareness, self-concept, and self-esteem are especially appropriate for patients in level three treatment.

As patients begin to develop responsibility and a sense of effectiveness in their environment, they can start to work with family members to repair damaged relationships. Treatment progresses, as patients solidify earlier treatment gains and look toward discharge. It is appropriate at this stage of treatment to focus on a return to work through the introduction of conflict resolution and job-stress management skills. Decision making, time management, and values clarification are also important skills to be gained in the rehabilitation process. See Table 8-7 for examples of useful interventions at all levels.

Group Treatment

Group treatment settings are especially appropriate for chemically dependent individuals since many people with alcoholic and addictive disorders

Table 8-7. Useful Interventions in Occupational Performance

Performance Areas

Self-Care	Work/School	Leisure
Instruction and practice in shopping, meal preparation, home maintenance, money management, budgeting, and community mobility.	Practice in developing job seeking, getting, and keeping skills; improvement of work habits such as punctuality, following directions, handling job stress, and seeking out community educational resources; assistance with resume preparation, interview techniques, and completion of job applications. Work skills task groups enable the therapist to observe and shape work-related behaviors.	Opportunities to try a variety of leisure activities, determine leisure time use preferences, and plan and implement rewarding leisure activities. Could include sports, games, hobbies, and community activities.

Performance Components

Sensory/ Perceptual-Motor	Cognitive	Psychological/ Psychosocial
Crafts and other tasks requiring fine motor coordination, group exercises to improve endurance flexibility, fitness and muscle tone. Introduce the patient to recreational activities that can potentially increase fine and gross motor coordination—dance, martial arts, hobbies, and sports.	Groups and activities requiring the development of concentration, time management, problem-solving, and decision-making skills—could be crafts, group projects or cooking activities. Psychoeducational approaches help the patient learn about the effects of drug use, healthy coping strategies, and available community resources.	Training and practice in anger management, stress management, assertive communication, and social interaction skills through topic and activity groups. Expressive modalities and creative activities promote increased self-awareness and -identification and the expression of feelings. Identify strengths and weaknesses, such as in art, writing, dance, drama, or music. Activities that increase self-esteem and self-confidence include crafts projects, volunteer work, and service to others through AA or other twelve step involvement.

tend to be socially and emotionally isolative, to drink and/or use alone, and to have great difficulty tolerating conflict or relating socially. Group settings can help create a sense of belonging and acceptance that puts the newly recovering individual at ease. Group treatment settings provide opportunities to decrease social isolation, learn new interpersonal skills, and practice reintegration into social settings such as family or work environments.

Relating in a group setting to others with addictions also facilitates the acceptance of a personal identification as a recovering alcoholic or addict and helps overcome the feelings of guilt, shame and denial that often accompany the illness. The support available at Alcoholics Anonymous and other twelve step meetings can help keep the patient focused on the value of abstinence and the benefits of social support. A willingness to follow through with aftercare recommendations has been shown to be essential to maintaining ongoing abstinence and preventing relapse (Zimberg et al., 1985).

Useful group structures include thematic and task groups with either a parallel or a cooperative structure. Groups can address deficits specific to the addictive process. They are particularly useful if they are both cognitive and behavioral, that is, if they address both thoughts and actions concerning various themes or topics.

Task groups, both parallel and cooperative (such as crafts, expressive therapy, cooking, and community events) have a special place in the treatment of chemically dependent (CD) individuals (Stensrud & Lushbough, 1988). Patients report finding the aspects of socializing and task engagement helpful and enjoyable, especially as most CD treatment programs are instead very verbally and cognitively focused. Task groups also provide opportunities for patients to tap into creative and symbolic aspects of the self and increase self-esteem, concentration, handling frustration, problem solving, and error recognition skills.

Structure and predictability are important aspects of recovery programs. Occupational therapy groups designated with a descriptive title (e.g., "communication skills") help patients more easily focus on the group and also educate other staff regarding the contributions of OT to the treatment process. Table 8-8 describes a typical treatment program structured specifically for those who are chemically dependent.

Individual patients benefit from individual occupational therapy interventions as needed for specific functional deficits. These could include parenting skills, money management, meal planning and preparation, accessing public transportation, or home management skills.

Occupational therapists are also working as case managers in many settings, coordinating patient care from initial intake procedures through treatment coordination to discharge. This is a new and challenging role, but one that is supported by the theoretical and philosophical foundations of the profession, especially as it directs occupational therapists to consider the treatment of the whole person.

Table 8-8. Prototype Occupational Therapy Program

Time	Group	Staff	Purpose	Group Type
7:30 A.M.	Fitness	OT	Increase flexibility, coordination, endurance; decrease depression, anxiety	Parallel
8:30 A.M.	Community meeting	All	Establish group milieu, review patient goals, go over daily schedule	Task
9:00 A.M.	OT task group: crafts, cooking, work projects	OT	Develop abilities to increase concentration, cooperative work skills, task completion	Parallel or cooperative
10:00 A.M.	Group therapy	Social Work, Nursing, CD counselor	Explore issues and feelings related to substance abuse, relationships, family	Mature, cooperative
11:30 A.M.	Individual counseling	Varies/case manager	Address individual treatment issues	
12:00 noon	Lunch	Sometimes prepared cooperatively		
1:00 P.M.	Psycho-education group	OT or other staff	Address knowledge deficits of patients in areas such as stress management, assertive communication, leisure skills	Instrumental
2:00 P.M.	Chemical dependency lecture	CD counselor	Focus on recovery process, including relapse prevention, twelve step groups, family systems	Instrumental, mature
3:00 P.M.	Free time			

(continues)

Table 8-8. Prototype Occupational Therapy Program (continued)

Time	Group	Staff	Purpose	Group Type
5:00 P.M.	Dinner	Sometimes prepared cooperatively		
6:00 P.M.	Family support group or leisure skills	OT/Recreation Therapist/CD	Involve family in recovery	Cooperative
8:00 P.M.	Wrap-up	Varies	Reflect on treatment day, progress toward goals	Mature

Source: Group structure is based on that developed by Mosey (1970, 1981)
Note: The structure of the daily program is designed to promote the normalizing of life patterns, regulation of routines, and incorporation of cognitive, affective, and behavioral elements (thinking, feeling, and doing) into each day's treatment.

CASE ILLUSTRATION: JILL— DUAL-DIAGNOSIS OCCUPATIONAL THERAPY

Jill is a 48-year-old female admitted to a psychiatric partial hospitalization program after a brief stay on an inpatient unit for acute depression and suicidal ideation, which was partly precipitated by conflicts with her adult daughter and difficulties in her new part-time job. Jill has been sober (off alcohol) for 6 years, but she is clinically depressed, has a pattern of binge eating, abuses prescription pain medications, and is frequently suicidal or self-destructive. Jill was sexually abused by her stepfather as a child and has been in several abusive relationships as an adult. She used to work as a massage therapist but has been on disability for the past year. She is not currently attending AA groups, although she has done so in the past, and she does see an outpatient therapist once weekly.

Jill's expected length of stay in the program is five weeks, on a schedule of decreasing days of attendance. The first week, Jill will attend five days; the second week, four days; and so on. The overall treatment goals for Jill are to stabilize her on antidepressant medications, have her withdraw from addictive pain medications, teach her pain management techniques, decrease her depression and suicidal ideation, improve her overall coping skills, and reconnect her to community supports.

According to the occupational therapy assessment, Jill has problems in her instrumental activities of daily living, including money management, eating and fitness routines, stress management, and time management. In the interpersonal area, Jill has poor communication skills and responds either passively or aggressively in conflictual situations. She also has great difficulty accurately identifying and expressing feelings, especially "difficult" ones like anger, sad-

ness, and hurt. Her responses in the structured interview and task observation portions of the OT assessment indicate low self-esteem and a pattern of highly critical self-talk. Jill is unable to function effectively in the work sphere, partly because of these functional deficits.

As the patient progressed in treatment, she was able to attend most scheduled days, participate in milieu groups and activities, and meet as planned with the OT. She identified being asked to baby-sit her infant granddaughter as stressful, and practiced assertively setting limits with her daughter on this issue. She also learned progressive relaxation techniques to use when feeling more anxious or in physical pain, as she had tended to binge-eat or abuse medications at these times. She learned about healthy eating, started carrying healthy snacks with her to the program, and reported intermittent success with meal preparation at home.

Jill began the process of exploring vocational options. She decided that her current job of telephone solicitor was too much pressure and that returning to massage therapy work while dealing with her sexual abuse issues was not a good idea. She decided instead to take a career exploration class at the local junior college and do volunteer work while living on disability compensation. She also tried to schedule more frequent meetings with friends for social events such as walks, coffee, or movies, and she began attending a weekly women's AA meeting. At discharge, she was seeing her outpatient therapist once weekly, was off pain medications, was no longer suicidal, and had daily scheduled activities four days a week.

Discussion

Occupational therapy goals and interventions are as follows.

1. *Patient will learn and practice two new techniques to reduce stress and manage pain without medications by the end of the first week. Techniques: fitness group, diaphragmatic breathing, progressive relaxation, distracting activity (see Chapter 12, which also discusses stress management techniques for anxiety)*
2. *Patient will make and follow a weekly schedule of activities designed to increase daily structure and opportunities for socialization with friends by the end of the second week. Techniques: weekly goals group, daily log of activities, regular check-in with OT and peers, attendance at twelve step meetings*
3. *Patient will plan, shop for, and prepare one nutritionally balanced meal per day by the end of the third week. Techniques: nutrition group, community lunch, individual meeting with OT, shopping trip to the supermarket*
4. *Patient will identify and express feelings accurately to peers and staff at least one time per treatment day, as evidenced by an "I feel" statement, by the end of the third week. Techniques: expressive art therapy activities, journal writing, assertive communication role-plays*

Summary

The abuse of alcohol and other substances in the United States is a major social and health problem, contributing to illness, injury, and disability. Many theories exist regarding the causes of substance abuse, including the biological, genetic, psychological, and sociocultural. Treatment approaches include cognitive-behavioral, psychodynamic, medically based, and social rehabilitation models.

Occupational therapists play a vital role in the treatment of individuals with chemical dependency, from assessment to discharge planning. The occupational therapist provides a focus on improving the function of the individual to live a more productive and satisfying life, which is free of drugs and alcohol, through activity-based aspects of treatment.

Review Questions

1. Name three categories of psychoactive substances and some of their effects on behavior.
2. Describe three treatment approaches. How do they differ? How are they alike?
3. Name three functional deficits typical of chemically dependent individuals.
4. Name three treatment interventions that you could use to address the deficits named in (3).
5. What are some interpersonal issues that may arise in treating chemically dependent individuals? How would you deal with them?
6. What performance components or areas would be addressed by a fitness group? A stress management group? A task group? What other types of groups or activities would be helpful for this population?

Learning Activities

1. Attend an open Alcoholics Anonymous or other twelve step meeting. Listen as people share their stories. Especially note when they describe the "unmanageability" of their drinking lives. How do these stories relate to functional impairments? As an occupational therapist, how could you be of help to such individuals?
2. Visit a chemical dependency program in your area. Talk with staff and clients and try to get a sense of how functional deficits are addressed.
3. Think of some of your own addictive behaviors or obsessive thinking, such as eating chocolate, drinking coffee, or smoking. What would it be like for you to stop right now? How could a group support you in quitting?

4. What image do you form when you hear the words "substance abuser" or "addict"? Do your images and views match common stereotypes? How could you challenge your own biases?
5. Visit some local bookstores and browse through the sections on self-help and recovery.

References

Alcoholics Anonymous. (1955). *Alcoholics Anonymous: The story of how many thousands of men and women have recovered from alcoholism* (Rev. ed.). New York: Alcoholics Anonymous World Services.

American Occupational Therapy Association (AOTA). (1994). *Uniform terminology for occupational therapy* (3rd ed.). Rockville, MD: AOTA.

American Psychiatric Association (APA). (1994). *Diagnostic and statistical manual of mental disorders* (4th ed.). Washington, DC: APA.

Blume, S. B., Neider, J. R., Suemnick, S., & Westermeyer, J. (1991). Introduction and overview. In J. Westermeyer & R. S. Krug (Eds.), *Substance abuse services: A guide to planning and management* (pp. 1–20). Chicago, IL: American Hospital Publishing.

Brehm, N., Khantzain, E. J., & Dodes, L. M. (1993). Psychodynamic approaches. In M. Galanter (Ed.), *Recent developments in alcoholism. Ten years of progress: Social and cultural perspectives, physiology, and biochemistry clinical pathology: Vol. 11. Trends in treatment* (pp. 453–469). New York: Plenum Press.

Brown, S. (1985). *Treating the alcoholic: A developmental model of recovery.* New York: Wiley.

Butters, N., & Cermak, L. S. (1980). *Alcoholic Korsakoff's syndrome: An information processing approach to amnesia.* New York: Academic Press.

Davies, V. E., & Walsch, M. J. (1970). Alcohol, amines and alkaloids: A possible biochemical basis for alcohol addiction. *Science, 167,* 1005–1007.

Deitrich, R. A. (1993). Physiology and biochemistry. In M. Galanter (Ed.), *Recent developments in alcoholism. Ten years of progress: Social and cultural perspectives, physiology, and biochemistry clinical pathology: Vol. 11. Trends in treatment* (pp. 167–178). New York: Plenum Press.

Friehlich, J. C., & Li, T. K. (1993). Opiode peptides. In M. Galanter (Ed.), *Recent developments in alcoholism. Ten years of progress: Social and cultural perspectives, physiology, and biochemistry clinical pathology: Vol. 11. Trends in treatment* (pp. 187–199). New York: Plenum Press.

Goldman, D. (1993). Genetic transmission. In M. Galanter (Ed.), *Recent developments in alcoholism. Ten years of progress: Social and cultural perspectives, physiology, and biochemistry clinical pathology: Vol. 11. Trends in treatment* (pp. 232–244). New York: Plenum Press.

Gomberg, E. L. (1991). Alcoholism: Psychological and physiological aspects. In E. L. Gomberg, H. R. White, & J. A. Carpenter (Eds.), *Alcoholism, sci-*

ence and society revisited (pp. 186–204). Ann Arbor: University of Michigan Press.

Goodwin, D. W. (1991). Alcoholism and heredity: Update on the implacable fate. In E. L. Gomberg, H. R. White, & J. A. Carpenter (Eds.), *Alcoholism, science and society revisited* (pp. 160–170). Ann Arbor: University of Michigan Press.

Herman, J. (1992). *Trauma and recovery.* New York: HarperCollins.

Inaba, D. S., & Cohen, W. E. (1993). *Uppers, downers, and all arounders: Physical and mental effects of psychoactive drugs* (2nd ed.). Ashland, OR.: CNS Productions.

Keller, M. (1991) . Alcohol, science and society: Hindsight and forecast. In E. L. Gomberg, H. R. White, & J. A. Carpenter (Eds.), *Alcoholism, science and society revisited* (pp. 1–17). Ann Arbor: University of Michigan Press.

Mann, W., & Talty, P. (1991). Leisure activity profile measuring use of leisure time by persons with alcoholism. *Occupational Therapy in Mental Health, 10* (4), 31–41.

Morgenstern, J., & Leeds, J. (1993). Contemporary psychoanalytic theories of substance abuse: A disorder in search of a paradigm. *Psychotherapy, 30*(2), 194–206.

Mosey, A. C. (1970). The concept and use of developmental groups. *American Journal of Occupational Therapy, 24,* 272.

Mosey, A. C. (1981). *Occupational therapy: Configuration of a profession.* New York: Raven.

Moyers, P. (1988). An organizational framework for occupational therapy in the treatment of alcoholism. *Occupational Therapy in Mental Health, 8,* 27–46.

Moyers, P. (1991). Occupational therapy and treatment of the alcoholic's family. *Occupational Therapy in Mental Health, 11*(1), 45–64.

Moyers, P. (1992a). Occupational therapy intervention with the alcoholic's family. *American Journal of Occupational Therapy, 46*(2), 105–111.

Moyers, P. (1992b). *Substance abuse: A multi-dimensional assessment and treatment approach.* Thorofare, NJ: Slack.

Myers, R. D. (1978). Tetrahydroisoquinolines in the brain: The basis of an animal model of alcoholism. *Alcoholism: Clinical and Experimental Research, 2,* 145–154.

Nace, E. P. (1993). Inpatient treatment. In M. Galanter (Ed.), *Recent developments in alcoholism. Ten years of progress: Social and cultural perspectives, physiology, and biochemistry clinical pathology: Vol. 11. Trends in treatment* (pp. 429–499). New York: Plenum Press.

National Institute on Alcohol Abuse and Alcoholism (NIAAA). (1978). *Alcohol and Health.* Rockville, MD: NIAA.

Pires, M. (1989). Substance abuse: The silent saboteur in rehabilitation. *Nursing Clinics of North America, 24*(1), 109–120.

Rothschild, D. E. (1992). Treating the substance abuser: Psychotherapy throughout the recovery process. In B. Wallace (Ed.), *The chemically de-*

pendent: *Phases of treatment and recovery* (pp. 82–91). New York: Brunner/Mazel.

Royce, J. E. (1981). *Alcohol problems and alcoholism.* New York: Free Press.

Schuckit, M. A., & Hagland, R. (1978). An overview of the etiologic theories of alcoholism. In N. J. Estes & M. E. Heinman (Eds.), *Alcoholism: Development, consequences and interventions.* St. Louis: Mosby.

Stensrude, M. K., & Lushbough, R. S. (1988). The implementation of an occupational therapy program in an alcohol and drug dependency treatment center. *Occupational Therapy in Mental Health, 8* (2):1–15.

Stoffel, V., Cusatis, M., Seitz, L., & Jones, N. (1992). Self-esteem and leisure patterns of persons in a residential chemical dependency treatment program. *Occupational Therapy and Psychosocial Dysfunction,* 69–85.

Tarter, R. E. (1983). The causes of alcoholism: A biopsychosocial analysis. In E. Gottheil, K. Druley, T. Skoloda, & H. Waxman (Eds.), *Ethological aspects of alcohol and drug abuse.* Springfield, Ill: Charles C. Thomas.

Van Deusen, J. (1989). Alcohol abuse and perceptual-motor dysfunction: The occupational therapist's role. *The American Journal of Occupational Therapy, 43* (6), 384–390.

Wallace, B. C. (1992). Multi-dimensional relapse prevention from a biopsychosocial perspective across phases of recovery. In B. Wallace (Ed.), *The chemically dependent: Phases of treatment and recovery* (pp. 82–91). New York: Brunner/Mazel.

White, H. R. (1991). Sociological theories of the etiology of alcoholism. In E.L. Gomberg, H.R. White & J. A. Carpenter (Eds.), *Alcoholism, science and society revisited* (pp. 205–232). Ann Arbor: The University of Michigan Press.

Zimberg, S., Wallace, J., & Blume, S. E. (1985). *Practical Approaches to Alcoholism Psychotherapy.* New York: Plenum Press.

Zweben, J. E. (1992). Issues in the treatment of the dual-diagnosis patient. In B. Wallace (Ed.), *The chemically dependent: Phases of treatment and recovery* (pp. 298–309). New York: Brunner/Mazel.

Suggested Reading

Alcoholics Anonymous. (1976). *The story of how thousands of men and women have recovered from alcoholism* ("The Big Book"). New York: Alcoholics Anonymous World Services, Inc.

Alcoholics Anonymous. (1984). *Pass it on.* New York: Alcoholics Anonymous World Services, Inc.

Black, Claudia. (1981). *It will never happen to me.* New York: Balantine Books.

Black, Claudia. (1985). *Repeat after me.* Denver: M.A.C. Printing and Publications.

Inaba, Darryl S., & Cohen, William E. (1993). *Uppers, downers, and all arounders.* Ashland: CNS Productions, Inc.

Johnson, Vernon. (1980). *I'll quit tomorrow*. New York: Harper and Row.

Milam, James R., & Ketcham, Katherine. (1981).*Under the influence*. New York: Bantam Books.

Moore, D. T. (1986). Reversal of alcohol effects, acute and chronic conditions. *Alcohol world, health and research, 11*(78), 52–59.

Schizophrenia

Anne MacRae

Key Terms

cognitive deficits
negative symptoms
positive symptoms

psychosis
psychotropic

Chapter Outline

Introduction

Schizophrenia is a common disorder affecting approximately 1 in every 100 people. According to the National Institute of Mental Health (NIMH), approximately 2 million people will develop schizophrenia in their lifetime.

The disorder of schizophrenia has probably existed as long as humankind, but it has been interpreted in various physical, emotional, and spiritual ways by different generations and cultures. Even after the condition was recognized as a specific disease entity, diagnostic criteria have varied historically as well as geographically. In other words, depending on when and where diagnosticians were trained, they may or may not agree on the diagnosis of schizophrenia. Kraeplin (1919/1971) was one of the first European clinicians to recognize schizophrenia as a specific disease process. He called the condition Dementia Praecox because of its relatively early onset (usually in young adulthood) and its tendency to produce cognitive and behavioral changes in the individual. Bleuler (1911/1950) concluded that the term Dementia Praecox was essentially inadequate because there was not always cognitive deterioration and the disorder was not necessarily degenerative, as had been thought by Kraeplin. It was Bleuler who first suggested that schizophrenia was really one of several possible diseases that present in similar fashion. Therefore, he suggested that the term Dementia Praecox be replaced with *the group of schizophrenias*. Current diagnostic criteria have been strongly influenced by Kurt Schneider 's (1959) identification of "first rank" symptoms of schizophrenia. These symptoms primarily consist of hallucinations (auditory especially), delusions, and bizarre behavior. This emphasis on the psychotic, or "positive," symptomatology of the disorder may not give an accurate representation of the functional level of people with schizophrenia.

Schizophrenia is referred to as a thought disorder, but not all forms of the disorder include long-term **cognitive deficits**. It is also referred to as a psychotic disorder, yet **psychosis** may be present only for some period during the course of the disease, not as a chronic condition. Both the terms *psychotic* and *thought disorder* could be applied to other conditions and lack the specificity needed to accurately identify schizophrenia.

MYTHS AND MISCONCEPTIONS

To this day, the term *schizophrenia* is often misused and the concept is frequently misunderstood. The misconceptions regarding this condition are rampant and must be dispelled before any meaningful understanding can be reached.

Eight Common Myths

Myth no. 1: "Split personality." A person suffering from schizophrenia does not have a split personality. This is an unfortunate, and essentially inaccurate, description. Schizoprenia is not a personality or dissociative disorder. The concept of split personality more accurately describes multiple personality disorder, which is now called, in the DSM-IV, dissociative identity disorder (American Psychiatric Association, 1994).

Myth no. 2: Bad parenting. People with schizophrenia are not a product of bad parenting. No one can cause another person to have schizophrenia. It is caused by a combination of factors, including hereditary predisposition. If someone who inherits the predisposition to schizophrenia is in a particularly stressful environment, the illness may manifest itself earlier, may have greater severity and frequency, and may lead to poorer outcome, but environment alone is not believed to cause the disorder. The vast majority of people who experience even catastrophic levels of stress do not develop schizophrenia. Although the popularity of this myth is waning, it still persists and is particularly damaging and painful to families—the very people who might best support people with schizophrenia.

Myth no. 3: Drug experimentation. Schizophrenia is not caused by taking drugs. It is a complicated disease, not the result of drug experimentation. People who have schizophrenia may have an acute exacerbation if they use certain drugs because of the disinhibiting effect of many substances. Moreover, a prime time for drug experimentation is adolescence and young adulthood, which happens to coincide with the usual onset of schizophrenia. It is not uncommon for people with schizophrenia to have a coexisting diagnosis of substance abuse. In many cases, people with schizophrenia use drugs and alcohol in an maladaptive attempt to control their symptoms and the related distress.

Myth no. 4: Lack of motivation. People with schizophrenia do indeed try to get better. No one wants to have a disorder such as schizophrenia. People who take their prescribed medication and maintain psychosocial support usually fare better, but dysfunction may persist regardless of the level of treatment. **Psychotropic** medications typically dampen or reduce the severity of the more obvious symptoms, but they often fail to eliminate them (Falloon & Talbot, 1981). Recently, a groundbreaking group of atypical antipsychotic agents, including clozapine and risperidone, have been introduced, but even these medications cannot be tolerated by all individuals and are not universally effective (Grace et al., 1996; Menditto et al., 1996; Peuskens, 1995). Maxmen and Ward (1995) state that clozapine and risperidone are effective in about one-third of people with schizophrenia who exhibit resistance to other antipsychotic medication. In other words, there remains a significant minority of people with schizophrenia who continue to display symptoms while taking medication.

There are a variety of reasons why someone may not be compliant with treatment. In some cases, appropriate treatment is simply unavailable. People with schizophrenia benefit the most from consistent and maintained intervention, yet community and outreach programs are scarce. The consequence is a "revolving door" syndrome whereby people decompensate and are recurrently hospitalized. (Further discussion of this dilemma can be found in Chapter 19, "Case Management.")

Myth no. 5: Rising incidence.   The incidence of schizophrenia is not on the rise, and there is no evidence to support the myth that it is increasing. However, modern Western society is stressful, particularly in the urban areas, so there may be a trend for people with schizophrenia to be more seriously disabled by the condition. Moreover, the deinstitutionalization movement created a situation in which people with schizophrenia are more visible in the community. This has had some positive effects but also many negative ones. The National Mental Health Association estimates that 25 to 35 percent of homeless people in the United States have schizophrenia.

Myth no. 6: Institutionalization and disability.   People with schizophrenia do not always live in institutions and are not always profoundly disabled. While it is true that in the past there were greater numbers of people who were institutionalized, they never constituted the majority of people who have schizophrenia. Most people with the disorder live with families, in residential care facilities in the community, or independently. The disorder has the potential for being gravely disabling and it is a serious mental illness. However, the actual functional deficits are highly variable, and it is possible for some people to work, go to school, and raise a family.

Myth no. 7: Low intelligence.   People with schizophrenia do not have below-average intelligence. Instead, the actual range of IQs of people with schizophrenia is highly variable. It is possible to have schizophrenia and be quite brilliant; it is also possible to have a coexisting developmental disability. Many, but not all, people with schizophrenia have a variety of cognitive deficits, but these do not necessarily include decreased intelligence. Rather, the cognitive deficits may include poor abstraction, judgment, and processing time, which can be misinterpreted as low intelligence.

Myth no. 8: Danger and violence.   People with schizophrenia are generally not dangerous and violent. This is a persistent and highly damaging myth largely fostered by the media. The sensationalization of stories such as accounts of the "Son of Sam" murders in New York and assassinations of prominent figures have distorted the facts. People who are actively psychotic, particularly if they are paranoid, sometimes do become very violent, and this can be understandably frightening. Statistically, however, people who have schizophrenia are no more likely to commit a serious crime than people in the general population.

People with psychotic symptoms are more likely to hurt themselves than someone else (MacRae, 1993). Self-inflicted violence includes a wide variety of injuries, including mutilation and starvation. It also unfortunately includes successful suicide attempts. The APA estimates that 10 percent of people with schizophrenia commit suicide (1994). It is also true that family members or significant others may sometimes be the target of violent outbursts (discussed by Calkins and Roth in Chapter 2).

Several recent reports have indicated that violent crimes committed by people with serious mental illness are on the rise. One explanation for this is the increased number of people with dual diagnoses. Clearly, violence related to drug and alcohol use is a significant problem, regardless of whether there is concurrent schizophrenia (see also Chapter 8).

Another explanation for this increase in violence is the shortage of appropriate treatment. As cutbacks in mental health and social services continue, people are forced to do without necessary treatment, become more disenfranchised, and experience both acute exacerbations and gradual decompensations of their illness. It could well be true that if the present trends continue, what started out as a myth about violence may become a self-fulfilling prophecy.

ETIOLOGY OF SCHIZOPHRENIA

Ideas regarding the cause of schizophrenia are constantly changing, but it is now generally accepted that there is some level of organic involvement, and many believe that at least a predisposition to the disease is hereditary. Stress may play a role in the onset of episodes and the severity of the disorder, but it is not the single causative factor.

Much of the neurological information about people with schizophrenia is due to the development of technology, including computerized tomography (CT) and magnetic resonance imaging (MRI) (Kaplan, Sadock, & Grebb, 1994). Unfortunately, however, understanding of the findings lags behind the information explosion created by these new technologies. The list of hypothesized causes of schizophrenia is somewhat daunting and may, on the surface, seem contradictory, but it highlights the need for much further research. Currently in the United States, research dollars available to study schizophrenia are only a small fraction of the money spent to research other diseases. According to NIMH statistics, the government spends $43 for research per person diagnosed with schizophrenia. Six to seven times that amount is spent for each person diagnosed with cancer. Also complicating the research efforts is the awareness that schizophrenia, like many other diseases, is probably caused by a combination of many factors. One of the criticisms of neurologic, and particularly structural, theories of etiology is that they cannot account for the episodic nature of the disease in some people or for its highly variable clinical outcome. Future research will most likely focus on the interaction of many variables rather than a single entity.

Many different structural anomalies have been discovered in the brains of people with schizophrenia. These include lesions in the brain stem, enlargement of the ventricles, brain atrophy, and abnormalities in the limbic structures, cerebellum, and corpus collosum. There is a growing body of evidence that frontal lobe dysfunction, possibly related to the basal ganglia, plays a role in the development of negative symptoms (Talbott, Hale, & Yudofsky, 1994). Structural abnormalities in the brain are clearly more common in people with schizophrenia than in the general population. However, the clinical significance of these findings is far from understood.

One of the most prevalent theories of etiology concerns the role of the neurotransmitter dopamine. It is hypothesized that people with schizophrenia have either an excess of dopamine or an excessive quantity of dopamine receptors, making the neurotransmitter more effective. No reliable measure presently exists to determine specific amounts of neurotransmitters in the brain, but it is known that antipsychotic medication, which often decreases overtly psychotic symptoms, affects dopamine levels. Therefore, it might be assumed that excessive dopamine is particularly related to positive symptoms. Although there has been a tremendous amount of emphasis placed on the role of dopamine, other neurotransmitters, specifically norepinephrine, serotonin, and glutamate, as well as certain neuropeptides, are also being studied.

Another promising area of research is the role of a virus or viruses in the development of schizophrenia. There are viruses that stay inactive for many years and then start to grow slowly. Thus, it is hypothesized that a possible cause of schizophrenia is exposure to certain viruses prenatally while involved areas of the brain are being developed (Coleman & Gillberg, 1996). The person's subsequent deterioration in adolescence or young adulthood may be the direct result of a virus or an autoimmune reaction triggered by a virus. Evidence to support this theory is limited, but certain demographic data on people with schizophrenia is suggestive. For example, there is a higher than average incidence of people with schizophrenia who are born in the winter or spring months, which coincides with the epidemiological patterns of many viruses. Moreover, low birth weight is more common than average in people with schizophrenia, possibly suggesting a viral infection in utero.

Deficiencies in diet and vitamins have been examined as possible causes of schizophrenia, but so far the results have been largely discounted or considered to be anecdotal. Nevertheless, considering what is still unknown about neurochemistry, these avenues of study may still hold promise.

DIAGNOSIS OF SCHIZOPHRENIA

There is criticism that schizophrenia tends to be overdiagnosed, particularly with people demonstrating bizarre or flagrant behaviors. Some societies more than others appear to tolerate "eccentric" behavior without necessarily considering it pathological. For a person to act "odd" or "different" does not necessarily mean that he or she has a disease. Even with the presence of obvious psychosis, it cannot be assumed that a pathological condition exists. For example, it has been well documented that hallucinations can occur as part of specific religious and cultural rituals, drug-induced behavior, or even within the realm of "normal" experience (MacRae, 1991).

For the purposes of this chapter, schizophrenia is considered a group of disorders that meet the minimum criteria as described in the DSM-IV (APA, 1994). These criteria are as follows:

A. Characteristic symptoms: two or more of the following, each present for a significant portion of time during a one-month period (or less if successfully treated):

1. delusions
2. hallucinations
3. disorganized speech (i.e., frequent derailment or incoherence)
4. grossly disorganized or catatonic behavior
5. negative symptoms (e.g., affective flattening, alogia, or avolition)

B. Social/occupational dysfunction: for a significant portion of the time since the onset of the disturbance

Clinicians should be aware, however, of the limitations of the DSM. As Andreason and Carpenter state: "Somehow, the existence of such criteria gives the sense that we know what schizophrenia is when in fact we do not. Schizophrenia remains a clinical syndrome comprising an unknown number of disease entities or pathologic domains" (1993, p. 203).

Another way of classifying schizophrenia is to differentiate distinct syndromes based on the predominance of either **positive symptoms** or **negative symptoms**. Two syndromes of schizophrenia have been identified by Crow (1985). Type 1 is characterized by positive symptoms, and Type 2 is characterized by negative symptoms. Table 9-1 further describes the differences between these two syndromes. It remains controversial as to whether these syndromes are distinct entities. Moreover, the prevalence of a mixed type syndrome is unclear. Although the DSM-IV does recognize the significance of negative symptomology, further research on the specific syndromes is needed.

Not all conditions presenting with psychosis are schizophrenia. There are many disorders that may present where psychosis is transient but is not a defining feature of the disorder. The DSM-IV also recognizes several disorders as being primarily a type of psychotic disturbance, including the following:

- schizophreniform disorder
- schizoaffective disorder
- delusional disorder
- brief psychotic disorder
- shared psychotic disorder

Table 9-1. Syndromes of Schizophrenia: A Comparison of Types 1 and 2

Type	Symptomology	Prognosis	Response to Treatment
1	Predominance of positive symptoms with minimal or no cognitive deficits	Characterized by a fluctuating course of exacerbations and remissions. Usual onset involves a full-blown psychotic episode	Generally responds well to antipsychotic medication. May need little or no other therapeutic intervention between psychotic episodes providing there is a stable environment
2	Predominance of negative symptoms, typically with some degree of cognitive deficits	Usually a chronic course. Onset may be insidious but is generally identified by early adulthood	Responds poorly to antipsychotic medication other than some benefit from sedation.° Typically needs ongoing supportive therapy for both rehabilitation and maintenance of living skills

°There is some evidence that negative symptoms may be reduced by some of the new antipsychotic medications such as clozapine or risperidone, or with the use of an antidepressant such as Trazadone along with an antipsychotic.

- psychotic disorder due to a general medical condition
- substance-induced psychotic disorder
- psychotic disorder not otherwise specified

POSITIVE SYMPTOMATOLOGY

auditory - most common

The most common positive symptoms associated with schizophrenia are delusions and perceptual distortions, especially hallucinations. However, various other perceptual and behavioral disturbances may also present as positive symptoms. Abnormal affect, such as uncontrolled laughing or silliness, is particularly common with the disorganized type of schizophrenia. Language disturbances may include bizarre speech, echolalia, and, more frequently, circumstantiality, tangentiality, loosening of associations, incoherency, and pressured speech. Changes are possible in motoric responses, including pacing, rocking, restlessness, and lethargy, as well as disturbances of sleep patterns. It is important to recognize that the range and severity of symptoms varies with the individual.

Delusions

Delusions vary in content. Typical delusions found with schizophrenia are considered bizarre in that they are implausible within the context of the individual's environment and culture. William Bowden, a man diagnosed with schizophrenia, paranoid type, described the intractable nature of delusional thinking in this first-person account: "My belief has withstood attack from anyone I've shared it with. It is also something that I truly wish would stop. I also wish, even if this phenomenon is true, that I did not believe it" (1993, p. 165).

Paranoid delusions are certainly not limited to schizophrenia, but they do partially account for the suspicious and guarded behavior sometimes seen with the disorder. The delusions of schizophrenia also take various forms of presentation. For example, a delusion may be in the form of thought broadcasting, which occurs when the individual believes that his or her thoughts can be transmitted. Thought insertion and thought withdrawal are the beliefs that someone or something is responsible for either putting thoughts into one's brain or removing one's thoughts (and ability to think). Thought control is also attributed to someone other than the person having the delusion and usually also implies action control (for example, someone who commits a crime and attributes the action to the force of a spirit or devil).

Presentations of thought broadcasting, insertion, withdrawal, and control are relatively consistent throughout different cultures and in historical reports of suspected delusions. What does change is the individual's rationale for what is happening. Thus, descriptions of these phenomena are remarkably similar throughout the world except for the individual's explanation for the phenomena. For example, a person who experienced a delusion of thought control in the European Middle Ages would have typically explained the control as coming from a demonic force, while in the decade of the 1950s in the United States, when the Cold War was raging, it was common for "the communists" to be blamed for thought control delusions. It is understandable that people would attempt to explain something happening to them that is out of the realm of the ordinary; therefore, these rationales are usually common themes found in the culture. The forms of the rationale may be political, religious, supernatural, scientific, or pseudo-scientific.

Perceptual Distortion

People with schizophrenia may experience many different kinds of perceptual disturbances, which also vary in severity. Hallucinations are probably the most common, particularly in acute phases of the disorder. However, illusions are also possible, as well as other perceptual disturbances indicative of sensory-integrative dysfunction (Blakeney, Strickland, & Wilkinson, 1983; King, 1974). These deficits may include poor body schema and personal boundaries, tactile defensiveness, distorted figure-ground (Eimon, Eimon, & Cermak, 1983), spatial, and time relations.

Distemporality does not fit neatly into a description of positive or negative symptoms, as it includes perceptual distortion and disorientation but also behaviorally presents as avolition. People with schizophrenia often report a sense of being stuck in present time, living only in the moment and unable to process the events of the past or determine a future course. Moneim El-Meligi stated that change in subjective time is "by far the most neglected area in both psychiatric evaluation and psychodiagnostic testing" (1972, p. 226).

Hallucinations are considered one of the hallmark symptoms of schizophrenia, but it has often been inaccurately considered that only auditory hallucinations are found in this disorder. Auditory hallucinations are probably the most common presentation, and they may lead to the greatest personal distress, possibly causing them to be reported with greater frequency. However, it is the phenomenon of multiple presentations of hallucinations that probably causes the greatest level of dysfunction. In other words, the more senses are involved with hallucinatory experiences, the more difficult it is for an individual to stay oriented to reality (MacRae, 1993).

Interestingly, the vividness or frequency of the hallucinations is not necessarily indicative of the severity of the disorder. Some people with quite pronounced perceptual distortion manage to develop adequate coping skills, while others with only a minimal disturbance remain severely impaired. In schizophrenia, the presence of negative symptoms, cognitive deficits, and a poor ability to manage environmental stimuli decreases the ability to cope with hallucinations, therefore creating a greater level of dysfunction.

CASE ILLUSTRATION: MAUREEN—POSITIVE SYMPTOMS

Maureen is a 23-year-old college student who was accompanied by her roommate to the Emergency Psychiatric Services at the county hospital. She arrived in a wildly agitated state, claiming, "They are all trying to kill me." During an initial interview, Maureen admitted that she had been hearing voices commanding her to kill herself. The voices had apparently worsened over the last several days to the point where she was unable to sleep or concentrate on any activities. It was decided that Maureen was a danger to herself, and she was admitted to the acute inpatient locked unit. Further interviews revealed that Maureen had a history of repeated psychotic episodes starting in high school. Six years ago she had been diagnosed with schizophrenia, paranoid type. When she took her medication, her symptoms remained under control and she was able to function relatively well. However, her attempts to finish college had been hampered by acute exacerbations of her illness at times when she stopped taking her medication.

Discussion

Maureen's behavior is characteristic of someone with predominantly positive symptoms, minimal cognitive deficits, a fluctuating course of exacerbations and remissions, and good response to antipsychotic medication, which aids her functioning.

NEGATIVE SYMPTOMATOLOGY

Many researchers and theorists have recently concentrated on negative symptomology in schizophrenia. This effort has been strongly influenced by the work of Nancy Andreason, who developed the Scale for the Assessment of Negative Symptoms (1984). The scale includes the following broad categories:

- affective flattening or blunting—a limited ability to express emotions and feelings
- alogia—impoverished thought process that is manifested in speech patterns
- avolition—a lack of interest or energy unaccompanied by depressed affect
- anhedonia—an inability to experience pleasure or sustain interest in activities
- inattention—an inability, of which the person may be unaware, to sustain concentration or attention

Because these deficits are most often observed during sustained and social activity, the occupational therapist has a critical role in the accurate assessment of negative symptoms. Moreover, the occupational therapy emphasis on activities of self-care, work, and leisure makes it essential that the therapist understand the nature of negative symptoms. A meaningful treatment plan reflects an awareness of these symptoms and efforts to be made to help the individual cope with, and compensate for, existing deficits.

CASE ILLUSTRATION: JAMES—NEGATIVE SYMPTOMS

James has lived in a residential care facility for the past seven years. He has not been hospitalized since living in this home but had several hospitalizations in the five years prior to this move. James takes antipsychotic medication, which seems to completely control the hallucinations he experienced in the past. Nevertheless, even in the absence of psychosis, James remains unable to function independently. He reports that he does nothing all day but has no plans for changing his lifestyle. He has been enrolled in several rehabilitative programs, including sheltered workshops, but was unable to follow through with their recommendations. James also attempted to complete an associate's degree at the local community college but dropped out during his first semester. Poor attendance and difficulty attending to tasks were the primary reasons for this cycle of failure. James also has great difficulty in social situations. He tends to be passive, avoiding conversation and relationships even though he states he is lonely.

Discussion

James's functioning is severely influenced by his negative symptoms of avolition, anhedonia, and inattention.

PROGNOSIS

Schizophrenia is a serious and persistent mental illness, but data on its prognosis is unreliable. "Because of the variability in definition and ascertainment, an accurate summary of the long-term outcome of schizophrenia is not possible" (APA, 1994, p. 282). In the past, prognosis was based on a "rule of thirds," meaning that one-third of the people with schizophrenia would remain chronically ill, one-third would have intermittent bouts of illness, and one-third would recover completely. This "rule" is now considered too optimistic and therefore is obsolete. The criteria for schizophrenia have been clarified and narrowed considerably in recent years. Therefore, many people who would have formerly been diagnosed with schizophrenia are now receiving a variety of psychotic and nonpsychotic diagnoses. The result is that the population currently diagnosed with schizophrenia has a more serious and globally dysfunctional illness with a much poorer outcome. It is now considered uncommon for people to have a complete remission of the disorder. Some researchers go so far as to suggest that if recovery occurs it means that the diagnosis of schizophrenia was inaccurate, but this assertion is not generally accepted at this time.

[handwritten margin note: still used.]

The severity and prognosis of schizophrenia may be affected by cultural and environmental influences. For example, the World Health Organization (WHO) concluded that schizophrenia has a more benign course in the Third World. This may be explained by different family structures and types of treatment, a less urban environment, or the possibility that the disorder found in the Third World may have a different biological basis (WHO, 1979).

Because of the changes in diagnostic criteria and the variability of treatment, there is a shortage of long-term studies on people with schizophrenia. It has been suggested, however, that some people with schizophrenia may have a natural remission after two to three decades. In other words, recovery rates may actually be much higher than previously estimated, but only after a prolonged course of illness (possibly 20 to 30 years). According to Liberman and Kopelowicz:

> Long-term follow-up studies of persons who had experienced severe forms of schizophrenia earlier in their lives have discovered that over 50 percent of these individuals are living what may be considered "normal" lives—working, socializing, playing, living without close supervi-

sion and with little or no psychotic symptoms—20 to 30 years after their illness began. These "recoveries" have been documented in Japan, Germany, Switzerland, Scotland, France, and the USA. (1994, p. 67)

These studies have many ramifications for treatment. Hypothetically, if a young man developed schizophrenia at the age of 17, by the time he was 40 years old the disease might have run its course, but by that time his identity will also be firmly entrenched as a "disabled person." Many functional deficits would continue because of lifestyle, habits, and societal expectations and, most important, because of the missed developmental milestones of adolescence and young adulthood. Role dysfunction, which is considered an integral part of schizophrenia, may be minimized if aggressive rehabilitation is provided early in the course of illness. "The onset of psychotic disorder often disrupts a person's ability to perform competently in occupational and social roles, thus adolescents with psychotic disorders are appropriate candidates for occupational therapy intervention" (Henry & Coster, 1996, p. 171).

It also must be acknowledged that poor prognosis may be linked to inadequate treatment. It has been repeatedly documented that outcome is improved when people with schizophrenia are given comprehensive and consistent long-term treatment. It is possible that if such treatment were universally available, there would be a higher incidence of full recovery. It is certain that, given comprehensive and consistent treatment, functional outcome and quality of life would be improved even should the course of the disease remain chronic.

INTERDISCIPLINARY TREATMENT

In the acute phase of illness, hospital treatment may be necessary and beneficial, but typical hospitalization stays have shortened considerably over the last decade, and in the United States they are often only three to seven days in length. The hospitalization of people with schizophrenia usually only occurs when the individual has a severe psychotic episode, has grossly decompensated in function, and is considered either a danger to the self, a danger to others, or gravely disabled. The primary goal of acute hospitalization is to provide a thorough evaluation and stabilize the person on medication. Acute care hospitalizations also help stabilize patients by providing a safe environment with adequate rest and nutrition. This is becoming especially pertinent as the incidence of homelessness among people with schizophrenia increases. Depending on the length of stay, the beginnings of a rehabilitation program may be commenced, but it is unrealistic to assume that brief hospitalizations will serve as sufficient intervention. People with schizophrenia require consistent treatment, typically of long duration, with a combined interdisciplinary approach. "Psychopharmacologic and psychosocial treatments appear to be additive in their efficacy. Combining social skills training with maintenance of antipsychotic medication yields better social functioning while minimizing relapse" (Liberman & Kopelowicz, 1994, p. 69). Treatment should include psychotropic medication, supportive services, and rehabilitation that includes both verbal and activity-based therapies.

Goal Setting

A key component of an interdisciplinary treatment plan is setting the goals of treatment. Ideally, these goals are determined by the individual in conjunction with the team. It is highly desirable to also include the family and significant others, provided the person in treatment consents. Unfortunately, there are many constraints to this ideal situation. The trend toward managed care has placed great limits on the amount of services that can be provided, and too often, services are predetermined by agency mandate. Moreover, Western society has a long history of an authoritarian approach to health care, whereby professionals are viewed as "experts" who know what is best for the patient. Although the "expert" model is changing to a more collaborative one, vestiges of the authoritarian health care system remain in practice.

Cooperative goal setting can also be hampered by the individual's pathology. People with delusions, poor insight, concrete thinking, or avolition may be incapable of healthy and realistic goal setting. Nevertheless, within the person's capabilities, every effort should be made to seek out and honor his or her expressed interests and desires, even if they sometimes conflict with the team's opinion.

CASE ILLUSTRATION: DIAMOND— GOAL-SETTING CONFLICT

Diamond, 38, has been diagnosed with schizophrenia, undifferentiated type. She has a long history of repetitive decompensations while living in the community. During her most recent hospitalization, the team recommended that she be placed in a residential care facility to help monitor her symptoms and medication. Diamond strongly objected, stating that she likes living alone in an apartment and that her goal is to return to independent living. After repeated discussions with the team, Diamond reluctantly agreed to the placement. Two weeks later, Diamond walked out of the facility and has not gotten in touch with her therapist in the ensuing month.

Discussion

This scenario might have been avoided if more effort had been made to comprehend Diamond's goals. While a residential care facility may be a safer alternative than independent living, it cannot be a feasible alternative without the individual's cooperation. Negotiation about follow-up care in the community, including day treatment and case management options, might have addressed the team's legitimate concerns while allowing Diamond to remain in an independent living situation.

Agreement as to what are "realistic" goals is not an easy task. The goals of the treatment team members may be quite different from the person with schizophrenia, whose ideas may also differ from the goals and expectations of the family. Professionals have been accused of contributing to chronicity by fostering dependency on the system and discouraging individuals from pursuing goals of independence in housing, employment, or school. On the other hand, for some people the demands of independent living exacerbate their symptoms, leading to a cycle of failure. "The patient with schizophrenia . . . is often walking a tightrope between exposure to understimulating or overstimulating environments" (Lukoff, Liberman, & Nuechterlein, 1986, p. 579). Either overestimating or underestimating a person's potential can have adverse effects, so it is essential that goal setting not be based on diagnosis or preconceived ideas of outcome but rather be founded on an assessment of the particular individual's strengths, deficits, interests, needs, and level of support.

Psychotropic Medication

A significant part of the treatment of schizophrenia involves antipsychotic medication prescribed by a physician. However, the role of drug therapy has often been misunderstood. Antipsychotic medication does not cure schizophrenia. It typically decreases symptoms, but treatment that involves only drug therapy is inadequate. The primary benefit of **psychotropic** drugs is to stabilize the individual sufficiently that he or she may benefit from other treatment. Commonly used antipsychotic medications are listed in Table 9-2.

Table 9-2. Commonly Used Antipsychotic Medications		
Compound	*Trade Name*	*Comments*
Chlorpromazine hydrochloride	Thorazine	The first antipsychotic drug developed. It is still used
Fluphenazine enanthate	Prolixin Enanthate	Can be time released and therefore given in injection form at two-week intervals
Trifuoperazine hydrochloride	Stelazine	High incidence of EPS but less sedating effect than Thorazine
Thiothixene	Navane	Low sedation but high risk of EPS
Haloperidol	Haldol	Extremely potent antipsychotic agent, often used in acute episodes
Clozapine	Clozaril	Low danger of EPS and low sedation. It appears to block seratonin as well as dopamine. Risks are seizures and agranulocytosis.
Risperidone	Risperdal	Low danger of EPS, low sedation, and low risk of other side effects. Currently expensive.

Side effects do occur with antipsychotic medication, including extrapyramidal symptoms (EPS), autonomic nervous system signs, endocrine side effects, and skin changes. Therefore, it is important that drug trials be closely monitored to determine the best choice of drug and optimum dosage. In the medical model, there is often an overemphasis on decreasing symptoms, even at the expense of overall function. For example, a person on relatively high dosages of medication may experience a complete elimination of hallucinations but be too sedated to engage in meaningful activity, while a lower dose may cause some of the positive symptoms to persist but allow the individual to continue functioning while coping with the symptoms.

It is theorized that antipsychotic agents primarily act as antagonists of dopamine. Their therapeutic effect is believed to come from blockage of dopamine in the frontal cortex and limbic system, which is responsible for behavior and affect. However, the traditional antipsychotic drugs (excluding clozapine or risperidone) also block dopamine in the basal ganglia, causing unwanted extrapyramidal symptoms. Antipsychotic medication tends to readily cross the blood-brain barrier and eventually attain a higher concentration in the brain. Because of this process, systemic side effects of antipsychotic medications will usually appear before the therapeutic effects.

The systemic side effects associated with antipsychotic medication are highly variable but can include the autonomic nervous system symptoms of dry mouth, stuffy nose, irregular heartbeat, fainting, dizziness, sedation, constipation, blurred vision, and difficulty in urination, as well as pigmentary changes and photosensitivity. Symptoms often disappear after the first few weeks of treatment, but persistent problems may require a change in medication. Education about symptom management is essential, including information on adequate diet and hydration and the use of sunscreen. Side effects also include medication-induced movement disorders (described in Table 9-3). The treatment of movement disorders typically consists of changing medications and dosages and prescribing additional medication such as antiparkinsonian agents, however, these agents are ineffective for tardive dyskinesia.

A major concern in drug therapy for people with schizophrenia is a relatively high incidence of noncompliance. Given the extent of side effects experienced with these medications, it should not be a surprise that people may not want to take their medication, but there are many additional reasons for noncompliance. People with schizophrenia find themselves in a paradoxical situation in that the very symptoms that need treatment may prevent them from taking their medication. These symptoms may include delusional thinking regarding the harm of the drugs or lack of insight regarding their illness. Moreover, people with schizophrenia often have cognitive deficits such as forgetfulness, confusion, and poor time orientation, making it difficult for them to independently manage medication.

Noncompliance can be minimized by providing education and supportive interventions to help the individual manage both symptoms and side effects. Moreover, people with cognitive deficits can benefit from simplified drug

Table 9-3.	Medication-Induced Movement Disorders
Acute dystonia	Acute muscular rigidity, especially in the neck, tongue, face, and back. Subacute symptoms include subjective reports of tongue "thickness" or difficulty swallowing. May impair speaking or breathing
(Neuroleptic-induced) parkinsonism	Bradykinesia, rigidity, tremor, masked facies, stooped posture, shuffling gait, and drooling. If severe, it can develop into akinesia
Neuroleptic malignant syndrome	An acute and severe muscular rigidity and elevated temperature, with the possibility of dysphagia, diaphoresis, confusion, and elevated blood pressure. May be fatal
Akathesia	Restlessness, agitation, inability to sit or stand still, and pacing. Subjectively described as an intensely unpleasant need to move
Tardive dyskinesia	Involuntary choreiform and athetoid or rhythmic movements involving the tongue, jaw, trunk, or extremities. Symptoms may be worsened by stress; particularly severe in the elderly

regimes, and time and memory management techniques. However, the most important predictor of compliance is the therapeutic relationship and level of trust the individual feels with the prescribing physician and treatment team as a whole. Unfortunately, the current state of mental health care makes it difficult for a consistent treatment team to follow people, who frequently become "lost in the system."

OCCUPATIONAL THERAPY INTERVENTION

Team treatment of people with schizophrenia is common and, depending on the model of treatment used, various disciplines may be involved. For the purposes of this chapter, discussion is limited to the role of the occupational therapist. It must be acknowledged, however, that in some team approaches, several disciplines may overlap with occupational therapy or conduct evaluation and treatments typically viewed as occupational therapy. In some cases, occupational therapists may also take on roles outside their traditional domain. Regardless of the model of intervention, the needs of the patient or client should dictate the services provided.

Evaluation

The choice of assessment tools is influenced by the therapist's theoretical frame of reference. One such theory-bound evaluation is Allen's Cognitive Levels test, which is based on Claudia Allen's model of cognitive disability (Allen, 1985). The information derived from this evaluation is helpful in structuring the environment and interactions to best compensate for the person's cognitive limitations.

Another commonly used formal evaluation for people with schizophrenia is the Kohlman Evaluation of Living Skills (KELS) (Kohlman Thomson, 1992). This is an easily administered evaluation, which provides information on an individual's ability to perform a variety of tasks necessary for independent living. The KELS is not intended as a diagnostic tool, as it does not give specific information on the causes of dysfunction. For this reason, it is not a sufficiently sensitive tool for treatment planning. However, it is very valuable for discharge planning, especially if placement of the individual is in question. For example, when a patient is being prepared for discharge from an acute care hospital, it is crucial that the treatment team have a clear understanding of the level of assistance needed. Based on the information provided by the KELS, recommendations may be made for independent living or a range of assisted living environments.

Another functional evaluation is the Assessment of Motor and Process Skills (AMPS) developed by Anne Fisher. "The AMPS is an observational assessment that permits the simultaneous evaluation of motor and process skills as a person performs two or three complex or instrumental activity of daily living (IADL) tasks (e.g., meal preparation, home maintenance, laundry) of his or her choice" (Fisher et al., 1992, p. 878). The AMPS is not specific to any diagnosis, but considering that people with schizophrenia often have both cognitive and sensorimotor deficits that result in dysfunction, it is very useful for this population. As stated by Pan and Fisher,

> Limitations in function of clients with psychiatric disorders are a major factor affecting their independence and need for service...[and] therefore, occupational therapists need to use valid, reliable, and sensitive functional assessment instruments that can guide the intervention process and measure change. (1994, p. 775)

Occupational therapists also use a variety of informal evaluation techniques. For example, the interview may be used to build a therapeutic relationship, determine interests and skills, and develop goals. The interview also discloses much information regarding symptoms related to thought processes, but it is not the most effective method of determining function. A more useful tool for evaluating the functional skills of people with schizophrenia is task analysis. The observation of an individual engaged in routine activities provides a wealth of information about functioning that could not be uncovered through an interview.

Treatment

Group work is the most common approach used by occupational therapists in mental health. Groups are especially effective for building social skills, but the importance of one-to-one personal contact should not be underestimated, especially in the early stages of treatment, when it aids in developing a relationship and performing evaluation. Unfortunately, occupational therapists working with budget and time constraints often must forgo individual treatments. One-to-one contact is vital for individuals who are withdrawn or are too psychotic to benefit from a group approach. The stimulation of an activity group may place undue demands on some people and exacerbate their symptoms. In addition, individual contact is often a prelude to group involvement. It is helpful if the occupational therapist in a one-to-one interaction explains the purpose of the available groups, and personally invites the individual to join. Attendance and participation in group activities is much more likely if the person already has a relationship with the group leader and knows what to expect.

Individual intervention is often thought to be too expensive, but in fact it is possible to meet specific objectives in a time- and cost-effective manner. For example, Figure 9-1 shows an occupational therapist visiting individual rooms on an inpatient unit with a cart stocked with grooming supplies. In this way, the OTR engages in one-to-one contact with the patients while providing evaluation and treatment. This activity gives the therapist an opportunity to check in with the patients at the beginning of the day. Introductions and orientation to occupational therapy occur simultaneously with activity of daily

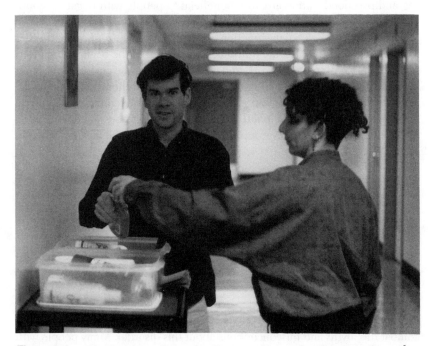

Figure 9-1.   The Grooming Cart on an Inpatient Unit at San Francisco General Hospital

living (ADL) evaluation and treatment. The actual contact may be quite brief, yet this form of individual treatment paves the way for more sustained one-to-one and group activities.

Although occupational therapists structure their interventions on the individual's strengths, understanding the pathology of the illness is also essential. People who display positive symptoms, especially hallucinations, benefit from activities that divert attention from their symptoms. In the process, the individual can learn self-help coping strategies to minimize the intrusiveness of positive symptomology. However, it is only when people can clearly identify activities with *personal meaning or purpose* that they are able to see them as a viable method of symptom management. While random applications of activities sometimes provided a temporary distraction from hallucinations, it is the use of activities that bolsters the sense of personal achievement and mastery that are consistently deemed as most successful in coping with hallucinations and other positive symptoms (MacRae, 1993).

Negative symptoms have a more profound effect than positive symptoms on an individual's overall ability to function. Understanding that negative symptoms are part of the disease process and not necessarily a learned maladaptive behavior can help the clinician structure interventions to compensate for these deficits. Individuals who display negative symptoms often need highly structured activities with concrete expectations and goals. Specific skill training and psychoeducation are very beneficial to people with negative symptoms, but many individuals need ongoing support to utilize their skills.

Considering the global dysfunction associated with schizophrenia, there is a wide range of possible interventions, which address the occupational performance areas of self-care, work, and leisure as well as the performance components of motor, sensory-integrative, cognitive, psychological, and social functioning. Most activities can address more than one component or area, and the therapist must adapt and grade the activities to best meet the needs of the individual patient or group. Treatment goals may be accomplished in many different ways using a variety of individual and group techniques. Table 9-4 describes some of the specific treatment formats used with this population by occupational therapists.

Summary

Schizophrenia is a complicated disorder affecting over a million people throughout the world. Its effects can be devastating on a person's ability to function but, moreover, individuals with schizophrenia additionally experience dysfunction from society's reaction to them for being ill. Schizophrenia is largely misunderstood by the general public, and clinicians have a responsibility to combat the myths and misconceptions about this disorder. Many people with schizophrenia can lead productive, meaningful lives, but only with consistent and comprehensive treatment. A knowledge of the underlying pathology of the

Table 9-4.	Occupational Therapy Treatment Formats for People with Schizophrenia
Types	*Comments*
Structured tasks	Provide habit training, diversion, coping skills, and time management training. Potential for leisure skill development. May also build self-esteem through successful completion
Expressive activities	Nonverbal communication, emotional and creative outlets. Potential for leisure skill development. May also build self-esteem through successful completion
Functional living skills	May include basic self-care, including hygiene, grooming, and dressing. Also includes independent living skills such as meal preparation and money management
Psychoeducation	Can be used to teach living skills but is also used for teaching symptom management, health and safety awareness, and assertiveness training
Social skills training	Especially effective in groups; includes verbal and nonverbal communication. Role-playing is one technique used
Vocational training	Includes basis skill preparation as well as time management and social skills. Vocational pursuits must be carefully graded and may require ongoing support

illness, an ability to work with a team approach, and a willingness to relate to the person with schizophrenia are essential for successful intervention.

Review Questions

1. Why is schizophrenia commonly misunderstood?
2. What is believed to be the cause of schizophrenia?
3. What can be done to minimize noncompliance with antipsychotic medication?
4. How does the presence of positive symptoms affect occupational therapy intervention?
5. How does the presence of negative symptoms affect occupational therapy intervention?
6. How does occupational therapy intervention for people with schizophrenia differ from other mental health professions?

Learning Activities

1. "Interference" is an interactive board game designed to help educate people working in mental health about the barriers to treatment experienced by people with serious mental illnesses such as schizophrenia. Play the

game with four to six people and allow yourself at least ninety minutes. The game is available through the following source:

Project Life
Interference Game
University of Missouri
623 Clark Hall
Columbia, MO 65211

2. Research the available services in your community for people with schizophrenia. Volunteer at a day treatment center or homeless shelter.
3. Find 5 to 10 examples of the term *schizophrenia* used incorrectly in the media.
4. Develop occupational therapy group protocols for each type of group listed in Table 9-4.

References

Allen, C. (1985). *Measurement and management of cognitive disabilities.* Boston: Little, Brown.

American Psychiatric Association (APA). (1994). *Diagnostic and statistical manual of mental disorders* (4th ed.). Washington, DC: APA.

Andreason, N. (1984). *Scale for the Assessment of Negative Symptoms (SANS).* Iowa City: University of Iowa.

Andreason, N., & Carpenter, W. (1993). Diagnosis and classification of schizophrenia. *Schizophrenia Bulletin, 19* (2), 199–213.

Blakeney, A., Strickland, L. R., & Wilkinson, J. (1983). Exploring sensory integrative dysfunction in process schizophrenia. *American Journal of Occupational Therapy, 37* (6), 399–407.

Bleuler, E. (1950). *Dementia praecox, or the group of schizophrenias* (J. Zinkin, Trans.). New York: International Universities Press. (Original work published 1911)

Bowden, W. (1993). First person account: The onset of paranoia. *Schizophrenia Bulletin, 19*(1), 165–167.

Coleman, M., & Gillberg, C. (1996). *The schizophrenias: A biological approach to the schizophrenia spectrum disorders.* New York: Singer.

Crow, T. J. (1985). The two-syndrome concept: Origins and current status. *Schizophrenia Bulletin, 11,* 471–486.

Eimon, M., Eimon, P., & Cermak, S. (1983). Performance of schizophrenic patients on a motor-free visual perception test. *American Journal of Occupational Therapy, 37*(5), 327–332.

Falloon, I., & Talbot, R. (1981). Persistent auditory hallucinations: Coping mechanisms and implications for management. *Psychological Medicine, 11,* 329–339.

Fisher, A., Liu, Y., Velozo, C., & Pan, A. W. (1992). Cross-cultural assessment of process skills. *American Journal of Occupational Therapy, 46*(10), 876–885.

Grace, J., Bellus, S., Raulin, M., Herz, M., Priest, B., Brenner, V., Donnelly, K., Smith, P., & Gunn, S. (1996). Long-term impact of clozapine and psychosocial treatment on psychiatric symptoms and cognitive functioning. *Psychiatric Services, 47*(1), 41–45.

Henry, A., & Coster, W. (1996). Predictors of functional outcome among adolescents with psychotic disorders. *American Journal of Occupational Therapy, 50*(3), 171–183.

Kaplan, H., Sadock, B., & Grebb, J. (1994). *Kaplan and Sadock's synopsis of psychiatry* (7th ed.). Baltimore, MD: Williams & Wilkins.

King, L. J. (1974). A sensory-integrative approach to schizophrenia. *American Journal of Occupational Therapy, 28*(9), 529–536.

Kohlman Thomson, L. (1992). *The Kohlman Evaluation of Living Skills*. Bethesda, MD.: American Occupational Therapy Association.

Kraeplin, E. (1971). *Dementia praecox and paraphrenia* (R. M. Barclay & G. M. Robertson, Trans. & Eds.). Edinburgh, Scotland: E. & S. Livingstone. (Original work published 1919)

Liberman, R. P., & Kopelowicz, A. (1994). Recovery from schizophrenia: Is the time right? *Journal of the California Alliance for the Mentally Ill, 5*(3), 67–69.

Lukoff, D., Liberman, R. P.. & Nuechterlein, K. H. (1986). Symptom monitoring in the rehabilitation of schizophrenic patients. *Schizophrenia Bulletin, 12,* 578–597.

MacRae, A. (1991). An overview of theory and research on hallucinations: Implications for occupational therapy intervention. *Occupational Therapy in Mental Health, 11*(4), 41–60.

MacRae, A. (1993). *Coping with hallucinations: A phenomenological study of the everyday lived experience of people with hallucinatory psychosis*. Ann Arbor, MI: University Microfilms.

Maxmen, J., & Ward, N. (1995). *Essential psychopathology and its treatment* (2nd ed.). New York: W. W. Norton & Co.

Menditto, A., Beck, N., Stuve, P., Fisher, J., Stacy, M., Logue, M. B., & Baldwin, L. (1996). Effectiveness of clozapine and a social learning program for severely disabled psychiatric inpatients. *Psychiatric Services, 47*(1), 46–51.

Moneim El-Meligi, A. (1972). A technique for exploring time experiences in mental disorder. In H. Yaker, H. Osmond, & F. Cheek (Eds.), *The future of time* (pp. 220–271). Garden City, NY: Anchor Books.

Pan, A. W., & Fisher, A. (1994). The assessment of motor and process skills of persons with psychiatric disorders. *American Journal of Occupational Therapy, 48*(9), 775–782.

Peuskens, J. (1995). Risperidone in the treatment of patients with chronic schizophrenia: A multi-national, multi-centre, double blind, parallel-group study versus haloperidol. *British Journal of Psychiatry, 166,* 712–726.

Schneider, K. (1959). *Clinical psychopathology* (M. W. Hamilton, Trans.). London & New York: Grune & Stratton.

Talbott, J.A., Hales, R. E., & Yudofsky, S. C. (1994).

World Health Organization (WHO) (1979). *Schizophrenia: An international followup study.* New York: John Wiley.

Suggested Reading

Andreasen, N. (1984). *The broken brain: The biological revolution in psychiatry.* New York: Harper & Row.

Beers, C. (1981). *A mind that found itself.* Pittsburgh: University of Pittsburgh Press. (Original work published 1907)

Bouricius, J. (1989). *Drugs and their effect on mentally ill persons.* Arlington, VA: National Alliance for the Mentally Ill.

Burrows, G., Norman, T., & Rubenstein. G. (Eds.). (1986). *Handbook of studies on schizophrenia.* New York: Elsevier.

Donaldson, K. (1976). *Insanity inside out.* New York: Crown.

Marneros, A., Andreasen, N., & Tsuang, M. (Eds.). (1991). *Negative versus positive schizophrenia.* Berlin: Springer–Verlag.

Sullivan, E., Shear, P., Zipursky, R., Sagar, H., & Pfefferbaum, A. (1994). A deficit profile of executive, memory, and motor functions in schizophrenia. *Biological Psychiatry, 36,* 641–653.

Torrey, E. F. (1988). *Nowhere to go: The tragic odyssey of the homeless mentally ill.* New York: Harper & Row.

Mood Disorders

Elizabeth Cara

Key Terms

cyclothymia
depression
dysthymia
mania

melancholia
mood
referential thinking

Chapter Outline

Introduction

Mood disorders have been described throughout history. Descriptions of depressive episodes are found in the Old Testament and in classical Greek literature. Originally, in ancient times, they were thought to be a curse of the gods, and therefore, sufferers were treated by priests. In the sixth century B.C., Hippocrates, "the father of physicians," introduced the terms **melancholia** and **mania** in clinical descriptions that are still accurate today. He also placed mental functioning, or malfunctioning , in the brain rather than in the spirit. Therefore, the mentally ill became the domain of the medical doctor rather than the priest. Although the disorders continued to be recognized throughout different periods of history, it was not until recently, in the nineteenth century, that the current diagnostic properties of manic and depressive illness were formally categorized (Kaplan & Sadock, 1995).

Many people living in the twentieth century can identify with the term **depression** because they have some idea of what it feels like to be sad, blue, or "under the weather" or to temporarily lose a sense of meaning in their lives. Many people can also identify with the term *mania*, because, due to today's fast-moving society, they have some idea of what it is like to feel "pressured," "pressed," "speedy," or "hyper." Perhaps because of our general ability to experience a range of emotions, depression and mania (to a lesser extent) have become household words.

Perhaps because these terms have become familiar and because, generally, people can identify the emotions associated with each term, beginning clinicians are often not prepared for the depth of the symptoms or for how extremely and strongly mood and behavior are affected. Although recognizing that there is a range of severity of symptoms accompanying depression and mania, this chapter will refer mostly to the extreme syndromes or symptoms of mania and major depression.

DIAGNOSTIC OVERVIEW

The DSM-IV (APA, 1994) describes a group of disorders with the essential feature of a disturbance in **mood** that is not due to any other mental or physical disorder, medication, substance use, or other psychiatric condition. These disorders are classified as *mood disorders*. Former classifications described the same disorders as *affective disorders*, so this term may be used interchangeably (Kaplan & Sadock, 1995).

The DSM-IV uses three groups of criteria to diagnose problems regarding mood: episodes, disorders, and specifiers that describe a most recent episode and a recurrent course (Morrison, 1995). DSM-IV divides mood disorders into bipolar disorders and depressive disorders. The essential feature of a bipolar disorder is the presence of one or more manic episodes (often with a history of at least one major depressive episode). The essential feature of depressive disorders is one or more periods of depression, but not necessarily with a manic episodic history. **Dysthymia** is a milder form of major depressive episode, but it lasts for a longer period of time. **Cyclothymia** is a milder form of bipolar disorder, and it also has a longer duration. Bipolar and depressive disorders range from mild to severe and may include psychotic features. They usually cause considerable distress and/or impairment in all occupational areas of functioning.

Episodes

A mood episode refers to any time at which a client feels abnormally happy or sad. The mood disorders are constructed from these episodes, that is, the episodes are the foundation from which the disorders are arranged (Morrison, 1995).

Major depressive. At least five of the following symptoms must be present for two weeks and represent a change from previous level of functioning. At least one of the symptoms is either depressed mood or loss of interest and pleasure.

1. daily depressed mood, indicated by subjective report or the observation of others. In children or adolescents, the mood can be irritable.
2. very marked decrease of interest or pleasure in most daily activities
3. significant weight loss (when not dieting) or weight gain or significant increase or decrease in appetite. For children this could be represented by failure to gain expected weight through normal growth.
4. inability to sleep or sleeping most of the day
5. psychomotor agitation or its opposite, psychomotor retardation
6. extreme fatigue or loss of energy
7. feelings of extreme worthlessness or inappropriate guilt nearly every day
8. indecisiveness or lack of concentration
9. recurring thoughts of death, suicidal ideas, or a suicidal plan or attempt

Manic. There is a distinct period of abnormal, elevated, expansive, or irritable mood lasting at least one week. During this period at least three or more of the following symptoms are significantly present. There may be psychotic features or hospitalization may be necessitated to prevent harm to the self or others.

1. grandiosity or overinflated self-esteem
2. decreased need for sleep
3. talking more than usual or pressured talking
4. the experience that thoughts are racing
5. extreme distractibility

6. increase in goal-directed activity (this can take form in different areas, e.g., socially, at work or school, or sexually) or psychomotor agitation
7. excessive involvement in pleasurable activities that have the potential for later painful consequences (such as buying sprees, imprudent investments, or indiscreet sexual activity)

Hypomanic.   The elevated mood must last at least four days, be observably different from the usual nondepressed mood, and include three of the symptoms of mania. The episode does not cause marked impairment in occupational or social functioning, call for hospitalization, or include psychotic features.

Mixed.   The criteria for both manic and major depressive episodes are met nearly every day for at least one week. The impairment in functioning is identical to that of the manic and major depressive episodes.

Disorders

A disorder is a pattern of illness due to an abnormal mood. Most people who have a mood disorder experience depression at some times, and some also have high moods. Most mood disorders are diagnosed on the basis of a mood episode (Morrison, 1995).

Major depressive disorder.   A major depressive disorder, single episode, is diagnosed if there is a single major depressive episode and there has never been a manic, mixed, or hypomanic episode. A major depressive disorder, recurrent episode, is diagnosed if there have been two or more major depressive episodes at least two months apart and there has never been a manic, mixed, or hypomanic episode. A dysthymic disorder is a depressed mood that lasts most of the day for a majority of days over at least two years. In children and adolescents the mood can be irritable, and symptoms need be present for at least one year. To qualify for diagnosis, during the period of symptoms, the person should not have been symptom free for more than two months at a time and he or she should have experienced no major depressive, manic, mixed, or hypomanic episode or cyclothymic disorder. There also must be at least two of the following symptoms:

1. poor appetite or overeating
2. insomnia or too much sleeping
3. fatigue
4. low self-esteem
5. poor concentration or difficulty with decisions
6. hopelessness

Bipolar Disorders. The various bipolar disorders are distinguished by the presence of either a manic episode or a major depressive episode. They are classified as either bipolar I or bipolar II depending on which is the dominant mood. Bipolar I features a dominant manic mood, and bipolar II features a dominant depressed mood. As with the other disorders, the symptoms cause significant distress or impairment in important daily areas of functioning, they are not the result of use of a substance, medication, or medical condition, and they cannot be better accounted for by positing the existence of other disorders.

In bipolar I, single manic episode, there is the presence of a manic episode and there have been no major depressive episodes in the past. In bipolar I, most recent episode hypomanic, there is currently a hypomanic episode and there has been at least one manic, or mixed episode in the past. In bipolar I, most recent episode manic, there is a manic episode and there has been at least one major depressive, manic or mixed episode in the past. In bipolar I, most recent episode mixed, there is a mixed episode and there has been at least one major depressive, manic, or mixed episode in the past. Finally, in bipolar I, most recent episode depressed, there is currently a major depressive episode and there has been in the past at least one manic or mixed episode.

In bipolar II, there is one or more major depressive episodes and at least one hypomanic episode in the past, but there has never been a manic or mixed episode. In cyclothymic disorder there have been periods of hypomanic symptoms with periods of depressive symptoms for at least two years and the person has not been symptom free for more than two months. Moreover, there has been no major depressive, manic, or mixed episode during that time (APA, 1994).

Specifiers

Specifiers are descriptors that help qualify disorders or episodes. One set describes the most recent major depressive episode and manic episode. "Atypical features" describes individuals who eat and sleep a lot, feel weighted down and almost immobile, and are extremely sensitive to rejection. "Melancholic features" describes what can be considered the classic features of depression: early morning awakening with a mood that improves later in the day, loss of appetite, guilt, and feeling slowed down or agitated, with loss of interest and pleasure in those events and experiences that usually bring pleasure. "Catatonia" describes features of either extreme motor hyperactivity or extreme inactivity. "Postpartum onset" describes either a manic or a depressed episode experienced by a woman within a month of giving birth.

The other set of descriptors describes the overall course of a disorder. "With or without full interepisode recovery" describes the presence or absence of symptoms between episodes. "Rapid cycling" describes a person who has had at least four episodes within a year. "Seasonal pattern" describes those who become ill with regularity at the same time each year.

CAUSES, OCCURRENCE, AND THEORIES OF MOOD DISORDERS

In all industrialized countries, major depression is twice as common in females as in males (Kaplan & Sadock, 1991, 1995). Reasons for this difference include hormonal and endocrine system involvement and other gender-related stresses, such as childbirth and social conditions related to women's sex roles (see also Bracegirdle, 1991; Feder, 1990, 1991). Bipolar disorder is reported to be equally common among males and females. Major depression is 1.5 to 3 times more common among relatives of people with the disorder than in the general population. Bipolar disorder clearly occurs at a much higher rate in first-degree relatives. Up to 1.2 percent of the adult population is estimated to have bipolar disorder. The prevalence of major depressive disorder ranges from 4.5 to 9.3 percent for females and approximately half that for males. An interesting statistic is that the incidence of depression has increased among individuals who matured after World War II.

Causes and Occurrence

The causes of mood disorders are unknown; however, genetic, social and biologic factors are all indicated and are currently being researched. (Table 10-1 lists those factors). Various theories have been proposed over the years.

Social factors for depression center on loss, such as that of a parent or a spouse, though to date, no data supports these factors for the onset of mania. Genetic factors center on attempts to isolate some biologic characteristic associated with a tendency toward depression or to study genes for depression or bipolar illness that may be inherited along with other genes. Both bipolar and depressive disorders run in families. At least 50 percent of those with bipolar illness have a parent with a mood disorder. Biological factors center on:

a. the firings and interactions of brain neurons and their neurotransmitters (e.g., norepinephrine and serotonin)

Table 10-1.   Mood Disorders: Origins and Theories

Origins	Theories
Genetic	Behavioral
Biologic	Environmental
Social	Biologic-Environmental
	Cognitive
	Psychoanalytic

b. endocrine disorders and "misfiring" of neurohormones (e.g., melatonin, vasopressin, peptides, endorphins)
c. psychophysiological causes or studies of waking and sleeping cycles. It is thought that mood disorders involve problems with the limbic system, basal ganglia and hypothalamus.
d. speculation that affective disturbance is associated with daylight (called seasonal affective disorder). Some people tend to be depressed in fall and winter and to be normal or hypomanic in spring and summer (Templer, Spencer, & Hartlage, 1994).

Physical diseases such as Addison's and Cushing's disease, thyroid disorders, diabetes, syphilis, multiple sclerosis, and chronic brain syndromes related to arteriosclerosis may induce depression. Other physical disorders are associated with depression, including mononucleosis, anemia, malignancies, hypoglycemia, colitis, congestive heart failure, rheumatoid arthritis, and asthma. Some medications are also associated with depression, including antiparkinsonian agents, hormones, steroids, and antihypertensives (Kaplan & Sadock, 1995).

Theories

There are various ideas of why people have mood disorders. Different theories become more or less popular in different eras and in different countries. Ideas concerning mood disorders closely parallel broad theories of psychological functioning (see Chapter 3 for a discussion of psychological models). Personality theorists (e.g., Millon, 1996) discuss how personality disorders and depressive illnesses relate to, and interact with, each other. One approach postulates that some features of a personality disorder may make an individual vulnerable to the psychosocial stresses that, in turn, are implicated in depression. Conversely, another hypothesis postulates that the experience of depressive disorder will influence personality. Still another hypothesis states that constitutional factors, in conjunction with environmental variables, may lead to both symptoms of personality disorders and depressive disorder.

Early psychoanalytic theories were based on structural theories of the ego, id, and superego. Depression and mania were considered in view of an intrapsychic, or internal, makeup of the mind. In other words, dealing with the loss of a "libidinal" or pleasurable internal representation or "object" became a drama played out in the internal structure of ego and superego. Freud noticed that depressed people were often critical of themselves. He hypothesized that the criticism was really a disguise for another person for whom the patient felt affection. When this other, loved object was symbolically lost, the patient felt despair. Any anger at the lost other or object is redirected inward, to the self, and results in depression. Later theories (notably those of Melanie Klein) looked at developmental infant stages and powerful angry feelings towards the symbolic losses or deprivation of the parent that must be overcome. Klein discussed the depressive and manic positions that resulted. Perhaps the common adage that "depression is anger turned inward" stems from these early psychoanalytic theories. Other explanations concerned influences on self-esteem (Gelder, Gath, & Mayou, 1989), while more contemporary theories elucidate the alternating patterns of grandiosity/euphoria and self-deprecation/depression, which better relate more to the personality in contemporary society (Kaplan & Sadock, 1995; Mitchell & Black, 1995).

Behavioral theories have also been advanced to explain depression. The learned helplessness theory connects depression a to continual failure to control one's environment. In this formulation, the continual lack of control leads to passivity and helplessness. Reinforcement theories explain depression as related to receiving few positive reinforcements and many negative reinforcements and punishments throughout life (Kaplan & Sadock, 1991).

Cognitive theories suggest that distorted thinking is central to depression. Accordingly, a faulty type of thinking is developed in childhood and leads to later susceptibility to depression. The distorted thinking follows the themes of seeing the world as cruel, the self as deficient, and the future as hopeless (Beck, 1976, 1979; Kaplan & Sadock, 1991).

Environmental or life events that cause a disruption in the usual patterns of living and, therefore, call for adaptive responses have been found to correlate with depression (mostly) and also mania. These include psychosocial stresses that concern loss and separation, are beyond one's control, or are severely threatening (Kaplan & Sadock, 1995). There is some evidence that depression occurs in the majority of people who experience harsh life events (Templer et al., 1994; see also Centoni & Tallant, 1986; Boswell, 1989).

Biological and environmental theories of depression and bipolar disorders currently are popular. Depression, mania and bipolar disorders are considered disorders in the regulation of neurotransmitters in the central nervous system. They are considered conditions that are genetic and that can be inherited. However, environmental events are often considered along with biological factors. An individual may be born with a vulnerability to depression or mania that combines with environmental events to precipitate the disorder (Gelder et al., 1989; Millon, 1996; Templer et al., 1994).

CLINICAL PICTURE

Most people experience varying moods at different times in their lives. Generally, moods can be described as ranging from happiness, elation, and joy to sadness, despair, and hopelessness. The usual feelings that one experiences in daily life should not be confused with the syndromes of mania and depression. Most happy, energetic people do not have a manic disorder, and unhappiness or sadness does not signal a depressive disorder. Both the manic and depressive disorders can be viewed according to the degree and duration of symptoms. Like other disorders they have to be viewed in the context of how an individual usually functions and to what degree and how long a change in function occurs.

Individuals experiencing a manic episode present themselves with a very elevated mood and their behavior is generally very expansive and irritable. There is heightened psychomotor activity, and they speak, think, and move very rapidly. Usually they have seemingly boundless energy. Often they feel very creative, and indeed, they are usually flooded with some ideas that are imaginative. Popular lore would have us envy those who are manic for their creative qualities. However, although there may be heightened motor activity, there is usually little productivity. An individual who is manic rarely finishes projects through to completion; attention is fragmented and activity has a purposeless quality to it. Increased activity often takes the form of sexual provocativeness and promiscuity, exaggerated political and religious concern, or purchasing many expensive items regardless of their affordability. Essentially, all activities are carried out with a gross lack of judgment.

An individual who is manic may be euphoric and have an infectious quality, but there is also an accompanying quality of being "driven." He or she may be humorous but, due to a low frustration tolerance, may also easily become irritable and angry. The grandiose behavior and sense of importance may give way to psychotic delusions. It is not unusual to think that one is God, and an individual may show considerable contempt for other people. Due to this grandiosity; frequent, loud speech; and an interruptive manner accompanied by poor social judgment, those with manic behavior are often socially rejected (Kaplan & Sadock, 1989, 1991). Often, beginning professionals find it difficult to simply "be with" someone who is manic, and therefore should seek out clinical supervision for assistance in tolerating this behavior and working effectively.

In my clinical experience, in the realm of occupational therapy, their heightened activity, difficulty concentrating and attending to tasks, distractibility, and intrusiveness often make individuals experiencing a manic episode candidates for individual treatment with engagement in simple concrete tasks or movement. Working with those who are manic often calls on one's best idea of the therapeutic use of self and the use of a full repertoire of interpersonal skills. At the same time, it also calls for the use of concrete and simple tasks or activities. The seeming contradiction involving requirements of simplicity, on one hand, and the use of complex interpersonal skills, on the other, is often confusing and difficult for new clinicians. Again, this is a time to seek out clinical supervision. Table 10-2 lists major symptoms of mania and depression.

Major depression is characterized by a triad of symptoms: the reduced capacity to experience pleasure (often called anhedonia), reduced interest in the environment (described as withdrawal), and reduced energy (sometimes called anergia) (Kaplan & Sadock, 1989). Often, the person feels hopeless and helpless. Depression often seems more than a mood disorder (Beck, 1973) because it affects all areas of life and produces symptoms in many realms. In

Table 10-2. Clinical Picture: Major Symptoms of Depression and Mania

Symptoms	Depression	Mania
Emotional	Depleted mood Hopelessness Decreased sense of humor Lack of pleasure	Euphoric mood Grandiosity
Cognitive	Negative thinking Decreased concentration and attention Indecision	Grandiose, expansive thinking Decreased concentration and attention
Motivational	Decreased energy Paralysis of will and initiation Avoidance or escapist wishes	Increased energy Agitation Distraction Low frustration tolerance
Self-Concept	Worthlessness Guilt	Inflated sense of worth and power
Vegetative	Loss of appetite Sleep disturbance Loss of sexual desire	Loss of appetite Sleep disturbance Increased sexual preoccupation

fact, life is usually described as, and felt to be, empty, remote, and without meaning or potential. The following symptoms are associated with depression:

- Emotional symptoms include hopelessness, depressed mood, lack of pleasure, and a decreased ability to experience humor.

- Vegetative symptoms are often present, such as inability to sleep or sleeping too much, psychomotor agitation or retardation, loss of appetite, and loss of interest in sexual activity (loss of libido).

- Cognitive symptoms are decreased concentration and attention, and difficulty organizing or "thinking straight." Sometimes there is an overwhelming feeling of being burdened by even the simplest task. Indecision is a hallmark. Even the most minor decisions are difficult to make (ambivalence).

- Symptoms in the area of self-concept include a negative sense of self and feelings of worthlessness. Often the person feels an overwhelming sense of guilt for real or imagined crimes. This often becomes **referential thinking**, as the person imagines that he or she is the cause of someone else's misfortune. Suicidal thoughts are often present.

Suicidal thoughts are experienced by some people who suffer from depression (Beck, 1973; see also Hemphill, 1992). The most dangerous periods often are in the beginning, usually when the person is most anxious and help is not present, and in the later remission period, when the person begins to feel better and then may become frightened of a relapse. At this time, he or she will have regained energy and be able to think straight enough to commit suicide. It is important to take suicidal statements seriously and inquire if an individual has the means (usually a gun or pills) and a formulated plan. All statements and other information should be immediately reported to the primary therapist and the treatment team.

It is my clinical experience that in the occupational therapy clinic, people who are depressed may have difficulty initiating any task or may protest often that they can do nothing. They may require much prompting and activities that are concrete and simple. They may take a very long time to complete a task or obsess over a perceived error. An individual who is manic may display the opposite behavior, initiating too many tasks, stating that he or she can do everything and anything, flitting from task to task, denying any errors, and requiring much attention and prompting to contain or stop behavior.

COMMON EVALUATION AND MANAGEMENT

There are some common strategies of evaluation and management for depressive and manic disorders that are recognized by most disciplines working in psychiatric settings.

Evaluation

The intensity, severity, and duration of symptoms are obtained by observation, interview, and history taking. Some scales are used by other professionals, most notably, the Beck Depression Inventory (Beck, 1978) and later, similar versions (Burns, 1989), which are lists of easily answered questions referring to symptoms. Due to biological research there are also tests that measure depression by various biological means (Kaplan & Sadock, 1991), However, they are expensive and their use and diagnostic efficiency are still questionable.

Usually, symptoms of mania, such as pressured speech, psychomotor agitation, and grandiosity, are easily observable. An interview and a recent history usually supplement the evaluation. Often, family members may aid in the history. The task is to differentiate the types of bipolar illness from major depressive disorder and other psychotic disorders.

Management

Psychotherapy and medications are common methods of managing depression and bipolar disorders (Gelder et al., 1989; Kaplan & Sadock, 1995; Templer et al., 1994). Interpersonal therapy focuses on social and interpersonal relationship functioning. It deals with disturbances between the depressed or manic person and others in the environment and current life situations. Family therapy aids in maintaining support for the individual in the environment. Behavioral therapy for depressive disorders is designed to alter behaviors that may be keeping a person isolated or defeatist. It also deals with changing life patterns or situations in the environment that may be negative reinforcers. It may involve skills training, such as assertiveness, self-monitoring, and systematic desensitization (Templer et al., 1994). Cognitive therapy is designed to change negative thinking processes that contribute to depression. Distorted thinking is targeted, and the here-and-now therapy interactions and current life situations are the focus for changing thinking.

Psychoanalytic theories attempt to change personality structure. This means targeting for change an individual's experience of trust, intimacy, dealing with loss, coping mechanisms, and recognition of a range of emotions. Short-term psychodynamic therapy has been developed for depression. Usually problems are thought to stem from relationships in early childhood. The therapy process utilizes *transference*; that is, the client transfers perceptions and feelings about important childhood figures and events to the therapist and the therapy situation. These are then interpreted by the therapist and discussed and explored together. In the short-term versions, the therapist quickly points out transference reactions and immediately uses the present session to explore and correct behavior carried over from the past. In managing bipolar disorders and mania, psychotherapy is usually short term with a focus on immediate management, coping with the effects of manic behavior, and preventing future manic responses or episodes.

The traditional medicines for depression are tricyclic antidepressants, monoamine oxidase (MAO) inhibitors, and lithium. Newer classes of antidepressants, including selective serotonin reuptake inhibitors (SSRIs) or serotonin and norepinephrine reuptake inhibitors (SNRIs) influence the amount of serotonin and norepinephrine in the brain. Medicines with the trade names of Prozac, Zoloft, Effexor, and Paxil have been designed to affect the level of neurotransmitters in the brain. These newer drugs, which are sometimes described as "atypical," are considered safer, have fewer side effects than traditional tricyclics, are more specific to neurotransmitter brain functioning, and are used with a wider number of people.

Lithium is the treatment of choice for the manic phase of bipolar disorder. It is used as a maintenance drug to prevent or reduce future episodes. However, it can be toxic, so that it is monitored very closely by daily tests of the level of the mineral in the blood. For those who do not respond to lithium, the treatment of choice may be a mild dose of an antipsychotic or antianxiety medicine (Kaplan & Sadock, 1995).

The use of electroconvulsive therapy (ECT) has stirred controversy for many years (Gelder et al., 1989; Kaplan & Sadock, 1989). Some claim it caused a permanent loss of memory, while others claim that ECT was the only intervention that aided their recovery. Some people claim that the practice should be outlawed, and it is illegal in several states. Others point to recent advances in administration of the treatment that make it less harmful. The method of delivery includes giving a general anesthetic along with a muscle relaxant and then placing electrodes, usually bilaterally, which causes a seizure consisting of muscular contraction in face, jaw, and plantar extensions for about 30 to 60 seconds. ECT can be extremely effective when there are very severe symptoms, such as psychomotor retardation, early morning awakening, agitation, decreased appetite and weight, psychotic symptoms, or little response to other antidepressant medications. It is indicated when there is a high risk of suicide or danger to physical health. The mode of action of ECT is thought to be brought about through physiological and biochemical changes in the brain, brought about by the seizure. Neurochemical changes are thought to produce changes in neurotransmitter function. Physiological changes are thought to be affected by the reduction of activity in the brain following the seizure.

Studies show an immediate loss of memory shortly after treatment, though patients are back to their baseline memory six months later. Unwanted effects of ECT include anxiety and headache immediately afterwards; confusion, nausea, and vertigo a few hours afterwards; and some muscle pain. The contraindications include respiratory infections, heart disease, aneurysms, and certain other drugs, such as reserpine. Obviously, the procedure's benefits and risks should be adequately and clearly explained, and the patient must sign a standard consent form. Other forms of medicine, such as the newer neurotransmitter drugs, are less controversial (Kaplan & Sadock, 1995) but nevertheless, ECT remains a topic of popular discussion (Kramer, 1993).

OCCUPATIONAL THERAPY TREATMENT

Various occupational therapy evaluations may be used depending on which context or performance area and components are being assessed or which occupational therapy model is followed (see Chapter 4 for a discussion of occupational therapy models; see also Devereaux & Carlson, 1992). There is not yet an occupational therapy assessment specific to depression. Not withstanding that fact, the therapist should always evaluate a client according to the severity of the mood disorder. A person's behavior and statements will indicate the stage of functioning on a continuum (see Figure 10-1). The following case illustrations demonstrate the difference in people's symptoms, whether severely depressed or severely manic. However, despite different symptoms, their behavior fits on the far ends of the continuum and therefore necessitates a similar approach and treatment.

CASE ILLUSTRATION: TAE—SEVERELY DEPRESSED

On Tuesday, Tae did not show up for the partial hospitalization occupational therapy group, "About Depression." When he was called by his therapist, he reported that he was still in bed, he had been there since Friday, and this was the first time he had answered the phone in three days. He reported that he had been ruminating about his life and obsessively thinking that he had hurt another client because of his remarks in a community meeting at the program. He felt as if he could hardly move from his house. However, after reassurance that he was missed and was expected at the program, he said he would try to make it. With prompting from the therapist that she was counting on him, he agreed to come in the next day.

Discussion

Tae had difficulty initiating any task and required much prompting to follow through. He obsessed over remarks that he perceived as wrong. He responded to concrete and structured behaviors by the OTR.

CASE ILLUSTRATION: MARIA—HYPERMANIC

Maria entered the occupational therapy group early, bringing five other inpatients with her. She proceeded to walk around the room, taking something from every cabinet and announcing how she would lead the group. Before the therapist caught up with her, she commented coquettishly on how sexy the occupational therapist looked and suggested that maybe they could get together since she was available. While thanking her for her willingness to assist and her flattering comments, the OTR assured her that he could aptly lead the group and asked her to take a seat.

Discussion

Maria initiated too many tasks, and did so in a grandiose and expansive manner, in addition to making inappropriate remarks to the therapist. Even though her symptoms were quite the opposite of Tae's, she, too, responded to a direct approach by the OTR.

Occupational therapists' training in analyzing and grading activities means that interventions can, and should, be tailored for anyone at any stage of the mood continuum. Moreover, an occupational therapist's approach should also be tailored to stages of the mood continuum (see Figure 10-1).

At the extreme ends of the continuum, represented by severe depression and hypermania, the therapist's focus is on providing structure and meeting demands. Interventions should be concrete and tangible, and activities should be short-term, simple, and success enhancing. The surrounding environment should be carefully arranged so as not to be too distracting. The therapist also should make decisions, provide clear expectations and parameters for activities, and provide limits on expansive behavior and validation for depressed behavior. The therapist's focus is on creating an external structure for the clients. Craft and exercise activities in short segments of 30 to 45 minutes can be most useful at this stage.

	severely depressed	maintenance	hyper manic
Structure	Increased	Decreased	Increased
Tasks	Repetitive Simple Tangible	New steps More complex More abstract	Repetitive Simple Tangible
Time	Short term	Longer term	Short term
Limits	Consistent Often Direct Understandable	Less required	Consistent Often Direct Understandable
Directions	Simple Demonstrable	More complex More abstract	Simple Demonstrable

Figure 10-1. The Mood Continuum

As a person improves and moves towards the middle, maintenance stage of the continuum, more abstract activities with more complex steps that require more time can be incorporated. Activities can include more client decision making and fewer limits. Clients can be expected to take more responsibility for functioning and for reflection on their behavior and thoughts. The therapist's focus is to assist the client to realize his or her internal abilities and resources. Useful groups are daily living and vocational, problem solving, and expressive activities; these can be an hour or longer.

The occupational therapy emphasis on independent functioning often leads beginners to insist on independent functioning and decision making from all people at all times. However, occupational therapy also advocates meeting a person at his or her particular level. If an individual clearly is unable to make independent decisions or to engage in daily activities, the occupational therapist should adjust to meet the demands of the person and the environment. Following the concept of the mood continuum helps a therapist know when to focus on the external or internal environments. It allows the OTR to flexibly provide treatment according to whatever the person (internal environment) and stage of the disorder (external environment) require.

Interpersonal Approach

Many occupational therapists may find themselves charmed by an individual who is manic and drawn to take inordinate responsibility for the individual who is depressed. They may be overwhelmed by overactive, expansive behavior or extreme depression. They may become impatient and frustrated. Beginners often make the mistake of expecting too much and therefore frustrating their clients.

When working with someone who is depressed, it is essential to relate with understanding and empathy. The client will not benefit from a "snap out of it" attitude. The depressed individual already feels sad, worthless, humorless, and, often, guilty. Depressed individuals may subject themselves to mental punishment because they are depressed and have been unable to change their condition. They may be stuck in a cycle of negative ruminations. If depressed people could benefit from badgering, they would not be depressed and would certainly help themselves. Often, the tendency is to treat them in an authoritarian manner, and sometimes staff members are unable to tolerate ruminating or negativistic behavior. Some find it difficult to work with people who may not respond immediately or may not be expressive. Although the tendency may be to "encourage independence" and limit setting or to help people see the brighter, often reality-based, alternative, one should provide the opposite: understanding and empathic responses and a validation of the client's feelings or thoughts. Particularly in the early stages of the disorder, one should permit dependence in the form of information about the depressive process and assurance that the person will get better although he or she may not know or feel it now.

CASE ILLUSTRATION: LIZZIE— HANDLING DEPRESSED BEHAVIOR

Initially, when Lizzie came to the occupational therapy group she would often sit alone and refuse to work on anything. She felt as if she could hardly move— as if she had a 100-pound pack on her back. To think about making a decision precipitated panic. She worried that she would never get better and would continue to fall into what she described as a "black hole." When approached she would only ruminate about the "black hole," and most interactions were negative statements about herself and her past, present, and future life. People on the unit stayed away from her, and the staff avoided her or attempted to provide reality testing by reviewing how her life "really" was. She became more depressed and hopeless, certain that others hated her, did not understand her, and maybe were unable to help her.

The OTR provided a different approach. She validated Lizzie's statements of how she felt, acknowledged that her state was indeed painful and difficult, and stated that although it seemed there was no light at the end of the tunnel, Lizzie would indeed get better. The therapist shared the information that she had worked with many people who had been severely depressed and had felt similarly hopeless, and that through treatment they did return to former functioning. The OTR was not put off by negative statements and continued to initiate contact. She continued to provide empathic responses and to invite Lizzie to participate in structured groups that included movement and working on very short-term activities. Lizzie's ruminations did not completely stop; however, they decreased. She felt that someone seemed to understand her, did not reject her, and was competent to help. She attempted to participate in groups and began to sense some hope.

Discussion

Lizzie demonstrated symptoms and behaviors of depression, negative rumi-nations, immobility, and hopelessness. These often are responded to with a positive manner that is not perceived as genuine. However, when the thera-pist responded in an understanding and validating manner and with struc-ture in activities, Lizzie's behavior changed for the better.

When working with an individual who is experiencing a manic episode, it is also essential to relate with understanding and empathy. For this behavior, empathy means being present and able to tolerate manic behavior while at the same time clearly providing limits or parameters for acceptable behavior. This client will also not benefit from a heavily authoritarian approach, but he or she will benefit when a therapist consistently demonstrates the ability to be with the client and is not "turned off" by the individual's often-overwhelm-ing behavior. In addition, the client will benefit from direction and an honest appraisal of behavior presented in a gentle yet firm, matter-of-fact way.

CASE ILLUSTRATION: JEREMY— HANDLING MANIC BEHAVIOR

Jeremy entered the occupational therapy evaluation group with expansive, grandiose behavior, talking about why he did not need the group. He spoke in a nonstop, stream-of-consciousness manner, with pressured speech. He was unable to remain in one place and was distracted by almost everybody and anything in the room. When approached by the OTR, he proceeded to tell her how attractive she was, asked if she was married, and told her how "good" he could be with women. The OTR asked him to begin the assessment. He did not think that he needed to be assessed and stated that, in fact, he could prob-ably "assess" and help her. She stated that she understood that he felt won-derful and probably wanted to make a connection with her, but his behavior was out of line, and, indeed, would distance her, which was probably oppo-site of what he wanted. Jeremy did begin the assessment but after two min-utes, he became distracted in an agitated way and declared to all that this was childish and the OTR "did not have a clue." The OTR gently asked him to return to the activity and continued. Occasionally she validated how agi-tated and disconnected his behavior made him feel.

When Jeremy's manic behavior subsided, following two weeks of hospital-ization and lithium treatment, he thanked the OTR for giving him directions and reminders to return to his activity at a time when he became distracted every few minutes. He also apologized for any behavior that was offensive or insulting, adding that he actually liked the therapist because she was able to tolerate and withstand sexual innuendoes by pointing out what was not ac-ceptable and did so without becoming angry or withdrawing from him.

Discussion

The OTR's approach to Jeremy's manic behavior was also empathic, direct, and consistent, demonstrating her ability to tolerate his behavior and, therefore, conveying that she valued him.

Intervention

Occupational therapy addresses all symptoms—emotional, cognitive, motivational, self-concept, and vegetative. See Table 10-2 for symptoms of depression and mania.

Particularly when addressing motivational symptoms, occupational therapy provides interventions that directly relate to changing behavior. For an individual who is depressed, it provides evidence of the ability to continue with occupations of everyday life and provides concrete proof, often through working with and mastering crafts, of a continued ability to function. For an individual who is manic, it provides concrete structure through which to focus attention. Concrete evidence of a remaining ability to function combats helplessness and distractibility with hope and defense, which are key motivational symptoms.

Occupational therapy can experientially contract or disprove negative thoughts through its focus on functioning in the everyday occupations and activities of daily life. Occupational therapy can intervene in the depressed person's negative cycle of misconstruing experiences as defeating, regarding oneself as deficient or morally defective, and viewing the future in a negative way. Through its focus on the activities of daily life, occupational therapy can intervene in the manic person's expansive and grandiose cycle by providing a structured environment and activities through which to organize and monitor behavior. Tables 10-3 and 10-4 outline the symptoms, problems, and interventions involved in depression and mania (see also Boswell, 1989; Centoni & Tallant, 1986; Devereaux & Carlson, 1992; Feder, 1991; Meyers, 1991; Stein & Smith, 1989).

Table 10-3 focuses on interventions for depression. Pervasive symptoms of depression lead to problems in all performance areas and all performance components, particularly cognitive and social. Treatment focuses on changing behavior, changing the environment, or changing internal appraisals. The most prevalent emotional symptoms of depression will manifest in a loss of interest in formerly valued activities or the pursuit of only one interest in an exclusive and or compulsive manner. The individual will tend to withdraw from others and become isolated. Some common interventions are to engage the individual in activities that he or she values or has valued in the past and to provide opportunities to engage in different activities or in activities within a group setting. Sometimes an individual will be reluctant to engage in any activities or group; however, the therapist should maintain an approach that is inviting and confident without being authoritarian and overly demanding. Providing activities that do not require too many choices or steps to com-

Table 10-3. Interventions for Depression		
Symptoms	*Problems*	*Interventions*
Emotional	Loss of interest in formerly valued activities or pursuit of narrow or single interests exclusively and in a compulsive manner	Engage in valued activities Expand opportunities to engage in other than one activity
	Tendency to isolate oneself and withdraw from others	Monitor value and pleasure while doing or completing activities and engage in values clarification activities. Engage in group activities
Cognitive and Motivational	Indecision and ambivalence Inability to concentrate and attend to usual daily activities Negative attitudes that predominate in all usual activities Inability to initiate or sustain activity Tendency to isolate	Initially provide occupations and do not require too many choices Provide opportunities to successfully accomplish short-term, simple, concrete activities Set realistic, step-by-step goals and behavioral "to do" lists, grading activities and environment for successful completion Reestablish normal routines: structured planning of daily occupations, simple behavioral lists Engage in cognitive therapy, i.e., recognizing, monitoring, and changing thoughts Perform reality testing and question unrealistic beliefs. Engage in psychoeducational groups concerning symptoms and behavior, such as recognizing precursors to mood changes and managing medicines.
Self-Concept	Worthlessness Guilt	Provide opportunities to successfully accomplish short-term, simple, concrete activities

(continues)

Table 10-3. Interventions for Depression (continued)		
Symptoms	*Problems*	*Interventions*
		Set realistic, step-by-step goals and behavioral "to do" lists, grading activities and environment for successful completion
		Perform cognitive therapy, challenge distorted ideas.
		Engage in activities that focus on self-exploration, such as recognizing and dealing with emotions, self-expression, and self-exploration through creative media and expanding coping styles.
Vegetative	Failure to sustain basic needs for food, rest, etc.	Provide external structure

plete, and perhaps allowing a person to work while in the presence of others but not necessarily interact will enhance engagement. A more behavioral intervention is to ask the client to monitor the pleasure or value received from working on, and completing, an activity. This can be a self-report, and it often is more effective if a simple, concrete scale is constructed. When a person is less severely depressed (on the mid-stage of the mood continuum), values clarification activities may be introduced.

Cognitive and motivational symptoms will manifest in indecision and ambivalence, difficulty concentrating and attending, difficulty initiating or sustaining activities, and the expression of negative thoughts predominantly rather than positive ones. Activities or occupations that do not require too many choices, can be accomplished successfully in a short time, and are tangible may enhance a person's motivation and self-concept. More behavioral interventions of setting and listing step-by-step, easily achieved goals and crossing them off when accomplished will enhance motivation. Cognitive interventions, such as recognizing and monitoring negative thoughts, changing the internal "tapes" one plays over and over, and questioning unrealistic beliefs can be directed towards cognitive symptoms. Psychoeducational groups concerning symptoms, behavior, recognizing precursors to mood changes, managing medicines, and expanding coping strategies can also address cognitive problems.

Symptoms that relate to one's self-concept are expressed as feelings or thoughts of worthlessness or guilt. Again, short-term concrete activities that

Table 10-4. Interventions for Mania

Symptoms	Problems	Interventions
Emotional	Over inflated or exaggerated interest and meaning attributed to all areas of life	Offer an honest, realistic appraisal of behavior and end products while engaging in activities or occupations.
		Elicit clients' appraisals and reflection regarding their behavior and end products after engaging in activities.
Cognitive and Motivational	Increased energy resulting in distractibility, initiation of too many activities, and inability to sustain activity	Provide opportunities to engage in concrete, short-term activities that include more than two steps
	Inability to concentrate and attend to usual daily activities	Provide clear expectations for behavior and end products
	Inability to follow through on decisions	Arrange a distraction-free environment
	Unrealistically positive attitudes that predominate in all usual daily activities	Assist client to return to goal-directed action whenever distracted
		Eventually assist in goal setting and planning and in anticipating the consequences of actions by monitoring behavior during activities
Self Concept	Inflated, unrealistic sense of worth and efficacy	Display an accepting, tolerant attitude
	Failure to take responsibility for consequences of behavior	Offer an honest, realistic appraisal of behavior and end products while engaging in occupations
		Engage in activities that focus on self-exploration, such as recognizing and dealing with emotions, self-expression, and self-exploration through creative media and expanding coping styles
Vegetative	Failure to sustain basic needs	Provide external structure

can be quickly mastered and completed will add to a person's sense of self. In addition, behavioral interventions that show that goals have been achieved usually also enhance self-esteem. Cognitive interventions that directly challenge self-distortions and expressive interventions that focus on self-awareness, self-expression, and self-exploration will model the power of self-reflection and -expression. Self-exploration can also include exploring and changing styles of coping. Again, it is important to be aware of where a person is located on the mood continuum when introducing interventions that require energy, initiation, imagination, and problem solving.

Table 10-4 focuses on interventions for mania. Emotional symptoms of mania will usually manifest in a person having an overinflated or exaggerated interest in various activities and perhaps attributing excessive meaning to all objects and people in life. Interventions can center around engagement in activities or occupations. The occupational therapist can offer honest, realistic appraisals of an individual's behavior while engaged in working on activities or can make honest realistic appraisals of end products. The therapist may elicit the client's appraisal and reflection concerning his or her own behavior and products. Sometimes reality testing (e.g., Socratic questioning) utilizing an appropriate tone may be productively employed, even though this may not bring about an immediate change of behavior. Again, the approach depends on where the behavior is located on the mood continuum.

Cognitive and motivational symptoms may result in distractibility, inability to concentrate and attend, and a desire to initiate too many activities, usually all at once. Once activities have been initiated there may be difficulty following through, and in spite of this inability, there may also be an unrealistic appraisal of the person's abilities. Just as with an individual who is depressed, it is important to provide opportunities to engage in concrete, short-term activities that do not contain many steps. It is also important to provide an environment with few distractions, including noises and visual stimulation. In addition, whenever possible the OTR should provide clear expectations for behavior and assist the client to return to the goal whenever he or she becomes distracted.

Symptoms involving one's concept of self will usually result in the expression of inflated, unrealistic ideas about oneself and one's effectiveness, often accompanied by a failure to assume responsibility for any consequences related to one's behavior. An approach that is genuine, authentic, and accepting, even while offering clear limits, is suggested, along with an honest, realistic appraisal of the person's behavior and the end products. It is particularly important to assess where a person with mania is located on the mood continuum. Those on the farther ends may have difficulty being in, and may indeed disrupt, a group setting. Engaging in self-exploration and -expression can be helpful for symptoms relating to self-concept and for expanding coping styles, but these interventions are usually most helpful when a person has moved to the middle of the mood continuum.

Following is the treatment process that was designed for Lizzie, which illustrates occupational therapy interventions.

CASE ILLUSTRATION: LIZZIE—TREATMENT PROCESS

An Allen Cognitive Levels evaluation (Allen, 1985; Allen & Allen, 1987; Allen, Earhart, & Blue, 1992; Allen & Reyner, 1994) indicated a cognitive function level of approximately 6.0. This indicated that Lizzie did not have a cognitive impairment. However, observation while performing crafts from the Allen Diagnostic Module (1996) indicated that Lizzie was slow to engage, and many comments indicated a lack of interest in what she was doing. A self-refport checklist adapted from the Burns Depression Checklist (Burns, 1989) indicated a high score of 40, indicating particularly that Lizzie felt very sad, discouraged, worthless, inferior, guilty, and unattractive. She was indecisive and irritable, had lost interest in life, and was generally unmotivated. An interview indicated a history of being newly divorced. She worried about losing her job due to downsizing and feared she would not be able to support her two children. She had become isolated, stopped going to work, and attempted suicide. She felt guilty that she was now hospitalized.

Lizzie liked to cook and bake; she had formerly enjoyed tennis and running and had belonged to a book club. Since her marital separation she had not pursued any of these activities. She reported that she had a few close friends but had withdrawn from them because she felt she was a burden and was generally not presentable to people. She did not see the point in participating in occupational therapy groups since she was feeling hopeless and negative about the present and future. However, she agreed to attend some groups.

Initially she attended a movement/exercise group after being sought out by the leader every day. It was difficult for her to follow the simple exercises, though she eventually did look forward to the group and expressed relief that she could just follow directions and did not have to initiate interactions. At the same time she attended a parallel group where people worked on individual craft projects, and after a few days she finally agreed to start a project after admiring another member's finished work. She found that, although she generally had negative things to say about the project, she actually felt some sense of accomplishment. She also was relieved that she did not have to make decisions or "process her feelings." Within a week she had become an active member and finished projects for both herself and her children.

After a few days, she attended a "Learning about Depression" workshop. She enjoyed receiving a handout about depression, and she was surprised at what she learned from the different theories. She gave the handout to her family and they were able to discuss their concerns about her.

Lizzie was discharged to a partial hospitalization program. She attended a medication management group, a "Learning about Feelings" group, and a group titled, "Preventing Depression/Coping Differently" three times a week in the occupational therapy program. In addition, she participated in a sports group and a community resource group, in which she identified resources in the community, such as Parents without Partners and a twelve step group addressing self-confidence. The OTR worked individually with her to help her learn vocational skills and interests. She completed a vocational assessment (APTICOM®), consisting of aptitude, interest and skills tests (Vocational Research Institute, cited in Asher, 1996). She began to focus on obtaining a job and to explore alternative careers. She eventually attended the partial program one day a week while she began to work at a new job three times a week. Eventually she began to work full time and was discharged from the day program. She enjoyed a continuing education group sponsored by the partial program, which focused on self-exploration through creative media.

Discussion

Initially, Lizzie was severely depressed but without cognitive impairment, as indicated on the assessments. She responded initially to structured interventions that did not require too much independent decision making and would demonstrate her ability to continue to function. She was able to utilize information regarding her disease, and later, as she improved, to utilize interventions that required more thought and independent decision making. She also responded to a reasoned approach of empathy and validation of her experience.

Summary

Mood disorders have been described throughout history. Initially, melancholia and mania were thought to be curses of the gods. Over the centuries, environmental and biological theories have emerged and mood disorders were classified as depressive and bipolar disorders. Research on, and treatment of, mood disorders address biology, personality, behavior, cognition, and life events.

Mania and depression represent opposite ends of what can be considered more than a mood disorder because both include multiple symptoms, which may be emotional, cognitive, motivational, or vegetative. Occupational therapy treatment consists of changing behavior, arranging the environment, and changing internal appraisals. One should tailor the therapy according to the severity of the mood disorder. Occupational therapy is particularly important for mood disorders because of its use of tangible concrete activities and its focus on everyday occupations and motivation.

Review Questions

1. What are some reasons for the prevalence of depression in females?
2. Which theories of mood disorders are addressed in occupational therapy treatment?
3. Explain the mood continuum. Why is it important?
4. Name one intervention for cognitive and motivational problems for an individual who is manic.
5. Name one intervention for emotional problems of depression.

Learning Activities

1. Think of a time when you were "blue" or sad. How did you want people to treat you?
2. Complete a short project: assess your mood before you start each day for seven days. Monitor your thoughts or feelings during work and after each project is completed (write them down or use a measurement scale). Assess your mood at the end of a week.
3. Any time a friend says something negative about her- or himself or about something she or he owns, try validating or agreeing with the statement while also expressing your concern.
4. For fictional descriptions of the many forms of depression, read *The Bell Jar* by Sylvia Plath, *Ordinary People* by Judith Guest, *Beloved* by Toni Morrison, or *The Color Purple* by Alice Walker. For an autobiographical description of depression, read *On the Edge of Darkness* by Kathy Cronkite.
5. For a biographical description of bipolar disorder, read *An Unquiet Mind: A Memoir of Moods and Madness*, by K. Redfield Jamison, and *A Brilliant Madness: Living with Manic-Depressive Illness*, by Patty Duke.

References

Allen, C. K. (1985). *Occupational therapy for psychiatric diseases: Measurement and management of cognitive disabilities*. Boston: Little, Brown & Co.

Allen, C. K., & Allen, R. A. (1987). Cognitive disabilities: Measuring the social consequences of mental disorders. *Journal of Clinical Psychiatry 48,* 185–191.

Allen, C. K., Earhart, C., & Blue, T. (1992). *Treatment goals for the physically and cognitively disabled.* Bethesda, MD: American Occupational Therapy Association.

Allen, C. K., & Reyner, A. (1994). *How to start using the cognitive levels: A guide to introducing Allen's theories into your practice* (2nd ed.). (Available from S & S Worldwide, P.O. Box 513, Colchester, CT 06415–0513.)

American Psychiatric Association (APA). (1994). *Diagnostic and statistical manual of mental disorders* (4th ed.). Washington, DC: APA.

Asher, I. E. (1996). *Occupational therapy assessment tools: An annotated index* (2nd ed.). Bethesda, MD: American Occupational Therapy Association.

Beck, A. (1973). *Depression: Causes and treatment: The diagnosis and management of depression.* Philadelphia: University of Pennsylvania Press.

Beck, A. (1976). *Cognitive therapy and the emotional disorders.* New York: International Universities Press.

Beck, A. (1978). *Beck Depression Inventory*. San Antonio: Psychological Corporation.

Beck, A. (1979). *Cognitive therapy of depression*. New York: Guilford Press.

Boswell, S. (1989). A social support group for depressed people. *Australian Occupational Therapy Journal* 36(1), 34–41.

Bracegirdle, H. (1991). The female stereotype and occupational therapy for women with depression. *British Journal of Occupational Therapy, 54*(5), 193–194.

Burns, D. (1989). *The feeling good handbook: The new mood therapy*. New York: Plume/Penguin.

Centoni, M., & Tallant, B. (1986). The projective use of drawings as a treatment technique with the depressed unemployed male. *Canadian Journal of Occupational Therapy, 53*(2), 81–87.

Devereaux, E., & Carlson, M. (1992). Health policy: The role of occupational therapy in the management of depression. *American Occupational Therapy Association, 465*(2), 175–180.

Feder, J. (1990). Occupational stress and the depressed female client. *Work: A Journal of Prevention, Assessment and Rehabilitation, 1* (2), 55–62.

Feder, J. (1991). Women, depression and work: Treatment strategies for the depressed patient. *Occupational Therapy Practice, 2* (4), 58–67.

Gelder, M., Gath, D., & Mayou, R. (1989). *Oxford textbook of psychiatry* (2nd ed.). New York: Oxford University Press.

Hemphill, B. (1992). Depression among suicidal elderly: A life-threatening illness. *Occupational Therapy Practice, 4*(1), 61–66.

Kaplan, H., & Sadock, B. (1989). *Comprehensive textbook of psychiatry* (5th ed.). Baltimore: Williams & Wilkins.

Kaplan, H., & Sadock, B. (1991). *Synopsis of psychiatry: Behavioral sciences: Clinical psychology* (6th ed.). Baltimore: Williams & Wilkins.

Kaplan, H., & Sadock, B. (1995). *Comprehensive textbook of psychiatry* (6th ed.). Baltimore: Williams & Wilkins .

Kramer, P. (1993). *Listening to Prozac*. New York: Penguin.

Meyers, J. (1991). Clinical differentiation between dementia and depression. *Gerontology Special Interest Section Newsletter (American Occupational Therapy Association), 14*(1), 5–6.

Mitchell, S., & Black, M. (1995). *Freud and beyond: A history of modern psychoanalytic thought*. New York: Basic Books.

Millon, T. (1996). *Disorders of Personality: DSM-IV and beyond* (2nd ed.). New York: John Wiley & Sons.

Stein, F,. & Smith, J. (1989). Short-term stress management programme with acutely depressed in-patients. *Canadian Journal of Occupational Therapy, 56*(4),185–191.

Templer, D., Spencer, D., & Hartlage, L. (1994). *Biosocial psychopathology: Epidemiological perspectives*. New York: Springer.

Suggested Reading

Popular Books about Depression and Mania

Berger, D., & Berger, L. (1991). *We heard the angels of madness: A family guide to coping with manic depression.* New York: William Morrow.

Gold, M. (1995). *The good news about depression: Cures and treatments in the new age of psychiatry.* New York: Bantam Books.

Ingersoll, B. D. (1995). *Lonely, sad and angry: A parent's guide to depression in children and adolescents.* New York: Doubleday.

Rosen, L. (1996). *When someone you love is depressed: How to help your loved one without losing yourself.* New York: Free Press.

Salmans, S. (1995). *Depression: Questions you have—Answers you need.* Allentown, PA: People's Medical Society.

Popular Self-Help Books

Colgrove, M., Bloomfield, H., & McWilliams, P. (Eds.). (1991). *How to survive the loss of a love.* Los Angeles: Prelude Press.

Copeland, M. E. (1994). *Living without depression and manic depression: A workbook for maintaining mood stability.* Oakland, CA: New Harbinger Publications.

Emery, Gary. (1988). *Getting un-depressed: How a woman can change her life through cognitive therapy* (Rev. ed.). New York: Touchstone.

Greenberger, D., & Padesky, C. A. (1995). *Mind over mood: Change how you feel by changing the way you think.* New York: Guilford.

Lange, A., & Jakubowski, P. (1976). *Cognitive behavioral procedures for trainers.* New York: Research Press.

U.S. Government Publications

U.S. Department of Health and Human Services. (1993). *Depression is a treatable disease* (AHCPR Publication No. 93-0553). Rockville, MD.

Resource Catalog

New Harbinger Publications Self-Help Titles, 5674 Shattuck Avenue, Oakland, CA 94609; 800-748-6273.

Dementia

Carolyn Glogoski-Williams, Ph.D., OTR
Assistant Professor, Department of Occupational Therapy and
   Program in Gerontology
San Jose State University

Diane Foti, MS, OTR
Senior Occupational Therapist
Kaiser Permanente, Hayward, California
Lecturer, San Jose State University

Mark Covault, MS, OTR
Occupational Therapist
Rehabilitation Institute of Santa Barbara, California

Key Terms

agnosia

apraxia

caregiver

executive functions

memory

respite care

Chapter Outline

Introduction

"Imagine finding yourself in a strange train terminal. Dozens of people are moving about. You search in vain for a familiar face, a sign you can understand—a way out. Desperately, you realize you don't know where you are or how you got there—or how to get out" (HLadik, 1982, p. 2).

Such an experience of disorientation may be a frequent occurrence for persons in the mid-to-late stages of dementia, triggering fear and confusion. At times life may seem frightening, overwhelming, and as if everything were spinning out of control (Lewis, 1989).

Experiences such as the one just described are secretly feared by many adults as they age and begin to encounter minor **memory** problems when unsuccessfully trying to recall a name or date involving a past event. They may wonder whether they are senile or whether this kind of memory problem may mean they are developing dementia. Occasional memory problems involving recall may be more likely to affect persons in positions that are mentally demanding. It is highly unlikely that this type of minor memory problem signals dementia. It has been found that healthy persons over age 50 typically score lower than younger adults on tests of memory (Crook et al., 1986, 1991). Memory does show some normal deterioration as individuals age, but unlike dementia, this type of memory loss does not progress rapidly or interfere with the individual's ability to function in daily life.

The incidence of dementia does, however, increase with age. It is estimated that 1.5 million Americans suffer from severe dementia. The incidence for people over the age of 65 ranges from 2 to 4 percent (American Psychiatric Association [APA], 1994). According to some studies, the incidence rises steadily for older generations until it reaches approximately 20 percent for those in their 80s (George et al., 1988) and close to 50 percent for those aged 90 years and above (Evans et al., 1989). However, these estimates are seen as too high by other researchers (e.g., Johansson & Zarit, 1994). After age 60 the prevalence of Alzheimer's doubles every 5.7 years and then levels off after age 90, according to Ritchie, Kildea, and Robine (1992), who reviewed the rates of dementia across several studies. As the current cohort of elderly persons lives longer, into the late 70s, the 80s, and the 90s, these figures may rise accordingly.

Dementia is often first noticed by persons in the affected individual's social network. Less often, individuals themselves become aware of changes in their social and occupational functioning; indeed, as the severity of dementia increases, minimal awareness of one's deficits and decreases in insight and judgment become increasingly common. The prevalence of this disorder in the later stages of life often creates additional, and sometimes overwhelming, responsibilities for a remaining aged spouse or for other family members who must assume the role of caregiver. This disorder presents occupational therapists with numerous challenges, as they will encounter persons with dementia and other cognitive disorders in a variety of treatment settings (including inpatient, rehabilitation, long-term care, outpatient, and home care).

Dementia involves multiple cognitive deficits primarily involving problems with learning and in memory, but also including disturbances in at least one of the following areas: language, the ability to execute motor tasks, recognition of familiar faces and objects, and other **executive functions** in persons who previously functioned at a much higher level. These impairments seriously affect a person's social relationships and the ability to successfully perform daily living tasks (e.g., money management, shopping, employment, meal preparation, house cleaning, planning activities, reading the newspaper, transportation, personal hygiene).

Dementia can be caused by a number of general medical conditions, the persistent effects of a substance, or a combination of etiologies (APA, 1994). While all the dementias share common symptoms, they are categorized according to the identified or suspected cause. Some of the medical conditions that cause dementia are treatable, but others are not. For example, thyroid disease or a subdural hematoma may cause a dementia that is reversible or resolved with the proper medication or medical intervention. However, in some potentially treatable dementias, the condition may not be fully reversible, especially when the condition is not treated early enough, or structures of the brain have been damaged. This potential for treatment highlights the importance of a proper diagnostic evaluation (Katzman, Lasker, & Bernstein, 1988).

Much confusion has occurred over the years about the word *dementia*, and there are many associated myths and stereotypes. Contrary to popular belief, dementia is not the end result of aging. Many older adults experience episodes of forgetfulness or difficulty in thinking of the name for an object, and in some cases they may take longer to recall information, but the ability to perform daily tasks and roles remains intact. Forgetting, even on a frequent basis, where one has put the car keys is not a sign of dementia, but forgetting what the car key is for may indeed indicate this type of severe cognitive disorder.

With dementia, cognitive and other related deficits increasingly disrupt the individual's ability to manage in social situations, at work, and at home. Settings in which occupational therapists provide treatment to the persons with dementia and offer support and identify resources for the **caregiver**, include home care, adult day services, and long-term care settings. The goal of occupational therapy treatment is to promote the highest quality of life possible for the person with dementia in the safest and least restrictive environment available, while decreasing confusion and managing behavior problems (Wheatley, 1996). Occupational therapy focuses on enhancing the abilities of the individual and on adapting and modifying meaningful activities and the context in which they are performed in order to achieve these goals (American Occupational Therapy Association [AOTA], 1994).

DIFFERENTIAL DIAGNOSIS

The differential diagnosis of dementia can seem perplexing, even to experienced clinicians, especially early in the clinical course or when multiple etiologies are suspected. Sometimes depression-induced cognitive impairments, termed "pseudodementia" (APA, 1994, p. 139) (including problems with memory, thinking, concentration, and daily functioning), may mimic the symptoms of dementia and prove very difficult to differentiate. Sometimes depression and dementia coexist, whereupon both will be diagnosed (APA, 1994), though only one, the depression, can often be treated and resolved. To be diagnosed with dementia, an individual must meet the diagnostic criteria as described in the DSM-IV (APA,1994) (see Figure 11-1). These criteria are similar for most dementias. For criteria on specific dementias, refer to DSM-IV.

The cause of the dementia is also recorded on Axis III (see Chapter 5 for further explanation), along with codes for different general medical conditions and substance-induced persistent disorders (e.g., for dementia due to a general medical condition like thyroid deficiency, the code is 244.9, hypothyroidism, on Axis III). Performing a differential diagnosis, including identification of the cause of the dementia on Axis III, can be critical because the specific etiology of dementia often dictates the treatment and suggests the course the disorder might follow (APA, 1994).

The following criteria are similar for most dementias. For criteria on specific dementias, refer to the DSM-IV.

A. The development of multiple cognitive deficits manifested by both
   1) Memory impairment (impaired ability to learn new information or to recall previously learned information)
   2) One (or more) of the following cognitive disturbances:
      a) Aphasia (language disturbance)
      b) Apraxia (impaired ability to carry out motor activities despite intact motor function)
      c) Agnosia (failure to recognize or identify objects despite intact sensory function)
      d) Disturbance in executive functioning (i.e., planning, organizing, sequencing, abstracting)
B. The cognitive deficits in Criteria A1 and A2 each cause significant impairment in social or occupational functioning and represent a significant decline from a previous level of functioning.

Figure 11-1. Diagnostic Criteria for Dementia

Source: Reprinted with permission from *Diagnostic and Statistical Manual of Mental Disorders, Fourth Edition.* Copyright 1994 American Psychiatric Association.

Many conditions cause dementia, including the following:

- degenerate disorders of the central nervous system
- metabolic disorders
- cerebrovascular disease
- nutritional deficiency disorders
- toxins and drugs
- brain tumors
- trauma
- infections

The dementia disorders share a common symptom pattern but differ in etiology. This chapter will, out of necessity, focus briefly on the types of dementia categorized in DSM-IV (APA, 1994) that are irreversible dementias and most commonly encountered in the clinical work of occupational therapists (AOTA, 1994). Those discussed include dementia of the Alzheimer's type, vascular dementia, and dementia due to other general medical conditions (focusing on Parkinson's disease, Huntington disease, HIV disease). While other dementias due to general medical conditions, substance-induced persisting dementia, dementia due to multiple etiologies, and dementia not otherwise specified are not discussed in great detail in this chapter, it is important to realize that these dementias are also seen in the clinical practice of occupational therapy.

Dementia of the Alzheimer's Type

Dementia of the Alzheimer's type is the most common form of dementia. It accounts for 65 percent of dementias in the elderly and affects as many as 2 to 4 percent of the Americans over the age of 65 (APA, 1994). Late onset is more common than early onset. The signs and symptoms of dementia are described in Figure 11-2, but the reader must remember that the presentation of the disease is variable and follows no precisely set pattern. The degenerative process is characterized by a shrinking of the brain and enlargement of the cerebral ventricles caused by destroyed neurons in the cerebral cortex, hippocampus, and basal ganglia. A number of microscopic changes are seen at autopsy, the most common of which include neurofibrillary tangles and senile plaques. These changes affect portions of the brain essential to memory, learning, and information processing. There appears to be a genetic component to the disease, especially with early onset dementia, which has been linked to specific chromosomes.

A conclusive diagnosis of Alzheimer's disease can be made only from brain tissue obtained via biopsy (which can only be performed after death), though there are other promising diagnostic advances currently being researched. Thus the diagnosis is considered "presumed" and is usually made by excluding all other syndromes. Progressive cognitive decline is inevitable, and the survival range is from 2 to 20 years, with an average of 8 to 10 years postdiagnosis (APA, 1994).

CASE ILLUSTRATION: DEMENTIA OF THE ALZHEIMER'S TYPE

Mrs. DelBiaggio is a 67-year-old Italian-American female in the severe stages of Alzheimer's disease. She no longer recognizes her grandchildren or remembers her own, long-standing phone number or address. She has begun leaving the home she shares with her daughter and wandering over to her other daughter's home, two blocks away, at 5:30 A.M. and wearing only her nightclothes despite freezing temperatures. She has lost 10 pounds in the past four months, as she often forgets to finish eating and has begun to pace restlessly. She requires moderate to maximal assistance with hygiene, and has begun to soil herself two or three times a week. She lapses into angry Italian when her daughter leaves her for even a short period of time and becomes agitated; she also accuses her sons, who visit daily, of never visiting. This behavior can quickly escalate into a catastrophic reaction of prolonged crying and agitation unless appropriate interventions are made.

Discussion

Mrs. DelBiaggio demonstrates behavior in stage 6 of dementia, severe cognitive decline.

Stage 1: No cognitive decline. — No reported or observed symptoms.

Stage 2: Very mild decline. — Complains of forgetfulness. Forgets names. Loses items. No deficits in employment or social situations observed. Individual displays appropriate concern.

Stage 3: Mild cognitive decline. — May remember little of passage read from a book. Decreased performance in demanding employment and social situations. Co-workers become aware of the individual's relatively poor performance. Difficulty finding words and names. May get lost when traveling to unfamiliar locations or lose objects of value. Anxiety is common. Denial is likely.

Stage 4: Moderate cognitive decline — Deficits are clear. Concentration deficits. Decreased knowledge of recent and current events. Difficulties traveling alone and in handling own financial matters. Remains oriented to time and person. Recognizes familiar persons and faces. Can still travel to familiar locations, e.g., corner drugstore. Withdraws from situations that may present challenges. Denial becomes dominant defense.

Stage 5: Moderately severe cognitive decline. (Early dementia) — Individuals need assistance in order to survive. May forget address, telephone number and names of close family members. Disorientation to time or place occurs frequently. Remembers own name and names of spouse and children. May clothe himself or herself improperly (e.g., weather or event). Assistance with eating or toileting is usually not necessary.

Stage 6: Severe cognitive decline. — Occasionally may forget spouse's name. Significant impairment for remembering recent events and past experiences in his/her life. Unaware of surroundings, season or year. Nighttime sleep patterns frequently disturbed. Assistance with A.D.L.'s required at times, occasional incontinence. Personality /emotional changes frequent (often occur at earlier stages) and may include delusions, repetitive behaviors, anxiety, agitation, occasional violent behavior, apathy and inability to initiate purposeful action.

Stage 7: Very severe cognitive decline. — Inability to communicate, grunting. Needs assistance with toileting, eating and dressing. May be unable to walk. General neurological signs and symptoms common.

Figure 11-2. Signs and Symptoms of Dementia of the Alzheimer's Type

Source: Adapted with permission from the Global Deterioration Scale (Reisberg, Ferris, & Crook, 1983, pp. 174–175).

Vascular Dementia

Vascular dementia (formerly known as multi-infarct dementia) is the second largest category of dementia. It is estimated that two-thirds of the individuals with a cerebrovascular disease in the United States have a resulting dementia. Vascular dementia does not typically result from a single stroke but rather from series of strokes occurring at different times (APA, 1994). Vascular dementia is more common in men than in women and generally occurs earlier in life than dementia of the Alzheimer's type.

The signs and symptoms of vascular dementia include memory impairment, aphasia, apraxia, agnosia, and cognitive deficits in the executive functions. However, the symptoms are variable and the pattern of cognitive deficits usually depends on the location and number of multiple infarcts (strokes) experienced. The onset of symptoms is often abrupt and usually progresses in a stepwise manner. This means that after a stroke, a person may experience a sharp decline in cognitive functioning followed by periods of apparent improvement as the brain gradually stabilizes from the trauma (APA, 1994). However, with repeated strokes, the changes and decline in functioning becomes more noticeable. The dementia may affect some cognitive functions and spare others; therefore, to employ a single, "typical" description may not give an accurate representation of any particular individual. There must be evidence of cerebrovascular disease for the diagnosis of vascular dementia. Lesions are often seen in both the white and gray matter structures of the brain. Neurological signs include pseudobulbar palsy, gait disturbances, extremity weakness, and exaggerated deep tendon reflexes, all of which that are related to the cause of the disorder.

The main cause of vascular dementia is a loss of brain tissue in the cerebral cortex and the underlying white matter due to the cumulative effects of many small infarcts. The dementia may be worse if all the strokes occurred in the same general area or bilaterally. Conditions that predispose individuals toward cerebrovascular disease are associated with an increased incidence of vascular dementia. The risk factors include hypertension, obesity, myocardial infarction (heart attack), transient ischemic attacks (TIAs), coronary artery disease, smoking, and diabetes (Whitehouse, Lerner, & Hedera, 1993). The detection of these risk factors is important because further deterioration may be prevented through the proper treatment of the primary cause of cerebrovascular disease. Agents that decrease clotting, anticoagulants, and antihypertensives all may limit the progress of the disease.

To distinguish between vascular dementia and dementia of the Alzheimer's type may be difficult, and the two often exist concurrently. A history of risk factors for vascular disease and/or an intermittent course in the clinical progression of symptoms can be helpful diagnostic conditions for distinguishing vascular dementia from dementia of the Alzheimer's type (Whitehouse et al., 1993). Computerized tomography (CT) and magnetic resonance imaging (MRI) scans may also be used to detect lesions in the brain, electroencephalograms (EEGs) may reveal focal lesions, indicating a cerebral vascular accident distinct from the degenerative changes, and increased cerebral ventricle size may appear on a brain scan, all of which differentiate vascular dementia from dementia of the Alzheimer's type.

CASE ILLUSTRATION: VASCULAR DEMENTIA

Mr. Jacobson is a 68-year-old Jewish male. He currently lives in a six-bed residential care home (RCH), where he has been residing over the last three years due to health problems and difficulties in managing his medication and other activities of daily living (ADLs). The RCH manager states that she has become increasingly worried about Mr. Jacobson over the last two months. He runs out of personal spending money by the middle of the month, and he has not purchased, or consistently used, hygiene products such as deodorant and shaving materials, all of which signal a decline in his usual level of functioning. Three times in the last week she has been called to come and retrieve Mr. Jacobson from the local grocery store because he has been unable to find his way home. Mr. Jacobson has been complaining of increased fatigue and seems somewhat more confused and forgetful. His physician recently changed his blood pressure (BP) medication as his blood pressure had become elevated and hard to control.

Discussion

Mr. Jacobson demonstrates behavior of dementia due to cerebrovascular disease. The onset of symptoms has occurred sometime after a stroke, but in a somewhat abrupt manner, and his memory has been affected.

Dementia Due to Parkinson's Disease

Parkinson's disease is the third most common neurological disorder, with a prevalence of approximately 1 in 100 people aged 65 and over manifesting some form (Joe, 1996). Dementia is more prevalent in older adults and those with more severe forms of the disease (APA, 1994). Clinical manifestations of Parkinson's disease include muscular rigidity, bradykinesia (slowed motor response), loss of postural reflexes, and "pill-rolling" tremors beginning in the fingers. In time, problems in speech, handwriting, and swallowing may become apparent. The muscle rigidity may extend to the face and produce facial expressions that appear fixed (flat affect). Individuals often have difficulty initiating movement and indeed may "freeze" when being encouraged to move. Cognitive impairments found with dementia include memory problems involving retrieval, significant mental slowing, and difficulty with executive functions, especially abstract thinking and the ability to shift thinking in response to environmental demands. Depression often worsens the cognitive deficits.

There is considerable speculation that Parkinson's disease may be caused by a degeneration of the neurons and by the presence of Lewy bodies in the substantia nigra, which interferes with the transmission of dopamine to the corpus striatum (APA, 1994). Through its influence on the basal ganglia, dopamine acts to inhibit movements. A deficiency of this neurotransmitter results in an imbalance of neurotransmitters to the motor system and thus in rigidity. No reliable laboratory test exists to establish a diagnosis. Brain tissue examined at autopsy often confirms the findings from physical examinations. Brain imaging may prove to be a helpful technique when causal factors are confirmed. Causal factors may include environmental triggers and hereditary factors (Joe, 1996). This disease is slowly progressive and degenerative, with a variable course. Treatment may involved levodopa, though its effectiveness is limited and it does not stop the progression of dementia.

CASE ILLUSTRATION: DEMENTIA DUE TO PARKINSON'S DISEASE

Mr. Jones is a 71-year-old African-American male who is currently in a **respite care** *program for one week while his wife is on vacation. He demonstrates a pronounced resting tremor and incoordination, which interfere with his self-care abilities. He has great difficulty initiating action, such as getting out of his chair and moving around the unit safely with his walker, for which he requires standby assistance. He remains sitting in his chair most of the day and does not participate in conversation or activity without considerable encouragement and direction from the staff. He responds slowly to questions, showing little enthusiasm or change in facial expression. Mr. Jones is not aware of his location at the present time and instead repeatedly states that his wife is making lunch and will serve it in "about 15 minutes"; this indicates impairments in orientation and short-term memory. He requires reminders and some minimal assistance to engage in self-care routines. Due to impairments in his memory and cognitive-processing abilities, he functions best on very structured tasks, which should be divided into two, sequenced steps accompanied by verbal and visual cues.*

Discussion

In addition to memory and cognitive-processing problems, Mr. Jones demonstrates muscle rigidity and movement difficulties typical of dementia due to Parkinson's disease.

Dementia Due to Huntington Disease

About 5 in 100,000 people are affected with Huntington disease, which was formerly known as Huntington chorea (Folstein, 1989). The disease is transmitted by an autosomal dominant gene, with offspring having a 50 percent chance of developing it (APA, 1994). Huntington disease is equally common in men and women and is characterized by cognitive deficits, emotional instability, and disordered movements. In the early stages the person may appear clumsy, fidgety, irritable, and anxious; half of those diagnosed experience affective disorders (Folstein, 1989). Cognitive deficits include problems in memory storage and retrieval, poor judgment, and difficulties with executive functions. As the disease progresses, memory deficits tend to become more severe and psychotic thinking and disorganized speech may emerge. Motor movements become increasingly exaggerated, making the afflicted person's walk resemble a bizarre, dance-like step (hence the term "chorea," meaning "dance").

The loss of neurons in Huntington disease results in atrophy of the corpus striatum, especially the caudate nucleus, and some loss in the cortex (Whitehouse et al., 1993). The neuron loss has the effect of decreasing the metabolic rate in the striatum and reducing gamma-aminobutyric (GABA) levels. To simplify, Huntington disease has been described as having the opposite effect of Parkinson's and thus resulting in increased motor activity. GABA is an inhibitory neurotransmitter within the dopaminergic system, so the reduction of its influence causes dopamine overactivity and increased motor activity.

The disease is often first diagnosed when individuals are in their late 30s or 40s, but it can be seen as early as 4 years or as late as 85 years of age (APA, 1994). An accurate genetic test is available to determine whether an individual carries the trait. Death usually occurs 10 to 20 years following the onset as a result of malnutrition, sepsis, pneumonia, or pulmonary embolus. There is also a high suicide rate in the early stages of the disease while the individual's insight is still preserved (Guberman, 1994).

CASE ILLUSTRATION: DEMENTIA DUE TO HUNTINGTON DISEASE

Mr. Kent is a 56-year-old Caucasian male with a diagnosis of Huntington chorea. He is currently living in the dementia unit of a residential long-term care facility. Early in his disease, Mr. Kent made several unsuccessful attempts at suicide. He is now confined to a wheelchair and is considered a "fall risk" due to the severity of his choreoform movements and cognitive deficits associated with the dementia component of his disease. He is unable to safely maneuver his wheelchair about the unit. He requires maximum assistance with toileting and dressing and moderate assistance with eating. Self-care is particularly problematic due to his swallowing problems, impaired lower and upper extremity function, poor judgment, and distractibility. Mr. Kent is frequently noncompliant with his self-care and medication requirements. He demonstrates outrage and occasional combativeness toward his caregivers, stating that he is the chief executive officer of "the company" and has the power to "fire" them.

Discussion

Mr. Kent's symptoms are opposite those of Mr. Jones. Mr. Kent is always active and directional in his movements, though he too demonstrates severe cognitive and memory problems and severe delusions.

Dementia Due to the Human Immunodeficiency Virus (HIV)

Estimates of HIV disease are changing rapidly. While men previously had higher prevalence rates of HIV than women, outnumbering them about 2 to 1, this statistic has changed (see Chapter 16). Symptoms of dementia due to HIV include impairments in memory, slowed thinking and movements, poor concentration, and difficulties in problem solving. Other changes include increased apathy and withdrawal from social situations, which may be accompanied by delusions, hallucinations, and delirium. Dementia occurs when the HIV virus infects the central nervous system, resulting in diffuse brain atrophy. Microglial nodules throughout the brain destroy the white matter and subcortical structures. Dementia may also occur as the result of other opportunistic infections. Blood tests are currently the most widely used means of diagnosing HIV. However, HIV can also be detected in cerebrospinal fluid, and brain changes can be seen at the time of an autopsy. For further information about neurological symptoms and opportunistic infections of HIV see Chapter 16.

The progression of the disease and that of the dementia depend upon the particular parts of the brain that become atrophied, the extent of lymphoma in the central nervous system, and the effectiveness of treatment of opportunistic infections. There is no cure for HIV, though many promising drugs have arrested the progression of the disease and there have been cases of long-term remission. Death occurs usually 7 to 10 years postdiagnosis.

CASE ILLUSTRATION: DEMENTIA DUE TO HUMAN IMMUNODEFICIENCY VIRUS (HIV)

Mr. Lindsey is a 42-year-old Caucasian male in the late stages of HIV disease. Significant impairment in short-term memory, general mental slowing, and word-finding difficulties have caused him considerable frustration and embarrassment when conversing with friends. Because of this, he has recently begun refusing treatment and isolating himself from his friends and family. He has been classified by the visiting nurse as demonstrating a "failure to thrive." His family fears that if he continues resisting in-home treatment, failing to eat, and isolating himself, he will need to be admitted to a nursing home for a higher level of care.

Discussion

Mr. Lindsay's dementia manifested in specific functions of memory and word finding difficulties. His general mental slowing is in contrast to the manifestations of the other dementias.

EVALUATION

Approximately 2 to 3 percent of persons with dementia have cognitive impairments related to substances or general medical conditions that can be managed with proper medical treatment. Unfortunately, some individuals are not evaluated early enough and do not obtain treatment until cognitive deficits begin to impede their functioning in daily life tasks. Stereotypes surrounding the idea of senility as a normal aspect of aging, lack of insight, and a fear of hearing that one has Alzheimer's disease may keep persons who are experiencing cognitive deficits and their family members from seeking a proper evaluation.

Evaluating individuals with cognitive complaints involves two phases. Initially, in the first phase, evaluation is aimed at recognizing cognitive impairments; classifying the disorder as a dementia, depression, or other cognitive disorder; and then, in the case of dementia, differentiating the specific type (Ramsdell, Rothrock, Ward, & Volk, 1995). This first phase utilizes a strong medical model. The second phase of evaluation involves determining to what degree the client's impairments interfere with functioning in activities of daily living. The occupational therapist assumes a strong role in this phase of evaluation by identifying the client's impairments and assets in underlying occupational performance components. These affect the level of function in the occupational performance areas, according to the client's occupational performance context (AOTA, 1994). Task performance is evaluated, and the need for adaptations or alterations in the social, cultural, and physical environments is determined.

Older adults in particular may present with confusing and complex symptoms that affect both physical and mental functioning. Thus, the older adult is particularly likely to be hard to classify according to the specific diagnoses described earlier in this chapter. Blazer (1995) suggests that the best approach to assessment with the geriatric population is to begin with the older adult's presenting functional problems (e.g., falling, incontinence, memory loss, or withdrawal from activities). He advocates conducting assessment and intervention with a broadened perspective involving a geriatric syndrome approach that considers the multiple systems that may cause and impact the functional problems presented by the older adult. Along with memory loss, older adults may present with depression, anxiety, sleep problems, and psychotic thoughts, which nonetheless fail to accord with the full criteria for a DSM-IV diagnosis. However, symptoms of frequent forgetfulness, persistent sadness, and restlessness can be caused by a number of medical and psychiatric conditions, all of which can seriously disrupt performance of the activities of daily living (ADL). Emphasizing the syndrome of functional impairment rather than seeking a diagnosis is a more effective approach, according to Blazer (1995), and certainly will prove more satisfying to the patient and family. There can be multiple reasons for cognitive deficits. Therefore, a thorough evaluation, a careful differential diagnostic process, and appropriate treatment can have a profound effect on the quality of life of individuals with dementia and their families.

Diagnostic Evaluation

All older adults should have their mental status assessed and be screened for cognitive impairments by their primary care physicians (Ramsdell et al., 1995) and by other health care professionals, both during initial visits and on a periodic basis. Reliance on the Mini-Mental State Exam (MMSE) (Folstein, Folstein, & McHugh, 1975) as a screen for mild dementia has only limited use according to Cullum, Filley, Kelly, and Schneck (1992), who also recommend the use of alternative brief tasks in place of parts of the MMSE. Lowered scores on mental status exams have been associated with losses in functional development and poorer performance on ADL tasks in the more severely impaired individuals, suggesting their usefulness as a monitoring instrument (Gurland, 1980; Nolen, 1987). There are a number of mental status questionnaires available for dementia-screening purposes (see Figure 11-3), though the Mini-Mental State Exam (MMSE) (assessing orientation, registration, attention, recall, three-stage commands, spelling, reading, writing, and copying) is used the most often. Cutoff scores suggestive of dementia should be viewed cautiously when used with older individuals with less than a high school education or cross-cultural populations (Wiederholt et al., 1993).

A standard assessment for differential diagnosis includes the evaluation of a variety of clinical domains, including functional status, mental health status, physical condition, environmental conditions, and socioeconomic resources. A suggested workup to more definitively diagnose cognitive deficits and functional problems includes making clinical observations and obtaining a careful history from the patient and family, which should identify the onset, nature, and progression of the signs observed and symptoms that have been experienced. Other components of the assessment include a full mental status exam, neuropsychological assessment, neurological exam, complete physical exam, chest x-ray, electrocardiogram (EKG), and complete laboratory testing (Breitner & Welsh, 1995). EEGs, CAT scans, MRIs, toxic screens, a lumbar puncture, and measures of drug levels are also used.

Specific areas of cognitive function evaluated by the treatment team include the assessment of: memory, language, **apraxia**, **agnosia**, perceptual behavior, attention span, orientation, concentration, ability to follow directions, problem solving, learning, abstract thinking, reasoning, judgment, affect, mood, executive functions (Whitehouse et al., 1993), and activities of daily living. Figure 11-3 identifies specific dementia assessments that determine degrees of cognitive impairment in a valid or generally reliable manner.

Occupational Therapy Evaluation

The occupational therapy evaluations typically begin by investigating the individual's functional levels in the instrumental activities of daily living (IADLs) connected with the occupational performance areas of work and productive activities (work tasks, community mobility, home management, and commu-

I. Clinical Dementia Assessment Tools (Multi-disciplinary)
   - Clinical Dementia Rating (CDR) (Berg, 1988) — assesses memory, orientation, judgment, problem solving, community affairs, home & hobbies, and personal care. Rating scale from questionable, mild, moderate to severe dementia .
   - Alzheimer's Disease Assessment Scale (ADAS) (Rosen, Mohs & Davis, 1984) — assesses memory, language, praxis, mood states and behavioral changes.
   - Global Deterioration Scale (GDS), (Reisberg, et al., 1983)

II. Mental Status Screens
   - Mental Status Questionnaire — (MSQ) (Kahn, Goldfarb, Pollack & Peck, 1960) brief mental status evaluation.
   - Mini-Mental State Exam (MMSE) (Folstein, et al., 1975) — brief screen of cognitive function

III. Occupational Performance Components — tests of cognition, perception, psychological, sensory, and motor and tasks performance.
   - Allen Cognitive Level test (ACL) (Allen, 1985) — determines cognitive levels through task performance.
   - Aphasia Language Performance Subscales (Keenan & Brasseil, 1975) — language
   - Assessment of Motor and Process Skills (AMPS) (Fisher, 1994)
   - The Boston Aphasia Evaluation (Goodglass & Kaplan, 1983) — language
   - Cognitive Performance Test (CPT) (Burns, Mortimer, & Merchek, 1994) — cognitive levels through task performance using ADL tasks.
   - Deuel's Test of Motor Apraxia (Deuel, Feely & Bonskowski, 1984)
   - Test of Orientation for Rehabilitation Patients (TORP) (Deitz, Beeman & Thorn,1986)
   - Rivermead Behavioral Memory Test (Wilson, Cockburn & Baddeley, 1985) — topographical memory and orientation
   - The Benton Visual Retention Memory Test (BVRT) (Benton, 1974) — memory
   - The Learning Efficiency Test (Webster, 1992) — memory
   - The Contextual Memory Test (Toglia, 1993) — memory
   - The Routine Task Inventory (RTI) (Allen, 1985; Allen, Earhart & Blue, 1992)
   - Trail Making Test (A & B) (Army Individual test battery, 1944) — perceptual, visual spatial, attention and mental flexibility

(continues)

Figure 11-3. Dementia Assessments

Source: Compiled from Baum (1993); Christiansen and Baum (1991); Levy (1996); Lewis (1989); and Wheatley (1996).

IV. Assessment—Includes elements of some or all of the following: occupational performance components, occupational performance areas, caregiver assessment and environmental conditions.
- Activity Profile (Baum, 1993c) — report of client involvement in activities in home and leisure activities
- Descriptive Home Evaluation (The Rehabilitation Institute, Kansas City, MO; in Davidson, 1991, p. 444)
- FROMAJE (Liblow, 1981) — a mental status evaluation with a brief functional evaluation of safety, Activities of Daily Living (ADL) and Instrumental Activities of Daily Living (IADL).
- Functional Behavior Profile (Baum & Edwards, 1993b) — caregiver report of client performance in tasks, social interactions and problem solving
- Functional Status Index (FSI) (Jette, 1980)
- Index of ADL (Katz, Ford & Moscovitz, 1963)
- Klein-Bell ADL Scales (Klein & Bell, 1979) — ADL scale can be used to instruct family members
- Memory and Behavior Problem Checklist (Zarit et al., 1982)
- The Kitchen Task (Baum & Edwards et al., 1993a)
- The Barthel Index (Mahoney & Barthel, 1965) — Basic ADL scale

Figure 11-3. Dementia Assessments (*continued*)

nity safety), which are often of the greatest importance early in the dementia process (AOTA, 1994). As the dementia progresses, the focus of evaluation shifts to activities of daily living (ADLs) that are connected with self-maintenance areas (leisure pursuits, communication, functional mobility, personal self-care, and home safety) and to the occupational performance components that support performance areas. Task performance, the balance of activity, social support networks, and the appropriateness of the work, leisure, and living environments are also evaluated when gathering the baseline data necessary for planning OT interventions (AOTA, 1994).

A general plan for the evaluation of individuals with dementia follows. Specific assessments of ADLs and IADLs used by occupational therapists in this evaluation process can be found in Figure 11-3. First, the occupational therapist evaluates function in occupational performance areas related to personal self-care, mobility, home management, and relevant work and leisure areas, along with the current occupational performance context (AOTA, 1994; Rogers & Salta, 1994). Attention is given to the specific tasks required in each performance area and the occupational performance components that enable task performance. The functional status of the individual is determined, and the skills, habits, and environmental features (physical and social) that interfere with, or support, the task performance of the person with dementia are identified. The level of assistance (independent, minimal, moderate, maximal, or dependent), type of assistance (supervision, type of prompt, modeling, guidance, or physical help), and adaptive equipment or environmental adaptations deemed necessary to complete tasks in ADLs and IADLs are specified. Functional outcomes identifying observable behaviors and necessary cues are then described (Reichenbach, 1993; Rogers & Salta, 1994).

Of particular importance in evaluating clients with dementia are the identification of deficits and abilities in cognition that influence the individual's task performance. For example, the presence of information-processing impairments that result in qualitative difference in the individual's functional capacity is an area that has been written about extensively by Levy (1974, 1986, 1987, 1988, 1992, 1996) and by Allen and colleagues (Allen, 1982, 1985; Allen, Earhart, & Blue, 1992; Allen & Robertson, 1993), who identified distinct hierarchical cognitive levels in sensorimotor information processing. The assessment of an individual's level of function (attention to sensory stimuli, goal orientation, and initiatiation of activity) is part of the Allen Cognitive Level Test (1985). Suggestions for specific intervention strategies, which include the selection and modification of activities and environments, are clearly identified and described based on Allen's cognitive disability model (for various assessments used with this model, see Figure 11-3).

Other occupational therapy and interdisciplinary assessments evaluate specific areas of cognitive function, sensorimotor abilities, and emotional-processing abilities that influence task performance and functional levels in the occupational performance areas (see Figure 11-3). Assessments are available to use in evaluating orientation, different types of memory, apraxia, aphasia, agnosia, and status of the executive functions. Memory can be evaluated in the following areas: visual, auditory, topographical (location), episodic (personal events/history), semantic (general learned knowledge), procedural (series of actions), and prospective (future time events) (Wheateley, 1996). Severe types of apraxia have been found in those in the later stages of dementia (Edwards, Deuel, & Baum, 1991). Problems with agnosia may involve an inability to recognize deficits in one's own abilities and behaviors (anosognosia), the failure to recognize objects by feel alone (stereognosis), the failure to recognize loved ones' faces (prosopagnosia), or disorientation in personal space (autotopagnosia); these impairments are often frustrating and difficult for caregivers to understand (Baum, 1993). The OT can often help identify other means of communicating with aphasic individuals, who can neither speak nor understand the spoken word. An assessment of executive functions can be done using complex batteries. They can also be assessed by observing poor performance in self-care tasks or productive work or the ability to maintain normal social relationships. Deficits in these areas due to global brain impairments occur because of a lack of initiation, poor self-control, changes in affect, lack of self-monitoring, poor motivation, and problems in planning and carrying out activity (Lezak, 1983).

The evaluation of sensorimotor function may include the assessment of gait, posture, balance, muscle tone, strength, gross and fine motor coordination, range of motion, and the smoothness and quality of movement. An evaluation of sensation (particularly tactile involving superficial pain, light touch, deep pressure, and position sense) should be considered in the overall assessment of the individual as it relates to safety and the potential for injury. It is important to be aware of impairments in the basic senses (taste, smell, hearing, and vision) that are associated with aging and can interfere with eating, safety, communication, and functional performance in other areas. The use of performance-based measures such as the Assessment of Motor and Process Skills (AMPS) (Fisher, 1994) provides information concerning motor and process functioning in the context of assessing IADLs.

Emotional changes occur insidiously as dementia progresses. Monitoring for signs of depression and denial is an important component to evaluate during the early stages of dementia. Depression, if it extends for too long a time and if it interferes with functioning, often should be treated with medications. An understanding of the nature and extent of depression and denial experienced by the individual will provide insight into the performance problems and stresses encountered in the family and caregiver relationships. During the latter stages of dementia, observing and asking about the presence of inflexibility to change, outbursts of uncontrolled crying or laughing, perseverative behaviors (repetitive, meaningless actions such as rubbing), and the display of regressive behaviors in the individual with dementia are of great importance in educating caregivers, effectively managing those behaviors in the future, and providing the appropriate environmental context to support optimal performance.

Finally, in the occupational therapy evaluation process, the appropriateness of the home environment is assessed for safety issues and to determine if modifications, adaptations, or alterations are necessary in order to support the highest level of independence with activities of daily living (AOTA, 1994). The individual's support network is assessed to determine available resources, become informed of the needs and opinions of the caregiver, and establish the caregiver's degree of availability, knowledge, skills, and health status.

Information about the client's ability to care for the self, relate meaningfully to others, and live safely in the community is usually obtained by interview, self-report, and a performance evaluation utilizing observation. An assessment based solely on an interview can sometimes be misleading. Some clinicians and researchers suggest that clients can overestimate their abilities (AOTA, 1994; McGlyn & Kazniak, 1991; Rogers, Holm, Goldstein, McCue, & Nussbaum, 1994) because of their cognitive deficits. It is thought by some researchers that caregivers may underestimate client abilities under certain circumstances (AOTA, 1994; Baum, 1993; LaRue, Watson, & Plotkin, 1992). Others, however, have found caregiver assessments to be quite reliable (Rogers et al., 1994; Watson et al., 1987). In some cases the caregiver perceives the individual as incapable, yet the therapist perceives him or her as having numerous capabilities. In addition, there are circumstances where the therapist assesses the client's performance as poor yet the caregiver reports that the performance is good. If the therapist's assessment is more accurate, potential safety problems can be prevented from occurring. Some individuals with dementia remain home alone during the early stages of the disease as they gradually lose the initiative and ability to engage in previous occupations. Over time, being home alone may pose a serious safety issue as the dementia condition progresses insidiously in ways that may not be noticed by family members.

It is crucial that, when assessing functional status, the occupational therapist directly observe the individual performing tasks. This will offer the most accurate information regarding the individual's level of independence, habit patterns, resources, and degree of safety in performing daily tasks. This information will help the therapist recommend the level of caregiver support and type of living situation that best meets the person's needs. For example, watching an individual make toast, as in the Cognitive Performance Test (see Figure 11-3), allows the therapist to observe his or her memory, language (ability to read and understand written material), problem solving, understanding of abstract concepts (i.e., heat), perceptual abilities (visual and auditory perception), and any motor deficits. Through observation, the underlying components for problem behaviors can often be identified as impairments related to memory, awareness, or judgment and the therapist can recommend specific environmental adaptations, caregiver training, or other treatment.

It is essential to identify the person's strengths in order to support or compensate for skill deficits resulting from the dementia. Occupational therapists assume a critical role in the assessment process and make major contributions to the interdisciplinary care plan, providing information about the individual's functional capabilities and not just the disabilities. It is important for the team to utilize a person's skills, such as those needed when dressing (memory, organization, and problem solving), and include them as an integral part of therapy rather than making deficits the primary focus of treatment. If approached in this way, the individual will be less threatened, be more enthusiastic, and more likely to comply with the treatment process.

Because of the progressive nature of some dementia disorders (such as dementia of the Alzheimer's type) and the stepwise deterioration of vascular dementia, the assessment must establish a baseline and then become part of an ongoing monitoring process. It is important to use assessments that record performance over time as the disease progresses so that treatment may be continually adjusted to compensate for changes in the individual's cognitive and other functional levels.

TREATMENT

The most valuable occupational therapy interventions for individuals with dementia and their families focus on maintaining the individual in the least restrictive environment while emphasizing his or her remaining skills, maintaining physical activity, and decreasing caregiver stress. Treatment planning for individuals with dementia must take into consideration their likely future decline in functional performance. The occupational therapist can be helpful in assisting caregivers and clients to develop strategies to cope with the decline in cognitive functions. Thoughts and feelings should be validated and skills taught so that tasks can be accomplished with the least amount of supervision and minimum frustration. Consequently, a variety of interventions may be required as the person's capacities change. For example, a person in the early stages of dementia of the Alzheimer's type may be able to take a walk in the neighborhood alone. However, in the middle or late stages of the disease, the individual's memory, reasoning, and spatial orientation may become so impaired that the same activity may result in the individual getting lost. The caregiver will then require education regarding methods to prevent the individual with dementia from wandering or in finding an alternative that is satisfying while still fulfilling the client's needs for competence.

Occupational therapists work in a variety of settings with individuals diagnosed with dementia. Several settings and treatment interventions are described in this chapter. Moreover, techniques and methods described in one setting may be adapted to meet the needs of an individual in a different setting. The American Occupational Therapy Association's (1994) position paper regarding the occupational therapist's role in regard to persons with dementia defines three primary intervention areas: (1) maintain, restore, or improve functional capacity; (2) promote participation in activities that optimize physical and mental health; and (3) ease caregiver activities (AOTA, 1994). This section of the chapter is divided into three similar areas of treatment: environmental adaptation, the use of purposeful activity, and caregiver education.

Environmental Adaptation

The occupational therapy evaluation that includes the concerns of the client and caregiver will help highlight areas of importance regarding the environment. The occupational therapist will then be able to make recommendations about environmental modifications to promote safety and independence and, possibly, reduce agitation and frustration. Proper environmental modifications allow the affected individual to focus more effectively on meaningful activities and improve function. Surroundings that help the person meet these goals have been called "prosthetic environments"; these environments compensate for some degree of lack of personal competence (Levy, 1987a, 1987b).

Simple adaptations can have significant results; for example, removing clutter can reduce agitation and promote cue recognition; clearly labeled cabinets and doors can reduce confusion and promote optimal independence; and simplifying of daily tasks can facilitate participation.

Purposeful Activity

Occupational therapists choose activities that are modified through the application of activity analysis to allow persons with dementia to succeed despite their impairments. Levy (1987b) explains that undertaking cognitive activity analysis (task analysis) enables therapists to match activities more accurately to the abilities and preferences of the cognitively impaired. Tasks are analyzed by the therapist to determine specific components in the procedure that the individual can and cannot manage. The task is then modified to maximize use of intact cognitive functions and to compensate for cognitive deficits. Previously learned skills can be tapped to engage the individual with dementia in productive behavior. This approach elicits a subcortical adaptive response through manipulation of the environment (King, 1978). Instead of depending on the individual's cognitive abilities, the environment is structured to elicit from the person the habitual responses of a previously learned activity. For example, a client whose previous occupation was as a carpenter could have a routine established whereby each day he or she did a very simple woodwork project, such as sanding a cutting board. Power tools would be removed from the work area and only those tools the client could still use safely would be available.

Borell, Sandman, and Kielhofner (1991) suggest the following approach when considering an activity for inclusion in treatment:

1. Identify the degree of difficulty the individual has in performing the activity and which impairments and capacities exist (e.g., cognitive, motor, sensory, or motivational).
2. Determine how much interest the individual has in the activity, how important it is to him or her, and the degree of satisfaction and pleasure it brings.
3. Determine how critical the activity is to the life role and sense of competence of the person with dementia.

This chapter stresses the importance of a structured, familiar, nonchanging environment in eliciting higher levels of performance from individuals with dementia. Without consistency, these individuals may experience frustration and often act out with disturbing behaviors. However, it should be noted that an overly structured environment, on the other hand, can constrain personal control and freedom, which can lead to low self-esteem, diminished self-concept, depression, and feelings of hopelessness and helplessness (Howe-Murphy & Charboneau, 1987). The goal of occupational therapy is to promote a balance between the client's cognitive abilities and the need for activities to involve structure and supervision.

Caregiver Education

Treatment of the individual with dementia not only focuses on the client's problems but also involves collaborating with the caregiver to determine his or her own concerns (Wallens & Rockwell-Dylla, 1996). The occupational therapist needs to understand the caregiver's perspective and cultural needs and the meaning of care giving to that individual. Gitlin, Corocoran, and Leinmiller-Eckhardt (1995) present an ethnographic approach to determine an understanding of the personal meaning of care giving, how care is provided, and how to assess care-giving problems from the family members' perspective. This study presents a collaborative approach intended to empower the caregiver while the occupational therapist plays the role of facilitator in establishing new caregiver strategies.

Baum and Edwards (1993b) present another collaborative method, the Functional Behavior Profile (FBP), which helps the caregiver focus on the presence of productive behaviors that can be useful in managing the cognitively impaired person and with developing care-giving strategies. This involves interviewing the caregiver to obtain information about the ability of the person with dementia to engage in tasks, interact socially, and solve problems. The FBP is not only designed for use with the caregiver in the home; an abbreviated version is designed for use in an institutional setting.

Once the caregiver's needs have been established, the occupational therapist collaborates to support his or her efforts to increase the knowledge, skills, and abilities needed to manage the individual with dementia. Caregiver education may include methods to modify the environment; strategies to manage problem behaviors and facilitate leisure, work, home management and self-care activities; and referral to community resources.

The treatment setting often shapes the role of occupational therapy intervention with caregivers. For example, if the individual is a resident of a long-term care facility, caregiver education will be directed to the nursing and activity staff members because they are the primary caregivers. Similarly, if the individual lives at home, efforts will be focused on a spouse, an adult child, or possibly an attendant. Because the nature of the treatment setting significantly affects the occupational therapist's role, treatment will be discussed in terms of various treatment locations and how the environment, purposeful activity, and caregiver education are used therapeutically in each situation.

MANAGING DEMENTIA IN THE HOME

Families provide close to 90 percent of the primary care for older adults diagnosed with dementia who live at home (U.S. Select Committee on Aging, 1990). Others with dementia may live alone with care provided by either an attendant, for a few hours each day, or by a live-in caregiver. The primary issues in home care are safety, promoting independence in self-care, increasing involvement in leisure activities, and caregiver education and support.

Safety is often a primary concern because individuals with dementia frequently have impaired memory and judgment, which can lead to such behaviors as wandering, unsafe use of household appliances, and improper use of medications (Trace & Howell, 1992). Important issues associated with self-care in the mid- to late stages of dementia include maintaining adequate nutrition, ambulating without falls, and continence.

Home safety is assessed through direct observation of the individual's activities around the house and from caregiver reports. An evaluation of the neighborhood environment will provide a broader understanding of safety issues, especially for individuals who continue to leave the house on their own. The home environment should be adapted to allow the individual as much mobility and freedom of function as possible without putting him or her at risk of injury. The following adaptations can help to facilitate safety in the home (adapted from Skolaski-Pellitteri, 1993):

- Assess the individual's ability to understand what the smoke alarm means and what he or she should to do in case of an emergency.
- Assess the individual's ability to use the telephone in case of an emergency.
- Lock up electrical tools, knives, medicines, guns, and car keys.
- Lock up household cleaning supplies that could cause poisoning.
- Install bells or alarms on doors or at the top of the stairs to alert the caregiver of the person's location.
- Remove control knobs from the stove and hide stove burners with covers (these are commercially available).
- Use child-proof doorknobs and cabinet locks.
- Put new locks on doors that lead outside to prevent wandering.
- Provide an identification bracelet that the individual will wear at all times.
- Install night-lights in halls and bathrooms.

These are just a few of the methods that can be implemented to improve safety in the home. Each person with dementia and caregiver confronts a unique situation, which requires a thorough assessment to determine which safety concerns are pertinent and which environmental adaptations will meet their needs.

The two areas of purposeful activity that need to be addressed in the home environment are self-care and leisure activities. The importance of the elderly adult contributing to the functioning of the household was highlighted in a study by Mindel and Wright (1992), which indicated that the more dependent the older adult was on the family, the lower was the family's level of family life satisfaction; however, when the older adult contributed to the household functioning, the family members' level of family life satisfaction rose.

Self-care and leisure activities should be within reach of the individual's physical and cognitive abilities, of interest, and perceived as valuable. Activities should always be presented in a nonthreatening manner and must not be overstimulating. Agitated behavior may occur if an individual is presented with too difficult a task or too much stimulation at one time, which can overwhelm his or her remaining cognitive skills and (already limited) ability to think or react and lead to an emotionally intense response, such as crying, verbal abuse, sudden mood changes, or possibly even physical violence.

Self-care activities can be prioritized according to the caregiver's and client's needs. The environment can then be adapted by use of the necessary safety equipment, the activity can be set up in the most appropriate fashion, the type of cues the individual best responds to can be determined (whether verbal prompts, gestures for the individual to imitate, or tactile cues such as guiding), and the activity can be structured to match the individual's capabilities. These adaptations will help the individual with dementia function as independently as possible and allow the caregiver to elicit the desired responses through appropriate cuing. These concepts will now be demonstrated in the case illustration of Mr. Baxter's morning routine.

CASE ILLUSTRATION: MR. BAXTER

Mr. Baxter was initially referred to occupational therapy for an in-home evaluation to assist his family with concerns about his self-care, wandering, incontinence, and the risk of falls, especially when he gets up at night. The occupational therapy evaluation involved observing of Mr. Baxter's performance with several self-care tasks and the Kitchen Task Assessment (Baum & Edwards, 1993a), interviewing the caregiver to determine her concerns, and conducting a home safety evaluation.

In collaboration with the caregiver, several recommendations were made. Mr. and Mrs. Baxter's bed was placed against a wall so that Mr. Baxter had to move across his wife in order to get out of bed. Mrs. Baxter also installed a bell on the bedroom door and shut this door when going to sleep at night. These two environmental adaptations increased the chance that Mrs. Baxter would be awakened should Mr. Baxter get up at night. It was also recommended that Mr. Baxter be guided into the bathroom at night as he has some difficulty maintaining his balance. Once in the bathroom, he is able to use the toilet independently. The shower includes a grab bar and a shower seat, which helps to prevent falls. A detachable shower hose allows Mr. Baxter greater independence with his bathing needs. With verbal cues, he is able to undress and partially wash himself. Mrs. Baxter assists with bathing the areas he does not wash adequately. He dries himself with minimal assistance from his wife.

Mr. Baxter was attempting to dress himself but frequently wore clothing inappropriate for the weather or wore items inside out. Apparently he lacks the cognitive ability to find the appropriate clothing to wear. (However, he requires more assistance on some days than on others.) The occupational therapist and Mrs. Baxter decided that Mrs. Baxter should set out the needed clothing and hand Mr. Baxter one item of clothing at a time.

Once he is dressed, Mr. Baxter goes to the kitchen table to have toast and coffee and read the morning paper. He is not able to comprehend written material, but as this has been his morning routine for many years, he continues to go through the routine. He assists with putting butter and jam on the toast as his wife hands him the items. He is not given the opportunity to use the toaster or boil water for coffee because he no longer has the problem-solving skills to decide what to do if the toast gets stuck or the memory capacity to remember to turn off the stove burners. Mrs. Baxter routinely places burner covers on the stove and removes the stove knobs when she is finished in the kitchen to prevent her husband from burning himself or setting a fire. Resources were provided to Mrs. Baxter to obtain respite care to be used on those occasions when she needs a break or has errands to run.

Discussion

Mr. Baxter's plan incorporated both his self-care needs and interests and those of his caregiver. This case study illustrates how the occupational can collaborate with the caregiver by teaching him or her to modify the environment for safety and adapt daily living tasks to promote independence. Mrs. Baxter had already shown her understanding of the importance of maintaining a regular routine by allowing Mr. Baxter to go through the ritual of pretending to read the newspaper, even though she knew he no longer comprehended the content. She also modified the kitchen for safety to prevent misuse of the stove and modified the demands she placed on Mr. Baxter to help with preparing his breakfast. She required assistance in preventing her husband's wandering and incontinence and maintaining his independence in dressing himself.

Understanding a person's skills and previous interests provides an opportunity for occupational therapists and caregivers to collaborate on promoting participation in leisure activities. Baum (1997) recommends the use of the Activity Card Sort to identify activities of past interest and those that the individual with dementia may be interested in resuming. The Activity Card Sort has pictures of people performing various activities, which serve to elicit the client's memories, whereas other interest inventories and checklists are generally language based or require recall without visual cues to elicit memories.

Like self-care activities, leisure activities can be modified either by altering the environment, simplifying the task, or determining the most appropriate type of cues required to promote successful participation in a given activity. Consider the individual with dementia who previously did complex woodworking but now often complains that he is frustrated with the activity. Rather than attempting to get him to do projects as elaborate as those he previously completed, the occupational therapist should work on a simplified form of the same activity. For example, by using woodworking kits with fewer pieces, directions with pictures, and glue instead of nails, the individual might be able to continue participating in enjoyable activities at which he was previously successful. For a client in the later stages of dementia, simply sanding a cutting board may provide the satisfaction of woodworking without the overwhelming challenge of completing a full woodworking project.

The primary caregivers in the home setting are often family members or friends who give their time and energy to look after loved ones, who may be incontinent, irrational, or unresponsive to their efforts. In order for treatment in the home to be successful, all the principal caregivers should be involved. Family involvement in treatment is important, not only to maintain consistency of care but also to give the family members skills for coping with their own reactions to the disease. Dementia impacts the quality of life for all members of the family, not just the person with dementia.

Occupational therapists play an important role in providing ongoing support and education for caregivers to help them develop the skills necessary to manage the dementia. Daily management issues may involve wandering, agitation, violence, aggression, and difficulties with self-care. Suggested approaches to the problem behaviors related to aggression, anger, catastrophic reactions, confusion, and depression are outlined in Figure 11-4.

Community Referrals

Under the present model of managed care, individuals with dementia are treated for short periods of time for a specific problem. Caregivers and persons with dementia often have ongoing needs that are not met through such short intervention periods or through the medical model. When developing a care plan for the client with dementia and his or her family, the professional must consider the types of services available in the community to provide the needed support. Referrals to community resources are provided by many different health professionals depending on the needs of the client. Some examples of community services that may be used by the client and family are family crisis centers, driving evaluation and consultation services, adult day health programs, home-delivered meals, home health services, and transportation (Baum, 1991).

Dementia caregiver support groups are offered on a regular basis by organizations such as the Alzheimer's Association and United Parkinson's Foundation. Some groups are structured with a goal to provide education to the caregiver about the progression of the disease or training in skills to manage the day-to-day demands of providing care. Other groups are less structured and instead provide a forum for the informal discussion of ideas and experiences, socializing, and referrals to service agencies.

Some communities offer short-stay **respite care** where the individual with dementia can live in a nursing home, board-and-care home, foster home, or other setting for a short period—a weekend or one or more weeks—while the caregiver takes a vacation, gets needed medical care, or simply rests (Mace & Rabins, 1991).

Aggression & Anger
- Assure individuals who behave aggressively that they are okay—that you understand that they cannot help themselves.
- Speak in a well-modulated voice.
- Offer food or drink (it is difficult to eat and be angry at the same time).
- Position yourself about four or five feet away.
- Sit or stand a little to the side rather than face them directly. You're less intimidating to them this way.
- Be prepared to accept some insults and verbal abuse.
- Ask yourself if too much is being expected of them.

Catastrophic reactions
- Reduce confusion with memory aids and highly structured routines.
- Simplify everything, e.g., decision-making, leisure activities.
- Assist them one step at a time. Reinforce each successful step.
- Stop and give those that are confused a chance to calm down.
- Reassure.
- Gently holding a person's hands, patting on the arm or gently rocking can be soothing, along with quiet music.
- Accept the behavior as a response to dementing illness, beyond the control of the impaired person.
- Distract, if possible.

Confusion
- Provide a nightlight to help the person see and locate familiar things and prevent falls in the dark; protect against wandering
- Consider the side effects of some sedatives and cold remedies as well as prescribed drugs.
- Encourage reminiscence. Gently assist with keeping facts reasonably accurate and related to the past.
- Use communication rich in reminders, cues, gestures and physical guiding (if appropriate) to increase personal awareness. Keep explanations simple.
- Avoid unrealistic promises.
- Keep your mood and responses consistent.
- Provide special personal space filled with familiar things where the confused person can go, rest and feel safe and secure.
- Ask permission if something must be moved or changed: This helps to establish feelings of trust and control.
- Overprotection leads to feelings of helplessness and boredom. Provide reminders, directions, adequate time and praise for self-care efforts on an adult level.

(continues)

Figure 11-4. Approaches to Problem Behaviors

Source: [Author unknown], [Handout on managing problem behaviors in people with dementia] (Presented at a workshop on dementia, Palo Alto Veterans' Administration Medical Center, Palo Alto, CA).

- Schedule respite care regularly in the caregiving routine so it becomes accepted and predictable.

Depression
- Respond to the impaired person with kind firmness.
- Try to rebuild self-esteem through reminiscence, participation in activities and decisions. Notice pictures and momentos. Ask about them and listen.
- Alert the person's doctor, medications may help.
- Spend time with them. Do not ignore quiet, uncomplaining people.
- Encourage them to talk freely.
- Be familiar with the factors that predispose people to depression. They include problems with: health, living situation, losses, and a family history of depressive illness.
- A gentle touch with a reassuring smile projects a caring attitude.

Hoarding, rummaging behavior — Because of memory loss, demented people frequently look for something that is "missing": rooms, clothes, personal items. These things may not look familiar so they are constantly looking for familiar things.
- Don't scold or try to rationalize with the person.
- Distract the impaired person when he/she is somewhere he/she is not supposed to be.
- Learn the impaired person's hiding places.

Sundowner's syndrome — This occurs when impaired people become confused, restless and insecure late in the afternoon and after dark.
- Set up a rigid daily routine. It will reduce anxiety about decision making and what happens next.
- Alternate activity with programmed rest.
- Reduce all stimuli during rest periods.
- Strive to keep daily activities within the person's coping ability.
- Prepare the impaired person for special events so it doesn't come as a shock.
- Take an inventory of the person's daily experience. Consider bright lights, noise from TVs, radios, and conversations, visitors and special events, odors from miscellaneous sources, and the stimulation of personal contact with the caregiver.

Suspiciousness, distrust — Occurs most often with people with dementia when they cannot make sense of what is happening.
- Be honest.
- Avoid grand gestures and promises that cannot be carried out.
- Go to the person when you have forgotten something and apologize.
- Do not argue about or rationally explain disappearances of the person's possessions.
- Offer to look for an item if the person says that it is missing.
- Learn the person's favorite hiding places.

Figure 11-4. *(continued)*

Because the occupational therapist in home-based care is treating the individual with dementia in his or her own environment, the therapist may identify family needs that have gone unnoticed. He or she then becomes the link between the family and the relevant community services.

MANAGING DEMENTIA IN ADULT DAY SERVICES

As the disease progresses, caregivers may seek other services to relieve some of the strain of providing care. Adult day service is a type of program that may relieve the caregiver of the stress resulting from providing continuous support and care. Programs such as these allow persons with dementia to remain in their own community setting, thus delaying permanent institutionalization. It also allows time for the caregivers to work or simply relax and refresh themselves so they can better care for their afflicted family member.

Adult day programs usually offer several hours a day of structured recreation in group settings plus a meal. These programs, much like special programs in long-term care facilities, offer activities such as exercise, arts and crafts, music, and discussions. They are designed to provide a meaningful, structured environment in which persons with dementia can be supported and helped to retain their cognitive and physical skills (Baum, 1991). These programs usually operate six to eight hours a day for two to five days per week. Clients are dropped off at the facility by their caregivers or specially arranged transportation.

Most activities in adult day programs and long-term care facilities are conducted in groups. Due to the similarities in developing activity programs in an adult day health program and a long-term care facility, these settings will be discussed together. In either setting, an occupational therapist may provide direct services or function as a consultant to the staff.

When working in a group setting, the life experiences of the person with dementia must be considered in structuring the group and setting the atmosphere of the activities. New activities can sometimes be perceived as a threat by persons with dementia, who may fear that others will recognize their inadequacies. By allowing individuals to have meaningful roles, whether singing along to an old tune, socializing with friends, or washing dishes, their self-confidence can be increased. The group leader structures activities appropriate to each individual's level of understanding and may model playful behavior to provide an atmosphere of acceptance and minimize the perceived consequences of failure (Glantz & Richman, 1996). Social contact has been shown to help those with dementia remain more involved and vital and should be encouraged through such activities as sing-a-longs, group games, and visitation programs. Without social contact it is thought that individuals with dementia decline at a much faster rate (Baum & Edwards, 1993b). An effective occupational therapist will find ways for people to succeed at little tasks so that they can feel better about themselves. Sheridan (1987) states that, when used appropriately, activities provide moment-to-moment satisfaction and raise self-esteem.

Group activities in adult day care and long-term care are variable, depending on the interests and needs of the clients. Some activities are designed for socialization and recreation, while others are medically oriented (Aitken & Goldstein-Lohman, 1996). Activities may include, but are not limited to, reminiscence, reality orientation, poetry reading, music, physical activity, grooming, and pet therapy (Foti, 1996). It is important to set up routines of exercise and to include meaningful engagement in exercise as a part of the daily program. Recent research indicates that people with Alzheimer's who are involved in exercise programs retain more memory function (Baum & Edwards, 1993b).

Other programs have utilized work activities for the clients. Burns and Bruell (1990), at the Minnesota Veterans' Administration Medical Center, developed a day care program structured around work tasks so that people could come in on a daily basis and continue to be productive workers. The occupational therapist set up work tasks such as folding towels, washing tables, and doing piecemeal work, which were available for two or three hours in each afternoon. Burns and Bruell (1990) report that people who participate in these work programs return home at night more calm and tranquil. They are less likely to wander or make extra demands on their families. Dementia deprives individuals of their ability to independently perform life role responsibilities. Without occupational roles to organize daily life, there may be no sense of structure or meaning in their daily existence, and feelings of incompetence, inadequacy, and low self-worth can result.

The cognitive disability treatment model developed by Allen (1985) may help streamline the assessment process and identify which type of groups are most appropriate for a particular client. The cognitive disability model involves determining the client's information-processing capacities to assess whether the individual can perform various functional activities safely and successfully. Once the therapist has determined the client's cognitive level on a hierarchical scale from six (highest) to one (lowest), environmental modifications can be implemented to ensure that the client is able to successfully participate in activities appropriate to his or her cognitive level (Allen, 1985; Levy, 1996). The model specifically describes observable behaviors, types of activities, and the nature and amount of cuing required to promote the successful completion of activities at each cognitive level.

Activity groups in either adult day care or skilled nursing settings need to include consideration of the individual's past and present interests and life roles in the design of a social and physical environment that will promote participation. Occupational therapists may train staff members in adult day programs and long-term care facilities in specific interaction skills to enable them to design more appropriate individual treatment programs for persons with dementia. The changes in personality and behavior seen in people with dementia can result in decreased social and interpersonal skills and they may become unable to behave appropriately in a social situation. Sometimes the person with dementia will be better able to interact socially in a one-on-one situation or in the home. Group activities that are not appropriately structured may overstimulate, distract, or frustrate the individual with dementia, resulting in acting-out and disturbed behaviors. Figure 11-5 identifies ways for caregivers to interact more effectively with individuals with dementia so as to enable them to participate fully in social activities.

Long-term care facilities have differed from adult day care service since the enactment of the Nursing Home Reform Section of the Omnibus Budget Reconciliation Act of 1987 (OBRA) was developed (in response to the failure of the long-term care industry to provide quality care for residents). The act changed the model of care from one with a medical emphasis to one with an emphasis on the quality of life for residents. Activities are included as a component of this emphasis, and long-term care facilities "must provide an on-

Methods to Facilitate Interactions with an Individual with Dementia
- Never approach a person with dementia from behind.
- Introduce yourself to them daily.
- Treat the person like an adult. Being talked down to is demeaning and dehumanizing.
- Make sure you have the person's attention before you begin to speak, e.g., say their name or gently touch them.
- When inviting an individual to an activity, use gentle assertion rather than a question that may be easily refused, for example, "Hello Mary, I'd love for you to join me in a sing-a-long."
- When possible, attempt all communication in a calm, relaxed, and quiet environment.
- Give short simple directions. Do not overwhelm them with too much information at once.
- Use short sentences and simple words. If they do not understand, repeat or rephrase.
- Do not shout, this will only serve to agitate them. Use a calm, natural voice when you speak.
- Do not rush them. Allow the impaired person enough time to answer questions, follow directions, and express themselves at the pace they choose to be most comfortable.
- Reduce distractions in the environment: turn the volume down on radios and TVs. Many people in a room can be over stimulating for just about anyone.
- Redirect to conversation or activities by asking questions or restating what you are doing with them when they become distracted or confused.

Figure 11-5. Caregiver Interactions to Help People with Dementia Participate in Social Activities

Source: Allen (1985).

going program of activities designed to meet the interests, and the physical, mental, and the psychological well-being of each resident" (U.S. Department of Health and Human Services, 1989). An important part of this legislation and its mandate for the provision of quality care is "empowering the long-term care resident with perceived control of important aspects of his or her daily life" (p. 5373). The following are suggestions for activity programming to enhance personal control of the resident in long-term care as outlined by Martin and Smith (1993):

1. Provide activities based on individual needs and preferences: activity programming should be individualized. Instead of fitting the individual into the facility's activity calendar; each activity should be planned with the individual's interests in mind. The Interest Checklist (Matsutsuyu, 1969) is useful in identifying personal preferences and should be reviewed with the caregiver for accuracy. Too often the only choice offered to the person with dementia who is residing in long-term care settings is to attend or not attend an activity. However, when individuals with dementia are given opportunities for increased choice, the amount and duration of their activity level has often been shown to increase (provided too many choices are not provided, which can be overwhelming).

2. Provide optimal levels of choices: providing too many choices may have a negative effect on some individuals with dementia. Rather than providing too much information, it is preferable to present a manageable number of choices. An example would be asking an individual, "Would you like to play checkers or cards?" instead of asking, "What would you like to play?"

3. Reduce or eliminate barriers to participation: barriers prevent or reduce an individual's ability to participate fully in activities. The occupational therapist and activity personnel should work with individuals with dementia to identify the particular barriers (e.g., social and physical) that limit their participation in activities.

4. Ensure that activities are age appropriate: participating in activities intended for children often feels demeaning to adults with dementia. All too often, personnel in long-term care facilities include children's games in their activity programming because they feel that anything else would be too complex. Occupational therapists have the training to analyze and match activities to the abilities and preferences of the demented individual to ensure successful experiences.

5. Normalize activities: if possible, activities should be performed in the same manner as if the person were not in long-term care. Promoting activity selection and participation based on previous interests is one way to accomplish this. One example of a normalized activity is a dining program that eliminates institutional trays and instead uses place settings, table cloths, and soft music. In these programs, staff members are encouraged

to eat with the residents, which helps to increase socialization and decrease the feelings of distance between 'them" (residents) and "us" (staff).

6. Emphasize active participation: research has indicated that most of a resident's waking hours are spent in passive activities (e.g., television viewing) (Gottesman, Baack, & Voelkl, cited in Martin & Smith, 1993). Active participation (e.g., discussions, dance, sing-a-longs, arts and crafts) can have a noticeable effect on self-perceptions of control. For example, some programs have been structured to be held in close proximity to a child care facility. In these settings, elders are given the opportunity to interact with the children (a familiar activity for many) under the supervision of a staff member.

MANAGING DEMENTIA IN RESIDENTIAL LONG-TERM CARE

The burden of providing continual care is sometimes too much for caregivers, who then must place the impaired person in a facility with more specialized care. Relocation to a residential long-term care facility is traumatic for any older person, but it can be especially devastating for a person with dementia. Long-term care usually refers to care that will be given for a minimum of three months (Lewis, 1989). Currently, only about 5 to 6 percent of the nation's elders live in long-term care facilities. However, of these people, approximately 60 to 70 percent have some type of dementia disorder (U.S. Department of Health and Human Services, 1991).

There are a variety of long-term care institutions available. These include nursing homes, veterans' hospitals, retirement communities, residential homes, and state mental hospitals. Individuals with dementia who are placed in one of these settings have been uprooted from the familiarity of their homes and their families and had their daily routines disrupted. To aid in their adjustment, the occupational therapist may provide direct evaluation and treatment to the individual with dementia or may consult with the staff regarding treatment approaches and activity programming in the long-term care setting.

The Environment

Often working in collaboration with an activity director and nursing staff, occupational therapists devise creative environments that make the transition to long-term care easier for persons with dementia. Environments are created that make it possible for them to reestablish and maintain their routines and to participate in meaningful activities on a daily basis.

Many individuals with dementia have lived in the same house or apartment for years, where they were surrounded by the evidence of a lifetime of memories. In order to personalize a resident's room, occupational therapists have recommended environmental adaptations such as painting the room the same color as the bedroom at home. Recommendations have also been

made to include a few items of the residents' furniture and personal possessions from home in an attempt to reconstruct a familiar, stable environment.
Pictures of the resident and his or her family members can also provide a basis
for reminiscence with the staff. Pictures also help the staff to perceive the
resident as an individual who had a rich and fulfilling life prior to admission
to the facility.

Caregivers in a long-term care facility include activity directors, registered
nurses, licensed vocational or practical nurses, social workers, and nursing assistants. Caregiver training should include an emphasis on the importance of
allowing for individual differences in personalizing the resident's environment, which should be structured to support the person's personal needs
while maintaining his or her safety. The following case illustration helps illustrate this point.

CASE ILLUSTRATION: MRS. LOGAN

*Mrs. Logan had been living alone prior to admission to the long-term care fa-
cility. She suffered from multi-infarct dementia with minimal physical deficits.
Mrs. Logan perceived of herself as being a good housekeeper. For example,
part of her routine at home was to make her bed immediately after rising each
day. One of her previous hobbies included sewing, and she had brought her
sewing machine with her to the long-term care facility. Initially Mrs. Logan
had difficulty finding her room at the facility, but once her sewing machine
had been set up, she was able to look in each room until she located her own
by her sewing machine. She also continued to make her own bed at the facility.*

*One day in an attempt to neaten Mrs. Logan's room, a nursing assistant re-
made her bed and put away the sewing machine, which was not being used.
However, when Mrs. Logan returned from the dining room, she became quite
frustrated because she could not locate her room or find her possessions.*

Discussion

*When cognitive skills, and especially memory, start to decline, individuals with
dementia often can arrange their environments to cue themselves: for example, placing certain things in a particular location can guide them through
the performance of daily tasks. When the nursing assistant put away her possessions, Mrs. Logan lost her environmental context cues, and thus her ability to maintain her independence.*

Occupational therapists must help the caregivers engaged in the care of the
individual with dementia to understand the significance of their routines and
environmental cues. If significant changes are made in the environment, procedural memory may be impaired and the person's capacities may, as a result,
undergo further decline.

Prior to the enactment of OBRA (1987), physical and chemical restraints were used to manage troublesome behaviors exhibited by persons with dementia. When residents wandered they were physically restrained in wheelchairs even though they were ambulatory. When residents became agitated, medications to sedate them were prescribed. Today, however, restraints can no longer be used indiscriminately to manage problem behavior; instead, the staff must consider creative alternatives to modify an agitated person's behavior (Trace & Howell, 1992). This has facilitated the inclusion of the occupational therapist to evaluate a resident's level of functioning and to make recommendations regarding the use of less restrictive interventions (Aitken & Goldstein-Lohman, 1996).

SELF-CARE ACTIVITIES

Maintaining independence with self-care tasks can be an important part of a coordinated care plan. The occupational therapist needs to work jointly with the staff to consider what the individual is mentally and physically capable of doing independently. Nursing staff may require in-service education on the rehabilitative approach of encouraging clients to become more self-sufficient. Indeed, a nursing assistant may incurrectly assume that to adequately perform her job he or she must do everything for the resident. The occupational therapist must also be sensitive to the size of the nursing staff workload to understand how recommendations can best be integrated into the daily patient care workload. A consistent approach using constant environmental cues will provide the most positive results.

The occupational therapist may serve as a model for nursing assistants to help them facilitate resident independence in self-care. Individuals with dementia living in long-term care settings are frequently physically helped out of bed, washed by a nursing assistant (possibly wheeled to the shower or a commode instead of walking), and dressed. The occupational therapist may demonstrate the following techniques for nursing assistants to promote greater dignity and independence for the residents with dementia:

- Use tactile cues and minimal verbal cues to help the individual get out of bed.
- Provide a bathrobe for walking to the shower.
- Cue the individual with the steps for bathing if he or she is capable of participation.
- Offer the individual two choices of clothing for the day. For example, a nursing assistant should not ask, "What do you want to wear today?" Instead, he or she may ask, for example, "Do you want to wear the pink or the blue dress today?"
- Provide a setup in the bathroom for oral hygiene, hair care, and shaving or applying makeup. Offer only the minimal supplies needed for each

task. The occupational therapist or nursing assistant can demonstrate the task that is to be completed.

Not all individuals with dementia are capable of participating in self-care. Those who are should be encouraged by supportive, well-trained staff and provided with a consistent environment. Individuals who have been institutionalized for an extended period of time may be overwhelmed by changes in routine that suddenly require them to participate in self-care activities if, in the past, they were dependent on others to perform these tasks. On the other hand, newly admitted individuals who previously resided in their own home or a board-and-care facility may be more independent with daily activities. These individuals may benefit the most from techniques to facilitate independence in self-care.

Other roles for the occupational therapist in the long-term care facility involve direct care. In the later stages of dementia, individuals may have neurological deficits resulting in mobility limitations and dysphagia. In the case of mobility limitations, there may be the need to consider the positioning of the client in a wheelchair. If dysphagia is present, the occupational or speech therapist will complete a clinical swallowing evaluation and then make recommendations regarding food and fluid consistencies and positioning techniques.

The presence of individuals who occasionally act out in bizarre ways can be very disturbing to the more cognitively intact individuals in the facility as well as to those staff members who have little training or understanding of the problems that individuals with dementia face. Such behaviors can disrupt an entire unit, occupy a great deal of the staff's time, and prevent or reduce the ability of the individual with dementia to participate fully in activities. According to Zarit, Zarit, and Rosenberg-Thompson (1990), staff members in long-term care facilities tend to be particularly troubled by individuals with dementia who persistently present their personal, distorted views of reality. Among the solutions that have been attempted for such behaviors are reality orientation, going along with the individual's beliefs, and viewing his or her beliefs as a metaphor for an unexpressed need or wish and responding accordingly. It was found that reality orientation did not work in these situations and, in fact, often upset the individual even more. It is difficult to win an argument with an individual with dementia concerning what is or is not real because he or she has lost the ability to evaluate incoming information accurately. The other two approaches—going along with an individual's beliefs and viewing personal beliefs as a metaphor—accept the person's view of reality, are more responsive to his or her underlying need, and are generally more effective (Zarit et al., 1990).

CASE ILLUSTRATION: MR. JUNIPER

Mr. Juniper was a former high school teacher who insisted that he wanted to leave the long-term care facility to teach his class. The staff first tried to ori-

*ent him to reality, but that did not work. They then told him that the class
had been canceled due to a school holiday and that they needed him at the facility to help with an activity class that day. Since there were frequent school
holidays throughout the school year, this response sounded realistic and, by
addressing his need to feel productive, it caused him to calm down.*

Discussion

*This case example illustrates an approach that validates the individual's be-
lief system (Zarit et al., 1990). Instead of trying to reason with Mr. Juniper by
convincing him that he was in a long-term care facility and no longer worked
as a high school teacher, the staff member supported his beliefs by providing
a response to his concerns in a framework to which he could relate.*

These examples clearly demonstrate that there is no rigid formula for treatment: different solutions are needed for different patients and situations.
The occupational therapist working in the residential long-term care setting
must work with staff to devise solutions to enable them to be more responsive to the needs and the problems faced by individuals with dementia.

Summary

It is expected that as the current tremendous growth in the number of very
old individuals (85 years or older) in our country continues, there will be a
similar growth in the population of individuals with dementia as well (an estimated 7.4 million individuals by the year 2040) (U.S. Congress, Select Committee on Aging, 1987). Dementia is a mental disorder characterized by
impairments in memory, language, recognition, planned motor movements,
and other executive functions that represents a significant decline in the person's social and occupational functioning. Occupational therapists will increasingly encounter persons with cognitive impairments in hospital settings
and in the expanding areas of practice in home care, long-term care, and outpatient services.

This chapter examines the cognitive deficits of persons diagnosed with dementia and the criteria used to differentiate the dementias into more specific
diagnostic categories based on etiology (physiological effects of general medical conditions, substances, or multiple etiologies). Several common types of
dementia were described and illustrated, including dementia of the
Alzheimer's type, vascular dementia, and dementias due to other, general medical conditions. Symptoms of dementia can be caused by a variety of medical
conditions that may be responsive to treatment, but in most instances no treatment is available and the condition is characterized by continuing cognitive
decline.

The concept of a geriatric syndrome (Blazer, 1995) was introduced to alert
us to the unusual presentation of physical and mental symptoms displayed in

older adults. This concept provides a basis for guiding assessment and treatment using functional problems and highlights the importance of identifying, when possible, the cause or underlying etiology of the cognitive deficits. The general assessment approach to dementia includes first identifying individuals with cognitive impairments by using screening measures such as a mental status exam. When indicated, this is followed by a comprehensive multidisciplinary assessment that is multidimensional and encompasses a wide range of systems (clinical and cognitive evaluations, psychosocial history, reports of the family, medical history and workup). Occupational therapy evaluation focuses on accurately determining the person's capabilities and limitations in occupational performance areas and the accompanying everyday tasks. The importance was highlighted of establishing a baseline of the client's functional level, assessing the safety and appropriateness of the social and physical environment, identifying resources, supporting caregivers, and specifying functional outcomes.

Due to the nonreversible and often progressive nature of many dementia disorders, occupational therapy interventions focus on managing the individual in the least restrictive environment and maximizing his or her remaining skills, satisfaction, and competence. Because the treatment setting affects the occupational therapist's role so significantly, interventions in this chapter were discussed in terms of various treatment locations. The locations identified include home-based care, adult day service programs, and residential long-term care. The role of purposeful activity, activity analysis, caregiver education, and environmental supports and adaptations used for intervention in these different settings were explained.

The primary objective for the occupational therapist is to carefully assess each individual's capabilities and weaknesses, adapt the tasks of daily living accordingly, and design and organize environments and caregiver interventions that provide opportunities for self-reinforcing, competent performance (AOTA, 1994; Levy, 1987a & b). Effective adaptations of the physical and social environment and task adaptation (following activity analysis) can help to reduce overstimulation and minimize confusion and to reduce agitation and frustration. This allows individuals with dementia to focus more effectively on the activities that retain meaningfulness, which simplifies learning and enhances their functioning.

Caregiver involvement in treatment is important, not only to maintain consistency of care but also to give families skills for coping with their own reactions to the impact of the disease. Occupational therapists may act as consultants to the staff in long-term care facilities. In these settings, occupational therapists collaborate with, and guide, staff in the management of disruptive behaviors, create effective groups, and provide instructions on how to cue individuals or change their environments to promote maximum function in the occupational performance areas and in specific task performance.

Occupational therapists find mutual benefit in working collaboratively with the client, family members, nursing staff, activity directors, physicians, rehabilitation staff, and other occupational therapists whenever possible. Occupational therapists, in collaboration with caregivers and families, assume a role in promoting effective and efficient caregiving. They enable individuals with dementia to maintain the highest level of independence possible, thus promoting a better quality of life in the least restrictive environment.

Review Questions

1. Choose a case study found in this chapter. Using the Clinical Course of Alzheimer's Disease Scale shown in Figure 11-2, identify the approximate stage of dementia you believe has been attained by the person in the case illustration. What additional information and further evaluations are required?

2. A 79-year-old woman living alone has come to seek advice concerning her increasing problems with short-term memory. She reports difficulty finding things at the grocery store and problems with attention and concentration, especially when driving or cooking. These cognitive problems began in the last four months. She was recently in a car accident and has frequent complaints of dizziness and fatigue. How urgent are these complaints? What diagnoses would you hypothesize as part of the clinical-reasoning process? Would you refer the woman, and what additional information is important to obtain?

3. The prevalence rate of dementia in the elderly population is expected to continue to grow at a rapid rate. Describe why this is the case. What impact will this have on occupational therapy practice?

4. Imagine that your family has made the decision to admit a relative with dementia to a residential long-term care facility. Explain the ideal facility—including environment, activities, and caregiver characteristics—to ensure the optimal care of your relative. Identify resources in the community that could help with this important decision. What alternatives could your family consider besides residential long-term care?

5. Imagine you are developing an education program for families in which a member has recently been diagnosed with dementia. What are the major components of your education program? What specific areas would you target in your planning?

Learning Activities

1. Attend a dementia support group (the Alzheimer's Association and United Parkinson's Foundation offer frequent meetings), spend a weekend at a family respite camp program for a person with dementia (the Family Caregiver's Alliance or the Alzheimer's Association can help you find one), or visit a local adult day service program that provides services to individuals with dementia and their families. How do your observations compare

to what you have read in this chapter? Write a summary and be prepared to discuss your experience.

2. As a group discussion activity, imagine you are in the middle of running an activity group at a day care facility, when suddenly, a client stands up and says it is time to go home. He starts walking toward the door, saying: "I have to go to work. I'm going to my car." The client does not have a job, nor has he driven a car in several years. Through group discussion, and also based on what you have read, identify the most effective approach in a situation such as this. Explain the steps you would use to calm the person down, keep him in the immediate area, and help him refocus on the group.

3. Identify some one-to-one and small group activities that might be used at a senior center for well elderly and that incorporate a cognitive, sensorimotor, or psychosocial focus. Conduct a brief activity analysis and explain what modifications might be required to accommodate a client in the moderate, moderately severe, or severe stage of dementia who lives in a residential, long-term care facility or attends adult day services.

4. View the video "Complaints of a Dutiful Daughter," directed by Deborah Hoffman, available from Women Make Movies, 462 Broadway, New York, NY 10013, or visit your local health library for other films about families and persons with dementia.

References

Aitken, M., & Goldstein-Lohman, H. (1996). Health care systems: Changing perspectives. In O. Larson, R. Stevens-Ratchford, L. Pedretti, & J. Crabtree (Eds.), *Role of occupational therapy with the elderly* (pp. 53–96), Bethesda, MD: American Occupational Therapy Association (AOTA).

Allen, C. K. (1982). Independence through activity: The practice of occupational therapy. *American Journal of Occupational Therapy, 36*, 731–739.

Allen, C. K. (1985). *Occupational therapy for psychiatric diseases: Measurement and management of cognitive disabilities*. Boston: Little, Brown.

Allen, C. K., Earhart, C. A., & Blue, T. (1992). *Occupational therapy treatment goals for the physically and cognitively disabled*. Rockville, MD: AOTA.

Allen, C. K., & Robertson, S. (1993). *Study guide for occupational therapy treatment goals for the physically and cognitively disabled*. Rockville, MD: AOTA.

American Occupational Therapy Association (AOTA). (1994). Statement: Occupational therapy services for persons with Alzheimer's disease and other dementias. *American Journal of Occupational Therapy, 48*(11), 1029–1031.

American Psychiatric Association (APA). (1994). *Diagnostic and statistical manual of mental disorders* (4th ed.). Washington, DC: APA. (3rd ed. rev. published 1987).

Baum, C. (1991). Addressing the needs of the cognitively impaired elderly from a family policy perspective. *American Journal of Occupational Therapy, 45*(7), 594–606.

Baum, C. (1993). *Managing cognitively impaired older adults.* Paper presented at the meeting of the Occupational Therapy Association of California conference, San Jose, CA.

Baum, C. (1997, Feb. 1–2). *Managing cognitive deficits in older adults.* Workshop presented in San Jose, CA.

Baum, C., & Edwards, D. F. (1993a). Cognitive performance in senile dementia of the Alzheimer's type: The Kitchen Task Assessment. *American Journal of Occupational Therapy, 47*(5), 431–436.

Baum, C., & Edwards, D. F. (1993b). Identification and measurement of productive behaviors in senile dementia of the Alzheimer's type. *Gerontologist, 33*(3), 403–408.

Benton, A. L. (1984). *The Revised Visual Retention Test* (4th ed.). New York: Psychological Corporation.

Berg, L. (1988). Clinical dementia rating. *Psychopharmacology Bulletin, 24,* 637–639.

Blazer, D. G. (1995). Geriatric syndromes: An introduction. *Psychiatric Services, 46*(1), 31.

Borell, L., Sandman, P. O., & Kielhofner, G. (1991). Clinical decision making in Alzheimer's disease. *Occupational Therapy in Mental Health, 11*(4), 111–124.

Breitner, J. C. & Welsh, K. A. (1995). Diagnosis and management of memory loss and cognitive disorders among elderly persons. *Psychiatric Services, 46*(1), 29–35.

Burns, T., & Bruell, J. (1990). Work program serves veterans with Alzheimer's disease. *OT Week, 4*(44), 7, 14.

Burns, T., Mortimer, J. A., & Merchak, P. (1994). Cognitive Performance Test: A new approach to functional assessment in Alzheimer's disease. *Journal of Geriatric Psychiatry and Neurology, 7*(1), 46–54.

Christiansen, C., & Baum, C. (1991). *Occupational therapy: Overcoming human performance deficits.* Thorofare, NJ: Slack.

Crook, T., Bartus, R. T., Ferris, S. H., Whitehouse, P., Cohen, G. D., & Gershon, S. (1986). Age associated memory impairment: Proposed diagnostic criteria and measures of clinical change. *Developmental Neuropsychology, 2,* 261–276.

Crook, T. H., Tinglenberg, J., Yesavage, J., Petrie, W., Nunzi, M. G., & Massari, D. C. (1991). Effects of phophatidylserine in age-associated memory impairment. *Neurology, 41,* 644–649.

Cullum, C. M., Filley, C. M., Kelly, J. P., & Schneck, S. A. (1992). *Utility of cognitive screening tasks in patients with mild Alzheimer's disease.* Paper presented at the 20th Annual Meeting of the International Neuropsychological Society, San Diego, CA.

Davidson, H. (1991). Assessing environmental factors. In C. Christiansen & C. Baum (Eds.), *Occupational therapy: Overcoming human occupation deficits* (pp. 427–454). Thorofare, NJ: Slack Publishing.

Deitz, J. C., Beeman, C., & Thorn, D.W. (in preparation). The Test of Orientation for Rehabilitation Patients (TORP).

Edwards, D. F., Deuel, R. K., & Baum, C. M. (1991). Constructional apraxia in senile dementia: Contributions to functional loss. *Physical and Occupational Therapy in Geriatrics, 9,* 53–59.

Elliot, S. (1996). Non-traditional patient in long-term care: What can we offer? *OT Practice, 1*(9), 31–37.

Evans, D. A., Funkenstein, H. H., Albert, M. S., Scherr, P. A., Cook, N. R., Chown, M. J., Herbert, L. E., Hennekens, C. H., & Taylor, J. O. (1989). Prevalence of Alzheimer's disease in a community population of older persons: Higher than previously reported. *Journal of the American Medical Association, 262,* 2551–2556.

Fisher, A. G. (1994). *Assessment of Motor and Process Skills.* Unpublished Manual, Department of Occupational Therapy, Colorado State University.

Folstein, M. F., & McHugh, P. R. (1975). Mini-Mental State: A practical method for grading the cognitive state of patients for the clinician. *Journal of Psychiatric Research, 12,* 189–198.

Folstein, S. E. (1989). *Huntington disease: A disorder of families.* Baltimore, MD: Johns Hopkins University Press.

Foti, D. (1996). Gerontic occupational therapy: Specialized intervention for the older adult. In O. Larson, R. Stevens-Ratchford, L. Pedretti, & J. Crabtree (Eds.), *Role of occupational therapy with the elderly* (pp. 629–645). Bethesda, MD: AOTA.

George, L. K., Blazer, D. F., Winfield-Laird, I., Leaf, P. J., & Fischbach, R. L. (1988). Psychiatric Disorders and mental health service use in later life: Evidence from the Epidemiologic Catchment Area program. In J. Brody & G. Maddox (eds.), *Epidemiology and Aging* (pp. 189–219). New York: Springer.

Gitlin, L., Corcoran, M., & Leinmiller–Eckhardt, S. (1995). Understanding the family perspective: An ethnographic framework for providing occupational therapy in the home. *American Journal of Occupational Therapy, 49,* 802–809.

Goodglass, H., & Kaplan, E. (1983). *The assessment of aphasia and related disorders.* Philadelphia: Lea & Febiger.

Guberman, A. (1994). *An introduction to clinical neurology.* Boston: Little, Brown.

Gurland, B. (1980). The assessment of mental status in older adults. In J. E. Birren & R. Sloane (Eds.), *Handbook of mental health and aging* (pp. 671–700). Englewood Cliffs, NJ: Prentice-Hall.

HLadik, P. (1982). *Once I have had my tea: A guide to understanding and caring for the memory-impaired elderly.* Syracuse, NY.

Howe–Murphy, R., & Charboneau, B. G. (1987). *Therapeutic recreation intervention: An ecological perspective*. Englewood Cliffs, NJ: Prentice-Hall.

Jette, A. M. (1980). The functional status index: Reliability of a chronic disease evaluation instrument. *Archives of Physical Medicine and Rehabilitation, 61*, 395.

Joe, B. E. (1996, Nov. 7). Parkinson's disease: The disabler. *OT Week*, p. 18.

Johansson, B., & Zarit, S. H. (1994). *Incidence of dementia in the oldest old for a 6 year period*. Paper presented at the 12th Nordic Congress in Gerontology, Jonkoping, Sweden.

Kahn, R., Goldfarb, A., Pollack, N., & Peck, A. (1960). Brief objective measures for the determination of mental status in the aged. *American Journal of Psychiatry, 117*, 326–328.

Katz, S., Downs, T., Cash, H., & Grotz, R. (1970). Progress in the development of the Index of ADL. *Gerontologist, 10*, 20–30.

Katzman, R., Lasker, B., & Bernstein, N. (1988). Advances in the diagnosis of dementia: Accuracy of diagnosis and consequences of misdiagnosis of disorders causing dementia. In R. D. Terry (Ed.), *Aging and the Brain* (pp. 17–35). New York: Raven Press.

Keenan, J. S., & Brasseil, E. G. (1975). *The assessment of aphasia and related disorders*. Murfreesboro, TN: Pinnacle Press.

King, L. (1978). Toward a science of adaptive response. *American Journal of Occupational Therapy, 32*, 572–581.

Klein, R. M., & Bell, B. (1982). Self-care skills: Behavioral measurement with the Klein-Bell ADL scale. *Archives of Physical Medicine and Rehabilitation, 63*, 335–338.

LaRue, A., Watson, J., & Plotkin, D. A. (1992). Retrospective accounts of dementia symptoms: Are they reliable? *Gerontologist, 32*(2), 240–245.

Levy, L. L. (1974). Movement therapy for psychiatric patients. *American Journal of Occupational Therapy, 28*(6), 354–357.

Levy, L. L. (1987a). Psychosocial intervention and dementia, part 1: State of the art, future directions. *Occupational Therapy in Mental Health, 7*(1), 69–105.

Levy, L. L. (1987b). Psychosocial intervention and dementia, part 2: The cognitive disability perspective. *Occupational Therapy in Mental Health, 7*(4), 13–37.

Levy, L. L. (1988). Cognitive treatment. In L. J. Davis & M. Kirkland (Eds.), *The Role of Occupational Therapy with the Elderly* (pp. 289–323). Rockville, MD: American Occupational Therapy Association.

Levy, L. L. (1992). the use of the cognitive disability frame of reference in rehabilitation of cognitively disabled older adults. In N. Katz (Ed.), *Cognitive Rehabiliation: Models for intervention in occupational therapy* (pp. 22–50). Boston: Andover Medical Publishers.

Levy, L. L. (1996). Cognitive integration and cognitive components. In O. Larson, R. Stevens-Ratchford, L. Pedretti, & J. Crabtree (Eds.), *Role of occupational therapy with the elderly* (pp. 569–586). Bethesda, MD: AOTA.

Lewis, S. C. (1989). *Elder care in occupational therapy*. Thorofare, NJ: Slack Publishing.

Lezak, M. D. (1983). *Neuropsychological assessment*. New York: Oxford University Press.

Liblow, L. (1981). FROMAJE. In L. Liblow & S. Sherman (Eds.), *The core of geriatric medicine* (pp. 85–91). St. Louis: CV Mosby Co.

Mace, N. L., & Rabins, P. V. (1991). *The 36-hour day: A family guide to caring for people in the home*. Baltimore, MD: Johns Hopkins University Press.

Martin, S., & Smith, R. W. (1993). OBRA legislation and recreational activities: Enhancing personal control in nursing homes. *Activities, Adaptation & Aging, 17*(3), 1–14.

Matsutsuyu, J. (1969). The interest checklist. *American Journal of Occupational Therapy, 23*(4), 323–328.

McGlyn, S. M., & Kazniak, A. W. (1991). When metacognition fails: Impaired awareness of deficits in Alzheimer's disease. *Journal of Cognitive Neuroscience, 3*, 183–189.

Mindel, C. H., & Wright, R. (1982). Satisfaction in multi-generational households. *Journal of Gerontology, 37*, 483–489.

Nolen, N. R. (1988). Functional skill regression in late-stage dementia. *American Journal of Occupational Therapy, 42*, 666–669.

Ramsdell, J. W., Rothrock, J. F., Ward, H. W., & Volk, D. M. (1995, Jan.–Feb.). Evaluation of cognitive impairment in the elderly. *Journal of General Internal Medicine, 5*, 55–64.

Reichenbach, V. R. (1993). Documentation in home care: Functional outcomes. *Gerontology Special Interest Section Newsletter, 16*, 5–6.

Reisberg, B., Ferris, S. H., & Crook, T. (1983). Global deterioration scale. In B. Reisberg (Ed.), *A guide to Alzheimer's disease*. New York: Free Press.

Ritchie, K., Kildea, D., & Robine, J.-M. (1992). The relationship between age and the prevalence of senile dementia: A meta-analysis of recent data. *International Journal of Epidemiology, 21*, 763–769.

Rogers, J. C., Holm, M. B., Goldstein, G., McCue, M., & Nussbaum, P. D. (1994). Stability and change in functional asssessment of patients with geropsychiatric disorders. *American Journal of Occupational Therapy, 48*(10), 914–918.

Rogers, J. C., & Salta, J. E. (1994). Documenting functional outcomes. *American Journal of Occupational Therapy, 48*(10), 939–945.

Rosen, W. G., Mohs, R. C., & Davis, K. L. (1984). A new rating scale for Alzheimer's disease. *American Journal of Psychiatry, 141*(11), 1356–1364.

Sheridan, C. (1987). *Failure-free activities for the Alzheimer's patient*, Oakland, CA: Cottage Books.

Skolaski–Pellitteri, T. (1983). Environmental adaptations which compensate for dementia. *Journal of Physical and Occupational Therapy in Geriatrics, 3*(1), 31–44.

Toglia, J. P. (1993). *The Contextual Memory Test Manual*. Tucson, AZ: Therapy Skill Builders.

Trace, S., & Howell, T. (1992). Occupational therapy in geriatric mental health. *American Journal of Occupational Therapy, 45*(9), 833–839.

U.S. Army individual test battery. (1944). *Trail making test.* Washington, D.C.: War Department, Adjutant General's Office.

U.S. Congress. Office of Technology Assessment. (1987, April). *Losing a million minds: Confronting the tragedy of Alzheimer's disease and other dementias* (Publication No. OTA-BA-323). Washington, DC: U.S. Government Printing Office.

U.S. Congress. Select Committee on Aging. (1987). *Exploding the myths: Caregiving in America* (U.S. House of Representatives Publication No. 99-611). Washington, DC: U.S. Government Printing Office.

U.S. Congress. Select Committee on Aging. (1990). *Sharing the caring: Options for the 90s and beyond* (U.S. House of Representatives Publication No. 101-750). Washington, DC: U.S. Government Printing Office.

U.S. Department of Health and Human Services (HHS). (1991, February). Mental health in nursing homes: United States, 1985. *Vital and Health Statistics* (Publication No. PHS 91-1766). Hyattsville, MD: HHS Publication.

U.S. Department of Health and Human Services. Health Care Financing Administration. (1989). Rules and regulations. *Federal Register, 54*(21), 5316–5373.

Wallens, D., & Rockwell-Dylla, L. (1996). Client- and family-practitioner relationships: Collaboration as an effective approach to treatment. In O. Larson, R. Stevens–Ratchford, L. Pedretti, & J. Crabtree (Eds.), *Role of occupational therapy with the elderly* (pp. 826–855). Bethesda, MD: AOTA.

Watson, J. S., Matsuyama, S. S., Dirham, P. M., Liston, E. H., La Rue, A., & Jarvik, L. F. (1987). Functional status in Alzheimer-type dementia: A comparison of retrospective and concurrent ratings. *Alzheimer's Disease and Associated Disorders, 1*, (98–102).

Webster, R. E. (1992). *The learning efficiency test* (2nd ed.). Novato, CA: Academic Therapy Publications.

Wheatley, C. J. (1996). Evaluation and treatment of cognitive dysfunction. In L. W. Pedretti (Ed.), *Occupational therapy: Practice skills for physical dysfunction* (pp. 241–252). St Louis: Mosby Year-Book.

Whitehouse, P. J., Lerner, A., & Hedera, P. (1993). Dementia. In K. M. Heilman & E. Valenstein (Eds.), *Clinical neuropsychology* (pp. 603–645). New York: Oxford University Press.

Wiederholt, W. C., Cahn, D., Butters, N. M., Salmon, D. P., Kritz-Silverstein, D., & Barrett–Connor, E. (1993). Effects of age, gender and education on selected neuropsychological tests in an elderly community cohort. *Journal of the American Geriatric Society, 41*, 639–647.

Wilson, B., Cockburn, J., & Baddeley, A. (1985). *The Rivermead Behavioral Memory Test.* Suffolk, U.K.: Thames Valley Test.

Zarit, J. M., & Zarit, S. H. (1982). *Measuring burden and support in families with Alzheimer's disease elders*. Paper presented at the annual meeting of the Gerontological Society of America, Boston.

Zarit, S. H., Zarit, J. M., & Rosenberg-Thompson, S. (1990). A special treatment unit for Alzheimer's disease: Medical, behavioral, and environmental features. *Clinical Gerontologist*, 9(3/4), 47–63.

Suggested Readings

Caulking, M. (1988). *Designs for dementia*. Owings Mills, MD: National Health Publishing.

Dowling, J. R. (1995). *Keeping busy: A handbook for persons with dementia*. Baltimore, MD: Johns Hopkins University Press.

Hellen, C. R. (1992). *Alzheimer's disease: Activity focused care*. Stoneham, MA: Butterworth-Heinemann.

Zarit, S. H., Orr, N. K., & Zarit, J. M. (1985). *The hidden victims of Alzheimer's disease: Families under stress*. New York: New York University Press.

Zogola, J. (1987). *Doing things: A guide to programming activities for persons with Alzheimer's disease and related disorders*. Baltimore, MD: Johns Hopkins University Press.

Anxiety Disorders

Vivian Banish Levitt, MA, OTR, ATR, LMFCC
Assistant Director, Rehabilitation Services
Stanford University Hospital, Palo Alto, California

Key Terms

autogenic training
benzodiazapenes
compulsions
depersonalization

derealization
obsessions
psychogenic
vasodilation

Chapter Outline

Introduction
Encountering People with Anxiety Disorders: Settings
    Acute Inpatient
    Outpatient
    Home Care
Description of Anxiety Disorders
Impact on Daily Functioning
DSM-IV Descriptions of Anxiety
    Agoraphobia
    Panic Disorder without and with Agoraphobia
    Specific Phobia
    Social Phobia
    Obsessive-Compulsive Disorder
    Post-Traumatic Stress Disorder
    Acute Stress Disorder
    Generalized Anxiety Disorder
    Anxiety Disorder Due to a General Medical Condition
    Substance-Induced Anxiety Disorder
General Treatment Strategies
    Psychopharmacology
    Psychotherapy
    Biofeedback
    Exposure Therapy
    Couples Therapy
Occupational Therapy and Self-Management Techniques
    Assessment
    Treatment Interventions
Summary

Introduction

The occupational therapist invites a patient on the psychiatric unit, a 35-year-old man who was found pacing the floors, to attend a stress management group. Wringing his hands, trembling as he talks, and speaking quickly, the patient refuses to attend the group and states he is too anxious to concentrate. This man has been diagnosed with generalized anxiety disorder and depression; he is a challenge to the occupational therapist, who wonders how to best intervene and make a therapeutic connection. People experience many kinds and degrees of anxiety, but only when anxiety markedly interferes with daily function is it called clinical anxiety.

The origin of the word *anxiety* lies in the Greek root *angh,* meaning both "to press tight" and "to be heavy with grief" (Taylor & Arnow, 1988), and more recently, in the Latin word *anxietas*, meaning "troubled mind" (Sims & Snaith, 1988). Anxiety disorders are often the most common psychiatric disorders and yet the least treated ones. Approximately 4 to 5 percent of the population can expect to have an anxiety disorder in his or her lifetime (Weissman, Myers, & Harding, 1978); women outnumber men two to one in this population (Sims & Snaith, 1988).

The number of words in the English vocabulary that describe anxiety highlights its pervasiveness—witness the words worry, edginess, panic, fright, alarm, terror, jitters, jumpiness, and uneasiness. Anxiety is linked to our primitive flight-or-fight response which, when activated, prepares the body biochemically for meeting possible danger. The heart rate and blood pressure rise, blood goes to the large muscles, adrenaline is secreted, and sensory functions such as sight and hearing become keener.

ENCOUNTERING PEOPLE WITH ANXIETY DISORDERS: SETTINGS

Anxiety is a concern that needs to be addressed in all practice areas, including home and physical rehabilitation settings, due to the related loss of function, uncertainty of prognosis, chronic pain, and other serious issues. It is a disorder that is not limited to any age group and is diagnosed in young children as well as older adults. In this chapter, anxiety disorders will be discussed in an adult psychiatric population and adult psychiatric settings; however, the interventions can be used with all ages and in any setting.

Acute Inpatient

The occupational therapist is likely to encounter patients with anxiety disorders on inpatient psychiatric units. Their symptoms are usually so severe that they are unable to function in their daily lives. This incapacitation may include suicidal thoughts or actual suicide attempts. In both instances, the safe and, perhaps, locked environment of a hospital meets the immediate need for structure and external control.

Outpatient

Patients are often referred to outpatient programs, usually called partial hospitalization programs, if (1) they require further intervention following hospitalization and are unable to immediately return to their former occupations or (2) they need considerable support and structure but are able to manage outside the hospital. In either case, people may be living at home, in halfway houses, or in other, special living arrangements. Patients with anxiety disorders as a primary diagnosis are usually able to function outside the hospital in spite of their distressing symptoms.

Home Care

Occupational therapists work in home care programs for patients with psychiatric as well as physical dysfunction. Isolated at home and too impaired to participate in a structured day program, people with anxiety disorders such as agoraphobia (fear of leaving the house) or obsessive-compulsive behavior (involving intrusive thoughts and ritualized behavior) may benefit from one-on-one programs in time management, activities of daily living, and community reentry.

Changes in health care are dramatically shortening lengths of stay in acute hospital settings. As a consequence of the reduction in patient care days, occupational therapists must now focus more on evaluation than on treatment and be ready to make recommendations for discharge early in the hospitalization. Anxiety, especially if it takes a chronic course, will usually not be fully resolved during an inpatient stay. Occupational therapists in these settings must be prepared to help identify problem areas in functioning, begin intervention, and solve problems related to the discharge environment with the patient and, often, with family members. The consideration of the entire continuity of patient care becomes a crucial piece in treatment so that gains made in one environment may be carried over to the next. Communication with professionals working with the patient in a prehospital or posthospital setting helps to both accelerate and consolidate treatment plans and recommendations.

DESCRIPTION OF ANXIETY DISORDERS

The *Diagnostic and Statistical Manual of Mental Disorders, Fourth Edition* (DSM-IV) (APA, 1994), describes a number of anxiety disorders, which may occur alone or concomitantly with other DSM-IV diagnoses. For example, obsessive-compulsive disorder may overlay another Axis I disorder, major depressive disorder. In this case, an individual may have an agitated depression manifested by sleeplessness, excessive motor activity, and extreme feelings of worthlessness (major depressive disorder) compounded by a compelling need to follow rigid behaviors, such as pacing a certain number of times around the halls of the hospital (obsessive-compulsive disorder). However, anxiety is also frequently a component of other psychiatric illnesses without necessarily meeting the definition of a true DSM-IV diagnosis of anxiety disorder.

Several different kinds of anxiety are defined in Figure 12-1. For example, people with diagnoses such as eating disorders, personality disorders, and schizophrenia are often highly anxious. Many have trait anxiety, or enduring personality patterns of anxiety. In addition, people without any history of mental disorders commonly experience acute anxiety—time-limited periods of anxiety—when, for example, undergoing uncomfortable and perhaps, life-threatening medical procedures. The mere prospect of dealing with an aversive event such as diagnostic testing, chemotherapy, radiation, or surgery may produce intense levels of anxiety (often called *anticipatory anxiety*). In these

Anxiety: unpleasant emotional, cognitive, behavioral, or physical experiences of stress

Trait Anxiety: enduring personality style that manifests persistent anxiety

Acute Anxiety: time-limited anxiety that diminishes with resolution of the problem

Anticipatory Anxiety: predictive anxiety in response to future actual or imagined situations

Chronic Anxiety: anxiety that persists, developing around new stressors after immediate problems are resolved

Free-floating Anxiety: generalized anxiety, which may be vague in origin

Clinical Anxiety: disruption in function due to anxiety

Figure 12-1. Definitions of Different Kinds of Anxiety

examples, the anxiety often diminishes with emotional support and the termination of the stressor. However, there are times when anxiety repeatedly arises around new stressors even after the resolution of the initial ones. In these circumstances the anxiety is labeled *chronic anxiety*. There are also circumstances when anxiety continues but is generalized and vague without an identifiable stressor. In this case, it is called *free-floating anxiety*.

There are certain medical diseases and conditions that are also likely to produce states or acute experiences of anxiety. However, these symptoms of worry, or even panic, often subside when the medical reason is resolved. Examples include hyperthyroidism, estrogen loss occurring in menopause, congestive heart failure, asthma, hypoglycemia, and temporal lobe epilepsy (Taylor & Arnow, 1988). A number of medications and nonprescription drugs may either cause or worsen acute anxiety symptoms. These include anticholinergic drugs, steroids, aspirin, cocaine, amphetamines, and hallucinogens (Taylor & Arnow, 1988). Caffeine and nicotine, two commonly ingested substances, may also produce symptoms of anxiety. Moreover, withdrawal from alcohol or other addictive substances presents a high risk for acute anxiety states.

The difference between normal anxiety (worry that propels one to act), and clinical anxiety (worry that disrupts function) is not always easily or clearly defined. Anxiety in a limited dose is universal, normal, appropriate, and adaptive as a protection from potential threat. It is almost always associated with the anticipation of future events accompanied by expected loss or pain (Sims & Snaith, 1988). It can be the force that propels people to act, cope, and even perform more efficiently. For example, most college students experience a normal level anxiety as they prepare for final exams, which usually helps induce studying.

On the other hand anxiety is often defined as abnormal when it hinders rather than helps the individual. If the individual's response to a stimulus is greater than one would expect, if his or her feelings of anxiety persist after the stimulus is removed, or if anxiety is ineffective in dealing with the threat of the stimulus, the state may be called abnormal (Sims & Snaith, 1988). Anxiety of this proportion has been likened to having a faulty burglar alarm that signals nonexistent danger (Agras, 1985).

Clinical anxiety is the name given to abnormal anxiety when it clearly affects and hinders daily function and is no longer serviceable. Anxiety becomes disabling when it persists without stimulating positive action to resolve the stressor or ward off distress. For instance, a woman with intense anxiety was so incapacitated by the feelings of terror associated with an upcoming job layoff that she was unable to develop an alternative survival plan for herself. Such clinical anxiety is seen in many people hospitalized on psychiatric units.

When action is taken to diminish the anticipated threat, there is a great possibility that the anxiety will be reduced. For example, patients who are preparing for discharge from the psychiatric hospital are often very anxious about responding to future inquiries about their hospitalization. They feel vulnerable to the feared onslaught of questions by friends and family and the (self-driven) expectation to reveal more personal details than they would like. If these concerns are effectively addressed in an assertiveness group led by an occupational therapist, anxiety related to this issue will likely decrease. Patients report feeling more prepared to encounter others after discharge when they have learned and practiced direct forms of communication.

Anxiety can affect a person physiologically, emotionally, behaviorally and cognitively. See Table 12-1 for a list of symptoms of anxiety in each area.

IMPACT ON DAILY FUNCTIONING

The impact of anxiety on a person's life may be dramatic and may affect all aspects of functioning, including work, social life, self-care, parenting, and leisure activities. Performance in all roles may dramatically decline as anxiety symptoms persist.

Employment may suffer because of cognitive impairment. Concentration, problem solving, and memory may all be markedly affected by episodes of acute anxiety, primarily because the individual's primary focus is directed toward combating unpleasant symptoms and not to the task at hand. Tardiness, inaccuracy in completing work, and distractibility are some of the problem behaviors that develop in people who experience persistent anxiety. For example, one patient with obsessive-compulsive disorder spent so many hours performing ritualistic hand and clothes washing that he was unable to maintain his required work schedule. Social relationships may decline as the person restricts activities and therefore becomes unavailable to others.

There is also the likelihood that others will be alienated by the rigidity and perceived self-involvement of the anxious person. For example, a woman with panic attacks stopped attending her church and volunteer activities and became reclusive in her small apartment. After some period of time, friends

Table 12-1. Symptoms of Anxiety

Emotional	Physiological	Cognitive	Behavioral
Feeling uneasy, off-balance	*Cardiovascular:* increased heart rate, tachycardia, chest pain and pressure	Confusion Poor memory Distractibility, poor concentration	Looks preoccupied Immobile, withdrawn
Feeling overwhelmed			
Feeling a sense of impending doom	*Gastrointestinatl:* diarrhea, constipation, nausea, vomiting, gas, cramps, and loss of appetite	Thought blocking Loss of perspective, cognitive distortion including catastrophic thinking and negative self-evaluation	Overactive, restless, agitated Excess consumption of substances and/or food
Feeling helpless and out of control			
Feeling one is going insane	*Respiratory:* dyspnea (shortness of breath) and choking sensations		
Depersonalization (having feelings of unreality, as if in dream)		Obsessive thoughts	
	Urinary: frequency and urgency of urination	Fears of loss of control, going crazy, injury, death, and not coping	
Derealization (feeling detached from one's surroundings)	*Genital:* loss of libido, premature ejaculation, and amenorrhea	Poor problem solving abilities	
	Autonomic: sweating, flushing, dry mouth, dizziness, and fainting		

Note: Some of the self-help behavioral methods sought to reduce discomfort may be unintentionally self-destructive and therefore not adaptive. For example, addiction to prescription medications and alcohol, extreme isolation, and regression are common secondary problems that develop from immediate, or nonadaptive, behavioral solutions.

and acquaintances associated with these activities no longer called her because of her continued self-imposed isolation and their experience of personal rejection.

Many persons with anxiety disorders experience marital stress as they curtail previously shared activities or become overreliant on the spouse for assistance. For example, the husband of a patient with agoraphobia became resentful of his wife's dependency when she began refusing to leave the house without him, even to complete the smallest task. The decrease in function may affect homemaking, grooming, and parenting activities, as well as leisure occupations. The agoraphobic woman described here sought to transfer responsibilities for transporting her children and shopping to neighbors and friends when her husband was not available. Another patient, an elderly man who was coping poorly with a generalized anxiety disorder, abandoned his avid avocational interest in the stock market because of difficulty in concentrating on the newspaper figures.

Depression commonly develops secondarily to anxiety symptoms. People often feel a sense of desperation as various forms of anxiety immobilize them or cause severe discomfort; therefore, the potential for suicide can be high. From a medical standpoint, patients are prone to certain physical diseases, such as heart problems, and gastrointestinal disorders such as ulcerative colitis and stomach ulcers. Figure 12-2 highlights the impact of anxiety disorders on daily functioning.

DSM-IV DESCRIPTIONS OF ANXIETY

There are ten major diagnostic groups related to anxiety in the DSM-IV (APA, 1994, pp. 394–444). A description of each group, with typical symptoms, follows.

Panic Attack

The term panic attack defines a limited period of intense fear or distress in which four or more of the following symptoms progress rapidly and peak within 10 minutes: cardiac symptoms (palpitations, pounding, rapid heartbeat), trem-

> *Work*: poor habits due to problems in concentration and time management
> *Social Relationships*: diminished due to restriction of activity and isolation
> *Marital Relationships*: decrease in shared activities, dependency on spouse
> *Activities of Daily Living*: homemaking, grooming, and parenting may be inadequate secondary to poor concentration, depression, and physical symptoms
> *Leisure Activities*: pleasurable activities may be neglected, primarily because of an inability to sustain sufficient attention
> *Depression*: feelings of low self-esteem and despair may result, hindering involvement in customary activities
> *Medical Status*: susceptibility to numerous diseases such as colitis, ulcers, heart disease, stroke, and respiratory disorders, which may decrease the ability to work, care for the self, and engage in pleasurable activities alone or with family and friends

Figure 12-2. Impact of Anxiety Disorders on Daily Functioning

bling, shortness of breath, feelings of suffocation, chest pain, sensations of choking, nausea or abdominal distress, dizziness or lightheadedness, **derealization**, fear of losing control or going crazy, fear of dying, paresthesias (numbness or tingling), and chills or hot flashes.

Agoraphobia

This state is included in the description of three of the anxiety disorders, although it is itself not a disorder. The primary features include: (1) avoiding situations where it might be difficult or embarrassing to leave or where assistance might not be available in the event of a panic attack and (2) avoiding or suffering through situations in which there is anxiety about having a panic attack or where a companion is needed.

Panic Disorder without and with Agoraphobia

Figure 12-3 reprints DSM-IV symptoms and diagnostic categories for panic disorder and agoraphobia, which occur in several of the anxiety disorders.

The person suffering from panic disorder without agoraphobia has repeated and unexpected panic attacks with at least one of the attacks followed by per-

---

A. Both (1) and (2):
    (1) recurrent unexpected Panic Attacks (see p. 395)
    (2) at least one of the attacks has been followed by 1 month (or more) of one (or more) of the following:
        (a) persistent concern about having additional attacks
        (b) worry about the implications of the attack or its consequences (e.g., losing control, having a heart attack, "going crazy")
        (c) a significant change in behavior related to the attacks
B. Absence of Agoraphobia (see p. 396).
C. The Panic Attacks are not due to the direct physiological effects of a substance (e.g., a drug of abuse, a medication) or a general medical condition (e.g., hyperthyroidism).
D. The Panic Attacks are not better accounted for by another mental disorder, such as Social Phobia (e.g., occurring on exposure to feared social situations), Specific Phobia (e.g., on exposure to a specific phobic situation), Obsessive-Compulsive Disorder (e.g., on exposure to dirt in someone with an obsession about contamination), Posttraumatic Stress Disorder (e.g., in response to stimuli associated with a severe stressor), or Separation Anxiety Disorder (e.g., in response to being away from home or close relatives).

Figure 12-3a.   DSM-IV Diagnostic Criteria for Panic Disorder without Agoraphobia

---

Source: Reprinted with permission from *Diagnostic and Statistical Manual of Mental Disorders, Fourth Edition.* Copyright 1994 American Psychiatric Association.

A. Both (1) and (2):
    (1) recurrent unexpected Panic Attacks (see p. 395)
    (2) at least one of the attacks has been followed by 1 month (or more)
         of one (or more) of the following:
         (a) persistent concern about having additional attacks
         (b) worry about the implications of the attack or its consequences
              (e.g., losing control, having a heart attack, "going crazy")
         (c) a significant change in behavior related to the attacks
B. The presence of Agoraphobia (see p. 396).
C. The Panic Attacks are not due to the direct physiological effects of a sub-
    stance (e.g., a drug of abuse, a medication) or a general medical condi-
    tion (e.g., hyperthyroidism).
D. The Panic Attacks are not better accounted for by another mental disor-
    der, such as Social Phobia (e.g., occurring on exposure to feared social
    situations), Specific Phobia (e.g., on exposure to a specific phobic situ-
    ation), Obsessive-Compulsive Disorder (e.g., on exposure to dirt in some-
    one with an obsession about contamination), Posttraumatic Stress
    Disorder (e.g., in response to stimuli associated with a severe stressor),
    or Separation Anxiety Disorder (e.g., in response to being away from
    home or close relatives).

Figure 12-3b.   DSM-IV Diagnostic Criteria for Panic Disorder with Agoraphobia

Source: Reprinted with permission from *Diagnostic and Statistical Manual of Mental Disorders, Fourth Edition.* Copyright 1994 American Psychiatric Association.

sistent worry about having additional attacks or dealing with consequences of the attack or by noticeable changes in behavior. When agoraphobia coexists, the individual will have developed avoidance behavior in response to panic attacks. People afflicted with this disorder restrict their activities by staying at home, traveling only with the company of other people, or limiting their destinations by avoiding long lines, bridges, or other potentially anxiety-producing situations. Panic attacks may be spontaneous, with no identifiable precipitant, or situationally bound with a known stressor, and can occur in clusters or sporadically, over longer periods of time.

Agoraphobia without History of Panic Attacks

In agoraphobia without history of panic attacks, the person has symptoms of agoraphobia alone. This is rarely found as agoraphobia usually occurs in the presence of panic disorder.

Specific Phobia

The specific phobia is characterized by recurrent illogical and excessive fear and anxiety, which is evoked during either the expectation of, or an actual encounter with, a particular stimulus, object or situation, which will be fiercely avoided even though the person realizes that the reaction is irrational. The anxiety responses dissipate if the stimulus is weakened or removed. A phobia in one subtype often leads to other phobias in the same subgroup.The degree to which a phobia impairs functioning appears to relate to the ease and success of avoiding the particular stressor. The diagnostic criteria for specific phobia are listed in Figure 12-4.

A. Marked and persistent fear that is excessive or unreasonable, cued by the presence or anticipation of a specific object or situation (e.g., flying, heights, animals, receiving an injection, seeing blood).

B. Exposure to the phobic stimulus almost invariably provokes an immediate anxiety response, which may take the form of a situationally bound or situationally predisposed Panic Attack. **Note:** In children, the anxiety may be expressed by crying, tantrums, freezing, or clinging.

C. The person recognizes that the fear is excessive or unreasonable. **Note:** In children, this feature may be absent.

D. The phobic situation(s) is avoided or else is endured with intense anxiety or distress.

E. The avoidance, anxious anticipation, or distress in the feared situation(s) interferes significantly with the person's normal routine, occupational (or academic) functioning, or social activities or relationships, or there is marked distress about having the phobia.

F. In individuals under age 18 years, the duration is at least 6 months.

G. The anxiety, Panic Attacks, or phobic avoidance associated with the specific object or situation are not better accounted for by another mental disorder, such as Obsessive-Compulsive Disorder (e.g., fear of dirt in someone with an obsession about contamination), Posttraumatic Stress Disorder (e.g., avoidance of stimuli associated with a severe stressor), Separation Anxiety Disorder (e.g., avoidance of school), Social Phobia (e.g., avoidance of social situations because of fear of embarrassment), Panic Disorder With Agoraphobia, or Agoraphobia Without History of Panic Disorder.

Specify type:
Animal Type
Natural Environment Type (e.g., heights, storms, water)
Blood-Injection-Injury Type
Situational Type (e.g., airplanes, elevators, enclosed places)
Other Type (e.g., phobic avoidance of situations that may lead to choking, vomiting, or contracting an illness; in children, avoidance of loud sounds or costumed characters)

Figure 12-4. DSM-IV Diagnostic Criteria for Specific Phobia

Source: Reprinted with permission from *Diagnostic and Statistical Manual of Mental Disorders, Fourth Edition.* Copyright 1994 American Psychiatric Association.

Social Phobia

An individual with a social phobia fears potentially humiliating social or performance situations in which there is the anticipation of examination or judgment by others. In most cases the disruption in the person's life is not debilitating, although there will undoubtedly be at least a mild impact on his or her work and interpersonal functioning. For example, the individual may restrict those activities that cause anxiety and thus compromise possible achievements. For example, one young woman with a social phobia resigned when her job duties were expanded to include conducting large monthly orientation meetings for all new employees. The diagnostic criteria for social phobia are listed in Figure 12-5.

Obsessive-Compulsive Disorder

Obsessive-compulsive disorder is characterized by recurrent **obsessions** and **compulsions** that cause anxiety or distress. Although the individual realizes that the compulsive behaviors, which are attempts to reduce tension, are ultimately fruitless and time-consuming, he or she feels unable to stop them and experiences surges of anxiety when attempts are made to do so. These odd behaviors often may lead to the alienation of others. The diagnostic criteria for obsessive-compulsive disorder are listed in Figure 12-6.

Post-traumatic Stress Disorder

Post-traumatic stress disorder (PTSD) occurs in individuals who have experienced a traumatic event. Natural disasters, combat, life-threatening diseases, rape, domestic violence, and accidents all may lead to the disorder. Sufferers reexperience the trauma in different ways. The symptoms most often occur in close proximity to the traumatic event, but they may also develop in the months or years that follow it. For example, a young male Cambodian refugee who had been hospitalized for PTSD had suddenly developed the symptoms many years after fleeing his homeland, while watching a movie about the war in Southeast Asia. People with this disorder may show a range of impairment. Substance abuse and violence, especially when related to combat stress, may lead to confrontation with the law. Depression may result in suicide attempts and difficulty with interpersonal relationships. The diagnostic criteria for post-traumatic stress disorder are listed in Figure 12-7.

Acute Stress Disorder

Acute stress disorder is similar to post-traumatic stress disorder in respect to the exposure to a traumatic event and the response of horror, terror, and powerlessness. However, the symptoms of this disorder develop within one month of the event and last only from two days to one month following the exposure. In addition to experiencing at least one symptom of each PTSD cluster

A. A marked and persistent fear of one or more social or performance situations in which the person is exposed to unfamiliar people or to possible scrutiny by others. The individual fears that he or she will act in a way (or show anxiety symptoms) that will be humiliating or embarrassing. **Note:** In children, there must be evidence of the capacity for age-appropriate social relationships with familiar people and the anxiety must occur in peer settings, not just in interactions with adults.

B. Exposure to the feared social situation almost invariably provokes anxiety, which may take the form of a situationally bound or situationally predisposed Panic Attack. **Note:** In children, the anxiety may be expressed by crying, tantrums, freezing, or shrinking from social situations with unfamiliar people.

C. The person recognizes that the fear is excessive or unreasonable. **Note:** In children, this feature may be absent.

D. The feared social or performance situations are avoided or else are endured with intense anxiety or distress.

E. The avoidance, anxious anticipation, or distress in the feared social or performance situation(s) interferes significantly with the person's normal routine, occupational (academic) functioning, or social activities or relationships, or there is marked distress about having the phobia.

F. In individuals under age 18 years, the duration is at least 6 months.

G. The fear or avoidance is not due to the direct physiological effects of a substance (e.g., a drug of abuse, a medication) or a general medical condition and is not better accounted for by another mental disorder (e.g., Panic Disorder With or Without Agoraphobia, Separation Anxiety Disorder, Body Dysmorphic Disorder, a Pervasive Developmental Disorder, or Schizoid Personality Disorder).

H. If a general medical condition or another mental disorder is present, the fear in Criterion A is unrelated to it, e.g., the fear is not of Stuttering, trembling in Parkinson's disease, or exhibiting abnormal eating behavior in Anorexia Nervosa or Bulimia Nervosa.

Specify if:
Generalized: if the fears include most social situations (also consider the additional diagnosis of Avoidant Personality Disorder)

Figure 12-5. DSM-IV Diagnostic Criteria for Social Phobia

Source: Reprinted with permission from *Diagnostic and Statistical Manual of Mental Disorders, Fourth Edition.* Copyright 1994 American Psychiatric Association.

(e.g., flashbacks, dreams, and avoidance of the stimuli), an individual must exhibit several dissociative symptoms, as numbing, derealization, **depersonalization**, and amnesia, in order to be diagnosed with this disorder.

For example, following the 1989 San Francisco earthquake, many cases of acute stress disorders were reported. One instance involved a woman who

A. Either obsessions or compulsions:

Obsessions as defined by (1), (2), (3), and (4):

(1) recurrent and persistent thoughts, impulses, or images that are experienced, at some time during the disturbance, as intrusive and inappropriate and that cause marked anxiety or distress

(2) the thoughts, impulses, or images are not simply excessive worries about real-life problems

(3) the person attempts to ignore or suppress such thoughts, impulses, or images, or to neutralize them with some other thought or action

(4) the person recognizes that the obsessional thoughts, impulses, or images are a product of his or her own mind (not imposed from without as in thought insertion)

Compulsions as defined by (1) and (2):

(1) repetitive behaviors (e.g., hand washing, ordering, checking) or mental acts (e.g., praying, counting, repeating words silently) that the person feels driven to perform in response to an obsession, or according to rules that must be applied rigidly

(2) the behaviors or mental acts are aimed at preventing or reducing distress or preventing some dreaded event or situation; however, these behaviors or mental acts either are not connected in a realistic way with what they are designed to neutralize or prevent or are clearly excessive

B. At some point during the course of the disorder, the person has recognized that the obsessions or compulsions are excessive or unreasonable. **Note:** This does not apply to children.

C. The obsessions or compulsions cause marked distress, are time consuming (take more than 1 hour a day), or significantly interfere with the person's normal routine, occupational (or academic) functioning, or usual social activities or relationships.

D. If another Axis I disorder is present, the content of the obsessions or compulsions is not restricted to it (e.g., preoccupation with food in the presence of an Eating Disorder; hair pulling in the presence of Trichotillomania; concern with appearance in the presence of Body Dysmorphic Disorder; preoccupation with drugs in the presence of a Substance Use Disorder; preoccupation with having a serious illness in the presence of Hypochondriasis; preoccupation with sexual urges or fantasies in the presence of a Paraphilia; or guilty ruminations in the presence of Major Depressive Disorder).

(continues)

Figure 12-6. DSM-IV Diagnostic Criteria for Obsessive-Compulsive Disorder

Source: Reprinted with permission from *Diagnostic and Statistical Manual of Mental Disorders, Fourth Edition.* Copyright 1994 American Psychiatric Association.

> E. The disturbance is not due to the direct physiological effects of a substance (e.g., a drug of abuse, a medication) or a general medical condition.
>
> *Specify* if:
>
> **With Poor Insight:** if, for most of the time during the current episode, the person does not recognize that the obsessions and compulsions are excessive or unreasonable

Figure 12-6. (continued)

could not recall how she had sustained cuts and bruises while trying to evacuate a store. Other San Franciscans confessed to waking up frequently during the night with cold sweats and a rapid heartbeat. Although it was very helpful at times for them to talk about the trauma, this was balanced by their need to stay distanced from the event and avoid discussing it or viewing the damage.

Generalized Anxiety Disorder

Generalized anxiety disorder occurs widely. It is described as persistent and excessive anxiety or worry, with difficulty controlling the worry, that lasts at least six months. Generalized anxiety disorder rarely occurs as a primary diagnosis but often accompanies depression. The diagnostic criteria are listed in Figure 12-8.

Anxiety Disorder Due to a General Medical Condition

Anxiety classified as due to a general medical condition is due to the physiological causes of a medical problem. Any of the symptoms common to the anxiety disorders may be present.

Substance-Induced Anxiety Disorder

The physiological effect of a drug medication or toxin causes substance-induced anxiety. The anxiety may be manifested in a variety of ways, as described thus far.

GENERAL TREATMENT STRATEGIES

A variety of treatments are used to diminish the symptoms of anxiety and promote more adaptive functioning. Treatments range from medications to self-management techniques. Figure 12-9 lists types of general treatment strategies.

A. The person has been exposed to a traumatic event in which both of the following were present:
    (1) the person experienced, witnessed, or was confronted with an event or events that involved actual or threatened death or serious injury, or a threat to the physical integrity of self or others
    (2) the person's response involved intense fear, helplessness, or horror. **Note:** In children, this may be expressed instead by disorganized or agitated behavior

B. The traumatic event is persistently reexperienced in one (or more) of the following ways:
    (1) recurrent and intrusive distressing recollections of the event, including images, thoughts, or perceptions. **Note:** In young children, repetitive play may occur in which themes or aspects of the trauma are expressed.
    (2) recurrent distressing dreams of the event. **Note:** In children, there may be frightening dreams without recognizable content.
    (3) acting or feeling as if the traumatic event were recurring (includes a sense of reliving the experience, illusions, hallucinations, and dissociative flashback episodes, including those that occur on awakening or when intoxicated). **Note:** In young children, trauma-specific reenactment may occur.
    (4) intense psychological distress at exposure to internal or external cues that symbolize or resemble an aspect of the traumatic event
    (5) physiological reactivity on exposure to internal or external cues that symbolize or resemble an aspect of the traumatic event

C. Persistent avoidance of stimuli associated with the trauma and numbing of general responsiveness (not present before the trauma), as indicated by three (or more) of the following:
    (1) efforts to avoid thoughts, feelings, or conversations associated with the trauma
    (2) efforts to avoid activities, places, or people that arouse recollections of the trauma
    (3) inability to recall an important aspect of the trauma
    (4) markedly diminished interest or participation in significant activities
    (5) feeling of detachment or estrangement from others
    (6) restricted range of affect (e.g., unable to have loving feelings)
    (7) sense of a foreshortened future (e.g., does not expect to have a career, marriage, children, or a normal life span)

(continues)

Figure 12-7.   DSM-IV Diagnostic Criteria for Post-traumatic Stress Disorder

Source: Reprinted with permission from *Diagnostic and Statistical Manual of Mental Disorders, Fourth Edition.* Copyright 1994 American Psychiatric Association.

D. Persistent symptoms of increased arousal (not present before the trauma), as indicated by two (or more) of the following:
   (1) difficulty falling or staying asleep
   (2) irritability or outbursts of anger
   (3) difficulty concentrating
   (4) hypervigilance
   (5) exaggerated startle response
E. Duration of the disturbance (symptoms in Criteria B, C, and D) is more than 1 month.
F. The disturbance causes clinically significant distress or impairment in social, occupational, or other important areas of functioning.

Specify if:
Acute: if duration of symptoms is less than 3 months
Chronic: if duration of symptoms is 3 months or more

Specify if:
With Delayed Onset: if onset of symptoms is at least 6 months after the stressor

Figure 12-7. (continued)

Psychopharmacology

Medications addressing the physiological component of anxiety are prescribed most often for the relief of acute attacks and are used in conjunction with other types of therapy, such as psychotherapy (Taylor & Arnow, 1988; Telch, 1982). Their aim is to reduce the level of arousal. Antianxiety drugs, such as **benzodiazapenes**, may lead to drug dependence and are therefore not suited to long-term use, though in the short term (4 to 12 months), they may be highly beneficial. Antidepressant medications are also commonly prescribed for panic disorder, generalized anxiety disorder, and obsessive-compulsive disorder. They are occasionally used for phobias and post-traumatic stress disorder. Antipsychotic drugs have proven successful in treating anxiety disorders in which symptoms are so debilitating as to prevent functioning or where delusions are present.

Psychotherapy

Psychotherapy includes many verbal approaches designed to help decrease anxiety in its maladaptive form. They range from intense, long-term treatment, such as psychoanalysis, to short-term, supportive treatment, such as cognitive therapy. Psychotherapy addresses the immediate relief of symptoms and has a direct focus on immediate, pressing issues; supportive psychotherapy enhances the ability to cope. Cognitive interventions help clients to identify faulty, irrational thinking regarding perceived dangers and to substitute more rational and realistic thoughts through various strategies.

A. Excessive anxiety and worry (apprehensive expectation), occurring more days than not for at least 6 months, about a number of events or activities (such as work or school performance).
B. The person finds it difficult to control the worry.
C. The anxiety and worry are associated with three (or more) of the following six symptoms (with at least some symptoms present for more days than not for the past 6 months). **Note:** Only one item is required in children.
    (1) restlessness or feeling keyed up or on edge
    (2) being easily fatigued
    (3) difficulty concentrating or mind going blank
    (4) irritability
    (5) muscle tension
    (6) sleep disturbance (difficulty falling or staying asleep, or restless unsatisfying sleep)
D. The focus of the anxiety and worry is not confined to features of an Axis I disorder, e.g., the anxiety or worry is not about having a Panic Attack (as in Panic Disorder), being embarrassed in public (as in Social Phobia), being contaminated (as in Obsessive-Compulsive Disorder), being away from home or close relatives (as in Separation Anxiety Disorder), gaining weight (as in Anorexia Nervosa), having multiple physical complaints (as in Somatization Disorder), or having a serious illness (as in Hypochondriasis), and the anxiety and worry do not occur exclusively during Posttraumatic Stress Disorder.
E. The anxiety, worry, or physical symptoms cause clinically significant distress or impairment in social, occupational, or other important areas of functioning.
F. The disturbance is not due to the direct physiological effects of a substance (e.g., a drug of abuse, a medication) or a general medical condition (e.g., hyperthyroidism) and does not occur exclusively during a Mood Disorder, a Psychotic Disorder, or a Pervasive Developmental Disorder.

Figure 12-8.   DSM-IV Diagnostic Criteria for Generalized Anxiety Disorder

Source: Reprinted with permission from *Diagnostic and Statistical Manual of Mental Disorders, Fourth Edition.* Copyright 1994 American Psychiatric Association.

Biofeedback

The goal of biofeedback is to decrease arousal by providing the client with objective data about, and then helping him or her gain control over, biological states that are normally involuntary. Biofeedback techniques target and attempt to alter changes in heart rate, blood pressure, sweating, and skin temperature by providing feedback through instrumentation (Davis, Eshelman, & McKay, 1988; Taylor & Arnow, 1988). Electrodes, blood pressure indicators, and finger sensors in contact with the body are examples of

Psychopharmacology
Psychotherapy
Biofeedback
Systematic Desensitization
Exposure Therapy
Couples Therapy
Self-Management Techniques

Note: These common strategies for treatment of anxiety disorders require expertise and training, and some are more likely to be utilized by certain professionals. For example, psychiatrists prescribe medication, psychologists may provide psychotherapy and exposure therapy, and social workers or marriage and family counselors often provide couples therapy.

Figure 12-9. Treatment Strategies for Anxiety Disorders

instruments used to provide data about a person's current biological states. Once information is received, the patient learns methods of altering the body functions to reduce anxiety. Biofeedback may be seen as a type of behavioral therapy in that objective, observable data is the focus.

Systematic Desensitization

Systematic desensitization attempts to systematically diminish anxiety related to specific fears primarily through the use of imagery and relaxation. Used most often with phobic disorders, the technique requires a trained therapist who helps the patient devise a hierarchical list of, usually, 10 items to break down the fear into steps according to the subjective rating of their intensity (Wolpe, 1973). For example, someone who fears rats would likely rank touching a rat as very challenging, while looking at a picture of a rat might be the least threatening. Starting with the least troubling item on the list and coupling progressive relaxation with visualization, the person advances up the hierarchy once each level is mastered (as evidenced by the absence of an anxiety response). A variation of this intervention is participant modeling (Bandura, 1977), whereby the therapist interacts with the feared object or situation and then encourages the patient to interact jointly before performing alone.

Exposure Therapy

Exposure therapy is a focused intervention (also called "programmed practice") (Agras & Berkowitz, 1994), that focuses entirely on real encounters with the objects of the individual's anxiety, while helping him or her to use a variety of techniques (i.e., cognitive and relaxation) to master the situation. This treatment is used primarily with persons with phobic, panic, and obsessive-compulsive disorders. Because of its in vivo (real-life) component, exposure therapy appears to be a highly effective and powerful treatment, which helps to weaken fear and the subsequent avoidant responses by combining cognitive and behavioral techniques in day-to-day situations.

Couples Therapy

How couples interact may greatly influence both the generation of anxiety and how it is managed. Marriage counselors and other psychotherapists help the client with anxiety and his or her partner to identify the dynamics of their relationship that trigger anxiety and to cope with a range of uncomfortable feelings such as anger, discouragement, and resentment. Improving communication, receiving mutual support, and understanding secondary gains (gains that may occur due to the cessation of usual activities) are other possible benefits of marital counseling.

OCCUPATIONAL THERAPY AND SELF-MANAGEMENT TECHNIQUES

Most of the anxiety disorders have a chronic course involving periods of remission. Therefore, the foremost task is learning how to manage anxiety in order to continue functioning and to face, rather than avoid, situations that irrationally generate fear. The avoidance of fear-producing stimuli is an attempt at self-protection, but it is maladaptive if it interferes with the fulfillment of environmental and internal needs (Depoy & Kolodner, 1991). Avoidant behavior also reinforces a sense of helplessness. Occupational therapists can help people develop a range of self-efficacy techniques that help to increase the feeling of influence or mastery over one's circumstances (Bandura, 1995). A problem-focused approach is especially useful with this population, for it helps people to respond rationally, rather than emotionally, to potentially fear-producing situations. Self-efficacy has been said to be a major factor in fear reduction (Taylor & Arnow, 1988). In fact, self-efficacy as a goal is a major tenet of the Model of Human Occupation (Kielhofner, 1995) (see Chapter 4, Occupational Therapy Models, for an explanation of the model).

Assessment

In order to develop strategies for improved functioning, the level of impairment of the person with anxiety must be assessed. The assessments serve to highlight the extent of the disorder's interference in daily life activities.

Interviews, surveys, observation of performance, role checklists (Figure 12-10), function questionnaires (Figure 12-11), self-assessment of activities (Figure 12-12), and activity configurations (Figure 12-13) elicit information about how anxiety impacts a person's life. For example, the role checklist (Figure 12-10) specifically targets roles that are valued but not being performed,

ROLE CHECKLIST

NAME _____ AGE_____ DATE_____

SEX: ☐ MALE ☐ FEMALE   ARE YOU RETIRED: ☐ YES ☐ NO

MARITAL STATUS: ☐ SINGLE ☐ MARRIED ☐ SEPARATED ☐ DIVORCED ☐ WIDOWED

The purpose of this checklist is to identify the major roles in your life. The checklist, which is divided into two parts, presents 10 roles and defines each one.

PART I

Beside each role, indicate, by checking the appropriate column, if you performed the role in the past, if you presently perform the role, and if you plan to perform the role in the future. You may check more than one column for each role. For example, if you volunteered in the past, do not volunteer at present, but plan to in the future, you would check the past and future columns.

ROLE	PAST	PRESENT	FUTURE
STUDENT: Attending school on a part-time or full-time basis.			
WORKER: Part-time or full-time paid employment.			
VOLUNTEER: Donating services, **at least once a week,** to a hospital, school, community, political campaign, and so forth.			
CARE GIVER: Responsibility, **at least once a week,** for the care of someone such as a child, spouse, relative, or friend.			
HOME MAINTAINER: Responsibility, **at least once a week,** for the upkeep of the home such as housecleaning or yardwork.			
FRIEND: Spending time or doing something, **at least once a week,** with a friend.			
FAMILY MEMBER: Spending time or doing something, **at least once a week,** with a family member such as a child, spouse, parent, or other relative.			
RELIGIOUS PARTICIPANT: Involvement, **at least once a week,** in groups or activities affiliated with one's religion (excluding worship).			
HOBBYIST/AMATEUR: Involvement, **at least once a week,** in a hobby or amateur activity such as sewing, playing a musical instrument, woodworking, sports, the theater, or participation in a club or team.			
PARTICIPANT IN ORGANIZATIONS: Involvement, **at least once a week,** in organizations such as the American Legion, National Organization for Women, Parents Without Partners, Weight Watchers, and so forth.			
OTHER:_____ A role not listed which you have performed, are presently performing, and/or plan to perform. Write the role on the line above and check the appropriate column(s).			

(continues)

Figure 12-10. Role Checklist

Source: Courtesy of Mrs. Frances Oakley, M.S., OTR, FAOTA.

as well as dysfunctional performance areas and components. The function questionnaire (Figure 12-11) indicates the individual's subjective level of anxiety and the degree to which it interferes with functioning. Accounting for daily activities by filling out typical schedules (Figure 12-12) reveals significant information in respect to productive activities as well as role functioning. It indicates, based on the client's perceptions, which daily life occupations he or she perceives as least and most troublesome. Someone with agoraphobia may stay indoors the majority of each day, during which time expected ac-

PART II

The same roles are listed below. Next to *each* role check the column which best indicates how valuable or important the role is to you. Answer for *each role,* even if you have never performed or do not plan to perform the role.

ROLE	NOT AT ALL VALUABLE	SOMEWHAT VALUABLE	VERY VALUABLE
STUDENT: Attending school on a part-time or full-time basis.			
WORKER: Part-time or full-time paid employment.			
VOLUNTEER: Donating services, **at least once a week,** to a hospital, school, community, political campaign, and so forth.			
CARE GIVER: Responsibility, **at least once a week,** for the care of someone such as a child, spouse, relative, or friend.			
HOME MAINTAINER: Responsibility, **at least once a week,** for the upkeep of the home such as housecleaning or yardwork.			
FRIEND: Spending time or doing something, **at least once a week,** with a friend.			
FAMILY MEMBER: Spending time or doing something, **at least once a week,** with a family member such as a child, spouse, parent, or other relative.			
RELIGIOUS PARTICIPANT: Involvement, **at least once a week,** in groups or activities affiliated with one's religion (excluding worship).			
HOBBYIST/AMATEUR: Involvement, **at least once a week,** in a hobby or amateur activity such as sewing, playing a musical instrument, woodworking, sports, the theater, or participation in a club or team.			
PARTICIPANT IN ORGANIZATIONS: Involvement, **at least once a week,** in organizations such as the American Legion, National Organization for Women, Parents Without Partners, Weight Watchers, and so forth.			
OTHER:_____ A role not listed which you have performed, are presently performing, and/or plan to perform. Write the role on the line above and check the appropriate column(s).			

Figure 12-10. *(continued)*

tivities will not be performed and roles such as hobbyist, homemaker, or worker will be lost.

Treatment Interventions

The primary occupational therapy interventions utilized with anxiety disorders are listed in Table 12-2 (p. 390). The selection of strategies will depend on the nature of the disorder, the setting in which the patient is being treated, and the environment to which the person will return. There is a broad application of principles, including approaches for people suffering more severe impairment (Stein & Nikolic, 1989). Most of the approaches listed in the table

WORK

The extent to which my work is impaired because of anxiety

0	1	2	3	4	5	6	7	8	9	10
Never		Slightly		Moderately			Markedly		Very Severely	

SOCIAL ACTIVITIES

The extent to which my social life is impaired because of anxiety
(going out with friends, dating, outings, entertaining)

0	1	2	3	4	5	6	7	8	9	10
Never		Slightly		Moderately			Markedly		Very Severely	

LEISURE ACTIVITIES

The extent to which engagement in leisure activities is impaired because of anxiety
(hobbies, use of free time)

0	1	2	3	4	5	6	7	8	9	10
Never		Slightly		Moderately			Markedly		Very Severely	

HOME, SELF-MAINTENANCE, AND FAMILY RESPONSIBILITIES

The extent to which my ability to care for myself and others is impaired by my anxiety
(cleaning house, meal preparation, carpooling, doing laundry, paying bills, grooming)

0	1	2	3	4	5	6	7	8	9	10
Never		Slightly		Moderately			Markedly		Very Severely	

Figure 12-11.   Function Questionnaire

Source: Adapted from the Fear Questionnaire in Taylor & Arnow, 1988.

have emerged from other disciplines, most notably from psychology and from health and wellness. However, they have become widely used by professionals of all disciplines who practice in mental health. Occupational therapists use the techniques to enhance occupational therapy goals and facilitate functioning in occupational performance. Naturally, it is assumed that, when employing any strategy, the therapist will become competent through education and training.

Relaxation training.   Relaxation training can be an effective intervention to help people with anxiety disorders diminish arousal states; the relaxation response and a feeling of well-being are incompatible with anxiety. Initially, patients usually require external direction, but the overall goal is to teach them to recognize and manage their own anxiety while it is "young" (still of short duration) to prevent major anxiety attacks, as well as to avert attacks if they occur. It is important to help people generalize from treatment sessions to the variety of life situations where anxiety is likely to occur. The Function Questionnaire (see Figure 12-11) targets these areas effectively. The patient rates the extent to which anxiety interferes with daily activities from a quan-

Self-Assessment of Activities

Name:_____

Date:_____

This checklist will be used to help develop an Occupational Therapy program for you. Mark the appropriate column for each item and add any comments you feel would be helpful.

Activity	Never a problem	Sometimes a problem	Always a problem	N.A.	Comments
Grooming					
Bathing or showering					
Preparing meals					
Food shopping					
Doing errands					
House cleaning					
Doing yardwork					
Caring for others					
Managing money					
Transportation					
Socializing					
Attending school					
Working					
Volunteering					
Exercising					
Concentrating					
Problem solving					
Communicating					
Coping with stress					
Managing time					
Managing impulses					
Doing leisure activities					

Figure 12-12.   Self-Assessment of Activities

titative and qualitative standpoint. The next step is to focus on these areas one at a time and strategize how relaxation techniques could be incorporated into the activities. For example, this method was successful with a construction worker who often became panicky when working on roofs. Utilizing abdominal breathing just before she went on the roof or while she was working on it greatly helped to reduce her symptoms of rapid pulse and queasiness.

Typically, occupational therapists teach a variety of relaxation skills (after they themselves have been sufficiently trained). These skills include deep breathing, progressive muscle relaxation, visualization, and **autogenic training** among others. As described by Benson (1976), who is a pioneer of relax-

Imagine that this circle represents your typical 24-hour day. Divide it up into pie-shaped wedges that correspond to the amount of time you spend in various activities such as sleeping, working, and managing the home. Label the activity and the number of hours devoted to it in each section.

Figure 12-13.   Activity Configuration

ation training, all relaxation interventions involve the following: (1) the person has a passive attitude, (2) there is a decrease in muscle tone, (3) the environment is quiet, and (4) a mental device is used, such as an image or sound. Anxious people often lack the ability to engage in all steps of the relaxation activity; therefore, it is helpful to teach specific relaxation exercises that have an action component in addition to the distraction of a mental device. Progressive muscle relaxation (discussed in a subsequent section) has this feature. Sessions usually last up to about 30 minutes. Because of the quiet atmosphere generated by the relaxation training, it is wise to include people with the same attention span and to exclude those who are extremely restless or distractible. People should be given the option of keeping their eyes open or closed and the choice of sitting in a chair or sitting or lying on the floor. A

Table 12-2. Occupational Therapy and Self-Management
Techniques

- *Relaxation Training*
  Breathing Exercises
  Progressive Muscle Relaxation
  Visualization
  Autogenic Training
- *Assertiveness Training*
- *Community Mobility/Reentry*
- *Expressive Activities*
  Journal Writing
  Craft and Art Activities
- *Functional Behavior Training*
- *Education/Lifestyle Alterations*
- *Rational/Cognitive Approaches*
- *Time Management*

protective covering such as a sheet should be available for hygienic reasons.
If an individual chooses to use a chair, the therapist should make certain that
there is back support by putting the chair against the wall. This will protect
the person's neck from possible injury should he or she fall asleep.

Each person will have a preferred technique therefore, it is helpful to
briefly introduce a variety of methods so as to gain feedback from the patient
as to which is the most useful. This can be accomplished by having people
rate their subjective levels of anxiety on a scale from 1 to 10 before and after
the exercises, by taking respiratory and heart rates before and after tasks, by
asking which exercise was the most effective, or by observing the person's apparent level of concentration during the exercises. Sampling a variety of relaxation techniques within one session has the advantage of addressing
problems of limited attention span and restricted opportunities for treatment
due to the increasingly short lengths of stay on inpatient units or treatment in
a home setting.

Making personalized audiotapes for relaxation can be extremely helpful,
but commercial tapes are also readily available. When making or selecting
tapes, it is essential to consider the concentration level as well as the particular needs of each person. If given a choice, most people will state a preference for either a male or female narrator; therefore, having both available is
useful. Once the individual learns and masters the selected techniques, he or
she should be helped to apply the skill to everyday barriers. For example, a
person with social phobia may learn to practice a few minutes of deep breathing before meeting coworkers for lunch, an individual with agoraphobia may
visualize a pleasant spot before leaving the house, and a person with PTSD
may engage in relaxation exercises to counteract insomnia.

People should also be encouraged to differentiate, and then apply, other resources they have previously used to enhance the relaxation process, such as music, meditation, lighting, warm baths, and humor.

Breathing exercises.　Abdominal breathing can effectively address relaxation, especially when people learn to self-monitor the technique by placing their hands on the abdomen and witnessing them rise on the inhalation. This is a logical first task for an individual with an anxiety disorder for it can be short in duration and requires limited direction. However, patients should be introduced to this technique slowly to avoid light-headedness from the increased oxygen consumption. Breathing exercises have been found to be a useful strategy to use during panic attacks (Clark, Salkovskis & Chalkley, 1985), with the addition of the patient counting to five between breaths. Under stress, many anxious people hyperventilate, causing blood chemistry changes that lead to unpleasant sensations, such as dizziness. It is this reaction that may actually precipitate the panic and fear. Respiratory control by means of slow, paced breathing counteracts the patterns of hyperventilation thought to contribute to acute anxiety attacks. Sometimes other types of breathing exercises are more effective or can be used in conjunction with abdominal breathing. Imagining the words, "I am," as one inhales, and, "relaxed," as one exhales helps to slow the breath and focus on breathing patterns. Synchronizing breathing with counting slowly or the visualization of color is also effective. Patients seem to respond favorably to imagining the inhalation of clear colors, such as yellow or blue, and the exhalation of gray.

Progressive muscle relaxation.　Progressive muscle relaxation, which was first described by Jacobson (1938), teaches patients to slowly and methodically tighten and release voluntary muscle groups in a progressive fashion, thereby contrasting the states of tension and relaxation. This technique offers a discharge of tension as a means to achieve a state of deep relaxation, with the underlying hypothesis that relaxation of the body leads to relaxation of the mind. For patients with limited concentration, the active involvement of tensing and relaxing can be more engaging and therefore more successful than pure mental activity. Daily sessions are recommended for practicing and mastering the technique.

Visualization.　Picturing a pleasant scene is another method used to enhance the relaxation response. It is easiest for people to activate images after anxiety has partially subsided; therefore, it is recommended to precede visualization with breathing exercises. Soothing music may also help to evoke images, but some people will still need guidance. If the therapist provides mental pictures for the patient such as floating or diving into water, it is important to know beforehand that the images selected are pleasant . Directions can include visualizing a leaf floating in a stream, walking in a meadow or strolling by a pond, returning to a pleasantly remembered childhood spot, imagining a fantasy place, or picturing a comfortable place in one's home. By presenting only a general direction and structure, such as saying, "Imagine a beautiful place you've seen," the therapist encourages the patient to fill in more of his or her personal experience. If the patient is unable to easily evoke images, simply picturing colors may provide a sufficient degree of pleasant sensation. Visualization exercises are contraindicated for patients experiencing perceptual distortions (hallucinations) or thought disorders (delusions) because these exercises can intensify the psychotic experience and become frightening. Before beginning the task, the occupational therapist should always inform patients to open their eyes if the exercise evokes unpleasant feelings. The therapist should assume this may be happening if he or she observes crying, restlessness, or the eyes suddenly opening. Visualization methods can also be adapted for use with children.

Autogenic training.   Autogenic training, which was developed by German neurologist H. H. Shultz, teaches the body and mind to relax through the person's own verbal commands. The intent is to relax the voluntary and involuntary muscles to provide vasodilation and help regulate the circulatory and respiratory systems (Davis et al., 1988). The occupational therapist can introduce several of the exercises, which are learned methodically over several weeks. They consist of imagining the limbs as heavy and warm, the heart as beating regularly and calmly, the lungs as operating regularly, the solar plexus as feeling warm, and the forehead as feeling cool. Since this method of relaxation has a strong effect on body physiology, it is not recommended for people with serious medical problems. In addition, it is contraindicated for children and for people with severe psychiatric disorders.

Assertiveness and general social skills training.   Patients with anxiety disorders often manifest passive behavior. This may be due in part to fears related to anticipated embarrassment in social situations in which they may feel they will have no control. This is particularly true of patients with social phobias and generalized anxiety disorder. For example, a young man with generalized anxiety and depression was exceedingly lonely. Terrified to attend social functions, where he could possibly meet a potential mate, he ruminated about rejection and humiliation. He was unsure of how to approach strangers, initiate conversation, or sustain friendships. The cycle continued as he further isolated himself in spite of craving social contact, which he did in part to manage his anxiety. This patient attended assertiveness groups while on a psychiatric unit and was referred to a community class at discharge. The OT group included the following stages: (1) understanding the components of assertive behavior, including differentiation between styles; (2) identifying personal styles and blocks to behaving assertively, including irrational beliefs and fears; and (3) practicing assertive communication and the principles and applications of good communication practices through role-play situations. Assertiveness training helped him to reduce anxiety and taught him to confront intimidating social situations in a way that offered more personal control.

Community mobility and reentry. Isolation is a serious problem for people with anxiety disorders, who may completely withdraw from friends, family, leisure activities, and work in order to curb their anxiety. Not only does such constraint lead to loneliness and depression, but the absence of physical and emotional outlets can also contribute to maintaining the anxiety cycle. With restricted activity, people may become even more focused on their thoughts, sensations, and other internal experiences. Clients with anxiety may benefit from locating community resources that draw on former or current interests and simultaneously provide contact with other people. Some feel most supported in activities provided by mental health agencies, such as support groups or social events, because here they can receive direct help with their anxiety while also engaging in the activity at hand. Other patients feel more comfortable in small classes such as private art, music, or bridge classes, which are offered in many communities. Many prefer noncompetitive enrichment classes over junior college courses such as those offered by adult education programs. The occupational therapist can help locate appropriate programs during an individual or group treatment session.

Expressive activities. Patients experiencing anxiety disorders may benefit from engaging in expressive activities, which provide an outlet and release for the physical and emotional turbulence associated with anxiety. Family members and friends may have limited tolerance for discussing the patient's repetitive concerns, so self-reliance techniques can help to preserve social relationships as well as promote independence.

Journal and diary writing. A journal can become a focus and receptacle for distressing thoughts. The symbolic act of writing down concerns and feelings may help the individual become better able to dismiss the troublesome emotions once the book is closed. Physiological symptoms usually are decreased by writing as well. When using a diary, a person has control over the expression of content and amount of time devoted to addressing symptoms. For example, a woman in her early 30s with obsessive-compulsive disorder annoyed her mother, who lived next door, by her persistent criticism of her mother's perceived lack of attention to home maintenance and safety. To improve their relationship, the daughter began to write these worries in a notebook rather than discuss them with her mother, who did not perceive that there was a problem.

Sometimes keeping a journal or diary is suggested by a psychologist or psychiatrist as a means for recording specific anxiety disorder symptoms such as those of panic attacks or phobias. The information included may concern the times during the day when the symptoms emerge, the nature and intensity of the symptoms, and events occurring prior to or after the attack. This data helps the person with anxiety achieve some control over the symptoms by recognizing their patterns, precipitants, and consequences.

Craft and art activities. Structured craft and expressive art activities both have a place in the treatment of anxiety disorders. In structured crafts, the limits of a repetitive and predictive project can offer reassurance to the fearful person and help to contain anxiety. Patients with anxiety disorders seem to prefer projects with true boundaries, such as plastic "stained glass," sophisticated coloring sheets, and mosaics. Simple greeting cards may have the same effect. Completing these tasks successfully also provides a sense of mastery through accomplishment and increases patients' perceived sense of effectiveness.

The more expressive activities involved in artwork may offer a release of tension through physical activity, such as ripping paper or using a stippling brush for painting designs on paper or cloth, and thus provide an acceptable substitute for an inappropriate expression of anxiety. For example, a client with multiple diagnoses including borderline personality disorder repeatedly burned herself with lit cigarettes in order to find relief from intolerable levels of anxiety. The occupational therapist provided her with a large body outline on which she was able to draw cigarette burns when she felt overcome by these impulses. Another client, a middle-aged man with schizophrenia and obsessive-compulsive disorder, was encouraged to draw with large felt pens whenever he began to frantically pace, wring his hands, or shake. His subsequent drawings were usually highly controlled, for example portraying multitiled houses and paved roads, but his obsessive behavior decreased (see Figure 12-14).

Expressive art activities may also stimulate self-understanding through the content that emerges. For example, in a group activity, a young mother with tenacious abdominal **psychogenic** pain and anxiety inadvertently drew a representation of her pain similar to the symbol she drew for her husband. When she discussed this likeness with her psychotherapist, she was able to connect the pain in her stomach to anger at her husband for not participating in any of the parenting responsibilities. All the expressive techniques discussed in this section are personally gratifying and increase the internal sense of control and self-mastery.

Functional behavioral training. A psychologist or psychiatrist may ask the occupational therapist to assist in carrying out behavioral programs that directly deal with improving functioning by decreasing symptoms as they relate to daily activities. For example, the plan may take the form of accompanying an agoraphobic patient on a community outing to combat anxiety symptoms while riding a bus or going to a store. This intervention (previously referred to as exposure therapy) addresses avoidant behavior and can be an effective approach in treating some of the anxiety disorders, particularly phobias.

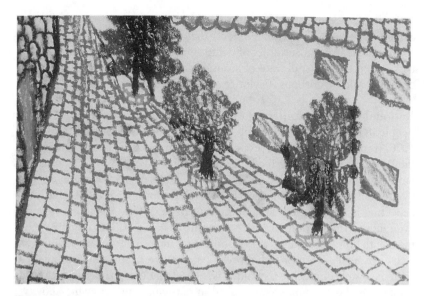

Figure 12-14.   Patient Drawing in Which Anxiety Is Expressed and Channeled

The occupational therapist may help the patient negotiate difficult tasks through instruction in breathing exercises, refuting irrational thoughts, or suggesting that he or she confront unpleasant sensations as if "riding the wave." More experienced occupational therapists may actually take part in devising the behavioral plan for decreasing symptoms. This might include helping the person identify target behaviors and then breaking them down into smaller, manageable steps. This is traditionally called *grading the activity* by occupational therapists. For example, one client with agoraphobia wanted to be able to go back to his favorite coffeehouse a few times a week. The occupational therapist guided him in making a plan—walking first one block from home with her, walking alone on the same route, buying a newspaper in front of the coffeehouse, and so forth. Another occupational therapist assisted a young woman with obsessive-compulsive disorder who had a fixation on soiled clothes and contamination of the washing machine, which prevented her from performing adequate hygiene routines as she felt impelled to wear the same, unwashed, clothes day after day. The occupational therapist helped her counteract these fears through relaxation training and visualization prior to, and during, the actual laundry activity, resulting in the patient being able to carry out the task and thus achieve adequate hygiene.

Education and lifestyle alterations.   The relationship between internal (inherent to an individual) and external (outside) factors and anxiety is often not understood by those experiencing anxiety disorders. In particular, reducing caffeine intake, eliminating nonmedically prescribed drugs, exercising regularly, eating a balanced diet, maintaining appropriate weight, sleeping sufficiently, lowering blood pressure, increasing leisure involvement, and managing time effectively are all elements that can positively affect one's ability to cope with anxiety. Sufferers of panic attacks tend to experience fewer attacks when their overall state of arousal is diminished by attending to some of these basic suggestions (Taylor & Arnow, 1988).

Rational-cognitive approaches. The occupational therapist may assist people in coping more effectively by utilizing cognitive interventions (Ellis, 1976) (provided he or she is properly trained in the techniques). Anxious patients are often highly perfectionistic and consequently self-critical of their current or anticipated behavior. They worry in the form of engaging in negative self-talk about their finances, health, job performance, and relationships, expecting failure in every area (Wright & Beck, 1994). The worry becomes even more magnified in obsessive-compulsive disorder. This negative thinking is both time-consuming and self-defeating and usually distorts reality. Cognitive strategies attempt to help replace negative self-talk statements with more favorable ones. One technique is to teach patients to make positive self-statements. For example, when asked to participate in a drawing activity, a good number of patients will disqualify themselves by saying: "I am a terrible artist. I can't do this." The occupational therapist can suggest a reframe of the statement such as, "It makes me nervous to draw but at least I'll give it a try." Another strategy is to help patients relabel internally directed, destructive emotions as more neutral and appropriate ones. For instance, anxiety at failing to meet work deadlines can be changed to "concern," feelings of worthlessness at being criticized can be changed to "annoyance," and guilt at criticizing a child can be changed to "regret" (Davis et al., 1988). These interventions seem to be most effective when they are presented as paper-and-pencil exercises, perhaps because problem solving through writing causes a delay in emotional response. The task can also be applied as a self-management strategy whereby the individual tracks responses over time.

Time management. Anxiety is often manifested by paralysis in goal-directed activity, which arises as a by-product of fears of failure, decreased concentration, or preoccupation with the stressor. Inactivity is further perpetuated by a lack of task mastery, which would likely enhance feelings of self-control and self-esteem. Instead, anxiety is often intensified by the failure to adequately meet personal and environmental demands. Patients may be surprised at the amount of nonproductive time they encounter in a 24-hour-day. This is effectively illustrated by an assessment of daily activities whereby patients account for their time hour by hour in either a graphic or a written format.

Learning effective time management techniques is a useful strategy for people with anxiety disorders. For example, the occupational therapist can teach how to prioritize tasks and break them down into manageable and attainable steps. People usually respond favorably to schedules and "to do" lists. Sometimes actually incorporating "worry time" into the daily routine helps to decrease the behavior. For example, one person was horrified that she had written down "worry" as a daily activity that consumed six hours a day. She was helped to plan more productive substitute activities during the vulnerable times of the day. This plan also provided her with access to her former hobbies; for example, she elected to write letters, knit, and practice computer graphics during those times.

CASE ILLUSTRATION: SHARMAN—OCCUPATIONAL THERAPY ASSESSMENT AND TREATMENT

A young, single woman reported problems in job performance following the development of a phobia and subsequent depression. Her usual route to work included driving on a particularly busy street where she had witnessed a catastrophic car accident. Shortly after the accident she developed acute anxiety when driving on this street, so she began to take a more circuitous route, which invariably made her late for work. She also became highly distractible, especially during the last hour of the workday as she mentally prepared to go home. In addition, she had difficulty organizing her various work tasks and had been counseled by her employer on several occasions. As her anxiety mounted about losing her job and her performance declined, she took a leave from work in order to attend a partial hospitalization program.

Assessment

Sharman's Role Checklist (see Figure 12-15) indicated difficulty in performing the worker role and the high value Sharman placed on it. The Function Questionnaire (see Figure12-16) indicated moderate to severe impairment in work because of anxiety. Sharman's Self-Assessment of Activity (see Figure 12-17) reported problems in concentration, job insecurity, excessive worry, poor coping strategies, and problem solving, and Sharman's Activity Configuration (see Figure 12-18) indicated that not enough time was allotted for commuting.

Goals

The overall goal of the occupational therapy program was to assist the patient in functioning more effectively in her role as worker, particularly through improved coping strategies. The objectives and interventions to reach this goal were as follows:

Objective

1. Client will have knowledge of alternative forms of transportation

Intervention

Community mobility through exploration of resources—bus routes, carpool accessibility, and alternative routes for driving

ROLE CHECKLIST

NAME S.T. AGE 26 DATE 2-24-95

SEX: ☐ MALE ☑ FEMALE ARE YOU RETIRED: ☐ YES ☑ NO

MARITAL STATUS: ☑ SINGLE ☐ MARRIED ☐ SEPARATED ☐ DIVORCED ☐ WIDOWED

The purpose of this checklist is to identify the major roles in your life. The checklist, which is divided into two parts, presents 10 roles and defines each one.

PART I

Beside each role, indicate, by checking the appropriate column, if you performed the role in the past, if you presently perform the role, and if you plan to perform the role in the future. You may check more than one column for each role. For example, if you volunteered in the past, do not volunteer at present, but plan to in the future, you would check the past and future columns.

ROLE	PAST	PRESENT	FUTURE
STUDENT: Attending school on a part-time or full-time basis.	✓		
WORKER: Part-time or full-time paid employment.	✓	✓	✓
VOLUNTEER: Donating services, **at least once a week,** to a hospital, school, community, political campaign, and so forth.	✓		
CARE GIVER: Responsibility, **at least once a week,** for the care of someone such as a child, spouse, relative, or friend.			✓
HOME MAINTAINER: Responsibility, **at least once a week,** for the upkeep of the home such as housecleaning or yardwork.	✓	✓	✓
FRIEND: Spending time or doing something, **at least once a week,** with a friend.	✓	✓	✓
FAMILY MEMBER: Spending time or doing something, **at least once a week,** with a family member such as a child, spouse, parent, or other relative.	✓		✓
RELIGIOUS PARTICIPANT: Involvement, **at least once a week,** in groups or activities affiliated with one's religion (excluding worship).	✓		
HOBBYIST/AMATEUR: Involvement, **at least once a week,** in a hobby or amateur activity such as sewing, playing a musical instrument, woodworking, sports, the theater, or participation in a club or team.	✓		✓
PARTICIPANT IN ORGANIZATIONS: Involvement, **at least once a week,** in organizations such as the American Legion, National Organization for Women, Parents Without Partners, Weight Watchers, and so forth.			
OTHER:___ A role not listed which you have performed, are presently performing, and/or plan to perform. Write the role on the line above and check the appropriate column(s).			

(continues)

Figure 12-15. Sharman's Role Checklist

Objective	Intervention
2. Client will plan daily schedule to ensure arriving to work on time	Training in time management—prioritization of activities and strategies to follow schedule
3. Client will learn and apply one method of relaxation to decrease general anxiety and to facilitate getting to work	Relaxation training—breathing and visualization exercises

PART II

The same roles are listed below. Next to *each* role check the column which best indicates how valuable or important the role is to you. Answer for *each role,* even if you have never performed or do not plan to perform the role.

ROLE	NOT AT ALL VALUABLE	SOMEWHAT VALUABLE	VERY VALUABLE
STUDENT: Attending school on a part-time or full-time basis.		✓	
WORKER: Part-time or full-time paid employment.			✓
VOLUNTEER: Donating services, **at least once a week,** to a hospital, school, community, political campaign, and so forth.		✓	
CARE GIVER: Responsibility, **at least once a week,** for the care of someone such as a child, spouse, relative, or friend.		✓	
HOME MAINTAINER: Responsibility, **at least once a week,** for the upkeep of the home such as housecleaning or yardwork.		✓	
FRIEND: Spending time or doing something, **at least once a week,** with a friend.			✓
FAMILY MEMBER: Spending time or doing something, **at least once a week,** with a family member such as a child, spouse, parent, or other relative.		✓	
RELIGIOUS PARTICIPANT: Involvement, **at least once a week,** in groups or activities affiliated with one's religion (excluding worship).		✓	
HOBBYIST/AMATEUR: Involvement, **at least once a week,** in a hobby or amateur activity such as sewing, playing a musical instrument, woodworking, sports, the theater, or participation in a club or team.			✓
PARTICIPANT IN ORGANIZATIONS: Involvement, **at least once a week,** in organizations such as the American Legion, National Organization for Women, Parents Without Partners, Weight Watchers, and so forth.	✓		
OTHER:_____ A role not listed which you have performed, are presently performing, and/or plan to perform. Write the role on the line above and check the appropriate column(s).			

© Copyright 1981 and Revised 1984 by Frances Oakley, M.S., OTR/L

Occupational Therapy Service, Department of Rehabilitation Medicine, Clinical Center, National institutes of Health

*U.S. GOVERNMENT PRINTING OFFICE: 1985-526-620:30339

Figure 12-15. *(continued)*

Objective	*Intervention*
4. Client will concentrate for 60 minutes on one task while at the program and for 60 minutes on one task at home.	Leisure and job simulation activities
5. Client will apply one strategy to neutralize fears that impede performance	Cognitive techniques focused on rational thinking

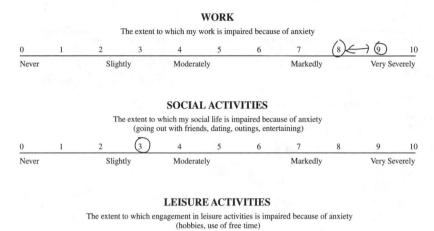

WORK

The extent to which my work is impaired because of anxiety

0	1	2	3	4	5	6	7	8	9	10
Never		Slightly		Moderately			Markedly		Very Severely	

SOCIAL ACTIVITIES

The extent to which my social life is impaired because of anxiety
(going out with friends, dating, outings, entertaining)

0	1	2	3	4	5	6	7	8	9	10
Never		Slightly		Moderately			Markedly		Very Severely	

LEISURE ACTIVITIES

The extent to which engagement in leisure activities is impaired because of anxiety
(hobbies, use of free time)

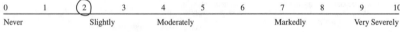

0	1	2	3	4	5	6	7	8	9	10
Never		Slightly		Moderately			Markedly		Very Severely	

HOME, SELF-MAINTENANCE, AND FAMILY RESPONSIBILITIES

The extent to which my ability to care for myself and others is impaired by my anxiety
(cleaning house, meal preparation, carpooling, doing laundry, paying bills, grooming)

0	1	2	3	4	5	6	7	8	9	10
Never		Slightly		Moderately			Markedly		Very Severely	

Figure 12-16.   Sharman's Function Questionnaire

Treatment

The occupational therapy program proceeded as follows:

1. Getting to work: this problem was approached from several perspectives, the intent being to provide Sharman with a variety of alternative methods of getting to and from her job. The occupational therapist guided the patient in exploring community resources. The patient contacted the county transit system for bus routes and schedules, and she sought information from her company regarding carpools. In addition, the OT helped her procure city maps and then locate alternative car routes should she elect to drive herself. This information enabled Sharman to feel less a "victim" to her anxiety and increased her feelings of personal control. On the other hand, it did not exclude directly confronting the phobia should she prefer—that is, driving on the dreaded street. Sharman worked on the two solutions simultaneously.

2. Arriving at work on time: Sharman's late arrival at work was generally the result of not allowing enough time for the task. She was used to her usual half-hour commute prior to the development of the phobia. The OT helped her to adjust other activities by reprioritizing them in order to ac-

Self-Assessment of Activities

Name: S T

Date: 2-24-95

This checklist will be used to help develop an Occupational Therapy program for you. Mark the appropriate column for each item and add any comments you feel would be helpful.

Activity	Never a problem	Sometimes a problem	Always a problem	N.A.	Comments
Grooming	✓				
Bathing or showering		✓			I tend to stay in too long-- 20 minutes
Preparing meals	✓				
Food shopping		✓			I don't like to drive to supermarket
Doing errands		✓			If I have to go down a particular street
House cleaning	✓				
Doing yardwork	✓				
Caring for others				✓	
Managing money	✓				
Transportation			✓		I am having difficulty driving-- very anxious
Socializing					
Attending school				✓	
Working			✓		Not as focused or organized as I used to be
Volunteering				✓	
Exercising	✓				
Concentrating			✓		I worry all the time about work, driving.
Problem solving		✓			I can't seem to figure out my problems
Communicating		✓			Most people o.k., but I avoid my boss.
Coping with stress			✓		I get overwhelmed by anxiety
Managing time			✓		Always a problem regarding getting to work
Managing impulses		✓			
Doing leisure activities		✓			Not as motivated as in past

Figure 12-17. Sharman's Self-Assessment of Activities

commodate the extra one to two hours (round trip) now needed when she drove herself by the longer alternate route. By categorizing her activities away from work from most valued to least valued (Lakein, 1973), she decided to decrease her evening time watching television ("least valued") and to wake up one hour earlier. To make the transition to the earlier wake-up time, she decided to prepare and lay out her clothes the night before, reduce her lengthy shower time, and read only half the newspaper over breakfast. As Sharman advanced in her partial hospitalization treatment program, she discarded television altogether and replaced it with a new hobby and therapy "homework."

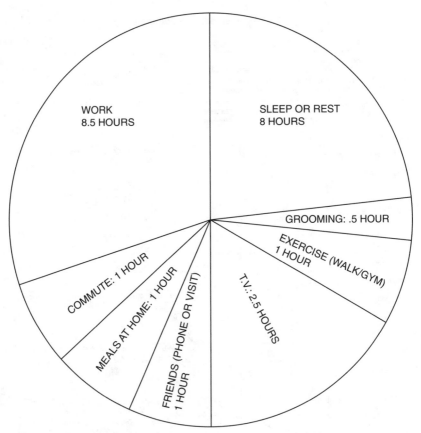

Figure 12-18. Sharman's Activity Configuration

3. Learning and applying relaxation techniques: Sharman's anxiety was focused primarily on the phobia as she thought about or actually commuted to and from work. However, merely thinking about the accident or about her work problems throughout the day caused rapid heartbeat, nausea, and poor concentration. The occupational therapist initially instructed Sharman in abdominal breathing during a group session. This method taught her to use her lungs more fully through deep breathing, since anxiety symptoms may be exacerbated with shallow breathing. She was trained to be aware of her abdomen rising as she took slow and deep breaths. Her position was supine on the floor on a blanket with her legs bent.

Sharman was told to practice this exercise once a day supine and one or two times a day in a sitting position. Each session was to last two minutes in the beginning and later to be expanded to about five minutes. In addition, she was coached to immediately make use of this technique while sitting in her chair whenever she experienced an initial sign of anxiety. She was also cautioned to return to her normal breathing patterns if she experienced any lightheadedness from increased oxygen flow. Sharman developed skill in using this breathing technique to combat her anxiety symptoms, such as nausea and poor concentration, and subsequently felt less helpless when symptoms appeared during the day.

Visualization and breathing were combined for the second phase. First, the occupational therapist, in an individual session, helped Sharman identify and visualize in her imagination a comfortable, safe place. To help guide the exercise, the OT encouraged her to describe places she had been that inspired a sense of well-being. Since Sharman particularly enjoyed the ocean, this was incorporated in the visualization. After first directing her in abdominal breathing, the OT instructed her to imagine being at the beach, while combining sounds, noises, and smells into the picture to strengthen the image. Two 10- to 15-minute sessions a day, to be done at home independently, were prescribed once Sharman had learned to concentrate and attain a state of relaxation with the therapist's assistance. After two weeks, she was able to perform this exercise independently and practiced it before going to the program, work, and bed.

The final phase of training focused on the patient visualizing, after completing the two previous steps, driving down the dreaded street in her car. When anxiety surfaced during this exercise, she was told to return to the calming image she had learned to picture. She reported difficulty mastering this aspect of treatment although she continued to practice regularly at home as well as deal with the phobia directly with a psychologist using desensitization techniques, by alleviating anxiety through controlled exposure to the scene of the accident.

4. Improving concentration: Sharman had reported difficulty attending to work tasks. Simulated leisure and work activities were introduced into the treatment program with the goal to work for 60 minutes uninterrupted in occupational therapy and then 60 minutes at home on predefined tasks. If she did work tasks in the program, she did a leisure activity at home, and vice versa.

In the past Sharman had enjoyed ceramics, and in particular, making necklaces. She readily accepted the idea of making jewelry using commercial beads and other materials. Sessions were initially 15 to 30 minutes long and involved uncomplicated techniques such as stringing beads for simple necklaces, but as her concentration improved, they were lengthened to 60 minutes and made to incorporate more complex tasks such as making fashion earrings and constructing beads from a quick-drying substitute clay material. She became so enthusiastic about this activity that she started going to yard sales to buy old, inexpensive jewelry to rework for her new hobby. She also found that engaging in this task helped to dissipate her anxiety at times when it surfaced at home.

Sharman's employment was as office assistant, and her workload consisted of a variety of clerical tasks. The occupational therapist was able to simulate some of these activities by requesting participation in a volunteer project the program had undertaken (assisting with a blood drive). Making up a flyer on the computer, writing letters to local businesses and organizations for support, and compiling blood donation packets were some of the tasks involved. Sharman also made a list of related jobs she needed to accomplish at home; specifically, reorganizing her financial files, working on her tax return, and updating her computer records. She made agreements with the occupational therapist as to the specific tasks and deadlines for jobs to be done at home.

In all these activities, the occupational therapist strategized with the patient on ways to stay focused on the task at hand. Creating an uncluttered work environment and removing distracting stimuli proved helpful. At home, Sharman turned off her telephone for one hour while she worked, and she agreed to get up from her desk only once during that time. If distracted, she was able to cue herself by saying, "I am able to focus on this task," and doing one minute of deep breathing. Sharman reported increased concentration and was able to meet her goals.

5. Overcoming irrational fears: Sharman reported worrying excessively about projected failures; that is, being shunned by her coworkers, being fired by her boss, having an anxiety attack while driving, and a host of other events. This response led to a heightened state of arousal and caused her either to avoid important activities or feel distressed while doing them. This negative thinking contributed to her depressive symptoms as well. With guidance from Sharman's psychologist, the occupational therapist helped her develop more realistic ways to perceive current and future events through changing her self-talk about the expected outcome. This was accomplished by first assisting Sharman in completing worksheets that helped to challenge her irrational thinking and then substitute more realistic thinking. For example, instead of telling herself that her life would come to an end should she be fired, Sharman learned to emphasize instead the immediate inconvenience of having to search for a job. She further reminded herself that many other people had lived through this experience and had even found the subsequent change rewarding.

Sharman stayed for four weeks in the partial hospitalization program and then returned to work, commuting by bus. She planned to join a carpool the following month, paying a small fee to members so that she would not be required to drive until her phobia was more resolved through continued work on this issue with her psychologist. She employed relaxation techniques and cognitive strategies to cope with anxiety throughout the day and reported a notable reduction in anxiety and improved concentration. Leisure activities also served as an outlet for her tension as well as a focus through which to override her irrational thoughts. Sharman made the transition into a new daily schedule in order to wake up earlier starting before her actual return to work and consequently was no longer late to her job. She became more self-confident as she showed improved performance in her worker role as well as a newly developed role as a hobbyist.

Summary

Occupational therapists work with people with anxiety disorders in a variety of treatment settings from acute psychiatric hospitals to home care programs. As changes in health care policies reduce the length of hospital stays, treatment is occurring more often in community settings.

Anxiety may be a mental disorder, as outlined in DSM-IV, or it may be a component of a physical or other psychiatric illness. The major disorders described in DSM-IV include panic disorder without and with agoraphobia, agoraphobia without history of panic attacks, specific phobia, social phobia, obsessive-compulsive disorder, post-traumatic stress disorder, acute stress disorder, and generalized anxiety disorder. When anxiety accompanies a physical illness, it may actually have been induced by a hormonal imbalance or other medical condition. On the other hand, anxiety may be the outcome of coping with a life-threatening illness and thus be likely to dissipate when the medical problem is resolved.

Differentiating between a true anxiety syndrome and normal anxiety is sometimes difficult. Anxiety is universal and often helpful, being related to the fight-or-flight response. However, when anxiety impairs rather than enhances functional performance, it becomes pathological. Anxiety symptoms fall into several categories: emotional, physiological, cognitive, and behavioral. Usually people experience some symptoms in each of these areas.

Treatment strategies aim to reduce symptoms, prevent relapse, and improve functioning. Approaches used by other health professionals include medications, psychotherapy, biofeedback, cognitive interventions, systematic desensitization, and couples therapy.

Occupational therapists work with individuals and families to improve functioning and adaptive behavior in everyday activities as well as the individual's perceived quality of life. Anxiety disorders are always accompanied by great emotional discomfort, which impacts both the patient and the family. Anxious people inevitably restrict their lives in order to accommodate the dysfunction. A parent may refuse to take family vacations because of a fear of crossing bridges or flying in an airplane. Another person may give up a satisfying job because of panic attacks. An older adult may drive away everyone in her support system with her excessive, relentless worrying. The challenge for the occupational therapist is to help the patient cope and therefore function productively. Improving effectiveness may be accomplished by actually reducing the level of anxiety, or it may be achieved by teaching the patient to grapple with life stresses in spite of anxiety. Both strategies involve the development of self-management skills. Empowering the patient through instruction in acquiring and developing these skills can be extremely beneficial.

Relaxation, assertiveness and general social skills training, community mobility, expressive craft and art activities, the functional behavior approach, education/life style alterations, rational/cognitive approaches, and time management are key strategies. Anxiety often takes a chronic course and requires much adaptation. Many people with anxiety are able to live productively when given the tools to cope more effectively.

Review Questions

1. What occupational therapy goals might be appropriate for a homebound elderly woman who has panic attacks when she attempts to leave the house to visit friends or do daily errands?
2. What types of community programs might assist someone who has not been able to work for several years because of flashbacks that impair concentration?
3. How could an occupational therapist simultaneously address a hospitalized student's stress disorder and depression following the sudden death of a parent?
4. Which types of relaxation training might be most successful with an adult with attention deficit disorder as well as generalized anxiety disorder?

Learning Activities

These activities are designed to help you understand what normal anxiety feels like by recalling situations that often evoke anxiety in people. (People with anxiety disorders may experience anxiety most of the time even when a specific event is not connected to it.)

1. Remember how you felt when (a) you had to give a presentation, (b) you sat for college entrance tests, (c) you anticipated a college or job interview, (d) you awaited your letter of acceptance into college, and (e) you prepared for an important social event. These are life events that all commonly provoke normal anxiety.
2. Imagine you are driving on the highway and you suddenly see the red, flashing light of a police car behind you and hear the siren blaring. Notice your body sensations and the thoughts that go through your head. Now picture the police car passing you and speeding ahead and note whether your level of arousal has decreased. If you refer to this lingering anxiety, you may better understand how anxious people feel in the absence of an immediate stressor.
3. Think of a time when your anxiety helped you to accomplish an important goal. Try to recall how your performance was enhanced by the limited amount of anxiety and remember the resultant feelings of achievement. Now recall a time when your anxiety was disabling and hindered your performance and adaptation.

4. Recall an encounter with a person who appeared very anxious. What were the signs indicating that this person was in distress? Were you drawn to or repelled by this person? Was your own level of anxiety affected by the experience?

5. Name one of your worries. Using a circle to represent the 24 hours of the day, fill in the percentage of time you spend focused on this worry. Now imagine being focused on this issue for 4 or more hours a day due to excessive anxiety and draw this condition on this circle. Try to imagine in what way this excessive worry might interfere with specific daily activities.

References

Agras, S. (1985). *Panic: Facing fears, phobias, and anxiety*. Stanford, CA: Stanford Alumni Association.

Agras, S., & Berkowitz, R. (1994). Behavior therapy. In R. E. Hales, S. C. Udofsky, & J. A. Talbott (Eds.), *Textbook of psychiatry* (2nd ed., pp. 1061–1081). Washington, DC: American Psychiatric Press.

American Psychiatric Association (APA). (1994). *Diagnostic and statistical manual of mental disorders* (4th ed.). Washington, DC: APA.

Bandura, A. (1977). Self-efficacy: Towards a unifying theory of behavioral change. *Psychological Review, 84*(2), 191–215.

Bandura, A. (1995). *Self-efficacy in changing societies*. New York: Cambridge University Press.

Benson, H. (1976). *The relaxation response*. Boston, MA: G. K. Hall.

Clark, D., Salkovskis, P., & Chalkley, A. (1985). Respiratory control as a treatment for panic attacks. *Behavior Therapy and Experimental Psychiatry, 16*(1), 23–30.

Davis, M., Eshelman, E., & McKay, M. (1988). *The relaxation and stress reduction workbook* (3rd ed.). Oakland, CA: New Harbinger Publications.

Depoy, E., & Kolodner, E. (1991). Psychological performance factors. In C. Christiansen & C. Baum (Eds.), *Occupational therapy—Overcoming human performance deficits* (pp. 304–332). Thorofare, NJ: Slack Publishing.

Ellis, A. (1976). *Growth through reason*. North Hollywood, CA: Wilshire Book Co.

Jacobson, E. (1938). *Progressive relaxation*. Chicago: University of Chicago Press.

Kielhofner, G. (Ed.). (1995). *A model of human occupation: Theory and application* (2nd ed.). Baltimore, MD: Williams & Wilkins.

Lakein, A. (1973). *How to get control of your time and your life*. New York: David McKay Co.

Sims, A., & Snaith, P. (1988). *Anxiety in clinical practice*. New York: John Wiley & Sons.

Stein, F., & Nikolic, S. (1989). Teaching stress management techniques to a schizophrenic patient. *American Journal of Occupational Therapy 43*,(3), 162–169.

Taylor, B., & Arnow, B. (1988). *The nature and treatment of anxiety disorders*. New York: Free Press.

Telch, M. J. (1982). *A comparison of behavioral and pharmacological approaches to the treatment of agoraphobia*. Unpublished doctoral dissertation, Stanford University, Stanford, CA.

Weissman, M., Myers, J., & Harding, P. (1978). Psychiatric disorders in a U..S. urban community: 1975–1976. *American Journal of Psychiatry, 135*(4) 459–462.

Wright, J. H., & Beck, A. T. (1994). Cognitive therapy. In R. E. Hales, S. C. Udofsky, & J. A. Talbott (Eds.), *Textbook of psychiatry* (2nd ed., pp. 1083–1114). Washington, DC: American Psychiatric Press.

Wolpe, J. (1973). *The practice of behavior therapy*. Elmsford, NY: Pergamon Press.

Suggested Reading and Other Resources

Expressive Art Activities

Capacchione, L. (1989). *The creative journal*. North Hollywood, CA: Newcastle Publishing Co.

Capacchione, L. (1990). *The picture of health: Healing your life with art*. Carson, CA: Hay House.

Progoff, I. (1992). *At a journal workshop*. New York: G. P. Putnam's Sons. (Originally published 1975).

Relaxation Training

Davis, M., Eshelman, E., & McKay, M. (1988). *The relaxation and stress reduction workbook* (3rd ed.). Oakland, CA: New Harbinger Publications.

Gawain, S. (1978). *Creative visualization*. San Rafael, CA: New World Library.

Relaxation Tapes

East West Book Shop
324 Castro Avenue
Mountain View, CA 94041-1297
(415) 988-9800
http://www.eastwest.com

Source (Tapes by Emmet Miller)
P.O. Box W
Stanford, CA 94309
(800) 52-TAPES

East-West Books
78 Fifth Avenue
New York, NY 10011
(212) 243-5994

Cognitive Training

Ellis, A. (1978). *A new guide to rational living*. North Hollywood, CA: Wilshire Book Company.

McKay, M., Davis, M., & Fanning, P. (1981). *Thoughts and feelings: The art of cognitive stress intervention*. Richmond, CA: New Harbinger Publications.

Wolpe, J. (1973). *The practice of behavior therapy*. Elmsford, NY: Pergamon Press.

Assertiveness Training

McKay, M., Davis, M., & Fanning, P. (1983). *Messages: The communication skills book*. Oakland, CA: New Harbinger Publications.

Time Management

Lakein, A. (1973). *How to get control of your time and your life*. New York: David McKay Co.

General Overview

American Occupational Therapy Association (AOTA). (1995). *Guidelines of occupational therapy practice in home health*. Bethesda, MD: AOTA.

Bonder, B. R. (1991). *Psychopathology and function*. Thorofare, NJ: Slack.

Hales, R. E., Udofsky, S. C., & Talbott, J. A. (Eds.). (1994). *Textbook of psychiatry* (2nd ed.). Washington, DC: American Psychiatric Press.

Korb, K., Azok, S., & Leutenberg, E. (1989). *Life management skills*. Beachwood, OH: Wellness Reproductions.

Korb, K., Azok, S., Leutenberg, E. (1991). *Life management skills II*. Beachwood, OH: Wellness Reproductions.

Korb-Khalsa, K., Azok, S., Leutenberg, E. (1994). *Life management skills III*. Beachwood, OH: Wellness Reproductions.

Oakley, F., Kielhofner, G., Barris, R., & Reichler, R. (1986). The role checklist: Development and empirical assessment of reliability. *Occupational Therapy Journal of Research, 6*, 157–170.

CHAPTER 13

Dissociative Disorders

Gwen Vergeer, MS, OTR
Occupational Therapist
George Miller Center West, Richmond, California

Elizabeth Cara

Key Terms

abreaction
alter personality
derealization
dissociation

host personality
multiple personality disorder
out
switching

Chapter Outline

Introduction

Dissociation refers to the act of separating or "splitting off" content from the conscious mind. It can refer to feelings, thoughts, information, or mental functioning that cannot be accessed consciously by a person for a certain period of time. Usually, the person who is dissociating experiences some alteration in sense of identity and there is a memory disturbance for events occurring during the period of dissociation. Batson and Stephens (1989) refer to dissociation as "confusion with a function" because it often serves to protect the individual against awareness of intense emotional pain. Other protective functions of dissociation (Putnam, 1991) include

- escape from conflict
- performing actions by rote without needing to focus conscious awareness on them
- soothing pain
- defying the constraints of reality
- altering one's self-concept

Dissociation is considered an adaptive response; it is a process used by individuals to handle extremely traumatic experiences. It is seen as serving an important function by attempting to ensure survival. Dissociative disorders are almost always induced by trauma that can be life-threatening, such as war-induced experiences and physical and sexual abuse. Although some researchers consider dissociation to be abnormal, others consider it a normal process that occurs in many people.

In fact, it is likely that all of us dissociate at times, even though we may be unaware. For example, a person may be anxious about taking a test and, even though he knows the material, may feel his mind "go blank" when the exam is placed on his desk. Someone else may cease to experience emotions after a loved one's death as a mechanism to help her carry out the tasks of planning the funeral and getting the financial and legal documents in order. After the tasks have been accomplished, the person may become immobilized with grief. Though it occurs normally, dissociation becomes a disorder when it interferes with daily functioning or becomes an unconscious way of regularly and consistently escaping situations that seem too difficult to face.

HISTORY OF DISSOCIATION AND DISSOCIATIVE IDENTITY DISORDER

The first case of **multiple personality disorder**, as dissociative identity disorder used to be called, is said to have been described in 1646. Scattered reports of cases occurred both in Europe and America up to the nineteenth century. From the period of 1880 to 1920 there was much interest in multiple personality disorder and many cases were reported in France and the United States. Physicians, psychologists, and philosophers described detailed cases, and there was lively discussion of dissociation and the nature of consciousness.

Pierre Janet (1859–1947), a French psychiatrist, is acknowledged for his extensive research and case histories delineating the nature of dissociation and multiple personality disorder. He acknowledged his debt to "pioneers" in the field who studied "magnetism" and "mesmerism," popular variations of hypnosis of the day, and also to Jean Martin Charcot, a well-known French physician. Contemporaries in America who elaborated on Janet's work included the psychologist and physician Morton Prince and Boris Sidis, a student of William James (Putnam, 1989).

Interest in dissociation declined after 1920; however, 50 years later it again became a popular topic. Different trends were responsible for the rebirth of interest in dissociation and multiple personality in the 1970s:

- Clinically, multiple personality disorder was being increasingly diagnosed.
- Public awareness of child abuse and post-traumatic stress syndrome was

directing professionals to look at dissociative phenomena.

- An explosion of information in the area of cognitive psychology, along with an increase in the use of hypnosis, led to a rebirth of interest in the nature of consciousness and the mind.

DSM-IV CATEGORIES

The *Diagnostic and Statistical Manual of Mental Disorders, Fourth Edition* (DSM-IV) (APA, 1994) characterizes dissociative disorders as disturbances or alterations in the normally integrative functions of identity, memory, consciousness, or perceived environment. It recognizes five different categories of disorders: dissociative identity disorder, depersonalization disorder, dissociative amnesia, dissociative fugue, and dissociative disorder not otherwise specified. Dissociative symptoms may be found in other disorders, such as acute stress, post-traumatic stress, and somatization disorders; however, if the dissociative symptoms occur exclusively during the course of those disorders, an additional diagnosis of dissociative disorder is not given. Since dissociative states may be a common accepted expression of cultural activity in other societies, one must use a cross-cultural perspective. However, dissociation is considered pathological in all societies when it leads to significant distress or impairment. There are other dissociative states not included in the DSM-IV, such as hypnotic states, sleepwalking, and out-of-body or near-death experiences; however, these are not a focus of clinical occupational therapy practice and so are not discussed in this chapter.

Dissociative Identity Disorder (DID)

Most people with DID are women, with about five times more women diagnosed than men. This may be because of the existence of different evolutionary styles of adapting to trauma in men and women (Perry, Pollard, Blakely, Baker, & Vigilante, 1995). Most cases are diagnosed between the ages of 29 and 40. There is little data on ethnicity and socioeconomic status, though case reports would lead one to believe that it can be found in all ethnic groups and economic backgrounds. The essential feature is the presence of two or more distinct personality states. There is an inability to recall important personal information, and this lack of recall cannot be attributed to ordinary forgetfulness. Each personality state is experienced as if it has a distinct personal history, self-image, and identity, and each state has a separate name. The identity states may differ in gender, age, affect, vocabulary, and general knowledge. The primary identity, or **host personality**, is often passive, dependent, depressed, or guilty. This personality may not have a good memory for past events and experiences. Each alternate identity, or **alter personality**, has qualities (e.g., provocativeness, brashness, hostility, aggressiveness) that seem to contrast sharply with the primary personality. Memories of experiences and events may be held separately by each personality. The alternate identities may have memories of more events and experiences than the host, yet it is these latter identity states (because of the qualities they possess) that interfere with activities of daily living. The personalities may deny knowing each other or may be in conflict with each other; they may gain access to consciousness and the outside world by what can be experienced as hallucinations, such as a voice giving instructions. Figure 13-1 lists the DSM-IV diagnostic criteria for DID.

Depersonalization Disorder

Depersonalization can be a symptom of many different disorders, including depression; other mood, anxiety, and personality disorders; schizophrenia; and even epilepsy. It is seldom seen as an isolated disorder, and despite its inclusion this way in the DSM-IV, the diagnosis of depersonalization is not made if it is secondary to a different disorder. Many people experience depersonalization during very stressful events; it is only diagnosed as a disorder if it occurs often and with intensity, affecting a person's ability to function and causing much distress. It is not known how many people experience depersonalization, although it tends to develop during adolescence or shortly thereafter. Clinically, to exhibit significant depersonalization may be a learned mechanism for coping with traumatic situations. Freud believed depersonalization was a defense against guilt and an attempt to distance oneself from the implication of negative feelings. More recently, depersonalization has been viewed as a nonspecific reaction to stress (APA, 1994; Putnam, 1989). Figure 13-2 describes the DSM-IV criteria for depersonalization disorder.

A. The presence of two or more distinct identities or personality states (each with its own relatively enduring pattern of perceiving, relating to, and thinking about the environment and self).

B. At least two of these identities or personality states recurrently take control of the person's behavior.

C. Inability to recall important personal information that is too extensive to be explained by ordinary forgetfulness.

D. The disturbance is not due to the direct physiological effects of a substance (e.g., blackouts or chaotic behavior during Alcohol Intoxication) or a general medical condition (e.g., complex partial seizures). **Note:** In children, the symptoms are not attributable to imaginary playmates or other fantasy play.

Figure 13-1. Diagnostic Criteria for Dissociative Identity Disorder

Source: Reprinted with permission from *Diagnostic and Statistical Manual of Mental Disorders, Fourth Edition.* Copyright 1994 American Psychiatric Association.

A. Persistent or recurrent experiences of feeling detached from, and as if one is an outside observer of, one's mental processes or body (e.g., feeling like one is in a dream).

B. During the depersonalization experience, reality testing remains intact.

C. The depersonalization causes clinically significant distress or impairment in social, occupational, or other important areas of functioning.

D. The depersonalization experience does not occur exclusively during the course of another mental disorder, such as Schizophrenia, Panic Disorder, Acute Stress Disorder, or another Dissociative Disorder, and is not due to the direct physiological effects of a substance (e.g., a drug of abuse, a medication) or a general medical condition (e.g., temporal lobe epilepsy).

Figure 13-2. Diagnostic Criteria for Depersonalization Disorder

Source: Reprinted with permission from *Diagnostic and Statistical Manual of Mental Disorders, Fourth Edition.* Copyright 1994 American Psychiatric Association.

Dissociative Amnesia

Dissociative amnesia is more pronounced than ordinary forgetfulness. It generally follows an emotionally traumatic situation and is often seen in combination with an environment that appears to the person to be difficult and inescapable. Sometimes the person experiencing dissociative amnesia fears physical injury or death. He or she may be able to function despite the amnesia and may be unaware of the memory disturbance. People who respond to severe emotional stress with dissociative amnesia may have more than one episode of this disorder, and the amnesia may be preceded, at times, by a headache (Gilmore & Kaufman, 1991).

There are several types of of dissociative amnesia. Localized amnesia involves the loss of memory for a short period of time, such as a few hours; it usually occurs immediately following an intensely traumatic event. Selective amnesia involves an inability to bring to mind some, but not all, of the events or information that occurred during a certain period of time. The most emotionally painful memories are the ones that remain hidden. Generalized amnesia is a total inability to remember past events and facts. This type of amnesia is the most rare (despite being favored by writers of soap operas). If the memory loss extends into the present time, it is referred to as continuous amnesia.

Gilmore and Kaufman (1991) point out that although the DSM-IV categorizes dissociative amnesia in these subtypes, the disorder often fails to appear in these subtypes clinically. Often two or three of these subtypes occur in one person as stages of a memory disturbance. For example, someone who experiences generalized amnesia immediately following a traumatic event may later remember his or her identity and past knowledge but retain localized amnesia concerning the event.

A. The predominant disturbance is one or more episodes of inability to recall important personal information, usually of a traumatic or stressful nature, that is too extensive to be explained by ordinary forgetfulness.

B. The disturbance does not occur exclusively during the course of Dissociative Identity Disorder, Dissociative Fugue, Posttraumatic Stress Disorder, Acute Stress Disorder, or Somatization Disorder and is not due to the direct physiological effects of a substance (e.g., a drug of abuse, a medication) or a neurological or other general medical condition (e.g., Amnestic Disorder Due to Head Trauma).

C. The symptoms cause clinically significant distress or impairment in social, occupational, or other important areas of functioning.

Figure 13-3. Diagnostic Criteria for Dissociative Amnesia

Source: Reprinted with permission from *Diagnostic and Statistical Manual of Mental Disorders, Fourth Edition.* Copyright 1994 American Psychiatric Association.

Dissociative amnesia is fairly rare; it is found more commonly in people who have experienced war, accidents, or natural disasters. The amnesia usually begins and ends suddenly. It is usually a temporary condition, which is followed by either a complete recovery or the recovery of all memories except those around the beginning of the amnestic period. However, it may recur, sometimes repeatedly, in susceptible individuals. Figure 13-3 describes the DSM-IV criteria for dissociative amnesia.

Dissociative Fugue

Dissociative fugue involves sudden, unplanned travel and the assumption of a new identity with no remembrance of the previous identity. (People who travel unexpectedly but retain their identity would not be given this diagnosis but rather that of dissociative disorder not otherwise specified, even though this situation is also seen in clinical settings.) Usually this condition has an abrupt onset and recovery, and typically, people do not remember events that occurred during the fugue.

Dissociative fugue is rare, although, like other dissociative disorders, it is diagnosed more frequently during war and following disasters. People often recover from a dissociative fugue without the benefit of treatment, and if they do seek psychiatric help it is generally after the fugue. Usually, people experiencing psychogenic fugue engage in brief, purposeful traveling with minimal social contacts and incomplete development of their new identity. Occasionally however, people with this condition develop complex new identities, which are usually more outgoing than their previous personalities. They may take on new names, residences, professions, and social networks, and they may not appear to be suffering from a psychiatric disorder. Figure 13-4 describes the diagnostic criteria for dissociative fugue.

A. The predominant disturbance is sudden, unexpected travel away from home or one's customary place of work, with inability to recall one's past.

B. Confusion about personal identity or assumption of a new identity (partial or complete).

C. The disturbance does not occur exclusively during the course of Dissociative Identity Disorder and is not due to the direct physiological effects of a substance (e.g., a drug of abuse, a medication) or a general medical condition (e.g., temporal lobe epilepsy).

D. The symptoms cause clinically significant distress or impairment in social, occupational, or other important areas of functioning.

Figure 13-4. Diagnostic Criteria for Dissociative Fugue

Source: Reprinted with permission from *Diagnostic and Statistical Manual of Mental Disorders, Fourth Edition.* Copyright 1994 American Psychiatric Association.

DISSOCIATIVE DISORDERS IN CHILDREN

It can be difficult to distinguish between normal and pathological dissociation in children and adolescents. This difficulty occurs because dissociative experiences that manifest as fantasy play and imaginary companionship are developmentally normal in children (Putnam, 1991). Children also typically have difficulty estimating time periods or the loss of time, so it is difficult to diagnose amnesia. Normal dissociation is most prevalent in late preschool–aged children; it then gradually declines until early adulthood. However, dissociative disorders do occur in children (Schwartz & Perry, 1994), and many cases of adult dissociative disorders can be traced to childhood or adolescence (Peterson, 1991). It is believed that children who are developing dissociative disorders repeatedly dissociate during times of extreme stress as a response to that stress, to the point where dissociation becomes a primary coping mechanism (Putnam, 1991). It is believed that extreme stress or trauma actually reorganizes the central nervous system and alters brain development in children so that traumatic states actually become traits that affect their later cognitive, emotional, and social functioning (Perry et al., 1995).

RELATED PROBLEMS

Clients who are diagnosed with DID often present with other major disorders or difficulties that play a part in the cause of the disorder or are its attendant consequences.

Abuse in Childhood

Over 95 percent of individuals diagnosed with dissociative identity disorder report a history of severe abuse beginning early in childhood and extending

The Abuse is:
- Sexual and/or physical,
- Begins at an early age,
- Physically intrusive and life threatening (objects, torture, or multiple perpetrators)
- Child has witnessed or has been brainwashed to believe that unspeakable acts have occurred (such as the murder of another child);
- Abusive pattern continues over an extended period of time.

The abuse and environment of abuse leads to a variety of internal psychological problems and external problems in daily living, most notably:
- Understanding the integrity of one's own body;
- Difficulties in believing one is ever truly safe in any environment no matter where living;
- Difficulties trusting in others;
- Difficulties in understanding one's own emotions, needs and desires in relationship to others resulting in communication problems;
- Difficulty considering oneself a lovable individual deserving of another's interest;
- Difficulty experiencing joy and happiness and corresponding ability to experience humor.

Figure 13-5. Psychological Problems Resulting from Severe Abuse

over a period of time. Since more females than males in our culture report, and are vulnerable to, abuse, it is not surprising that more women than men are diagnosed with DID. Due to recent empowering social movements (notably the feminist movement of the 1960s) and the attendant change or relative relaxation in sexual values, abuse has been more recognized and discussed over the last 20 years. The abuse reported to accompany dissociative identity disorder has been reported to be severe. Figure 13-5 describes psychological problems that may result from an environment of severe abuse.

Since it is commonly accepted that dissociation is a defense against trauma, it makes sense that children would easily use an adaptive coping mechanism that they are developmentally and, perhaps, genetically prepared to use. Utilizing this defense consistently at an early age, prior to the time when a cohesive personality has been formed, could lead to the development of dissociative identity disorder. The additional problems that result from any abusive situation will also be manifested in the person with DID.

Substance Abuse Disorder

Substance abuse is found commonly among people who experience dissociative disorders. Just as dissociation involves entering a state of lowered consciousness in order to separate from, and block out, painful feelings, using drugs and alcohol helps people to numb their consciousness and escape reality. Some side effects of substance abuse, such as "blacking out" after heavy drinking and being unable to remember one's actions or whereabouts during a period of time, are similar to symptoms of dissociative disorders.

Jacobs (1988) has found that people addicted to alcohol or gambling report an unusually high incidence of dissociative experiences while they are engaging in their addictive behaviors. The experiences his subjects reported frequently included feeling as if outside one's body and watching one's actions, experiencing memory blackouts or trance states, and feeling as though one has taken on a different identity. The fact that substance abusers often report these dissociative experiences concurrent with their addictive behaviors (while substance users who are not addicted may not have such experiences) may assist mental health practitioners in differentiating substance abusers from substance users. It is important to be aware that addicts who are hospitalized to undergo alcohol or drug withdrawal may experience alterations in reality ranging from dissociative symptoms to psychosis as part of their withdrawal reaction.

Eating Disorders

Eating disorders are also common among people who have dissociative disorders, and the two types of disorder may be interconnected. The three primary eating disorders are anorexia nervosa, bulimia, and overeating. These disorders most commonly begin in adolescence or early adulthood, as do dissociative disorders. Many people with eating disorders have a distorted body image, for example viewing themselves as fat when they are actually of average weight or less. They may also feel unable to control their eating or purging (vomiting) behaviors. It is as though people with these disorders had a deep-seated sense of depersonalization, which causes them to experience their bodies as alien and their actions as out of their conscious control.

In treating patients with any eating disorders or substance-abusing behaviors, it is important to remember that the destructive behaviors and addictions may have served the purpose of providing a sense of comfort and control while at the same time detaching the person from traumatic feelings. Hence, giving up the destructive patterns may be very difficult. It is not uncommon for people to experience depersonalization and other dissociative states as coping mechanisms when they stop their destructive patterns.

Self-Mutilation

Self-mutilation involves injuring one's own body. The behavior does not solely belong to the realm of dissociative disorders, as it may also be a symptom of a borderline, histrionic, or antisocial personality disorder (Favazza & Conterio, 1988) or may indicate autism or mental retardation.

Self-mutilation can include behaviors such as cutting, burning, hitting, head banging, biting, scratching, or other forms of bodily abuse. Most people who are self-mutilators and are not psychotic injure themselves many times and use multiple methods of self-abuse (Strong, 1993); some feel ashamed of their behavior. For example, when Judy, a woman who engaged in self-mutilation, was first admitted to hospital for routine exploratory surgery on her knee, she was asked about the many scars that horizontally crossed her left wrist and the deep round scars on her upper arm. Acting embarrassed, she stated that she had tripped and fallen on a glass.

It would be a mistake to believe that all self-mutilators are alike or that people with this disorder always try to manipulate others or kill themselves. In fact, self-mutilation differs from a suicide attempt in several important ways. For one, a self-mutilator typically uses methods which are not intentionally life-threatening. Instead, the mutilation may serve to reduce psychological tension so that the individual can continue to survive psychologically (Walsh & Rosen, 1988). Alternately, the self-destructive acts may be the only way in which a person can overcome a numbness of feeling.

A large percentage of self-mutilators were abused or molested as children. Many have eating or substance abuse disorders as well as dissociative disorders. Self-mutilation is more common in women, although in the prison population, many men have been diagnosed with this problem, and it has received more public attention with the increased acceptance of the cultural practice of tattooing (Strong, 1993). Self-mutilation sometimes occurs in "epidemics" in clinical settings such as inpatient hospitals and group homes. Walsh and Rosen (1988) state that the strongest predictor of this disorder among adolescents is body alienation (body image distortion and self-hatred), which can be a symptom of depersonalization.

Frequently, self-mutilation is a form of self-punishment for perceived wrongs or an attempt to escape extreme tension and emotional pain or numbness. People who mutilate themselves often describe episodes of intense depersonalization and **derealization**, in which they feel invisible, unreal, or dead or in which the external world appears to be caving in on, or suffocating, them. Frequently, their body parts may feel foreign or altered in shape or size. The mutilating act often serves to end an episode of depersonalization (Favazza & Conterio, 1988). The sight of blood, the pain, and the need to tend to the physical injury often serve to "jolt" the person back into reality. Moreover, by inflicting the injury, an individual may feel a renewed physical integration and be able to regain the sense of his or her body as whole and correctly proportioned (Walsh & Rosen, 1988).

Post-Traumatic Stress Disorder (PTSD)

Often, patients with DID will experience symptoms of PTSD—in particular, nightmares, intrusive thoughts and memories, and the reliving and recall of painful events from childhood. This makes sense considering the history of abuse of most patients. Often the symptoms will begin after a traumatic event, such as rape or the death of a parent (who may have been the perpetrator of abuse). The event experienced during adulthood sets off a chain of reactions in which dissociated material begins to come into consciousness.

INTERDISCIPLINARY CLINICAL INTERVENTION

Various evaluations and interventions are recognized by various disciplines in psychiatry. They may include structured interview scales, careful history gathering and observation, and psychotherapy.

Evaluation

In addition to the usual historical interview and mental status examination, the Dissociative Experiences Scale (DES) (Bernstein & Putnam, 1986) is more commonly used to learn the frequency with which dissociative or depersonalization experiences occur. It is a short, self-administered questionnaire that asks the taker to mark the frequency of dissociative or depersonalization experiences on a visual scale. This quick assessment tool may be particularly useful as professionals increasingly encounter clients in community and home health settings where they do not have the luxury of continuing contact and team support.

Dissociative identity disorder is often described as the ultimate dissociative disorder in that people with DID may have a variety or all of the other dissociative symptoms. Nonetheless, it is a difficult task to recognize and diagnose the disorder. There is professional skepticism about the existence of the disorder, and professionals have not received much information about it in their training (although this may be changing since DID has gained popularity with the general public). Often patients present with many psychiatric, neurological, and medical symptoms. A patient may have had a series of diagnoses and have received many different treatments. Because of the public controversy and increasing knowledge of the disorder, and in the interest of sound practice, thorough evaluation is important.

In taking a history from patients, certain lines of questioning can be helpful in distinguishing the dissociative disorders, especially dissociative identity disorder. Usually, questions concern time gaps and memories of important events in an individual's life, and how an individual has been viewed by others. Figure 13-6 lists an example of some specific questions.

Clinical Management

Psychotherapy, hypnosis, hospitalizations, and medicines (to a lesser extent) have traditionally been used in managing DID. Some of these forms of treatment, notably psychotherapy and hypnosis, have become sensationalized in

1. Have you ever looked at a clock at 10 in the morning and the next time you looked it was 4 in the afternoon and you don't remember anything in between?
2. Do you remember graduation from grammar or high school, the junior prom, a bar mitzvah or first holy communion?
3. Do people accuse you of lying about events or insist that you are purposely not remembering?
4. Have you ever found yourself dressed in clothes that you did not put on?

Figure 13-6. Example of Lines of Questioning for Dissociative Identity Disorder

media accounts of therapists whose licenses have been challenged and sometimes revoked. However, treating professionals still proceed according to ethical principles and the traditional methods of psychotherapy.

Psychotherapy. Psychotherapy is generally the treatment of choice for those with dissociative disorders. Psychotherapy can take from months to several years. Different therapies and techniques, including Jungian, psychoanalytic, cognitive, and behavioral approaches, have been used to treat dissociative disorders (Fike, 1990b).

In psychotherapy, the events, feelings, thoughts, sensations, or affects that are being dissociated are usually brought to conscious awareness. The psychotherapist can help the patient learn to cope with the emotionally painful experiences, memories, or thoughts that were being avoided by dissociating. For example, when asked to remember in therapy sessions, Jake initially dissociated but then gradually recalled frequent fist fights between his uncle and aunt prior to his uncle coming to tuck him in before bedtime. He remembered the fear and hurt he felt during those times.

In the case of dissociative amnesia, recovery of the lost memories is a secondary goal to that of helping the person understand and accept the feelings and conflicts that led to the loss of memory. For example, a mother who experienced dissociative amnesia after her daughter was kidnapped might, for example, be helped to acknowledge her fear, grief, and feelings of powerlessness. An acceptance of these feelings might help her cope with her situation and even avert further episodes of amnesia.

Another goal of psychotherapy for people with dissociative disorders is for them to recognize their tendency to cope with painful situations by retreating into altered states of consciousness. Realizing this fact, patients may be able to stop or diminish this pattern and therefore to deal with their problems more successfully by consciously facing their emotional conflicts.

In treating people with dissociative identity disorder, therapy generally involves helping patients become aware of their alter, or other personality, states; the roles that they serve; and the way they relate to one another; and then gradually assisting the patients in integrating their feelings and personalities into their primary, or host, personality. However, the full integration of all alter personalities is not always a therapeutic goal. The overall goals for people with dissociative identity disorder are inner cooperation and life satisfaction (Fike, 1990b).

Hypnosis.   This is sometimes used in the treatment of dissociative disorders, and it has shown some success in helping people recall lost memories after suffering from fugue or amnesia. It has been used to help people with dissociative identity disorder uncover their alter personalities or communicate between personalities. People with dissociative identity disorder tend to be able to enter hypnotic states very easily. However, the use of hypnosis in the treatment of dissociative disorders has been controversial for several reasons. First, it involves the patient turning control of her consciousness over to another person, which can be especially threatening to people who have a history of abuse and are prone to dissociative episodes. Hypnosis also, by definition, involves putting the patient into a dissociative state, which could foster the tendency to dissociate. Finally, the information brought to the patient's consciousness by hypnosis could cause extreme anxiety and thus prompt him or her to use a method of choice—more dissociation—for anxiety reduction. Hypnosis is still commonly used for therapeutic situations, especially in the treatment of dissociative identity disorder (Fike, 1990b). However, many health professionals are currently recommending more conservative methods, such as psychotherapy, because of the problems associated with hypnosis.

Hospitalization.   When people with dissociative amnesia, fugue, or depersonalization disorders are hospitalized, it is generally for psychological problems that threaten their lives or well-being, such as depression, suicidal feelings, or psychosis. Sometimes external events and problems or realizations of past abuse that have previously been hidden from their conscious memory will push patients into a state of crisis in which daily functioning seems very difficult, and they will be hospitalized to help them regain a sense of control. At times, in patients with dissociative identity disorder one of the personalities will try to harm or kill another, necessitating protective hospitalization. Occasionally patients will need hospitalization to protect themselves because of severe self-mutilation or other attempts at self-harm. Studies have shown that a significant percentage of psychiatric inpatients indicate depersonalization as one of their symptoms, although depersonalization was in no case the primary reason for admission (Brauer, Harrow, & Tucker, 1970).

In treating hospitalized patients who have dissociative disorders, the main concerns are to provide a safe environment in which they cannot harm themselves; to offer them a supportive and trusting therapeutic relationship; assist them in expressing their thoughts, feelings, and conflicts more directly; help them feel more in control of their lives; and begin the process of integrating personalities.

Pharmacological.   Medication has not proved effective as a primary treatment for any of the dissociative disorders. Some studies have shown that antipsychotic medications can even worsen dissociative symptoms and that minor tranquilizers do not seem to affect them (Brauer, Harrow, & Tucker, 1970). However, if symptoms such as anxiety or depression coexist with the dissociative disorder, antidepressants or antianxiety medication may help alleviate them. Once freed from these symptoms, the client will have more emotional resources available to focus on overcoming dissociative problems.

In patients with dissociative identity disorder, different personalities may have different physiological reactions to medications that are prescribed. For example, one personality may experience an increase in blood pressure from a medication that causes another person's blood pressure to fall. One alter may be allergic to a medication that does not affect another. As a result, medication is not a primary treatment.

OCCUPATIONAL THERAPY INTERVENTION

When working in the realm of multiple personalities, it is useful to consider traditional occupational therapy treatment in a pluralistic way. In other words, DID represents a creative way of coping that explores the furthest reaches of our minds. Consequently, it demands a creative and eclectic approach to treatment. Certain media and specific occupations (art and exploratory media, self-care, and leisure occupations) and certain theories (developmental) are "a natural" for working with DID, though others can be utilized, in particular when working with alters in addition to the host personality.

The Context of Adaptation

Dissociative disorders may be thought of in terms of adaptation. The dissociative response to stress has served an adaptive role in the patient's life in the past in that it has protected the person against the full-blown impact of intense emotional pain and trauma. By the time someone with dissociative problems is in treatment or is seen by an occupational therapist, the dissociation is no longer adaptive. It interferes with the person's ability to face and cope with reality, and thus with the ability to function.

CASE ILLUSTRATION: CECILIA— DISSOCIATION AND ADAPTATION

While Cecilia was being molested, she remembers being an observer floating above, but looking down on, the scene with detachment and, therefore, without experiencing physical or emotional pain. Throughout her molestation experience, which covered the time when she was ages 5 to 12, she successfully avoided any pain by dissociating almost effortlessly. The abuse stopped when she entered high school; however, now, at the age of 30, she cannot report any satisfying love relationships or relationships in which she feels passionate. She has begun to realize that she dissociates and "goes away" whenever she experiences strong feelings, particularly passionate ones. Her capacity to dissociate hinders her ability to form close relationships and, in fact, robs her of exhilarating and joyful experiences.

Discussion

Originally, dissociation was an adaptive defense that Cecilia used to help herself though intense traumatizing experiences. However, currently it interferes with important aspects of her life.

The occupational therapist can work with each person's strength and offer opportunities to learn new, more adaptive responses to what have been experienced as painful situations and emotions.

The Purpose of Treatment

The purpose of occupational therapy treatment for patients with dissociative disorders is twofold. Patients need first to recognize their fear of experiencing emotions and begin to allow and accept their feelings. They need to recognize formerly traumatic events that hold many conflicting, painful feelings for them. Occupational therapy and expressive and cognitive media can aid in an individual's exploration toward self-awareness. Second, occupational therapy can help people to learn new functional ways of coping when their fears interfere with functioning in daily life.

The acknowledgment and acceptance of painful emotions can be very frightening for patients with dissociative disorders, who, understandably, may have a difficult time choosing to face their difficult realities over choosing a more familiar and comfortable "escape." It takes time and the development of a trustworthy therapeutic relationship for patients to be willing to risk this change. Part of "accepting" feelings involves learning more effective ways to cope with the accompanying pain rather than escaping into an altered reality or different personality. This involves, first, learning to recognize personal patterns of dissociation—in other words, when, where, how, and under what circumstances dissociation tends to occur—in order to avoid using these old patterns when stress increases. Second, it involves relearning and learning specific new strategies for coping with stresses that may have induced the person to dissociate in the first place. The integrating of personalities means that some personalities will no longer exist as separate and distinct. Alters typically perform specific, compartmentalized functions. Talents and skills that may have resided with one alter may thus be lost, resulting in a loss of familiar ways of coping. Therefore, the newly integrated individual may have much to relearn. An individual will typically have learned to dissociate to the exclusion of learning other, adaptive ways of coping. In this case, unfamiliar, new ways of coping must be learned, and new roles may have to be taken over and learned by the remaining personality or personalities.

Occupational therapists, in conjunction with other members of the treatment team, can assist patients with dissociative disorders in all the ways described here.

The Therapeutic Approach

Occupational therapists can aid the therapy team by gathering historical information. This may often be expressed through a nonverbal medium (art, drawing, sculpting, crafts), and thus is more likely to be facilitated in the occupational therapy process than in other therapies. Through the same process, occupational therapists can learn general information about specific alter personalities, such as their names, ages, reasons why they were created, and functions they serve for the patient.

Working with patients who have dissociative disorders can be like filling in a puzzle as the therapist tries to piece together events during a period of amnesia or the personality characteristics of different alters (this is especially important in cases where an alter may be suicidal or want to harm one of the patient's other personalities). Acceptance, understanding, and avoidance of voyeuristic curiosity are essential. Coupled with a past history of severe abuse and inconsistent, unpredictable, and neglectful caregivers, demonstrating empathy, genuineness, reliability, consistency, and nondefensiveness is especially important. Working with such patients can also be personally demanding. Stories of past abuse may be difficult to hear, behaviors may confusing and slow to change, and there may be additional problems ranging from self-mutilation to substance abuse or additional character disorders. A cooperative team effort is therefore necessary to provide the best possible understanding and care of the patient while also supporting each staff member in his or her therapeutic interactions.

Methods of Intervention

Interventions include those that are generally shared by all treatment team members, such as contracting for safety, history gathering, communication with personalities, and working specifically with each personality. Interventions also may be designed according to a specific occupational therapy modality or media.

In addition to information gathering and projective evaluations, some occupational therapists will use specific occupational therapy measurements. They may follow a specific frame of reference (Fike, 1990b), or they may evaluate a specific occupational performance area or component. In the case of DID, the evaluations may be given to the host personality and other alters. Evaluating as many alters as possible not only helps fill in gaps in understanding the whole patient, it also provides information on the functional level of each alter. The occupational therapist who has this knowledge can more easily seek the cooperation of all alter personalities and can plan treatment utilizing those functions that the alters have in common.

Treating more than one personality.   An aspect of treatment unique to dissociative identity disorder is that the patient has not just one primary, encompassing, well-known personality but rather many personalities in one (some therapists, notably Milton J. Erikson, metaphorically treat alters as many different aspects of the self rather than defining them as separate personalities with distinct histories). Some therapists will ask alters to be included in treatment or in evaluations. Even if you do not specifically treat or evaluate various alters, you will no doubt meet them during **switching**, when a host personality changes into an alter. You may encounter other personalities besides the host when the person arrives at occupational therapy, or you may encounter an alter while the patient has an abreactive experience (an **abreaction** is an emotional release or discharge following recall of a painful experience that had been repressed because it was consciously intolerable). (APA, 1980, p. 1).

When an alter presents itself, there are various ways of responding, generally keeping in mind that your response and treatment should developmentally fit the age of the alter. For example, if a five-year-old alter arrives, your treatment response should be consistent with that for a five-year-old child. For example, a child alter may need simple activities that express feelings nonverbally, such as playing with dolls or coloring. If a teenage personality surfaces, you should treat him or her as you would any adolescent. For instance, crafting and tooling a leather belt would be a more appropriate activity for an angry and rebellious teenage personality. Whatever the chronological age of the alter, do not speak in a childish, demeaning way. In general, the different personalities of a patient with DID will require different occupational therapy activities.

Alters may emerge in a frightened state and not know where they are or recognize you. The occupational therapist should introduce him- or herself, explain where the patient is, and also state his or her intentions of helping the patient. Hornstein and Tyson (1991) suggest that the personalities can be addressed collectively. For example, saying, "You are all safe here," rather than just, "You are safe here," is an effective way of encouraging personality cooperation, decreasing dissociation, and validating the reality that the person remains the same no matter which alter is **out**. Similarly, if one of the personalities has superseded his or her limits and a consequence needs to be imposed, the consequence should be give even if that alter is no longer in charge of the person so that the client can be made to understand that he or she is responsible for all of the personalities and their behaviors. The occupational therapist who is familiar with the patient and comfortable doing so may ask if there are other alters who may be able to help a scared alter cope with the fear or may specifically ask for a certain alter and work with that personality. However, this may require levels of knowledge and experience not yet acquired by a new therapist; if this is not possible, it is customary to proceed with treatment for whichever alter is out. Each of these measures helps the patient feel accepted as a whole person and facilitates the integration of dissociated aspects of the self.

It is possible that occupational therapy treatment may not be able to accommodate alters in the ways suggested here. If not, as may be the case in a cooperative or verbal group of adults, the person who exhibits an alter personality who is not appropriate for this group should be safely escorted from it, usually with the aid of another staff member.

When working with people who have dissociative identity disorder, once the occupational therapist has established a therapeutic alliance and an awareness of some of the personalities, he or she can use this knowledge to help such individuals learn to cope more effectively. You can help them learn to deal with difficult situations, in which they might otherwise feel overwhelmed or unable to express certain thoughts and feelings, by calling on other, alter, personalities who can provide support and stability. If patients can internalize this skill and learn to call on the strong parts of themselves when needed, they will be well on the way to developing an integrated, whole personality.

Counteracting dissociation and depersonalization. Patients with dissociative disorders can be helped to develop a sense of control over their dissociative symptoms (including, for those with dissociative identity disorder, control over switching between alter personalities) by increasing their self-understanding and self-acceptance. As patients explore the thoughts and feelings that occur just before the dissociative episodes, they can gradually learn to tolerate those feelings and thoughts that once precipitated dissociation, which may cause their use of this response to decrease. This process may be facilitated in occupational therapy through the use of semistructured and unstructured art projects. For instance, a patient might be given an assignment to express her child alter in a clay mask or simply to draw how he or she is feeling at the time.

Patients who have experienced dissociative amnesia or fugue might be asked to express through an art medium the memories that they can access in an attempt to help them recall further. Patients who experience depersonalization might depict themselves as they feel when they are in a depersonalized state to develop better self-understanding and a reality orientation; this, in turn, will reduce fear. Often, feelings and memories will emerge for patients as they are working on creative projects. They can then share these feelings in psychotherapy, where they can be helped to accept and cope with them.

As with all patients, safety issues must be considered, particularly when working with sharp tools. Those with DID in particular may have self-destructive personalities or alters that tell them to harm themselves. They may be very sensitive to cues in their environment that may remind them of dangerous and threatening situations, and they may utilize self-harm as a way of coping with painful memories or abreactions. For example, a patient may notice that another patient always grabs for a tool when she is reaching for it, which may remind her of her older brother's domineering teasing and aggression when she was a child; she may then reach for the scissors and matter-of-factly start scratching herself with them, both to stop the memory of her brother's treatment and to vent hurt and angry feelings that she feels powerless to direct at either her brother or the other patient. Some occupational therapists will discuss these issues with patients and make contracts that specifically and concretely contract for their safety. These contracts, by virtue of their discussed and explicitly stated expectations, also enrich the context of safety, honesty, and consistency within the therapeutic relationship.

Treating self-mutilation.   Since body alienation is a strong trait in those who self-mutilate, treatment that focuses on this symptom is important. Occupational therapy can be especially useful in this area, and treatment might include training in grooming and hygiene, use of makeup, clothing selection, and overcoming distorted body images and self-hatred.

In treating self-mutilation, it is important to maintain a caring, yet matter-of-fact, attitude. A protective, worried approach that conveys either fear of the behavior or acceptance of responsibility for protecting the person from him- or herself is not effective. Equally ineffective is to take an angry, chiding approach or adopt a voyeuristic curiosity about the person's injuries (in other words, one does not need to ask to see the injuries or be told the details of how they were made). The therapist should convey the message that he or she cares about the person but knows the person is responsible for his or her own decisions and capable of making healthy ones.

A primary goal of treatment is to assist an individual to express needs more directly. Another goal is to assist those who self-mutilate to resist giving in to their impulse to hurt themselves when they feel like doing so. The first goal can be approached by role-modeling direct behavior or through assertiveness and communication training. The second goal can be addressed through developing behavioral contingency plans or by having the patient devise a list of alternative activities in which to engage when the desire to self-mutilate is strong. Sometimes a symbolic alternative, such as using a red pen instead of a sharp object to mark oneself, may counteract self-mutilation. Contracts to tell someone of the impulse can be made between a patient and trusted staff member. There are a few support groups—such as Self-Mutilators Anonymous and Self Abuse Finally Ends (SAFE)—and at the time of this writing, one inpatient hospital program exists (Hartgrove Hospital in Chicago, Illinois) for people who abuse themselves. Generally, occupational therapists can assist the individual to manage his or her behavior in these mentioned ways. However, overcoming self-mutilative behavior may require longer-term psychotherapy.

Learning new coping skills. As the personalities become more integrated and the functions of different personalities become integrated in one, the person with DID may need to learn coping skills that were formerly the province of the individual alters. Occupational therapy that addresses teaching ways of coping can be valuable. Since a primary coping method has been to dissociate in stressful or apparently life-threatening and dangerous situations, correctly identifying potential danger and discovering other adaptive methods of coping may lead to more adaptive living.

In clients with dissociative identity disorder, important life roles have often been filled by only one of the alters. For example, a woman with DID, Joan, had an alter named Hecuba who was the part of her who was employed and went to work each day, while another alter, Orestes, handled homemaking tasks. As Joan integrated the personalities, Orestes and Hecuba became less defined and it became difficult for Joan to carry out either of their functions. In the process of more effectively reintegrating personalities and roles, a patient may be expected to go through a period of even greater disintegration, extending even to social and self-care skills, as a precursor to better integration (Fike, 1990a). As an occupational therapist, you can assist patients with DID by helping them to relearn daily living skills at a more integrated level.

Expressive and exploratory. Occupational therapy group treatment for people with dissociative disorders often involves media that are expressive and symbolic, such as painting, drawing, sculpting, collage, assemblage, writing prose or poetry, and journal writing. Expressive media are useful for expression and self-exploration. Individuals with dissociative identity disorder have particular difficulty expressing themselves verbally due to having been threatened for speaking up or revealing secrets. Expressive media are helpful, especially to people with DID, because they provide a useful medium for nonverbal expression in the face of what may still be perceived as dangerous situations. Expressive media can be thought of as nonverbal or nonlinear ways of recovering and integrating memories and/or hidden or missing aspects of a person's life that had previously not been conscious or accessible. Expressive media can aid in exploring aspects of alter personalities and perhaps in sharing these aspects with other personalities. Expressive media provide a way to foster communication and to explore self-dispositions, roles, and values.

Play. Leisure occupations, which allow a person to have fun and experience a sense of well-being, are important for individuals with dissociative disorders. The occupations are closely allied with exploratory occupations in that both provide an opportunity for spontaneity and self-understanding. Most people with multiple personalities rarely experienced a safe or consistent environment while growing up or the joy and wonder of learning and growing. Due to being in therapy, such patients are also involved in very difficult work emotionally, which necessitates remembering very painful life events. Media that allow for spontaneity, play, and fun facilitate exploration and also allow the person with

DID to begin to learn that the environment can be safe and is not always threatening. Additionally, the person with dissociative identity disorder can experience the freedom and sense of competence that comes from mastery.

Self-care and activities of daily living.   Self-care occupations and activities of daily living (ADL) become important for patients with dissociative disorders as they become aware of past histories and traumas, begin to break down amnestic barriers and cope with multiple minds. Alters that have served self-care functions may be lost, and the patient may seem unable to perform adequate grooming or hygiene, appropriate dressing, and other functions. Sometimes more complex skills are lost, such as driving, managing money, or performing job-related tasks. These functions may have to be relearned by the host or other integrated personalities. The person may become depressed, confused, disoriented, or distracted because of these functional limitations. As in any activities of daily living (ADL) and self-care treatment, the occupational therapist may use various techniques to assist patients, such as practice and retraining in daily life tasks, adaptive techniques, and making schedules.

Educational.   Group treatment for people with dissociative disorders often takes a supportive educational approach in terms of teaching more effective methods for coping with stress. Such groups may teach techniques such as assertiveness training and conflict management. Self-regulatory techniques such as relaxation, managing negative thoughts with affirmations, and meditation can also be taught in a group setting. Some aspects of self-awareness training, such as developing an awareness of body movement, lend themselves to group treatment. Compared to dissociation, the exercise provided by these and similar groups can provide a more constructive outlet for some of a patient's anxiety and fear. Self-help groups, whether connected or not with occupational therapy, can also be useful treatment modalities for patients with dissociative disorders.

Trends and Research

No doubt the current debate over traditional (verbal analysis and exploration of life patterns) and nontraditional (hypnosis and altered states) treatment will continue. Perhaps future research will illuminate the success of each of these methods for specific dissociative disorders.

Perhaps because of the increasing public acknowledgment of childhood abuse, there will be fewer cases of dissociative identity disorder in the future. However, the current climate of cultural and political thinking in the last decade of the twentieth century threatens to unleash a conservative backlash against the public acknowledgment of strong feelings and events that counteract what are perceived to be American values. The current debate concerning whether patients are suffering from false memories when they make claims of childhood abuse emphasize the magnitude of the cultural forces affecting the debate.

Memories: True or false?   There has been much debate recently about recovered memories of atrocities such as child abuse and incest. One group has labeled so-called recovered memories as false memories and described a "false memory syndrome." This concept has been picked up and sensationalized by the media. Currently, patients who have accessed memories of sexual or other types of abuse through psychotherapy are confronting their parents, who often deny the abuse. The battle has reached the legal arena, with adult children suing parents for alleged abuse remembered during hypnosis or other therapeutic support and parents suing psychotherapists for allegedly encouraging their children (through suggestion) to concoct memories of mistreatment. Recently earning national attention are a number of cases in which patients reported recovering memories of repeated ritual abuse by their parents as part of a cult of satanic worship. Neither researchers nor the legislative or psychotherapeutic communities have yet demonstrated conclusively where the truth lies in these cases. As an occupational therapist it is important to avoid making judgments about patients or their family members if the whole picture is not clear, but rather to be supportive to your patients in their search for their own self-understanding.

Neural mechanisms.   It has been proposed by Peterson (1991), Li and Spiegel (1992), and Perry et al. (1995) that the development of dissociative disorders in children may include a neural selection process. Children's natural tendencies to dissociate and to use primitive defense mechanisms to avoid emotional conflicts may evolve into a preferred reaction pattern. On a physiological level, this may mean that certain nerve combinations in the brain are chosen often enough under a condition of stress that, without the person's conscious awareness, they become the preferred pathways on which impulses will travel during stress. It is possible that the brain can even form completely different neural networks for different sets of experiences without any conscious link between them. Traumatic, dissociated experiences may thus be stored in a separate network, which may be activated by stress (as when a Vietnam veteran with post-traumatic stress disorder experiences a flashback after hearing a civilian helicopter) but is not affected by conscious thought (Li & Spiegel, 1992). Further research is needed to explore this possibility in more depth. Other fruitful areas of research include investigating specific factors, such as age, gender, nature of the trauma, cognitive meaning of the event, possible presence of exacerbating or attenuating circumstances, and type of adaptive response (dissociative or hyperaroused) (Perry et al., 1995).

CASE ILLUSTRATION:
DID INPATIENT TREATMENT GOALS

Christina entered the hospital for evaluation because of a recent incident in which she had suddenly become aware of being in a strange city and was not sure how she had gotten there. She had no memory of a four-day period of time that had passed since her last memory of self-awareness.

Her primary therapist asked Christina to fill out the Dissociative Experiences Scale, which they then discussed together. During that time, the therapist also asked Christina about the continuity of her life, others' memories of her, and whether she ever heard internal voices. Christina reported significant gaps in time; for example, she was unable to remember anything about being in third grade or her graduation from high school. She acknowledged that she often experienced "people in her head" who talked to her and to each other. At these times she often would get a severe headache. She reported vague childhood memories of her uncle watching her, and she was uncomfortable around him to this day.

Christina was eventually diagnosed with dissociative identity disorder. Treatment consisted of psychotherapy with her primary psychologist, group therapy in a group for people with dissociative symptoms, family therapy, and occupational therapy groups. In her supportive group and in psychotherapy, Christina elaborated on her "people" and came to know them and be able to delineate each alter as a well-formed personality. In the occupational therapy group sessions she explored the role, functions, talents, and skills of her various alters through various expressive media. She often utilized supplies from the occupational therapy treatment space to independently explore with watercolor paints. As she participated in the occupational therapy group, Christina came to realize that an alter actually performed most of her life tasks, including her self-care. She therefore concentrated on teaching these skills to other, willing alters. In addition to integrating her alters around life tasks, through the expressive process, she became aware of, and filled in, gaps in her life history. Just before attending an occupational therapy group meeting that was to focus on one's abuse experiences and resulting dysfunctional behaviors, she became aware of the bodily sensations and thoughts that usually occurred when she dissociated. Now able to recognize and reveal these crucial sensations and thoughts, she told the OTR about them. She agreed that she would remain aware of herself in the here and now and invest herself in the occupational therapy group. Christina was now able, without dissociating, to successfully participate in the group, connect painful past abusive experiences to her current difficulties in taking care of herself, and receive some useful suggestions from the other group members.

Discussion

Inpatient treatment for Christina progressed through diagnosis and recognition and exploration of the similar aspects of her alter personalities. Occupa-

tional therapy assisted her in integrating aspects of her alters, filling in gaps in her history, and utilizing other coping mechanisms to replace dissociation.

CASE ILLUSTRATION: DID OUTPATIENT TREATMENT

Christina was referred to a partial hospitalization program upon her discharge from inpatient hospitalization. In an initial interview with the OTR, Christina stated that she had a Ph.D. in nursing science and currently managed the health department of a large corporation. She had been an effective and respected manager who was usually able to efficiently manage her time and job until the deterioration that she experienced over the last year. She also stated that she shared custody of two children from a previous marriage. She reported that she did not have many close friends but was acquainted with numerous professional colleagues. She also reported that she enjoyed outings with her family but spent most of her time working. She added that her two daughters had taken on much of the responsibility for home maintenance.

An initial occupational therapy evaluation consisted of an Allen Cognitive Level (ACL) evaluation (Allen, 1985; Allen & Allen, 1987) and an Occupational Performance History Interview. The ACL revealed no cognitive deficits: Christina scored at level 6.0, meaning she could abstractly plan and anticipate for the future. In the occupational therapy evaluation process, she indicated that she would like to become involved in some former pursuits, such as bridge. She also wished to learn new, relaxing activities, utilize the groups for learning to form friendships, and learn how to have fun and reestablish a better relationship with her children. She expressed goals of returning to work, learning how to cope with stressful situations and events, and learning how to be less of a workaholic and more social.

Christina reported that during her hospitalization she had become aware of some alters, including a child and an adolescent, a helper, and others of both genders and with various talents. With the aid of the Occupational Performance History Interview she revealed that her alters had learned some common self-care skills.

She attended the program four days per week for the first two weeks, then three days per week for the next two weeks, and finally two days a week at the program and two days at her job.

While in the program she attended group psychotherapy, individual psychotherapy, and occupational therapy. In occupational therapy she attended:

- *psychoeducational groups, which discussed the components of dissociative identity disorder and coping with dissociation and self-mutilation*

- *expressive groups, which utilized art (drawing and painting) and clay to express feelings and thoughts about various themes*

- *relaxation and stress management groups, which taught stress management techniques*

- *community task groups, which planned outings and agendas and where members provided support for each other*
- *leisure awareness groups, where she rekindled an interest in playing cards and explored various enjoyable activities with the other participants*
- *individual sessions with the occupational therapist to relearn home and family management and negotiate her return to work*

While in the program, Christina switched twice into a child alter. While her child alter was out, she was able to use occupational therapy modalities to engage in play therapy with puppets and toy figures. During the play therapy sessions, one puppet assumed Christina's emotional state and was comforted by the other puppet. Later she was able to discuss what had precipitated the experience, and the OTR reported her activities and actions to her afterwards.

At the conclusion of her program, Christina felt less overwhelmed in her life, was able to work a reduced workweek (three days), and was able to take over on home management tasks. As she became more competent at home and more sociable outside the home and workplace, her daughters worried less about her and became calmer, which caused family conflicts to decrease. She had more ideas of what situations precipitated dissociation and had developed more adaptive strategies, such as avoidance, drawing, or phoning key people who had agreed to be available to her. She also planned to attend yoga classes with her children.

Discussion

Outpatient treatment capitalized on what she had learned as an inpatient, and assisted Christina to make changes in her work, leisure, and self-care areas that included occupational components of developing intimacy in relationships and understanding herself and further expanding her ways of coping.

Summary

Dissociative disorders were first identified in the seventeenth century. Up to the present time, there has been much interest and controversy regarding the nature of dissociative disorders, particularly dissociative identity disorder. The DSM-IV lists dissociative disorders of dissociative amnesia (localized, selective, and generalized), dissociative fugue, depersonalization, and dissociative identity disorder. Often, the disorders are not distinct, and DID symptoms can also be found in other disorders. Problems that are frequently related to dissociative identity disorder include abuse, substance abuse, eating disorders, self-mutilation, and post-traumatic stress disorder.

Dissociation is an originally creative adaptation that has become obsolete and ineffective. Consequently, one purpose of treatment is to help the individual find more adaptive methods to cope with traumatic memories and events. Occupational therapy interventions focus on learning new coping skills and self-care activities of daily living through expressive and exploratory media, play, and education.

Review Questions

1. What situations or experiences may precipitate dissociation?
2. What are some methods of coping with, and preventing, dissociation?
3. What makes it possible for different alters to acquire different talents and skills?
4. What themes might be useful in expressive groups for people with DID?
5. What are some of the problems and disorders that correlate with DID? In your opinion, why are these problems or disorders prevalent in people diagnosed with DID?

Learning Activities

1. Read Lewis Carroll's *Alice in Wonderland* and *Through the Looking Glass*. Can you identify examples of depersonalization, derealization, and dissociative amnesia?
2. Read autobiographies of people with dissociative identity disorder. Note how they exerienced everyday life and what helped them function day-to-day, particularly while they were integrating their personalities.
3. Send $5 to SAFE (Self Abuse Finally Ends; c/o Hartgrove Hospital, 520 N. Ridgeway, Chicago, IL 60624) for a group outline and information on working with people who self-mutilate.
4. Empathy experiences: (a) Think of the times when you have dissociated. Was it when driving a long distance? When a conflict occurred that frightened you? When you witnessed an accident? (b) To get an idea of the concept of multiple minds, think of a time when you acted completely out of character or made statements that were totally out of character, as if someone else was talking. Think of times when you were so mad that you ran through different scripts in your head of how you would triumph over another person, while at the same time working at your desk or having lunch with friends.
5. Rent the movies *Sybil* and *The Three Faces of Eve*. If you were the occupational therapist in the inpatient treatment setting, what would you want to know about these individuals? What groups might you place them in? Which perfomance areas or components are problematic for each?

References

Allen, C. K. (1985). *Occupational therapy for psychiatric diseases: Measurement and management of cognitive disabilities*. Boston: Little, Brown.

Allen, C. K., & Allen, R. A. (1987). Cognitive disabilities: Measuring the social consequences of mental disorders. *Journal of Clinical Psychiatry, 48*, 185–191.

American Psychiatric Association. (1980). *Diagnostic and statistical manual of mental disorders* (3rd ed.). Washington, DC: Author.

American Psychiatric Association. (1994). *Diagnostic and statistical manual of mental disorders* (4th ed.). Washington, DC: Author.

Batson, R., & Stephens, G. (1989). Integrating a dissociative disorders curriculum into residency training. *Dissociation, 2*, 105–109.

Bernstein, E., & Putnam, F. W. (1986). Development, reliability and validity of a dissociation scale. *Journal of Nervous and Mental Disease, 174*, 727–735.

Brauer, R., Harrow, M., & Tucker, G. J. (1970). Depersonalization phenomena in psychiatric patients. *British Journal of Psychiatry, 117*, 509.

Favazza, A. R., & Conterio, K. (1988). The plight of chronic self-mutilators. *Community Mental Health Journal, 24*(1), 22–30.

Fike, M. L. (1990a). Clinical manifestations in persons with multiple personality disorder. *American Journal of Occupational Therapy, 44*(11), 984–990.

Fike, M. L. (1990b). Considerations and techniques in the treatment of persons with multiple personality disorder. *American Journal of Occupational Therapy, 44*(11), 999–1007.

Gilmore, M. M., & Kaufman, C. (1991). Dissociative disorders. In J. O. Cavenar (Ed.), *Psychiatry* (Vol. I, pp. 1–12). Philadelphia: J. B. Lippincott.

Hornstein, N. L., & Tyson, S. (1991). Inpatient treatment of children with multiple personality/dissociative disorders and their families. *Psychiatric Clinics of North America, 14*(3), 631–648.

Jacobs, D. F. (1988). Evidence for a common dissociative-like reaction among addicts. *Journal of Gambling Behavior, 4*(1), 27–37.

Kielhofner, G., & Henry, A. D. (1988). Development and investigation of an occupational performance history interview. *American Journal of Occupational Therapy, 42*(8), 489–498.

Li, D., & Spiegel, D. (1992). A neural network model of dissociative disorders. *Psychiatric Annals, 22*(3), 144–147.

Perry, B. D., Pollard, R. A., Blakley, T. L., Baker, W. L., & Vigilante, D. (1995, winter). Childhood trauma, the neurobiology of adaptation and "use dependent" development of the brain: How "states" become "traits." *Infant Mental Health Journal, 16*(4), 271–291.

Peterson, G. (1991). Children coping with trauma: Diagnosis of "dissociation identity disorder." *Dissociation, 4*(3), 152–164.

Putnam, F. W. (1989). *Diagnosis and treatment of multiple personality disorder*. New York: Guilford.

Putnam, F. W. (1991). Dissociative disorders in children and adolescents: A developmental perspective. *Psychiatric Clinics of North America, 14*(3), 519–531.

Schwartz, E. D., & Perry, B. D. (1994, June). The post-traumatic response in children and adolescents. *Psychiatric Clinics of North America, 17*(2), 311–326. (From PsychoInfo: Abstract No. 14)

Strong, M. (1993). A bright red scream. *San Francisco Focus, 40*(11), 58–65, 135–144.

Walsh, B. W., & Rosen, P. M. (1988). *Self-mutilation: Theory, research, and treatment.* New York: Guilford Press.

Suggested Readings

Hacking, I. (1995). *Rewriting the soul: Multiple personality and the science of memory.* Princeton, NJ: Princeton University Press.

Multiple personality disorder from the inside out. (1991). Baltimore, MD: Sidman Press.

Phillips, J. (1995). *The magic daughter: A memoir of living with multiple personality disorder.* New York: Viking.

Sizemore, C. C. (1989). *A mind of my own: The woman who was known as Eve tells the story of her triumph over multiple personality disorder.* New York: Morrow.

Personality Disorders

Elizabeth Cara

Key Terms

ego syntonic
"hardwired"
personality

splitting
traits

Chapter Outline

Introduction

For many beginning health care professionals, the term *personality disorder* strikes fear in their hearts, conjuring up images of manipulative people who are resistant to treatment. Students have heard negative stories of "borderlines" who leave a mass of angry and drained professionals in their wake, wreak havoc with the staff, and are untreatable by anyone. At the same time, in reading about the range of personality disorders, students often identify their own behavior. It is not uncommon when they encounter an individual with a personality disorder to wonder how the patient differs or why he or she needs treatment when they, presumably, do not. The difference between the myth and the real-life encounter adds to the confusion. Additionally, it is rare to find information specifically concerning personality disorders in the occupational therapy literature. It is no wonder that the treatment of individuals with personality disorders is often confusing, sometimes frightening, and frequently difficult to grasp.

There are other reasons why it is difficult to understand and treat people with personality disorders. Unlike most mental disorders, the varied personality disorders are defined solely based on behavior patterns and personality traits. Personality disorders do not represent a clear symptomatic picture or disease but rather are determined by interactive patterns, coping skills, and adaptive capacity (Millon, 1996). The main features of personality disorders are enduring and persistent personality traits. Moreover, the very terms **traits** and **personality** are abstract and ill-defined, and personality is still a vague and controversial concept (Ratey, 1995).

The term personality is a perilous one. Personality is one of the most abstract words in our language, and like any abstract word suffering from excessive use, its connotative significance is very broad, its denotative significance negligible. Scarcely any word is more versatile. (Allport, cited in Millon, 1996, p. 12).

An individual with a personality disorder may display fluctuating behavior. He or she may function with enough stability to manage everyday living, then quickly seem to become unstable and dysfunctional, and then, just as quickly, recover following an emotional crisis. This cycle occurs in a regular and periodic pattern. Because the problems often manifest in the social and interpersonal realm of living (as a result of ill-timed or maladaptive coping strategies), other people can quickly become part of the emotional crisis, even while remaining unaware of the underlying personality disorder. For example, you may wonder how your friend gets himself into such a bind, when anyone else would resolve it successfully or simply avoid the situation. You may feel resentful of your friend's continuing need for help yet respond because you believe that friends must help each other. Suppose, for example, that John often parks in no-parking lanes, has his car towed, and fails to pay the tickets, so that warrants are issued for his arrest. He often calls Ellen to ask for money or to borrow her car, as if he were unaware of his role in losing his own car. Ellen often feels annoyance over his demands and seeming lack of concern, but since she considers herself John's friend, she accedes to his demands.

Different types of information written about personality disorders is often presented as fact when it is actually based on the writers' varied theoretical concepts. "The totality of personality is today increasingly conceptualized through the lens of particular perspectives" (Millon, 1996, p. 3). The different concepts and theories help a reader to focus and integrate observations, but they are potentially confusing because they are not explicit. Table 14-1 lists various theories concerning personality disorders. This chapter presents a view primarily stemming from a biopsychosocial/evolutionary theory and utilizing cognitive, interpersonal, and behavioral interventions. Much of the information in the chapter pertains primarily to a specific disorder, borderline personality disorder, because this disorder is most likely to be encountered in mental health and other settings.

Individuals with personality disorders can indeed be treated, and occupational therapy, with its focus on adaptive functioning and behavior in everyday life, can be helpful. In fact, individuals with personality disorders often are bright, charming, and creative. Because of the challenges and opportunities for self-learning that may occur in treatment, they can be rewarding and gratifying clients.

Because occupational therapy focuses on adaptive function and behavior in everyday life, it is a very important aspect of treatment. The methods and

Table 14-1. Theories of Personality Disorders

Biophysical Anticipate that chemical deficiencies or other defects will be found that account for symptoms. Just as physical disease represents a disease of the organ system that manifests in the realm of the physical body, psychological disease reflects central nervous system disruptions that will manifest in the realm of behavior, emotions, and thought (Kaplan & Sadock, 1995).

Neuropsychiatric Recognize the influence of the neurobiological system on mood and behavioral symptoms. Neuroanatomical (functional) and neurochemical (operational) aspects are assessed to determine how they are causing or amplifying symptoms. It holds that intrinsic dispositions are modifiable by medicine, environments can be changed, and biological factors underlie some dimensions of personality disorders (Ratey, 1995).

Psychodynamic Emphasize the impact of early experiences and past events. Early theories were based on the idea of instinctual, dammed-up energy and conflict within the ego, id, and superego. Contemporary theories focus on the infant-caregiver environment. Problems in personality are due to unconscious defensive maneuvers that were originally protective and most likely result from deprivation (Kaplan & Sadock, 1995; Millon, 1996).

Behavioral Emphasize environmental influences and learning from the social environment (Kaplan & Sadock, 1995).

Cognitive Individuals react to the world depending on their perception of it. A person's way of construing the world determines behavior. Dysfunctional feelings and behaviors reflect biased schemas and result in repetitive interpersonal errors (Millon, 1996).

Interpersonal Personality is understood in terms of recurrent interpersonal tendencies that shape and perpetuate styles of behavior, thought, and feeling. There are maladaptive causal sequences between interpersonal perceptions, behavior and others' reactions. Sequences are often activated in inappropriate situations (Millon, 1996).

Biopsychosocial/Evolutionary An interaction of biology and environment determines whether traits become disorders. In the presence of psychological risk factors such as trauma, loss, or inadequate parenting, personality traits tend to be amplified. Also called predisposition stress theory (Paris, 1994). Newer theory looks at how disorders represent maladaptive functions due to inability to relate in the environment (Millon, 1996).

Neurobiological/Temperaments Biological constitutional dispositions are central to understanding personality disorders. Attempt to break down constituents of temperament that underlie personality traits (Millon, 1996).

strategies grounded in occupations provide opportunities to modify behavior. Because problems manifest in both the social and interpersonal realms, it is necessary for the therapist to be competent not only in occupational treatment methods, but also in the use of self and interpersonal communication. Therefore, a willingness to reflect and understand oneself, including one's conscious and unconscious motivations, values, thoughts, feelings, and responses, is vitally important for the occupational therapist (see Chapter 1, "The Occupational Therapy Process in Mental Health," for a discussion of the self and interpersonal skills).

THE PERSONALITY CONTINUUM

A brief review of what is entailed in the concept of personality will help to clarify what is meant by a "disorder" or "dysfunction" of personality. Personality could be considered to comprise a person's lifelong style of relating, coping, behaving, thinking, and feeling. The concept represents a network of traits that emerge from a matrix of biological dispositions and experiential learning, persist over extended periods of time, and characterize the individual's distinctive manner of relating in the environment (Millon, 1996).

Every individual possesses a small and distinct group of primary traits that persist and endure and that exhibit a high degree of consistency across situations. These enduring (stable) and pervasive (consistent) characteristics make up a person's personality. The personality pattern, that is, the repertoire of coping skills and adaptive flexibilities, will determine whether a person will master his or her psychosocial environments. Millon (1996) views personality as composed of three polarities: positive versus negative, self versus other, and active versus passive. These polarities represent an individual's survival mode. That is, people will be motivated by the type of reinforcement they seek, whether the pursuit of pleasure or the avoidance of pain, relying on self or others for support and nurturing, and behaving in an active and controlling, or more accommodating and reactive, way (Millon, 1996; Retzlaff, 1995).

Those people whose personality patterns do not permit consistent mastery of the psychosocial environment can be distinguished from their normal counterparts by:

- adaptive inflexibility and poor choices of behavior
- a tendency to foster vicious circles
- tenuous stability under stressful conditions

See Table 14-2 for a description of maladaptive personality patterns.

Problems of personality thus include stable and consistent traits that are not easily changed, are exhibited inappropriately and in situations in which they are not warranted, and foster vicious cycles of behavior that are difficult to stop and perpetuate and intensify already-present difficulties (Millon, 1981). Daily life activities and interactions cause overwhelming stress. This

Table 14-2.	Maladaptive Personality Patterns
Pattern	*Description*
Adaptive Flexibility	Interpersonal strategies for relating to others, achieving goals and coping with stress are limited and practiced rigidly. Choices of behavior often do not match the situation in which they are used.
Vicious Circles	Person's choices elicit similar rigid or extreme responses from others. Little understanding of poor choices and how the "wrong" behaviors have "pulled" for other's responses. Consequently, there is little awareness of responsibility for the interactions and inability to change behavior. This sets into motion additional poor choices of behavior and self-defeating sequences with others, which cause already-established difficulties not only to persist but to be aggravated further.
Tenuous Stability	Lack of resilience in conditions perceived as stressful, causing extreme susceptibility to new difficulties and disruptions and reversion to familiar, maladaptive ways of coping. There is lessened control over emotions and a tendency toward developing increasingly distorted perceptions of reality.

Source: Adapted from Millon (1981).

triggers maladaptive responses, which further heighten the stress and preclude obtaining support or help from others. Thus the vicious circle is put in motion (see Figure 14-1). The individual with a personality disorder lacks the flexibility to choose from a broad range of interpersonal behaviors. He or she may rigidly rely on the same interpersonal behavior or choose an extreme form of behavior that is not warranted in every situation. These poor behavioral choices in turn elicit constricted and extreme responses from others. Finally, the person with a personality disorder is unaware of his or her poor choices and does not understand how the "wrong" behaviors have elicited others' responses (see Figure 14-1). Consequently, there is little awareness of responsibility for the interactions and a resultant inability to change interpersonal behavior (Kiesler, 1986).

An important feature in the disordered personality that complicates understanding and treatment is that what therapists consider abnormal personality traits and patterns generally are perceived as appropriate by the individual. This is often described as an **ego-syntonic** feeling—it "feels right" to the individual. Most people would feel troubled if they were labile, persistently distorted reality, were involved in chaotic and troublesome interactions with others, failed to engage in or were neglected in relationships, and seemed unable to understand or express empathy for others. In these situa-

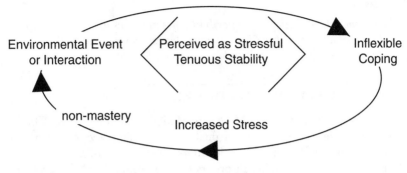

Figure 14-1. Vicious Circle

Source: Millon (1996). Reprinted by permission of John Wiley and Sons.

tions, most people would seek help or at least talk to someone they trusted. However, for an individual with a personality disorder, it seems that these traits and patterns are not overly disturbing, troublesome, or strange. Chaos may seem strangely untroubling and part of everyday life. This may be because an individual's strategies and behavior have been determined by haphazard and casual events in the environment to which he or she has been exposed. "The particulars and coloration of many pathological patterns have their beginnings in the offhand behaviors and attitudes to which the child is incidentally exposed" (Millon, 1996, p. 112). Moreover, some behaviors also feel as if they make sense because they are **"hardwired"** into an individual's neurological makeup (Ratey, 1995). If certain strategies and behaviors have been learned and have neurological substrates, they will tend to "feel right."

CASE ILLUSTRATION: ROBYN—BORDERLINE PERSONALITY DISORDER WITH DISABLING PROBLEMS

Robyn was pleased with her new love of four months, James. It seemed that this relationship was a dream come true. Since the two met they had spent almost every night together, sometimes going out, but often just spending time alone. Robyn said that she finally felt that she could trust someone.

About four months into the relationship, however, Robyn became enraged and hung up on James after he called to cancel a date because he was required to work overtime (environmental event). *She refused to answer his messages or to answer calls from friends. She even started refusing to leave her apartment for awhile* (maladaptive coping response) *and began thinking that maybe James was cheating on her* (distorted thinking). *Robyn began to doubt her perception of the previous four months. She experienced familiar feelings that she could only describe as painful. She began to think that cutting herself would be the only way to release the pain* (further aggravation of difficulties).

Discussion

Robyn demonstrated adaptive inflexibility, poor choices of behavior, tenuous stability, and a tendency to foster vicious circles. Her problems did not necessarily feel strange or "weird" to her.

THE DSM-IV PERSONALITY DISORDERS

The Diagnostic and Statistical Manual of Mental Disorders (DSM-IV)(APA, 1994) lists general criteria for a personality disorder and recognizes common features in some of the individual disorders (see Figure 14-2).

The individual personality disorders can be grouped or "clustered" according to similar features (see Table 14-3). OTRs specifically tailor interventions for the domains of expressive acts, interpersonal conduct, cognitive style, self-image, and regulatory mechanisms. The three clusters follow a dimensional perspective, that is:

> The personality disorders represent maladaptive variants of personality traits that merge imperceptibly into normality or into one another . . . [though] the relationship of the various dimensional models to the personality disorder diagnostic categories and to various aspects of personality dysfunction remains under active investigation. (pp. 633–634)

A. An enduring pattern of inner experience and behavior that deviates markedly from the expectations of the individual's culture. This pattern is manifested in two (or more) of the following areas:
  (1) cognition (i.e., ways of perceiving and interpreting self, other people, and events)
  (2) affectivity (i.e., the range, intensity, lability, and appropriateness of emotional response)
  (3) interpersonal functioning
  (4) impulse control
B. The enduring pattern is inflexible and pervasive across a broad range of personal and social situations.
C. The enduring pattern leads to clinically significant distress or impairment in social, occupational, or other important areas of functioning.
D. The pattern is stable and of long duration and its onset can be traced back at least to adolescence or early adulthood.
E. The enduring pattern is not better accounted for as a manifestation or consequence of another mental disorder.
F. The enduring pattern is not due to the direct physiological effects of a substance (e.g., a drug of abuse, a medication) or a general medical condition (e.g., head trauma).

Figure 14-2. General Diagnostic Criteria for a Personality Disorder

Table 14-3.	Expression of Personality Disorders across the Domains of Clinical Science				

Domain/ Disorder	Expressive Acts	Interpersonal Conduct	Cognitive Style	Self-Image	Regulatory Mechanisms
Paranoid	defensive	provocative	autistic	inviolable	projection
Schizoid	impassive	unengaged	impover- ished	complacent	intellectual- ization
Schizotypal	eccentric	secretive	autistic	estranged	undoing
Antisocial	impulsive	irresponsible	deviant	autonomous	acting-out
Borderline	spasmodic	paradoxical	capricious	uncertain	regression
Narcissistic	haughty	exploitive	expansive	admirable	rational- ization
Avoidant	fretful	aversive	distracted	alienated	fantasy
Dependent	incompetent	submissive	naive	inept	introjection
Obsessive- Compulsive	disciplined	respectful	constricted	conscientious	reaction formation

Note: Expressive acts are the observed verbal and behavioral actions of a person that reveal certain dimensions such as competence, incompetence, self-control or lack of self-control, and so forth.

Interpersonal conduct is a style of relating to others, methods in which others are engaged, and ways of coping with tension or conflict.

Cognitive style is how a person perceives events, focuses or allocates attention, encodes, and processes information, and organizes thoughts.

Regulatory mechanisms are usually unconscious processes determining how one gratifies oneself, resolves internal conflicts, and generally copes to maintain personal stability.

Self-image is the perception of self as distinct, ongoing, cohesive; self-identity involves having a consistent sense of who one is.

Domain/ Disorder	Object Representations	Morphologic Organization	Mood/ Temperament
Paranoid	unalterable	inelastic	irascible
Schizoid	meager	undifferentiated	apathetic
Schizotypal	chaotic	fragmented	distraught
Antisocial	debased	unruly	callous
Borderline	incompatible	split	labile
Narcissistic	contrived	spurious	insouciant
Avoidant	vexatious	fragile	anguished
Dependent	immature	inchoate	pacific
Obsessive-Compulsive	concealed	compartmentalized	solemn

Source: Adapted with permission from Millon (1996).

Note: Object representations are memories, attitudes, and affects that are organized and serve as a base for how one perceives and reacts to life events; they include representations of significant figures and relationships.

Morphologic organization refers to the overall cohesion of one's internal self.

Mood/temperament comprises an individual's affect and intensity and the frequency with which it is expressed in level of activity, speech, and physical appearance.

Personality disorder clusters have also been described based on other dimensions (Millon, 1996). These other clusters are also described in Table 14-4. (See Table 14-5 for a more detailed list of essential features, the clinical picture, and general interpersonal approaches for the individual disorders [Kaplan & Sadock, 1995] according to their DSM-IV clusters.)

Table 14-4. DSM-IV and Other Personality Disorder Clusters

DSM-IV Classifications

Odd-Eccentric (Cluster A)	*Dramatic-Emotional (Cluster B)*	*Anxious-Fearful (Cluster C)*
Paranoid	Antisocial	Avoidant
Schizoid	Borderline	Dependent
Schizotypal	Histrionic	Obsessive-Compulsive
	Narcissistic	

Other Classifications

Pleasure Deficient/Detached	Interpersonally Imbalanced	Structurally Defective	Intrapsychically Conflicted
Schizoid	Dependent	Schizotypal	Obsessive-compulsive
Avoidant	Narcissistic	Borderline	
	Antisocial	Paranoid	
	Histrionic		
Characteristic isolation from external support systems and few interpersonal sources of support; thus disposed to be increasingly isolated, preoccupied, and depressed.	Primarily oriented to others (referred to as dependent) or toward themselves and their own needs (referred to as independent). They either consistently seek out others or are oriented to behave always in their own favor.	Socially incompetent, difficult to relate to, and often isolated, confused and hostile; thus, they are unlikely to elicit support that can help them be more effective. Personality organization and behavior mitigates against adaptation.	Split between orienting themselves toward others or self and maintaining an independent or dependent stance. Consequently, they often reverse interpersonal behaviors and feel internally divided.

Source: Millon (1996).
Note: Millon (1996) groups the disorders according to dimensions that include both an internal and external perspective; that is, he views the person from what may be happening internally or intrapsychically as well as how he or she interacts with others and believes that both internal personality makeup and external interpersonal behavior combine to manifest the disorder.

Table 14-5. Essential Features, Clinical Picture, and General Approach for the Various Disorders

	Paranoid	*Schizoid*	*Schizotypal*
Essential Features	Long-standing suspicion and mistrust. Responsibility often refused and assigned to others.	Social withdrawal, discomfort in interactions. Eccentric, constricted emotions.	Strikingly odd and strange. Difficulty in close relationships. Closest to illusions, like schizophrenia, but not psychotic.
Clinical Picture	Very moralistic, hypersensitive. Can easily spot others' vulnerabilities. Personalizes coincidental events. Hypervigilant, tense, humorless. Fears both intimacy and rejection.	Aloof, reserved, reclusive in everyday events but may have imagined life of closeness.	Hypervigilant to others' feelings but not their own. Superstitious, unusual uses and meanings of words. Shun relationships. Diminished ability to experience pleasure.
General Approach	Courtesy, honesty, respect, serious, without defensiveness.	Courtesy, honesty, respect. Tolerance of silence and whatever degree of involvement they present. Initiating.	Respect, tolerant attitude. Curiosity but not confrontation or too much fascination with strange beliefs.

	Borderline	*Narcissistic*	*Histrionic*	*Antisocial*
Essential Features	Pattern of: unstable mood, behavior, relationships, self-image, impulsivity.	Lack of empathy, exaggerated sense of importance or specialness. Indifference to others' feelings. Alternate between idealizing and devaluing.	Flamboyant, dramatic, excitable, over emotional. Shallow relationships.	Disregard for or violation of rights of others. Often behavior results in imprisonment or court appearance. Lack of remorse Irresponsibility.
Clinical Picture	When in crisis may show anger, anxiety,	Depression not fitting to event.	Temper tantrums, accusations.	Seeming lack of anxiety or depression not

(continues)

Table 14-5. Essential Features, Clinical Picture, and General Approach for the Various Disorders (continued)

	Borderline	Narcissistic	Histrionic	Antisocial
	depression and expression of feelings of emptiness. Unpredictable behavior, self-destructive acts, dependent or hostile behavior. May perceive rejection when it isn't warranted. Difficulty being alone and desperate attachments.	Immature behavior indifference to others feelings. Tendency to overreact with rage or shame to perceived criticism. Preoccupation with own feelings of inferiority. Sudden attachment and rejection with others.	Seductive or provocative behavior, though seem unaware of it. Command the center of attention, and will be very disappointed if someone else is more noticeable.	fitting to the situation. Seem charming to the same sex, manipulative to the opposite sex.
General Approach	Support and reality testing in a cognitive-behavioral way. Provide calmness and consistency, without being drawn into rescuing or power struggles.	Setting firm limits, interpreting behavior or understanding and support of idealization. Consistency, matter-of-fact approach.	Identification of one's thoughts and feelings. Do not get caught up in the tendency to embellish emotions.	Limit setting, understanding, and acceptance when anxious. Group treatment with peers.

	Avoidant	Dependent	Obsessive-Compulsive
Essential Features	Extreme sensitivity to rejection, extreme shyness	Tendency to subordinate one's own needs to those of others. Get others to assume responsibility for major areas of one's life.	Constricted emotions, orderliness, perseverance, stubbornness, indecisiveness and rigidity, difficulty expressing warmth.
Clinical Picture	Lacks confidence Uncertain, hypervigilant re rejection. May have an ingratiating, waif-like quality.	Pessimism, self-doubt, fear of expressing feelings, passive. Avoid responsibility. Easier to initiate tasks for someone else than themselves.	Preoccupation with lists, details, minor problems. Few friends, fear of making mistakes, time spent with rituals. Boring conversation.

(continues)

			Obsessive-
	Avoidant	*Dependent*	*Compulsive*
General Approach	Respectful, honest, warm, accepting.	Accept initial dependency, but resist assuming responsibility. Gradually expect and require independent problem solving and actions. Use Socratic questioning method.	Accepting of frankly boring conversation. Interrupt when possible. Focus on feelings whenever possible and provide opportunities for spontaneity.

Table 14-5. Essential Features, Clinical Picture, and General Approach for the Various Disorders (continued)

Source: Information adapted from Kaplan and Sadock (1995).

Cultural Controversy

Controversies based on gender bias and cultural considerations surround some of the personality disorder diagnoses. For example, at least three times more women than men are diagnosed in inpatient samples. A continuing debate surrounds the issue of gender labeling. Some of the very negative criteria that enable one to make the diagnosis are often considered "normal" female behavior. An example is the following operative definition for inclusion in borderline personality disorder: affective instability, marked shifts from baseline mood to depression, irritability or anxiety. Borderline personality characteristics are accepted as more congruent with male sex roles and therefore more tolerable in men than in women (Gibson, 1990). At the same time, personality characteristics that are more congruent with male sex roles and less so with female sex roles, such as overt aggression, are not included in personality disorders. In other words, we have a diagnosis—borderline personality disorder—that is assigned to mostly women based on impulsive behavior and labile affect, which are traits usually ascribed to females rather than males, but there is no diagnosis (such as "overaggressive personality disorder") assigned to mostly men based on aggressive behavior and angry affect, the traits usually ascribed to males.

In other countries, some of the features of personality disorders may not be considered pathological (Alarcon & Foulks, 1995). Particularly since personality disorders are, by definition, based on interpersonal function, how one is perceived to behave in the social field brings into play cultural values. For example, in countries outside the United States, the features of schizotypal, avoidant, or dependent personality may have to be much more extreme to be considered deviant. The features are more deviant in the United States, where they are embedded in a more materialistic culture with strong values of individualism. Moreover, some diagnostic criteria, such as paranoia, may be the result of enculturation. For example, members of minority groups, immigrants, and political and economic refugees may act defensively to perceived indifference. Language barriers and general lack of knowledge of the rules of the majority may create guarded behaviors that are misperceived as suspicious. Similarly, a reaction to moving from a small rural area to a large urban one may involve emotional "freezing," which could be misperceived as a schizoid symptom. Alarcon and Foulks call for recognizing cultural contextualization when working with an individual with a personality disorder. This means " to put into a local and cultural perspective each and every behavior presented by a potential patient as well as each and every evaluative technique or clinical approach" (1995, p. 5).

Clinical Picture

Millon (1996) describes personality types according to various other domains (see Table 14-4) that give the clinician a better idea of the features of personality disorders. His system gives a comprehensive picture and enables disorders to be compared and contrasted with each other. It also allows the OTR to tailor interventions for the specific domains of expressive acts, interpersonal conduct, cognitive style, self-image, and regulatory (coping) mechanisms.

In a treatment setting the maladaptive patterns and characteristics of people with personality disorders, particularly those diagnoses listed in cluster B (Dramatic-Emotional) can evoke predictable, similar, and troubling responses from the treating therapist or staff. Due to inflexible responses to stress, seemingly minor events may be perceived as very stressful. The individual may respond to a nonexistent problem in what seems to be an immature way. This may happen repeatedly. See Table 14-5 for a description of clinical features for all the personality disorders.

Because cluster B disorders may be seen in a clinic setting more often than the others, the following discussion will focus on that cluster.

CASE ILLUSTRATION: JEAN, LOTUS, AND CASEY— INFLEXIBLE RESPONSES TO STRESS

When the occupational therapist ended a group 10 minutes early due to an impromptu meeting, Jean (diagnosis: narcissistic personality disorder) became teary and angry, protesting that she was overlooked, no longer felt safe in the group, and could not possibly return. Lotus (diagnosis: schizoid personality disorder) was nonchalant, said nothing, and left unnoticed. Casey (diagnosis: obsessive-compulsive personality disorder) talked about the necessity of cleaning up and ritualistically ordered and reordered the project he had been working on.

Discussion

Jean, Lotus, and Casey's reponses to stress were each inflexible, however, each person functioned differently in accordance with the symptoms of his or her specific disorder.

Individuals may display a capacity to "get under the skin" of others. People may find themselves caught up in the life of the person with a personality disorder. Others may feel "stuck" in thinking too much about the individual. All of which can lead to a sense of failure to help someone. For example, in the case of Jean, Lotus, and Casey, the occupational therapist found himself thinking about them for the rest of the afternoon. He questioned whether he should have ended the group early and if he had adequately explained why he was doing so. He wondered if his treatment was effective. He felt guilty concerning Jean, annoyed concerning Casey, and detached concerning Lotus.

In a treatment setting, the relationships with staff of a person with a personality disorder often become strained or conflictual. A parallel process may happen among the staff. This may be due to an individual's tendency to treat some staff in an idealized way, with intense admiration and complete cooperation, and to treat other staff in a denigrating way, showing disdain and avoidance and acting as if they were almost invisible. This may play into one professional's wishes to be helpful and saving or provoke rejecting behavior and attendant guilt from another for not being helpful enough. Conflict begins when unspoken feelings, such as envy, jealousy, or anger, prompt behavior in which some staff members defend a patient, while others complain about the him or her. Working relationships in the staff will be disrupted, and the staff members may turn away from the patient. This situation is especially likely to occur with a novice therapist due to lack of experience in understanding the situation, desire to be a "good" therapist and do the right thing, inability to examine his or her own personal motives and needs, or fear of appearing vulnerable when speaking with the other staff members.

When this situation manifests itself with more than one individual or with a staff member, it is called **splitting**. This can be counteracted if the staff members anticipate the splitting process, strive to understand the internal feelings of the client, and recognize that he or she is not acting in this way deliberately. (The neuropsychiatric approach discusses the difference between "can't," implying difficulties in biological structure and operations, and "won't," implying deliberate will [Fogel & Ratey, 1995]). Staff members must also remain aware of their own internal feelings and discuss them openly with each other. They may also model certain responses for the client. Responses should: (1) indicate that no one is all good or bad; rather, each of us has both strengths and limitations; (2) aid the patient in becoming aware of the tendency to categorize people in a black and white way; and (3) accept the expression of both positive and negative aspects in the patient, in oneself, and in other staff members. That is, it is important not to moralize or say that behavior is unacceptable or inappropriate, and rather to provide some understanding of the client's process.

Related Problems

Personality disorders are defined on axis II of the DSM-IV; however, there also exist relationships to axis I disorders and to other problems (Ruegy & Frances, 1995). For example, it is not uncommon to encounter a related diagnosis of major depression. In fact, Allen (1985) believes that personality disorders are social disorders that result from coping with lifelong depression. Studies have indicated that 36 to 76 percent of those with a remitted mood disorder had at least one personality disorder (Ruegy & Frances, 1995).

Other syndromes and symptoms commonly occurring with personality disorders are substance abuse or addiction, eating disorders, post-traumatic stress syndrome due to childhood abuse and neglect, anxiety disorders, and a tendency for self-abuse and mutilation. Currently, information points to childhood abuse and neglect as occurring in a high percentage (59–70 percent) of individuals with personality disorders. A large minority of those with eating disorders have a personality disorder, and 40 percent of those with a personality disorder also have bulimia. Between 36 and 76 percent of those with anxiety disorders are estimated to also have a personality disorder (mostly avoidant, dependent, obsessive-compulsive, schizotypal, or paranoid). In addition, some studies (listed in Ruegy & Frances, 1995) support a clinical impression that there is a connection of cluster B and chronic pain, conversion (symptoms that affect motor or sensory functioning that cannot be explained by neurological or physical conditions [APA, 1994]), and somatoform symptoms (a variety of physical complaints, such as chronic fatigue, gastrointestinal symptoms or loss of appetite, that cannot be explained by any known physical condition [APA, 1994]). Treatment may address problems or behavioral patterns that result from these symptoms (see Chapters 8, 10, 13, and 17 for further discussion). A knowledge of attendant factors in the etiology of personality disorders can also aid in further understanding behavior.

INTERDISCIPLINARY ASSESSMENT AND TREATMENT

Assessment usually consists of self-report inventories, projective techniques, and structured clinical interviews (Millon, 1996). Well-known psychological assessments include the Millon Clinical Multiaxial Inventory–III (MCMI-III), the Minnesota Multiphasic Personality Inventory (MMPI-2), the Rorschach Test, and the Thematic Apperception Test. Clinical interviews geared to the DSM criteria include the Structured Clinical Interview for DSM (SCID) and the Structured Interview for DSM Personality Disorders-Revised (SIDP-R) (cited in Millon, 1996).

Treatment generally consists of long-term or intense outpatient psychotherapy, group psychotherapy, day or therapeutic community treatment, and, possibly, inpatient treatment for times of crisis. More recently, short ter. therapy has been proven successful (Ruegy & Frances, 1995; Linehan, Armstrong, Suarez, Allmon, & Heard, 1991; Linehan, Heard, & Armstrong, 1993; Millon, 1996; Retzlaff, 1995). In the past these disorders were most prevalent in inpatient settings, but currently it can be expected that they will be encountered universally. Therefore, the treatment suggestions in this chapter apply to all settings. Crisis situations may be precipitated by troubles in relationships and adapting to life changes and also by resultant depression, suicidal thoughts, and impulsive behavior.

Although medicines may be in order if there are symptoms of major depression, anxiety, or psychotic episodes along with a personality disorder, psychotropic medicine is generally not helpful for alleviating enduring personality traits. In fact, drugs are given judiciously due to the potentials for suicide and polydrug abuse. Currently, neurotransmitter studies focus on serotonin, dopamine, and norepinephrine (Ratey, 1995; Ruegy & Frances, 1995). It is believed that serotonin deficits may be implicated in suicide and impulsively violent behavior and may be linked to impulsivity in general.

Due to the potential for staff splitting, maintaining a consistent approach and constant clear communication between and among all treating professionals is a necessity.

Interpersonal Approach

Table 14-6 lists general interpersonal treatment approaches that are useful guides for all practitioners, including occupational therapists, when interacting with individuals with character disorders (recognizing however, that each person and performance context is unique). In occupational therapy, activity and daily living groups promote a focus on here-and-now behavior, encourage thinking sequentially and anticipating consequences, and facilitate inter-

Table 14-6. General Interpersonal Treatment Approaches

Useful Concepts for Interaction

Establish a collaborative stance.

Provide understanding instead of giving advice.

Confront defensive behavior in a supportive atmosphere by focusing on the clients' demonstrated behavior instead of your judgment of it.

Provide consistency in the structure of your program and behavior and in limit setting.

Encourage membership in social support groups.

Whenever possible, assist the client to think through the consequences of actions.

Sincerely express pleasure in the individual's attempts to change and grow.

personal relating, adaptive coping, and realistic thinking. Because problems are manifested in the interpersonal realm, attention to the interpersonal approach is important.

OCCUPATIONAL THERAPY TREATMENT INTERVENTIONS

There are many character disorders, and each cluster is distinguished by certain features. Discussing treatment for each individual disorder is beyond the scope of this text, however, this section will discuss treatment directed towards the cluster B disorders, which are most often encountered in treatment settings. Generally, in addition to an interpersonal approach, treatment consists of making behavioral, cognitive, and social interventions, such as practicing adaptive coping strategies, learning to think before acting, paying attention to emotional style, learning to develop satisfying relationships, and developing a sense of effectiveness in the world—defined as personal causation (Kielhofner, 1995)—or sense of self-identity. These interventions correspond to the domains described by Millon (1996) and shown in Table 14-4.

A common general purpose of an occupational therapy treatment program is to create a safe, interesting, and playful context for treatment (Barris, Kielhofner, & Watts, 1988) through collaboration and establishment of a setting that makes clear, consistent, functional demands within a specific time frame. The program should allow for spontaneity in work and play and provide a predictable setting in which to practice adult roles, explore adult values and identity, and reflect on one's thoughts, feelings and behavior. Ultimately, the goal of occupational therapy is to facilitate clients' adaptation in their specific environment (performance context). The program should incorporate treatment that addresses problems in performance components stemming from concurrent symptoms (substance abuse, self-mutilation, etc.), as well as the essential features of personality disorders, particularly impulsive and rigid, maladaptive behavior patterns. Occupational therapy can address these issues in the standard occupational performance areas.

Leisure

Some individuals with personality disorders lack the ability to gain satisfaction from recreational or leisure pursuits. This may be due to rigid, narrow interests; paranoid or fearful behavior; or fear of closeness. It may be due to a background of growing up where any spontaneous or exploratory behavior was dangerous because it was not approved of by caregivers, or it may be due to an inability to regulate pleasurable feelings or guilt that one is feeling pleasure. It may be due to simply not learning that one can enjoy recreational pursuits because recreation may have involved social activities that patients have shied away from, the pursuits may have been inherently competitive and therefore avoided, or perhaps the clients were so perfectionistic that they held back out of fear they could not meet their own standards.

In other cases, recreational/leisure activities may be one area in which people with personality disorders can feel spontaneous, enjoy some sense of worth for their achievements, and perhaps feel relief from a relentless inner turmoil. For example, Jamal loved words, so he looked forward to playing the game "Dictionary," whereby he realized that he was articulate and had an advanced vocabulary. In this case, leisure activities may demonstrate a strength that can be utilized in treatment. Leisure occupations may also counteract various cognitive beliefs and statements that patients tell themselves, such as, "I enjoy doing things by myself," "I don't deserve to have fun," or "I can't let my guard down." Leisure occupations may provide opportunities to plan sequentially, sustain attention, and anticipate actions.

Psychologically, leisure occupations may provide specific responses to overwhelming feelings and help patients regulate their emotions. Leisure occupations may provide ways in which patients can feel worthwhile and enjoy a sense of accomplishment and competence. In this way they may realize that indeed, some activities can be intrinsically pleasurable and can provide pleasure and meaning even though they are not based on approval. For example, Anais worked out at the gym so that she could gain approval from others. However, in the occupational therapy leisure group, when she carefully monitored her thoughts and feelings while working out, she realized that she also enjoyed the feeling she got after finishing a hard workout.

Socially, leisure occupations can provide avenues in which people can be around others and develop casual relationships in a nonthreatening manner. They can relate to others in a reciprocal fashion, thereby developing a knowledge of empathy, while at the same time enjoying the opportunity to gain attention in an adaptive way.

Work

Work is often is a troublesome area due to a person's shyness and paranoid or fearful behavior on the job. Work may also be troublesome due to a person's difficulties in regulating the expression of emotions while on the job. For example, in a session discussing a return to work, Jill was unable to state why she had been fired from her previous three jobs except that she had had trouble meeting deadlines due to feeling overwhelmed about a new relationship. Trouble with work may be due to difficulties meeting concrete standards of performance or problems in sequencing and anticipating consequences of actions or in utilizing logical thinking. Work situations may seem difficult due to a person's lack of empathy and therefore lack of ability to "read" situations or unwritten rules. People with personality disorders may be underemployed, have jobs for which they are seemingly overqualified, or have an erratic work history. In spite of potential problems, work, like leisure, may be the one area where they may excel and learn to focus solely on objective tasks to the exclusion of other areas of life. For example, cognitively, vocational activities may provide arenas in which participants can learn to anticipate consequences of their actions, problem-solve, develop frustration tolerance, and accept responsibility. Alternately, work may provide opportunities for clients to learn how to regulate emotions, the appropriate times and situations in which to express them, and how to tolerate stress from performance standards. Work activities could provide arenas in which people can learn social appropriateness and how to get along with others in the workplace.

Self-care

Usually people with personality disorders are independent in self-care, except perhaps when undergoing acute crises. They possess self-care skills, although at times, due to personality patterns such as impulsivity, they may not use them and they may display poor judgment. For example, even though Jolene had an itemized budget, she felt deprived and so spent half of her one-year student loan on a wardrobe. She rationalized that she needed to have clothes for work when she graduated. Most treatment for self-care, then, would focus on how to utilize skills or on motivation and judgment strategies. Often this involves concrete planning and goal setting with built-in rewards or recognizing activities that are valued. It may involve learning how to handle impulsive behavior, such as simply stopping whatever one is doing, breathing deeply, or phoning a friend. It may be learning how to think before acting, such as focusing on self-talk and "changing the tape."

Inner self-care skills—those that concern taking care of the internal self (called the internal environment in other chapters of this book) in a psychological/emotional way by utilizing a knowledge of the self and psychological skills in a social environment—may be practiced. Cognitively, an individual focuses on how to think before acting and how to anticipate events in a step-by-step manner. Psychologically, an individual may assume a self-identity, learn values and interests, and practice how to recognize what is pleasurable and interesting for its own sake through exploration and mastery. Socially, being able to work with others helps to develop a capacity for empathy for oneself and others by learning that everyone has strengths and weaknesses. For example, in a group utilizing art media in which the task was to "draw your favorite place" and then tell others about it, Robert was able to patiently wait for his turn. As others discussed their work, he realized that he had similar emotions about his favorite place and that he could understand their statements. He also realized that he valued aspects of nature that brought him tranquillity.

Groups

Groups can be either nonverbal or verbal. Nonverbal groups that provide opportunities to work in the presence of others and relate in a casual way can be nonthreatening and motivating. Working in groups on concrete craft and art projects provides structured ways of utilizing one's strengths, resources, and talents while providing an engaging context in which to explore values and interests. Relaxation and restorative groups provide concrete ways to intervene in impulsive situations or when an individual has the experience of feeling overcome by overwhelming emotions. In addition, clients can explore activities that provide intrinsic pleasure. Verbal groups, particularly those that include action and then reflection on the action, can call on individual problem solving skills, accessing and delineating of emotions, and recognition of how they interfere maladaptively (such as in work). They can also provide training in social skills and communication and in how to be empathic with others.

CASE ILLUSTRATION: ROBYN—TREATMENT COURSE FOR BORDERLINE PERSONALITY DISORDER

Friends of Robyn who worked with her at a record store became concerned about her when she failed to show up for work for three days. When they went to her apartment, they found that she had not been eating or sleeping and that she had burned herself in two different places on her body. After evaluation in an emergency room, she agreed to psychiatric treatment.

An occupational therapy evaluation with the Allen Diagnostic Module (Allen, Earhart, & Blue, 1996) revealed cognitive functioning of 5.0 (able to cognitively explore the environment, but restricted to overt trial-and-error learning and unable to anticipate consequences). An Occupational Performance History Interview (OPHI) (Kielhofner, 1995; Kielhofner & Henry, 1988; Kielhofner, Henry, Whalens, & Rogers, 1991) revealed that Robyn perceived that she did not have control in any areas of her life, wished for a better job or career, and had a sense that she had troubled relationships. Although recently she had not engaged in hobbies or other forms of recreation, she enjoyed jewelry making and furniture refinishing and had worked out with weights. Based on this information, and in concert with her occupational therapist, Robyn chose to attend the following groups:

1. *The "Coping Skills" group addressed topics such as "stamping out impulsivity," "what to do when you want to hurt yourself," and "bringing tranquillity into your life." The group included education, discussion, paper-and-pencil exercises, and trying out of new behaviors while in the acute setting.*

2. *The "About Work" group included working on small jobs that were time limited and paid, learning about work behaviors and environments, discussing the "unwritten rules" of work, and analyzing and reflecting on each work session.*

3. *The " Becoming Creative with Crafts" group offered a variety of art and craft projects that could be learned and completed in short time frames.*

Robyn's chosen goals of treatment were to handle her self-mutilating and impulsive behavior, find another job and explore career options, and learn to feel better about herself. She worked individually with an occupational therapist to organize a workout schedule and further explore career options. After one week she had practiced some coping skills. Specifically, when she had the urge to burn herself, she learned that she could stop. At the same time, she began to experiment with making painted picture frames, which became popular on the unit. In the vocational group, she began to realize her problems in following through, which helped her to explore careers that would suit this trait.

Prior to discharge, the OTR assisted Robyn in exploring options in the community for continuing her interests and anticipated how she might handle setbacks when she was alone in her own home. In a predischarge review, Robyn stated that she "felt better about herself." She had learned that she could follow through in the art and craft group and, in fact, that she possessed some creativity and originality. She realized that perhaps she could indeed positively affect her environment. In fact, people had asked her to make craft projects for them and she had successfully practiced moderating her impulsive behavior. She also felt hopeful about finding a new job. Since she had explored her abilities and personality aspects in relation to her career, she realized that she could maintain more control of her own destiny and satisfaction.

Discussion

Robyn's course of treatment demonstrates how occupational therapy, individual and group, in all performance areas is a useful and creative aspect of treatment for a person with a personality disorder.

Summary

Understanding and treating personality disorders is difficult and often daunting to new students and clinicians for various reasons, including an unclear symptomatic picture, different classifications based on personality traits, behavior that alternates between functioning and instability, and problems that involve other people. However, treatment is possible based on an understanding of personality and the therapist's willingness to reflect on his or her own responses.

Disabling personality patterns—that is, adaptive inflexibility and tenuous stability—lead to vicious circles of self-defeating behavior in most areas of life. Occupational therapy includes an interpersonal approach (for example, a collaborative stance, consistency, and understanding) and interventions in leisure, work, and the personal, psychological, social, self-care area, all focusing on cognitive, social, and psychological aspects.

Review Questions

1. What are the negative stereotypes about personality disorders? Why are they inaccurate?

2. What are some of the reasons why understanding personality disorders is complicated?

3. What patterns in living distinguish the behavior of someone with a personality disorder from someone without the disorder?

4. What are useful ways of interacting in a clinical setting with individuals with personality disorders?

5. Why are the performance areas of work and leisure and the cognition, psychological, and social components particularly important for people with personality disorders?

Learning Activities

1. Think of a time when you planned a trip. Think of all the step-by-step activities and occurrences that you anticipated and planned for. Now, think about planning the same trip without being able to anticipate future occurrences.

2. Think of a time when you were impulsive. Now exaggerate that behavior and think about how it would influence your life if it occurred every two months.

3. Think of the activities or hobbies that you currently practice. How did you become interested in them? Do you receive comments from others? Would you continue them without any others commenting on them? If so, what is the nature of the intrinsic pleasure that they give you?

4. Practice telling a friend your expectations for a planned outing. After the outing, reflect on the experience. Did it live up to your expectations? If not, were you able to remain unperturbed?

5. Think of a time when you had a misunderstanding with a friend. What qualities in your friend, in you, and in your interaction enabled you to clear it up? (These qualities may be lacking in an individual with a personality disorder.)

6. Watch the movie *Fatal Attraction*. What characteristics remind you of borderline personality disorder in the female character? Read *Bastard Out of Carolina* by Dorothy Allison for a portrait of an antisocial character and abuse, and *A Thousand Acres* by Jane Smiley for a portrait of the shame that results from abuse. Read *Anne Sexton: A Biography* by Diane Middlebrook for symptoms of a personality disorder and adaptive coping for them.

References

Alarcon, R., & Foulks, E. (1995). Personality disorders and culture. *Cultural Diversity and Mental Health 1*(1), 3–17.

Allen, C. K. (1985). *Occupational therapy for psychiatric diseases: Measurement and management of cognitive disabilities.* Boston: Little, Brown.

Allen, C. K., Earhart, C. A., & Blue, T. (1996). *Understanding cognitive performance modes*. Colchester, CT: S&S Worldwide.

American Psychiatric Association. (1994). *Diagnostic and statistical manual of mental disorders* (4th ed.). Washington, DC.: Author.

Barris, R., Kielhofner, G., & Watts, J. (1988). *Occupational therapy in psychosocial practice*. New Jersey: Slack.

Gibson, D. (1990). Borderline personality disorder: Issues of etiology and gender. *Occupational Therapy in Mental Health, 10*(4), 63–77.

Kaplan, H., & Sadock, B. (1995). *Comprehensive textbook of psychiatry* (6th ed.). Baltimore, MD: Williams & Wilkins.

Kiesler, D. J. (1986). The 1982 interpersonal circle: An analysis of DSM-III personality disorders. In T. Millon & G. Klerman (Eds.), *Contemporary directions in psychopathology: Towards the DSM-IV*. New York: Guilford Press.

Kielhofner, G. (1995). *A model of human occupation: Theory and application* (2nd ed.). Baltimore, MD: Williams & Wilkins.

Kielhofner, G., & Henry, A. D. (1988). Development and investigation of an occupational performance history interview. *American Journal of Occupational Therapy, 42*(8), 489–498.

Kielhofner, G., Henry, A., Whalens, D., & Rogers, E. S. (1991). A generalizability study of the Occupational Performance History Interview. *Occupational Therapy Journal of Research, 11*, 292–306.

Linehan, M. M., Armstrong, H. E., Suarez, A., Allmon, D., & Heard, H. L. (1991). Cognitive-behavioral treatment of chronically para-suicidal borderline patients. *Archives of General Psychiatry, 48*(12), 1060–1064.

Linehan, M. M., Heard, H. L., & Armstrong, H. E. (1993). Naturalistic follow-up of a behavioral treatment for chronically parasuicidal borderline patients. *Archives of General Psychiatry, 50*(12), 971–974.

Millon, T. (1981). *Disorders of personality: DSM-III: Axis II*. New York: Wiley.

Millon, T. (1996). *Disorders of personality: DSM-IV and beyond* (2nd ed.). New York: Wiley.

Paris, J. (1994, November). The etiology of borderline personality disorder: A biopsychosocial approach. *Psychiatry, 57*, 316–324.

Ratey, J. J. (Ed.). (1995). *Neuropsychiatry of personality disorders*. Cambridge, MA: Blackwell Science.

Retzlaff, P. D. (1995). *Tactical psychotherapy of the personality disorders: An MCMI-III based approach*. Boston: Allyn & Bacon.

Ruegy, R., & Frances, A. (1995). New research in personality disorders. *Journal of Personality Disorders, 9*(1), 1–48.

Suggested Readings:

Effects of Childhood Abuse

Gil, E. (1983). *Outgrowing the pain*. San Francisco: Launch Press.

Herman, J. (1992). *Trauma and recovery*. New York: HarperCollins.

Miller, A. (1983). *For your own good*. Toronto, Canada: McGraw-Hill.

Williams, G., & Money, J. (1980). *Traumatic abuse and neglect of children at home* (abridged). Baltimore, MD: Johns Hopkins University Press.

Borderline and Narcissistic Disorders.

Gallop, R. (1985). The patient is splitting: Everyone knows and nothing changes. *Journal of Psychosocial Nursing, 23*(4), 6–10.

Hickey, B. (1985). The borderline experience: Subjective impressions. *Journal of Psychosocial Nursing, 23*(4), 24–26.

Kernberg, O. (1975). *Borderline conditions and pathological narcissism*. New York: Aronson.

Kohut, H. (1977). *The restoration of the self*. New York: International University Press.

Layton, M. (1995, May–June). Emerging from the shadows: Looking beyond the borderline diagnosis. *Networker*, pp. 35–41.

Miller, A. (1981). *The drama of the gifted child*. New York: Basic Books.

Miller, S. G. (1994). Borderline personality disorder from the patient's perspective. *Hospital and Community Psychiatry, 45*, 1215–1219.

Shapiro, D. (1965). *Neurotic styles*. New York: Basic Books.

Obsessive-Compulsive Personality Disorder

Rapoport, J. (1989). *The boy who couldn't stop washing*. New York: Penguin.

Treatment Strategies

Linehan, M. (1993a). *Cognitive behavioral treatment of borderline personality disorder*. New York: Guilford Press.

Linehan, M. (1993b). *Skills training manual for treating borderline personality disorder*. New York: Guilford Press.

Simon, S. (1993). *In search of values: 31 strategies for finding out what really matters most to you*. New York: Time Warner.

Tavris, C. (1982). *Anger: The misunderstood emotion*. New York: Simon & Schuster.

Literary Portraits

Allison, D. (1992). *Bastard out of Carolina*. New York: Dutton.

Middlebrook, D. (1991). *Anne Sexton: A biography*. New York: Houghton-Mifflin.

Smiley, J. (1992). *A thousand acres*. New York: Knopf.

Occupational Therapy Intervention

CHAPTER 15

Groups

Elizabeth Cara

Key Terms

activity group
group
group content
group dynamics
group process

group protocol
group structure
personhood skills
psychodynamic
psychoeducational

Chapter Outline

Introduction

Occupational therapists in the psychosocial arena conduct much, if not most, of treatment in **group** settings. Group treatment can be incredibly exciting, stimulating, and interesting. It is exciting to implement or to "lead" groups, and it is stimulating to develop or "create" them. Developing and implementing groups includes both artistic and scientific elements. The science is involved in developing the **group structure**, organizing a **group protocol**, recognizing the needs of the setting and the population with whom one works, applying a knowledge of occupations and occupational skills, and utilizing good communication and interpersonal skills. The art lies in being aware of the **group process**, using oneself in a therapeutic way, and knowing, and responding to, the here-and-now needs of the individual group participants and to the participants as a group—simultaneously. Both the art and the science can be learned through acquiring knowledge and practicing experientially. This chapter discusses groups in general and how to think about occupational therapy groups so that they can be developed and implemented creatively and competently, in any setting, and with any participants.

What Makes a Group a Group?

There are various definitions of groups, all of which include a situation in which two or more people come together and think of themselves as a group. A group can be thought of as an intentional coming together to produce change for the members (Borg & Bruce, 1991; Howe & Schwartzberg, 1995) and also as a microcosm of society, in which participants can learn about themselves and their relationships (Corey & Corey, 1992). There are common properties that characterize almost any group. These include:

- a background, history, and purpose
- a structure imposed by the group leader, which usually consists of preparations, expectations, a composition, and arrangements
- an interaction pattern, for example, member-to-member or member-to-leader
- communication or action taking place, whether verbal or nonverbal
- usually, a cohesion, or a "we" feeling
- standards or rules of acceptable behavior

The norms or standards of a group usually contribute to cohesion and a feeling of safety and trust. Norms can be explicit or implicit, verbalized or unstated, developed initially by the leader or based on the group interaction (Cole, 1993). Norms are often set and monitored by how the group leader models expected behavior and handles unwanted behavior. In addition to the leader, the environment—both physical space and how people react in and to it—and goals of the group also are responsible for the development of norms (Borg & Bruce, 1991). For example, a norm of talking to other group members and not to the leader is developed when the leader does not answer every question directed to him or her, but instead asks the group in general to answer the question. A norm of talking to, not about, each other is established when the leader asks an individual who is talking about another person in the group to direct his or her comments to the person about whom he or she is speaking. A norm of the members' acceptance and importance in the group is set when the group meets at a regular time, is held in a comfortable, distraction-free place that accommodates everyone and is identified as the space where occupational therapy happens, and supplies are made readily available. In addition, the therapist should make contact with the members individually each day to invite them to the group and should greet them warmly. It is also important to start the group on time and to always begin and end the meeting in a similar manner. When the group leader states the clear goals of the group and the purpose for the group to each new member—or asks participants to do so—a norm is established concerning how new members will enter the group and what individuals should learn in the group is made explicit.

Common norms necessary in any group are confidentiality, a here-and-now focus, respect for each individual, and participation—though each member has a right to choose how to interact, what to disclose, and what to do in the group (Corey & Corey, 1992).

Advantages and Limitations of Groups

Practically speaking, group treatment in mental health is time- and cost-effective. It costs less to treat people in groups than it does to treat them on an individual basis, and they allow more people to be seen in a shorter amount of time. Group treatment facilitates personal growth by virtue of providing more people with whom to interact. Participants can learn about themselves through identifying with others; observing, and being able to compare and contrast, their own experience with those of others; experiencing closeness and caring; and having opportunities to be around others in a safe or trusting context. Groups support experimentation and trying of new behavior, with a variety of feedback provided by different people (Corey & Corey, 1992). More specifically, occupational therapy groups facilitate learning new skills from others. Groups are like mini-laboratories in which one can practice skills for living in a simulated experience.

Of course, there are some limitations to group treatment. Not everyone is suited for groups. For example, an individual may be too disoriented, confused or too suspicious of others to be able to tolerate a group. A group may be too distracting or require too high a degree of abstract ability. Some clients may require individual treatment; for example, they may not be able to leave their room or setting due to precautions or illness. Last, some people may need the concentrated effort of individual treatment. The following section discusses some of the properties, norms, stages, and themes of groups.

OVERVIEW OF GROUP THERAPY

Studies of group behavior have been conducted in various fields, including business or psychology (Corey & Corey, 1992, Howe & Schwartzberg, 1995; Kaplan & Sadock, 1991, 1995). In the United States, group treatment was pioneered in the 1930s. In the mid-1940s, the understanding of group process became popular due as a result of World War II, which caused numerous psychiatric casualties at a time when there was a shortage of psychiatrists. Therefore, therapy in groups was born as a necessity. Therapy groups have taken various forms and been developed for various populations (Alonso & Swiller, 1993). The increasing use of group therapy techniques has paralleled the rise in popularity of different psychological models. For example, from the concept's inception through the 1950s, groups were based on a psychoanalytic model, which was popular in the United States during this period. Today, self-help groups and brief behaviorally oriented groups are popular because of the popular growth of behavioral and cognitive models and a community self-help movement.

Different concepts, techniques and leadership roles will be assumed depending on which model a group is grounded . A brief explanation of various psychological models of group therapy is presented in Table 15-1. Although one may pattern a group specifically on one model, in actuality many groups are implemented utilizing various principles. Each group developer and leader will generally blend what they feel to be the most effective concepts and techniques to create a unique group (Corey & Corey, 1992).

Table 15-1.	Models of Group Therapy		
	Psychoanalytic	*Humanistic*	*Behavioral*
Philosophy	Childhood Experiences	Self-Actualization	Changing Behavior
Emphasis	Make the unconscious conscious	Self-Awareness	Learning effective, eliminating maladaptive, behavior
Key Concepts	Work through resistance and transference	Understanding values and discovering meaning	Increasing effective, decreasing ineffective, behavior
Goal	Insight	Maximize climate of growth and awareness	Change behavior
Role of Leader	Interpret	Keep focus in the present; model authenticity	Organize, direct, teach new skills
Techniques	Interpret and analyze	Understanding, modeling, confronting, clarifying; coaching, role modeling	Learning principles: delineating, reinforcing, extinguishing

Group Content and Structure

The **group content** is the activity that is planned and carried out in the group (Denton, 1987) or what is said in the group (Howe & Schwartzberg, 1995). It can be either verbal or nonverbal. The way in which the activity is presented; the directions, procedures, techniques and time arrangements; and the way in which membership is organized comprise the group structure. The content and structure of a group will naturally flow from its purpose and the style of the leader. Group content and structures have been combined in various ways to produce many types of occupational therapy groups.

Group Dynamics and Process

Group dynamics are the forces that influence the relationships of members and the group outcome (Cole, 1993). Some important dynamics of a group are the process and stages of groups, leadership styles and leader behaviors, roles that members assume, norms and expected standards of behavior, the behavior and interaction of the group members, the group structure, and environment in which it is held.

The process consists of the patterns or stages that groups usually go through; these are characterized by recognizable feelings and behaviors that are usually unspoken or not made explicit (Corey & Corey, 1992). It refers to how the work of the group is carried out (Howe & Schwartzberg, 1995), including how participants relate to each other, who talks to whom, how tasks are accomplished, and how decisions are made. Group process involves two tiers (Yalom, 1995). On the first tier, it includes the here-and-now experience of the group members, who focus their attention on their feelings toward other group members, the therapist, and the group as a whole. The immediate events in the meeting take precedence. The second tier involves the group's focus on recognizing and understanding its own process. The group becomes self-reflective in looking at the here-and-now behavior that has just occurred. This two-tiered process is what facilitates learning and generalization as the group becomes a microcosm for the participants' outside lives. It becomes a personal laboratory in which to discover, study, and change one's life experience. In psychotherapy groups, "processing" about the group experience may occur during the meeting, whereby individuals may become reflective and analytical, which allows them to understand, integrate, and generalize their behavior from the group experience to their everyday life. Continual processing about the group does not usually occur as an **activity group** experience, although members may reflect and analyze their experience through the activity of the group or as it pertains to activities generally (Fidler & Fidler, 1969); moreover, group leaders may—and, in fact, should—analyze and reflect on each group meeting after its completion.

The stages and patterns of a group can be considered as happening over a length of time in different sessions or, with the advent of shorter treatment, within one session. Stages have been described primarily with traditional psychotherapy groups in mind; however, these stages and themes can be recognized in all types of groups, including activity groups. In fact, it appears that activity groups are often nonthreatening, causing stages to occur more rapidly. Although stages are written about as if they were linear, in fact, different stages can overlap. Group stages have been characterized in different ways according to certain themes that arise in each stage (cited in Borg & Bruce, 1991; Cole, 1993). The themes have been described as "forming, storming, norming, and performing"; "inclusion, control, and affection"; "flight, fight, unite, and orientation"; and "conflict, harmony, and maturity." The general themes describe or explain the participants' own thoughts and feelings about the group and the other group members, including the leader. They connote the process of coming together with unknown others and involve an unknown future process: (1) wondering if one will be accepted and liked, (2) deciding on standards for the group, (3) agonizing about the degree to which one wants to be in the group and whether one can follow the norms, (4) a cohesive stage of acceptance of the self and others and investment in using the group for the work that needs to be done, and (5) an ending and consolidation of growth and learning.

The stages of a group have been characterized as initial, transition, working, and final (Corey & Corey, 1992). In the initial stage, participants generally learn the norms and expectations, get acquainted, and attempt to determine whether they will be included or excluded. Members will decide whom they can trust and will like, how much they will be involved, and how deeply they with to disclose. Some tasks of the group member are to begin to behave in a way that will establish trust, learn how to express feelings (especially fears, concerns, and hopes for the group), being involved in the creation of the group norms, and establishing goals for themselves. The leader functions are usually to role-model active participation, develop the rules, assist members to establish a trusting atmosphere and establish goals, and structure the group so that it will have the right balance, discouraging both excessive dependence and excessive floundering. Possible problems involving group members are the failure to participate, an unwillingness to reveal themselves, and the refusal to accept a role of advice giver or problem solver.

In the transition stage there tend to be more feelings of anxiety on the part of group members. Participants may be concerned about being accepted, how safe the group is, and the leader's competence. They may struggle with ambivalence between choosing risk taking or compliance and, possibly, control or conflict and confrontation. Tasks may include recognizing and expressing negative feelings, learning how to deal with one's own personal resistances, and overcoming conflict with others. The leader functions so as to support the group through the transition so that members will accept and resolve conflict and personal resistances. The leader provides a model of tact and directness, assists members to recognize their personal resistances and interpersonal conflicts, and encourages them to "stay with" expressing reactions that pertain to the here-and-now happenings in the group. Problems may arise if members are categorized as problem types and scapegoated, refuse to express feelings or engage in handling conflicts, or form subgroups to discuss negative reactions outside of the group but not in the presence of the group as a whole.

The working stage is characterized by a high level of trust and cohesion. Members tend to openly communicate in a responsible way, the group shares leadership functions, there is a willingness to take risks, conflict is recognized and handled constructively, and participants generally feel energized to change their behavior outside the group. There is a general tone of high energy and hope. Members function as independent initiators, bringing topics that they are willing to openly express to the group, offering and accepting constructive feedback, and striving to be both more challenging and more supportive of each other. The leader functions as a role model who provides a balance of support and confrontation, interprets the meaning of behavior patterns so that members can engage in a deeper level of self-exploration, explores common themes to link the work of the individual members, and encourages members to practice new skills. Possible problems include members' tendency to challenge each other, the possibility of gaining insufficient insight in the group but to understand the necessity of behavior change on the outside of the group, and the risk of becoming more anxious because of the intensity of group meetings.

In the final stage group members may feel sadness and fear over the group's eventual ending, hopes and concerns for each other may be expressed, members generally ready themselves for dealing with the reality of the world outside the group, and there may be an evaluation of the group experience. Members' tasks are to deal with their feelings regarding separation, offer feedback to others, complete any unfinished business concerning others in the group, discuss changes still to be made and how to make them, and attempt to generalize what they have learned to everyday life. The leader assists the members in dealing with their feelings regarding termination, reinforces changes, and assists members to consolidate what they have learned in the group and understand how it might be applied to everyday life. Possible problems concern members' avoidance of reviewing their experience or putting it into a framework that enables generalization and the danger they may distance themselves from the other group members, thus limiting the possibility of expressing and consolidating feelings. Table 15-2 reviews group properties, norms, stages, and themes.

With the advent of shorter treatment duration, fewer groups will have the luxury of smoothly moving through the various stages to completion. Instead, groups may remain at one stage and fail to progress to the next. However, the various themes that characterize each stage may still become apparent. For example, in a short-term evaluation group, the theme of wanting to be accepted may be expressed by a group member refusing to participate in the assessment or, in a daily movement group, a member may only participate by watching from the sidelines. A theme of deciding how to be in a group may be expressed by a member attempting to take care of other group members or attempting to assume responsibility like the group leader. Harmony or affection may be achieved in a daily group that runs for a week, yet at the end some members may fail to show up for the last meeting or demean their accomplishments in the group.

The Group Leader

The role of the group leader may change somewhat according to the type of group, but there are also general leadership aspects that define the role, communication skills that can be utilized in the role, and general **personhood skills** (which translate into leadership skills) (Corey & Corey, 1992). Every group has properties and norms and goes through stages characterized by certain themes. Table 15-3 lists ideal roles, communication skills, and personhood traits of group leaders.

Table 15-2. Group Properties, Norms, Stages, and Themes

Properties	Norms
Background, history, purpose	Confidentiality
Structure	Here-and-now focus
Interaction pattern	Manner of participation
Communication	Activities
Cohesion	Individual respect
Rules and standards	

Stages	Themes
Initial	Learning expectations
	Getting acquainted
	Wondering about inclusion/exclusion; disclosure/involvement; trust
Transition	Wondering about acceptance/rejection; safety; leader competency
	Struggle with compliance versus risky behavior
Working	Trust and cohesion
	Responsible communication
	Constructive resolve
	Sharing of responsibility
Final	Evaluation of experience
	Feelings of ending/separation
	Completion of unfinished business
	Continuing change

Roles and style of leadership. Overall, the leader is the organizer of the group. He or she initiates action and interaction, directs the activities of the group, and establishes an atmosphere of trust and openness. The leader can be thought of as the "holder" of the group by virtue of his or her development, implementation, and overall investment (Yalom, 1995). Group leaders must remain aware that ongoing careful attention to the structure and content of the group through their interactions and directions continually establishes its tone and influences its success and the degree of member participation.

By establishing the norms and boundaries of a group through organization and attention, a group leader can assist members in feeling comfortable and motivated to participate. The group leader should strive to establish an "ambiance of safety." More specific aspects of the leader's role are:

- demonstrating by example
- setting rules and limits, such as confidentiality, not interacting in subsets, not interrupting
- providing orientation
- being tuned in to the mood of the group

Table 15-3. The Group Leader

Roles

Organizer	Sets and maintains norms, boundaries, and rules
	Establishes a tone, or ambiance, of safety and participation
Role Model	Demonstrates by example
	Provides orientation
Facilitator	Determines and directs or enables the group activity and participant interactions

Communication Skills

Active Listening	Absorbing the content, noting a person's gestures and changes in expression, sensing underlying messages (what a person is not saying) while simultaneously remaining fully present and concentrated in the moment for each interaction
Reflecting	Communicating back to a person the essence of what they have communicated to you
Clarifying	Recounting what a person has communicated
Blocking	Prohibiting, either directly or by your interpretation, types of communication that are destructive to the group process or members. Examples of destructive communication are gossiping, breaking another's confidence, and invading other's privacy
Facilitating	Inviting others to participate, that is, to express thoughts or feelings or to work on the activity of the group; to work or interact with other members or to make comments concerning other members' statements or products
Empathizing	Providing a response to indicate you understand a person and what he or she has wished to communicate; that you can "put yourself in another person's shoes"

Personhood Skills

Courage	The ability to admit mistakes, express fears, or act on hunches; to be direct and honest with members; to be genuine and not defensive in the face of criticism; to do what the leader expects others to do in that group situation
Willingness	To model or exhibit behaviors that one expects of group members
Being Present	Fully experiencing the group's activity or interactions and not being distracted from the purpose of the group
Belief in the Group	Believing in the value of what is being done or is happening in the group
Ability to Cope Nondefensively	Not personalizing, retaliating, or withdrawing from comments or actions that you perceive as critical of you or your performance
Self-Awareness	Awareness of personal goals, identity, motivations, needs, strengths and limitations, values and feelings
Sense of Humor	The ability to laugh at yourself and to see and understand the frailty of the human condition
Inventiveness	The capacity to be spontaneous and creative, often combined with the ability to learn from every experience in life

Source: Corey and Corey (1992).

Basically, as group leader, you are a role model. Through your behavior and attitude, you model the norms you would like to create in the group (Corey & Corey, 1992; Howe & Schwartzberg, 1995; Kaplan, 1988). This is true for all groups whether the members only work in the presence of others or interact with each other, the content is activity-based or psychodynamic, and the structure is verbal or nonverbal. This is true even though you may perceive your role as being simply an organizer or resource guide.

Your natural style of leadership may be broadly considered as active and directive in your involvement or as more facilitative and supportive. As a directive leader, you actively control or direct the group, usually choose the activity and direct the process, and actively direct interactions to motivate clients. A more facilitative leader will remain more in the background, perhaps supporting the members as they make their own decisions and interact among themselves. Often the structure of a group may dictate the leadership style; for example, the leader may be introducing a new or novel activity, the group members cognitively may require direction, or the goal of the group may be to increase motivation or interpersonal skills. In these cases, a directive and active leadership style is required. Another example is a group whose goal is to determine community resources that support finding a job. In this task, members should be more independent and can benefit from interacting with, and supporting, each other (skills that will be required in a job). In this case, the leadership style must necessarily be facilitative.

Communication Skills.   There are many communication skills that can be learned and become part of a group leader's repertoire of skills. Although there are many skills, some of the most important are active listening, reflecting, clarifying, blocking, facilitating, and empathizing. (These skills are explained more fully in Table 15-3.)

Personhood Skills.   Other skills sometimes are more difficult to explain or acquire because they often have to do with an individual's personality, or personal traits, temperament, and experience. These can be called personality traits, but the term "personhood skills" (Corey & Corey, 1992) better conveys that these are particular traits that positively influence how one person relates to another. They can sometimes be learned by observing the behavior of someone who has the traits and noting how he or she practices the skills in everyday life. (The personhood skills are listed and explained in Table 15-3.)

Problems in Groups

There is a temptation to label certain people as the source of problems in groups (such as the storyteller, the avoider, the monopolizer) instead of simply labeling their behavior (Cole, 1993; Corey & Corey, 1992). It seems very human to attribute a person's behavior in a particular situation to an enduring character trait. However, this can be a danger in groups (as it is in the practice of psychiatry) due to the tendency to then consistently characterize the person by a single instance of behavior, which in reality may not occur again or may be inconsistent and only happen in certain situations. In particular, a group situation should allow for testing of behavior, and often, participants are unaware that their behavior is considered a problem. With this caveat in mind, we will now review behaviors that may interfere with the normal development of groups if allowed to persist, and that may be addressed by the group leader in fundamental ways.

Although in some instances, problematic behavior may have to do with the participant's thoughts and feelings about the group leader, in general, "problem" behavior is not usually personally directed to the leader. Often, it is mostly unconscious and unintentional. (This is a basic assumption of psychiatry.) Generally, the best procedure to utilize in handling "problem" behavior is to (1) attempt to understand the meaning of the behavior for that specific time, group, and group members, (2) accept the behavior in a nondefensive way and address it in a manner appropriate to the situation, the functioning of the person, and the level of disruption (disruption either in the behavior itself or to the group), and (3) allow the person to "save face" and avoid power struggles whenever possible.

A group member's nonparticipation, silence, or withdrawal is not an overt problem, but it will influence the other group members if it continues and is usually not helpful for the individual participant. Natural silences do occur in individual or group treatment, and often they may define a therapeutic moment or positive transition point. Naturally occurring silence can be distinguished from silence that is more defiant or defensive. The latter, which will be discussed here, is ongoing and noticeable as a behavior pattern, and it is not necessarily spontaneous. It may occur because the individual is not cognitively competent to handle the demands of the group or because symptoms, such as hallucinations, may be a barrier to participation. The individual may fear looking foolish, or being rejected, feel unlovable and vulnerable, be paranoid or uncertain about how the group works, or not trust or want to be in the group. The leader should invite participation in the group, direct comments to the person, or make contact in some way, and if possible, he or she should directly explore what makes the person behave in that way. In an activity group, this is less problematic because clients usually will become involved. For example, a task can be adapted (e.g., graded to make the steps more simple) or the individual who does not want to participate can be asked to at least remain with the group. An extreme of nonparticipation is leaving a group before its completion. Again, the leader should consider whether the client may have been cognitively incompetent or too distracted for that specific group. Contact should be made with nonparticipants to assure their safety and let them know that their presence is valued. If appropriate, the leader should explore the reasons for departure. Sometimes clients are unable to consciously recognize or discuss their behavior. If that is the case, then the leader should either just make contact or provide a choice of reasons that they may agree to or at least think about.

Monopolizing behavior is at the opposite end of the spectrum, with story-telling, questioning, advice giving, and intellectualizing somewhere in between. A person's symptoms, such as symptoms of mania, may interrupt the group or the individual may be driven by the same fears and concerns that lead to unnatural silences. Monopolistic behavior can be more problematic than silence because it demands to be addressed and will eventually cause the other members to resent the person. If the behavior is part of a person's symptoms, the leader should continually address it by interrupting the person and redirecting him or her. The behavior can be confronted by gently describing the situation, stating, for example: "I don't know if you realize that you are taking up all the group's time. Your thoughts and feelings are important, but I think other group members would also like to participate." Alternately, the leader may attempt to deepen the person's self-understanding, as appropriate to the person and the situation, by saying, for example, "You seem to want a lot of attention, but I sense that the way you are asking for it is turning people off, which is not really what you want."

Hostile behavior can be direct or indirect. In the latter, it may come subtly in the form of sarcasm, jokes, seeming bored and detached, or arriving late. The individual may fear looking foolish, fear rejection, feel unlovable, be uncertain about how the group works, or not trust or want to be in the group. The person may be expressing him- or herself in a learned manner and may not recognize that this is distancing. The person may be disappointed and hurt, or he or she may be feeling angry and expressing it in an indirect way. A special case occurs often with activity groups and occupational therapists, whereby clients will denigrate an activity—or the occupational therapist who suggests it—as being too simple, childish, or totally unrelated to treatment or change. For some people, this may mean that the activity is too challenging and, perhaps, cognitively overwhelming. In that case, acknowledging the right to decline participation or changing the activity may take care of the situation. If the level of difficulty is not the apparent problem, gentle confrontation may be enough to change the behavior, such as by saying, "You seem upset today—is that so?" or "I don't know if you realize that your comment sounds somewhat angry—is that how you are feeling?" In the case of denigration of the activity, there may be different ways to approach the situation. A serious explanation of the rationale for the activity and how it may be helpful to the person will often defuse the situation. Alternately, an acceptance of the person's feelings and explanation that although the activity may appear overly simple it has additional benefits may defuse the hostility. Sometimes an exploration of how the person felt when engaged in the activity helps to shift or reframe the situation. In all instances of problem behavior, the leader's response will depend on the situation, the person's level of functioning, and the leader's understanding of the behavior's meaning.

CASE ILLUSTRATION:
HANDLING PROBLEM BEHAVIORS IN A GROUP

In a life skills group for young adults that met daily, participants at times discussed how to use cognitive techniques to quiet their minds and avoid distractions when asked to do group projects together with other students in their classes. They acknowledged that their anxiety, as demonstrated by obsessive and negative thoughts about themselves as individuals, often prevented them from even starting the projects. They were then labeled "lazy," ostracized from the class, and more than likely denied a grade indicative of their knowledge. After the first week of the group, Maria, the OTR, was feeling increasingly uneasy about the sessions. For the most part, the group was functioning, but two members often interfered with the process. The first, John, declined to comment when asked to share some pertinent cognitive problem or solution and often physically separated himself from the others. Most of his comments were aimed at interpreting other people's problems or offering solutions for others in the group. Another member, Louise, participated in group exercises and made comments but also often directed comments with subtle sexual innuendos to the therapist.

After careful consideration of each member's difficulties and circumstances in supervision, Maria decided to handle the two individuals in two different ways. Knowing John and observing him in other groups, she believed that he felt less intelligent than the others and feared they would find this out if he acknowledged his perceived shortcomings. Maria raised this fear as a group issue, not mentioning John but rather questioning whether others worried about rejection and acknowledging how difficult it is to reveal perceived weaknesses that have seemed hopelessly intractable. The group members, including John, were able to discuss their fears of seeming inadequate and thus to identify with, and support, each other.

Knowing Louise, the leader judged her comments to reveal a more personal issue—that Louise either liked the group leader and was expressing it in this indirect, almost unconscious, way or, perhaps, was expressing a fear about the leader's competency. She decided to discuss this with Louise personally and inquire whether Louise was aware of the nature of her comments. In fact, Louise was surprised and embarrassed to realize that she had made such comments; however, she also acknowledged her affection for Maria, who represented a healthy, strong model that Louise wished to emulate.

Discussion

Each instance of "problem behavior" meant something different for the individual participant and the group and was, therefore, handled differently. In each case, however, the therapist's reaction was congruent with her assessment of the group process, the meaning of the comment, and each person's individual process.

In addition to considering the individual's behavior as a personal problem, it is useful to consider whether one's own leadership style and manner of interacting or the group structure or content may be contributing (Howe & Schwartzberg, 1995). For example, is the activity matched with the person's ability? Is the person able to meet the demands of the group? Is the reason for the activity clear? Has the leader successfully created norms of safety and trust and interacted in a respectful and genuine manner? Has the leader assumed too much responsibility for the process of the group? Perhaps neither the leader, the interaction, nor the person is a cause of problem behavior and instead, some outside influence has affected the group or its members. For example, was there an incident on an inpatient unit, such as a suicide attempt or theft, or was the person just notified of a workplace review by his boss or social security audit? Perhaps visitors have just left. Indeed, there are many potential outside influences.

OCCUPATIONAL THERAPY GROUPS

Occupational therapy groups have much in common with groups based on other models. Often they borrow techniques, such as assertiveness training or role-playing, that originated according to other psychological models. Such a blending of methods and techniques is not uncommon in the field of mental health. However, occupational therapy groups tend to be unique in two ways. They are unique in their *focus on the activity,* which is the aspect that produces change. They are also unique in their *emphasis on occupations,* which involves changing occupational performance areas and components. These two emphases often dictate the purpose of occupational therapy groups; the required changes in occupational performance areas, components, or skills, and the leader's role in the group (which is often active and directive). This broad purpose can be incorporated in any occupational therapy model. Although people often erroneously assume that every group's purpose is interaction, the broad categories of activity groups listed in Table 15-4 show that the purpose of occupational therapy groups extends far beyond simply social interaction.

Activity Groups and Categories

Activity.   Activity groups have been defined in different ways in occupational therapy. A variety of activity groups are defined and practiced by occupational therapists and modeled after occupational therapy frames of reference, but no consensus has yet been reached on an inclusive, unique definition of the type of activity group employed exclusively by occupational therapists. Groups have been developed according to occupational therapy models (Kaplan, 1988; King, 1974); they generally follow the principles of other systems, especially the psychoanalytic and developmental approaches (Borg & Bruce, 1991; Fidler, 1969; Mosey, 1970, 1981), and they may delineate a specific struc-

Table 15-4.	Activity Groups	
	Focus	**Purpose**
Thematic	Topic or theme	Change attitudes Acquire knowledge and skills
Expressive	Creative media	Recognize, acknowledge Express feelings and ideas
Sensory	Sensory, bodily	Awareness of sensations Relaxation
Activity of Daily Living	Functional, everyday activities	Learn, perform activities of daily living
Vocational	Work activities	Acquire work-related knowledge skills

ture (Cole, 1993; Howe & Schwartzberg, 1995; Kaplan, 1988). What they all have in common is that the content focuses on activity, emphasizes occupation, and addresses occupational performance components and skills to aid in adaptation and functioning in the areas of occupational performance. All groups also share a common structure, which deemphasizes reflecting on the group process throughout the duration of the whole group.

Activity groups have been considered to have the properties of both psychotherapy groups and task groups (Borg & Bruce, 1991; Denton, 1987). A psychotherapy group usually emphasizes group process with a goal of resolving inter- or intrapersonal issues, whereas a task group usually emphasizes an outcome or product, which can be tangible, such as an art project, or intangible, such as a decision or recommendation. The goal of the task group is to accomplish a group task. An activity group falls somewhere in between the two types of groups. It may emphasize a group goal, yet the interaction concerning the group goal may be considered as important as the goal. Alternately, the interaction may occur through a medium of activity. The goal of the activity group is to enable change in skills, which may be either interpersonal (social) or intrapersonal (feelings, thoughts); the focus is always on interaction. Education is included as an activity group, but the parallel group is not, because group interaction is not a means of change in a parallel group. Activity groups are considered effective for promoting interaction through practicing interpersonal skills and social skills training in a group.

Activity groups have been defined (Howe & Schwartzberg, 1995) as those in which members are engaged in a common task directed toward occupational performance. The group focuses on function and replicates living in the community or family. The activity focuses the group's attention, and the group members learn from direct experience. The task provides form and organization and serves the needs of members in different ways, including utilizing purposeful activity in developing skills. A functional group has been proposed based on adaptation and occupation. According to this approach, groups enhance the use of occupations to help people adapt to the environment or vice versa, and groups utilize purposeful activities and active involvement (doing) so that members can maintain or develop skills in occupational performance areas.

Cole (1993) suggested a seven-step format for activity groups, involving introduction, the activity, sharing one's own product or experience, processing or reflecting and making sense of the experience, generalizing or summing up the responses to the activity, applying what was learned to everyday life, and summarizing the group experience. The steps can be adapted to maximize learning for any population according to the purpose of the group and the overall level of functioning of the group members.

Task. In the classic task-oriented group (Fidler, 1969), a task was defined as either an end product or a service, though task accomplishment was not the purpose of the group. Instead, the task provided a shared experience whereby the participants could reflect on the relationship between behavior, thinking, and feeling and explore their impact on others. What is demonstrated in the process of participating in the task and encountering problems in doing or interacting can be observed and thus become the focus of group problem solving and trying out alternative patterns. In this way the group becomes engaged in processing behavior and then trying out more adaptive modes.

Developmental. Group interaction skills have been described as a developmental sequence necessary for adaptation (Mosey, 1970, 1981, 1986). Five types of groups, from least to most developed, are (1) parallel, where tasks are done side-by-side and interaction is not required, (2) project, emphasizing task accomplishment and some interaction, (3) egocentric-cooperative, requiring more interaction and responsibility, (4) cooperative, requiring much interaction and taking care of others' needs, and, (5) mature groups where the members take on all necessary leadership roles to facilitate task accomplishment and caring for others' needs. In the hierarchy, initially task accomplishment is emphasized while interaction and meeting each others' needs are deemphasized. At each successive level, interaction becomes more important and the role of the therapist or leader becomes less primary. At the highest level, task accomplishment is emphasized equally with meeting the needs of other group members.

Directive. The directive group (Kaplan, 1986, 1988)—and also the focus group (Yalom, 1983), which was modeled on the directive group—meets the needs of the most severely and acutely mentally ill and most minimally functioning patients, representing a wide range of diagnoses, ages, and problems. The environment is actively structured in form, organization, and leadership to assure maximum participation. The directive group format is a consistent one involving orientation, introduction, a warm-up, selected activities, and a wrap-up, while the focus group format is orientation, warm-up, structured exercises, and review. The formats enable group goals of participation, inter-action, attention, and initiation; within this broad range, goals can be indi-vidualized.

Neurodevelopmental.   Neurodevelopmental groups (King, 1974; Levy, 1974; and Ross, 1987, cited in Cole, 1993) utilize movement activities often based on sensory integration theory and techniques. The movements are usu-ally imitative, gross motor movements and involve tactile, kinesthetic, and pro-prioceptive input. The groups are designed for persons with chronic schizophrenia who have been in the mental health system for a long time.

Occupational therapists develop and implement many activity groups. They may fall into broad categories based on the group's content, which usually ad-dresses occupational performance areas and components. Table 15-4 gives a brief explanation of activity group categories.

A thematic group (Mosey, 1981; cited in Denton, 1987) is organized around a topic or theme. The aim is to help the participants change or examine atti-tudes or acquire knowledge and skills in certain areas. Examples of thematic group titles are "Grieving and Loss," "What Do You Say after You Say Hello?" "On Depression," "On Anger," "On Guilt," and "Recognizing Feelings."

An expressive/projective group (Denton, 1987) uses creative media to fa-cilitate the recognition, acknowledgment, or expression of feelings and ideas. Examples of expressive groups are art or craft groups, play groups, and recre-ation or sport activity groups. A sensory group is one in which the activity in-creases the awareness of bodily sensations and responses or facilitates bodily relaxation. Examples include training in progressive relaxation, shiatsu, yoga, karate, or other Eastern forms of movement.

Activity of Daily Living (ADL) groups concentrate on learning daily func-tional activities. Examples include groups for grooming, self-care, using pub-lic transportation, and learning about community resources.

Vocational or prevocational groups offer work opportunities, which may be paid or unpaid. They may involve projects that are brought in for mem-bers to work on within their routine day or include discussions or experiences regarding the basics of job hunting or personal behavior expected in a job.

Although not strictly an activity group, the **psychoeducational** group also has a clear objective: to teach specific information or techniques. It is typically time limited and utilizes cognitive-behavioral and social learning theory (Alonso & Swiller, 1993). For example, a group for people with eating disor-ders may provide facts on nutrition and the social correlates and medical con-sequences of eating disorders. Due to the shorter duration of mental health treatment and the dictates of managed care, many professionals utilize the techniques of psychoeducation.

In all these categories, the structure of the group, pattern of interaction, leader's role and methods, and techniques utilized in the group are dictated by the group developer or implementer. In one sensory group the leader may demonstrate how to stretch and have the participants practice the technique. The only verbalization may be the leader's. In another sensory group, participants may share knowledge and demonstrate their own relaxation techniques. The leader's role may be simply as facilitator or the sessions may contain both elements.

In one expressive group participants may simply sit silently together in a room, working on their own, individual crafts. The role of the leader will be to help each person initiate and follow through. Alternately, in another expressive group participants may draw themselves in a certain setting and then discuss the emotions and thoughts that the drawing evoked. In this case, the role of the group leader is more active, that is, to help members interact with each other or make connections between their drawings and their thoughts and feelings.

In a thematic group, the group leader may provide education about a topic, such as, "How Thoughts Get in Our Way." Then participants might individually write down negative things they say to themselves and when they do so. Participants may then participate in an interactive discussion facilitated by the leader.

An ADL group on community outreach may consist of the group participants deciding who or what institution they would like to visit, discussing transportation and setting time schedules, and deciding who will use the phone book and phone to make the necessary arrangements. The group leader may facilitate by making resources available or giving advice when asked.

A vocational group may involve working on a clerical task on an assembly line. The role of the leader will be to set up the project, decide who will perform which roles, and monitor the work and the end products. Participants may interact and help each other or they may work only on their task.

Starting a Group

There are basic steps involved in starting a group (Rerek, 1966). At each step there are questions to ask to clarify your thinking and make the group development a smooth process. If you know the steps and questions, you will know how to think about groups, and consequently, you will be able to develop and utilize groups in any setting and with any population. You will be able to work alone as a group leader, effectively and successfully, to provide meaningful treatment. Table 15-5 reviews the steps to starting a group.

The first step is to survey the patient population. The questions to ask yourself are, "Who are the patients and what are their needs?" An inpatient acute setting where people of all ages stay for three days to be stabilized on medication will dictate a group setting that addresses here-and-now functioning or cognitive reorganization. An outpatient setting that provides service primarily to women who may be depressed would dictate a group for women that provides opportunities for success and mastery and addresses longer-term

Table 15-5.   Starting a Group: Tasks and Critical Questions

Therapist Task	Critical Questions
1. Survey of patient population	Who are they? What are their needs?
2. Setting	Short or long term? Inpatient or outpatient? Specific disorder or special services? Roles for other health professionals? Your job description?
3. Purpose	Why is this group necessary? What do you and the participants want to accomplish?
4. Selection criteria	How will you select participants? Who will and will not benefit? Why? Are evaluation and screening based on issues, problems, diagnosis, cognitive level, interests, gender, age?
5. Specific activities	Concrete or abstract? Simple or complex? Short or long duration? Based on a model? Easy to transport?
6. Your skills and knowledge	Are your skills adequate? Is a consultant, supervisor, or mentor available? Are you interested in this group? Is it a good fit for you?
7. Structure and logistics	Minimum and maximum allowable participants? Voluntary or required? Open or closed? When? How often? How long? Where? One or more leaders?
8. Outcome measure	How will you determine success, whether goals and purpose are being achieved?

Source: Rerek (1966).

occupational areas or daily functioning. A setting in which intense, **psychodynamic** work is the daily focus would dictate a group that provides relaxation/restoration or recreation.

The second step is to consider the constraints of your setting. Is your setting a short-term, acute unit where people who function differently are treated together? Is it a long-term setting where people live in the community and attend four days a week? Does the setting provide treatment for a specific disorder, such as addiction, or does it provide special treatment, such as vocational services? Does the setting include many other health professionals, such as psychologists, nutritionists, social workers, recreational therapists, or movement therapists, with specific roles? Are you the only health professional with a more generalized role? Is your job description specific or are you allowed some freedom?

An important step is to establish the purpose of the group. What do you want to accomplish? What do you want the participants to accomplish? What do the participants wish to accomplish? Why is this group necessary? These questions often translate into group goals. In some groups the purpose is not to change one's life forever but rather to increase one's recognition of the internal resources needed for a transition from the structured setting or a return home. Some groups may allow people to be creative and explore the meaning of their lives, while others may help people reorganize their thinking and decrease confusion. Another type of group may be designed to improve members' personal appearance and therefore will address grooming and self-care. The purpose of a group in a day treatment setting may be to provide a sense of belonging to a community, whereas the same group in an acute care center may be intended to provide a sense of community safety and comfort.

Another step is to consider selection criteria. How will you select participants? Who will benefit from this group and who might not? Some groups will evaluate and screen participants, while others will be open to anyone who wishes to attend. Some groups may require an ability to think abstractly and will therefore screen out individuals who are actively psychotic. Some may address retirement issues and therefore will not benefit adolescents.

A step that is often dictated by the purpose and goals of the group and the nature of its membership is the consideration of what activities to use. What will be the specific activities featured? Will they be tangible or abstract? Will they be short or long term? Will they vary? Will they be easy to use and transport? Stress management groups may use meditation, movement, and music or writing; activities of daily living groups may use discussion and demonstration; and craft groups may use specific modalities, such as clay, jewelry, or leather. Some groups may be nonverbal, while others may involve a great deal of talking.

A step that has been implied in discussing group development and implementation is for the leader to consider his or her skills and knowledge. Are your skills and knowledge adequate for this group? Is there someone who can consult or mentor you? Are you excited about this group? Is it a good fit for you (does it match your personality and strengths)? Although it is important to be aware of the members' needs, which should be paramount, some of the best groups are those that interest their leaders. In fact, if you are not excited or interested in some way by a group, you should not lead it.

The structural details of the group should be well thought out. How large will the group be? Will it be voluntary, or is it required in the program? Will it be open (that is, members may enter and leave at any time) or closed (that is, membership remains stable for a time period)? For how long should the group meet? When and how often will it meet? Where will it meet? Will it be led by the same person or persons? Who has primary responsibility for the group? How will participants be kept informed? Often, such structural details about the group are written down in a group protocol.

A final consideration is to determine a measure of effectiveness for the group. How will you determine if this group is successful and achieves its purpose and goals? Often therapists develop and implement groups and informally assess success, usually as based on attendance or comments of the group members. If at all possible, however, a more formal evaluation of the group's success—an outcome measure—should be established. This is not a requisite in most institutions and in many fields. However, outcome measures document the usefulness and utility of your group and the profession. An ongoing formal evaluation also gives feedback about what does and does not work. It guides the therapist in providing the most useful treatment.

Formal evaluation does not have to be complicated, perplexing, or time-consuming. It could simply involve consistently taking attendance and comparing it with your institution's census to learn the percentage of patients who attend. It could involve a questionnaire about the group to be filled out by the members at various times after their attendance. It could involve questions posed before, during, and after the group experience. It could mean posing the same questions about the group after trying out different activities or techniques. A professional who engages in research (your occupational therapy professor or consultant or a psychologist on staff) will usually assist you.

The Group Protocol

The group content and structure are often written in a protocol. Protocols vary in form but usually include similar content. They often include the group's: name, purpose, goals, content or methods, structure and logistics, method of entry, requirements, and referral criteria. They also generally cover who would and would not benefit, contraindications for membership, and name of the group leader. They often also include a short description or narrative about the group. Two examples of protocols are presented in Table 15-6. Protocols can be more extensive (Borg & Bruce, 1991; Cole, 1993; Howe & Schwartzberg, 1995) and include a more detailed description of the patient population, a rationale, a frame of reference, an outline of treatment sessions, and a listing of outcome criteria.

Writing a group protocol is a way of organizing your thinking about a group. In a narrow sense, it is an aid for yourself, while in a broader sense, it is an aid for others with whom you work. It provides them with a brief, useful description of the group and aids them in referring people to your group and knowing what type of treatment clients are receiving. In these different ways, the group protocol contributes to the functioning of the organization for which you work, in that it also aids the institution to describe its services to prospective clients. Sometimes, the group protocol serves to demystify psychological treatment.

Table 15-6. Group Protocols

Occupational Therapy MAC Group: Mastery and Accomplishment through Crafts

Purpose: Provide opportunities for participants to master concrete activities in a parallel group setting that is not threatening and nondemanding.

Goals: Long-term — Increase sense of effectiveness as demonstrated by participant self-report.

Short-term — Improve concentration and attention span and ability to plan sequentially, as demonstrated by daily assessment.

Group Content: Concrete activities (craft).

Group Structure: Therapist will present participants with crafts. Often all will be working on the same type of craft though each will have his or her own project. Crafts will be structured and graded according to Allen's Cognitive Levels. Therapist will prepare projects and client decision making will be minimal. Interaction will not be required or encouraged, although it often occurs.

Logistics:

Place:	CCB 209
Number of Patients:	Maximum of 8
Meeting Schedule:	Daily, Monday–Friday, 9:00–10:00 A.M.
Group Facilitator:	James Lopez, OTR

Occupational Therapy — Life Skills

Who: • Those who identify areas of daily life that are problematic or that they would like to change.
• Those who use few coping mechanisms or one for all situations

Goal: • Provide opportunities to learn a range of coping mechanisms or ways of adapting
• Provide opportunities to practice old skills of managing in new ways that are more satisfying
• Provide opportunities to clarify values and ways of being in the world, ultimately expanding choices.

Method: Occupational therapist will provide a theme or topic for each session and will provide specific experiential exercises for the group to follow.

Contraindications: Those who are presently actively psychotic or hypermanic, or those who have difficulty thinking abstractly.

Group Leader: Ahmad Wallace, OTR

You may also share your protocols with your clients or members of the group, particularly on entry, as a way of explaining the group. Providing this information can relieve the fears and satisfy the curiosity of new members. Often it favorably disposes the new member to the group and aids in the rapid cohesion and integration. In my clinical groups, group members have shared protocols with their families, often giving relief to worried or curious family members and providing a basis of discussion regarding the client's difficulties and experiences.

Documentation and Outcome

It is becoming increasingly important to document outcomes, and group outcomes can indeed be documented. A simple measurement of outcomes is self-report (Howe & Schwartzberg, 1995), whereby members are asked to evaluate a group either at the end of each session or at the end of a series of meetings. The form can be structured, providing forced choices such as "always," "sometimes," "rarely," or "never," or it can be unstructured, perhaps asking participants open-ended questions regarding their experiences.

Members can be asked to monitor their progress by filling out a behavioral assessment regarding their own behavior in the group. A behavioral observation form (Kaplan, 1988) can also be filled out by the group leaders. Assessment and observation should always tie in to the goals and the purpose of the group as a whole and the individuals in the group. This implies that an initial assessment has been performed to ascertain baseline functioning and that assumptions regarding the group and the frame of reference in which it is grounded will be explicit.

An ideal method of evaluating a group or the individual participants is goal attainment scaling (Ottenbacher & Cusick, 1990). This method employs operational goals and outcomes and explicit time sequences that are determined by the therapist, individuals, and others involved in treatment. It also includes a quantitative measurement of treatment effectiveness. It can be used both for the evaluation of group efficacy and for the evaluation of treatment efficacy for group members.

Documentation may cover the group process and content or discuss each individual in the group. It is generally written in the form of a narrative note; a more structured, problem-oriented or behavioral outcome format; or a list (Acquaviva, 1992; Borg & Bruce, 1991; Denton, 1987; Kaplan, 1988). Generally, a note regarding the group will contain a description of the activity and patients in attendance and a summary of the group experience, or what has occurred. This includes what has been accomplished, any changes since the previous group session, and any unusual occurrences. It may restate the purpose and goals of the group and whether the goals were accomplished. It may include the plan for the subsequent group meeting. A note regarding each individual in the group generally will include descriptions of the person's behavior in the group, how the person interacted and responded to interaction, how the individual participated in the activity, and changes in performance from previous group sessions. Goals may be reiterated, or the plan for an individual in the next group meeting may be stated. As with the group narrative, a baseline assessment and explicit grounding in a frame of reference are required.

CASE ILLUSTRATION:
DEVELOPING A GROUP, PROTOCOL, AND PLAN

Janice Nyugen is an OTR in a large psychiatric hospital that treats people of all ages and diagnoses. One of her roles is as evaluator of incoming clients. After six months of evaluating six to eight patients per week, she noticed that 70 percent had a diagnosis of depression. Of this group, 90 percent were female, 60 percent were between the ages of 25 and 40, and about 15 percent had accompanying problems, such as eating disorders or addictions, for which they were attending other groups or self-help programs based on the 12 steps of Alcoholics Anonymous.

At the hospital, no groups specifically targeted people with the diagnosis of depression. Janice had been interested in this topic in school and so welcomed the opportunity to learn more. She read about depression and spoke with her supervisor about her ideas for a group. She attended case consultations and interviews and spoke with her colleagues concerning how a group for people who were depressed might fit into the program. She attended communication workshops to supplement what she learned in her occupational therapy classes and observed other people whose traits and skills of group leadership she admired. She then developed a group protocol and an explanation of the group that she had designed. Table 15-7 shows the protocol she wrote for the group. Table 15-8 delineates the group leadership, activity, process, and desired outcomes of the group.

Discussion

Janice demonstrated the correct way to go about developing a group; that is, she noticed a need and a population that were not served in her organization, she sought consultation and more knowledge, she observed other leaders' styles, and she developed a logical group plan and description.

Summary

Much treatment in the psychiatric arena is provided in groups. Groups are cost-effective, facilitate personal growth, and provide feedback by more than one person (though not everyone is suited for group treatment). The content, the structure, and leadership contribute to the process of the group.

Occupational therapy groups often combine principles and techniques of psychological models, but they are unique in their emphases on activity and on occupational performance and components. Various types and models of activity groups have been proposed for occupational therapy. A theory of activity groups is evolving; currently, occupational therapy groups can be fit into broad categories based on content.

Certain steps can be followed to successfully start a group. Starting a group involves planning and writing a group protocol. A successful group combines following the appropriate steps while assuming leadership and modeling communication skills. Group outcomes can be subsequently evaluated.

Review Questions

1. What distinguishes occupational therapy groups from others?
2. What other groups might you encounter in a psychosocial setting?

Table 15-7. Protocol for a Group Dealing with Depression

Name: Making Friends with Your Demons: Dealing with Depression

Purpose: Increase opportunities for mastery and success, improve participants' strategies and tools to cope with depression, and educate participants regarding the warning signs of depression.

Goals: Given participation in the group daily for two weeks, the participants will be able to accomplish two concrete activities successfully, report improved mood as measured by the Beck Depression Inventory, state three strategies for coping with depressed mood, and state three warning signs of impending depressed mood.

Group Content: The group will include simple craft activities that can be worked on independently and finished successfully in one session, identification of thoughts and feelings relating to depressed moods, and identification of coping strategies and signs of impending depressed mood through written exercises, exploration, and discussions.

Group Structure: The leader will provide opportunities for engagement with concrete activities and assist members to complete them. The leader will actively direct written exercises and discussion and provide education regarding coping strategies and recognizing signs of impending depression. The sequence of the group is such that initially there will be little demand on the participants as they successfully complete activities, and then gradually demands will increase as exploration and discussion are introduced. However, participants do not have to initiate in this group, and interaction is initially mostly between the leader and individuals, gradually giving way to group discussion with other members, facilitated by the leader.

Who Would Benefit: This group would primarily benefit women between the ages of 25 and 40 with depressed mood who also are dealing with issues of addiction. They must be able to think abstractly and should demonstrate some capacity for self-reflection.

Who Would Not Benefit: Those who are unable to think abstractly or have psychotic thinking; those who are unable to attend to a group for at least one hour or concentrate on abstract concepts; those who are presently in a manic state.

Logistics: Monday–Friday, 9–10 A.M., 2/1–2/12.
The Rose Room, #200
Group Leader: Janice Nyugen, OTR

3. What are some categories of groups? Which do you believe would most interest you and why?
4. What are some questions you might reflect on as you develop a group?
5. Which leadership communication and personhood skills do you know or have? Which ones do you need to learn?

Learning Activities

1. Think of any organization to which you belong. Think of how you would start a group in that organization by utilizing the steps to starting a group.

Table 15-8. Making Friends with Your Demons: Dealing with Depression (Two-Week Process)

Day	Group Leadership	Group Activity	Group Process	Desired Outcome/ Rationale
1	Explains the group to the participants, giving them the group protocol and discussing it. Gives them self-report questionnaires to fill out. Solicits questions and concerns.	Reading and discussing thoughts and feelings regarding the group protocol; stating desired personal outcomes. Filling out the Beck Depression Inventory, a list of strategies each individual uses to cope with depression, and a list of behavioral and cognitive warning signs of impending depression.	The leader introduces herself and members introduce themselves to each other. Most interaction is between the leader and the members.	Introduction to each other. Developing rapport with leader and members. Beginning comfort among members. Completion of evaluative measures.
2–4	Provides categories of craft activities: ceramics, jewelry, or leather. Assists members in their projects.	Craft projects.	Members work independently and individually on their chosen craft projects, with assistance from the leader when necessary. They speak casually with each other, though this is not required. They display their finished projects on the last day.	Developing rapport and comfort in the group and with each other. Increased sense of ability and mastery and therefore awareness of self-effectiveness. Beginning group participation in a nondemanding way.
5	Provides a written handout, "On Depres-	Group discussion with a handout about	Members read and listen to the leader's	Beginning interaction.

(continues)

Table 15-8. Making Friends with Your Demons: Dealing with Depression (Two-Week Process) (continued)

Day	Group Leadership	Group Activity	Group Process	Desired Outcome/ Rationale
	sion," that describes the symptoms of depression and theories of its cause. Directs an active discussion by asking each participant to comment on various aspects.	various aspects of depression.	thoughts about depression. Members are asked to comment by the leader. The interaction is primarily leader-to-participant.	Education about depression. Beginning ability to identify specific, personal aspects of depression.
6	Provides written exercise, "Stressful Events." Directs participants how to do the activity. Directs a discussion of how everyday events cause more stress than one is likely to realize. Asks each member to share their stress test and validates thoughts and feelings. Points out similarities with other participants.	From a list of stressful events weighted from most stressful to least stressful, chooses those that have occurred in the last year and adds up the stress score. Discusses thoughts and feelings regarding the scores and the events.	Members complete the activity individually , and share their comments, at first to the leader, then to the other members	Recognition of stressful events. Realization of how each event may cause stress. Validation of thoughts and feelings. Decrease of isolation and guilt.
7	Provides written exercise, "Chalk Talk." Directs participants how to do the activity. Directs a discussion of how automatic negative thoughts contribute to depression. Asks	Introduces the concept that automatic, usually negative, thoughts contribute to depression. Introduces the concept of the "chalk talk," that is, that individuals are	Members write their "chalk talk" individually and share their comments, at first to the leaders and then to the other members. Members begin to validate and	Participants become aware of the effect of their internal, usually negative, thoughts. Participants become aware of how their thoughts interfere with behavior and

(continues)

Table 15-8.	Making Friends with Your Demons: Dealing with Depression (Two-Week Process) (continued)		

Day	Group Leadership	Group Activity	Group Process	Desired Outcome/ Rationale
	each member to share their "chalk talk," validates, and points out similarities with other members. Ends with a symbolic erasure or throwing away of the negative "chalk talk," while carefully saving the positive "chalk talk."	constantly coaching themselves as they go about daily life. Members choose an event from the previous day that causes moderate stress, then list the thoughts that usually occur before, during, and after that event.	initiate with each other.	occur with depression. Participants learn strategies for coping with the negative thoughts.
8	Provides written activity, "Practice." Directs participants how to do the activity. Directs a discussion of how automatic behavior contributes to depression. Asks each member to share their practice routines. Validates and points out similarities with other members. Asks members to work with each other in dyads to create a new practice routine.	Introduces the concept that automatic behavior often contributes to depression. Introduces the concept of automatic practice routines that need to be changed. Members choose the same stressful event from the previous day and list their behavior before, during, and after the event.	Members individually write their "practice routine." Members share their routine with others and validate others' comments.	Participants become aware of how their actions are automatic and can lead to depression. Participants learn new strategies to practice different behavior.
9	Provides written activity, "Creating Positive Chalk Talk and New	Written exercises, the "Next Chalk Talk" and "Creating New	Members individually choose and share the anticipated	Members anticipate events connected to depressed mood

(continues)

Table 15-8.	Making Friends with Your Demons: Dealing with Depression (Two-Week Process) (continued)			
Day	*Group Leadership*	*Group Activity*	*Group Process*	*Desired Outcome/ Rationale*
	Practice Routines." Directs members how to do the activity. Asks members to share their thoughts and feelings. Facilitates the group working together to help each other create new talk and new routines.	Practice Routines." Leader introduces the concept of anticipating events that lead to depression. Members choose one situation/event that will evoke depression in their environment. Members create new talk and new behavior to prevent depressed mood.	event and their automatic thoughts and behavior. Members work together designing new practice routines and chalk talks.	and create prevention strategies. Members cooperate with each other, decrease isolation, and learn how to accept help.
10	Group leader asks members to fill out the Beck Depression Scale and to list strategies to cope with and prevent depression. Group leader guides the wrap-up, in which each member says good-bye and expresses a message directly to every other member.	Each member individually fills out evaluative measures and comments on them. Each member directly interacts with the other members.	Each member has a chance to express any ending thoughts or feelings about the group, each other, and what they had anticipated, thereby having a chance to realize a positive sense of completion.	To have comparative outcome measures so that members may recognize personal change and progress. To have comparative outcome measures regarding group goals to evaluate the efficacy of the group.

2. Notice the leadership and personhood skills of your favorite teacher, friend, or parent.
3. Attend any short-term group offered at your college and observe your experience in the group. Keep a record or self-report of your moods and thoughts after each meeting. Did the group accomplish its goal?

4. For ideas for groups, review the lists of activities, sample groups, and plans listed in the reference books, particularly Borg and Bruce (1991), Cole (1993), Howe and Schwartzberg (1995), and Kaplan (1988).
5. Think of a group that you would like to join. What are the needs of the group? How would you like it to be structured? How would you like to be treated? How would you know if the group was successful for you?

References

Acquaviva, J. (Ed.). (1992). *Effective documentation for occupational therapy*. Rockville, MD: American Occupational Therapy Association.

Alonso, A., & Swiller, H. (Ed.). (1993). *Group therapy in clinical practice*. Washington, DC: American Psychiatric Press.

Borg, B., & Bruce, M. A. (1991). *The group system: The therapeutic activity group in occupational therapy*. Thorofare, NJ: Slack.

Cole, M. B. (1993). *Group dynamics in occupational therapy*. Thorofare, NJ: Slack.

Corey, G. (1991). *Theory and practice of counseling and psychotherapy* (4th ed.). Pacific Grove, CA: Brooks.

Corey, G., & Corey, M. S. (1992). *Groups: Process and practice* (4th ed.). Monterey, CA: Brooks/Cole.

Denton, P. L. (1987). *Psychiatric occupational therapy: A workbook of practical skills*. Boston: Little, Brown.

Fidler, G. S. (1969). The task-oriented group as a context for treatment. *American Journal of Occupational Therapy, 23*, 43.

Howe, M., & Schwartzberg, S. L. (1995). *A functional approach to group work in occupational therapy* (2nd ed.). Philadelphia: Lippincott.

Kaplan, H., & Sadock, B. (1991). *Synopsis of psychiatry: Behavioral sciences: Clinical psychology* (6th ed.). Baltimore, MD: Williams & Wilkins.

Kaplan, H., & Sadock, B. (1995). *Comprehensive textbook of psychiatry* (6th ed.). Baltimore, MD: Williams & Wilkins.

Kaplan, K. L. (1986). The directive group: Short term treatment for psychiatric patients with a minimal level of functioning. *American Journal of Occupational Therapy, 40*, 474–481.

Kaplan, K. L. (1988). *Directive group therapy: Innovative mental health treatment*. Thorofare, NJ: Slack.

King, L. J. (1974). A sensory integrative approach to schizophrenia. *American Journal of Occupational Therapy, 28*(9), 529–536.

Mosey, A. C. (1970). The concept and use of developmental groups. *American Journal of Occupational Therapy, 24*, 272.

Mosey, A. C. (1981). *Occupational therapy: Configuration of a profession*. New York: Raven.

Mosey, A. C. (1986). *Components of psychosocial occupational therapy*. New York: Raven.

Ottenbacher, K. J., & Cusick, A. (1990). Goal attainment scaling as a method of clinical service evaluation. *American Journal of Occupational Therapy*, *44* (6), 519–526.

Rerek, M. (1966). *The use of groups in occupational therapy*. Unpublished manuscript.

Yalom, I. (1983). *Inpatient group psychotherapy*. New York: Basic Books.

Yalom, I. (1995). *The theory and practice of group psychotherapy* (4th ed.). New York: Basic Books.

Suggested Reading

Bion, W. (1961). *Experiences in groups and other papers*. New York: Basic Books.

Kaplan, H., & Sadock, B. J. (1993). *Comprehensive group psychotherapy* (3rd ed.). Baltimore, MD: Williams & Wilkins.

PART V

Specialized Roles for OT in Mental Health

Psychiatric Issues in HIV Infection

Lynne Andonian, OTR
Formerly, Occupational Therapist
San Francisco General Hospital

Romy Falck, OTR
Clinical Director of Occupational Therapy
Sundance Rehabilitation Corporation
Emeryville, California

Key Terms

AIDS (acquired immune deficiency syndrome)
HIV (human immunodeficiency virus)

opportunistic infection
outed
seroconversion
universal precautions

Chapter Outline

Introduction

HIV (human immunodeficiency virus) and **AIDS (acquired immunodeficiency syndrome)** are currently among the most serious social, political, and medical issues of our time. Regardless of the setting, occupational therapists will treat patients with HIV and AIDS and, therefore, may observe changes or symptoms that may not be the primary reason for referral. This chapter mainly addresses the psychological aspects of the disease; however, due to the many ramifications of HIV and AIDS, it is also necessary to encompass basic information regarding the HIV/AIDS disease process and its psychopathology, legal and ethical issues, clinical treatment, and caregiver issues.

HIV DISEASE PROCESS

Humans begin life with an inborn immune system consisting of dermal tissue or skin, mucosal linings and cilia of the digestive and respiratory systems, stomach enzymes and gastric fluids, and, finally, phagocytes, all of which help keep harmful microorganisms out of the body. There is also a second line of immunological defense involving acquired immunities to specific harmful microorganisms, which begins developing in utero and continues throughout life.

For the purpose of this chapter, it is acquired immunity that is of particular interest. When a pathogen enters the body, this cell-mediated system of immunity dispatches macrophages to organs in the lymphatic system. It is here that they phagocytize and digest all but a fragment of the pathogen. This fragment remains and protrudes from the cell surface, where it is identified by the B cells and T cells. T cells are lymphocytes produced in the bone marrow whose primary function is to mediate cellular immune responses. The two T cells of main concern here are the suppressor T cell (CD8) and the helper T cell (CD4+). When CD4+ cells identify the antigen fragments on the cellular surface, they stimulate production of additional lymphocytes to destroy the foreign matter. Once they have completed their job, the CD8 cells signal for the T and B cells to stop, thereby protecting noninfected cells from destruction (Le Cocq, Bonck, & MacRae, 1995). Figure 16-1 provides a visual representation of the HIV transmission process, which shows the immune system's response to the entrance of HIV into the bloodstream.

HIV is a member of the retrovirus class, which means that it carries its genetic material in the form of ribonucleic acid (RNA) as opposed to deoxyribonucleic acid (DNA). HIV infects some B cells but primarily targets lymphocytes, especially macrophages and CD4+ cells. After binding to a lymphocyte, HIV enters the cell nucleus, where a copy of the virus is made. The

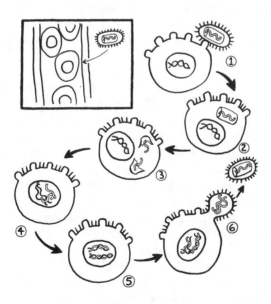

Once in the bloodstream, the virus, in (1) and (2), attaches itself to, and then enters, a T-cell; in (3) and (4), the viral RNA unites with the T-cell DNA. After a period of dormancy (5), the T-cell buds off a new HIV virus (6).

Figure 16-1. HIV Transmission Process: The T-cell As HIV Factory

lymphocyte then begins replicating the virus and releasing it to infect other cells (Le Cocq et al., 1995).

Seroconversion occurs within 3 to 12 months. In retrospect, many people have described nonspecific flu-like symptoms, including fatigue, diarrhea, muscle ache, and fever during this time, followed by an asymptomatic period in which the individual tests seropositive (Flaskerud, 1992).

Transmission

It seems that one can hardly exist in society today without having some degree of knowledge regarding the transmission of HIV; however, this is not necessarily a valid assumption. Much of the information circulating in the lay community is based on myths or outdated information. Quite simply, the only way that one can contract the virus is by coming into direct contact with infected bodily fluids or fluids that have been recognized by the government Center for Disease Control (CDC) as linked to the transmission of HIV, such as blood and blood products, semen, vaginal secretions, and cerebrospinal fluids. While the virus has also been found in saliva, tears, and sweat, the concentration is markedly lower than in blood, semen, or vaginal fluids.

There is also a risk for infants born to mothers who have the virus as it can be contracted through bodily fluids such as blood and vaginal secretions at and around the time of birth. In addition, some research points to transmission of the virus after birth via breast milk (Chorba, Holman, & Evatt, 1993; Segal, 1993).

One of the greatest concerns among health care professionals is that of contracting HIV while performing job-related tasks. Occupational (accidental) exposures can occur in the form of needle sticks and splashes or sprays of contaminated bodily fluids. Statistics released from the CDC in Atlanta, Georgia, on September 30, 1992, reported 32 documented cases of occupationally acquired HIV infection in the United States and an additional 69 cases of possible HIV infection from occupational exposure ("Surveillance," 1992). Of the 32 cases of occupationally acquired HIV, 7 individuals (22 percent) developed AIDS, and of the 69 cases of possible occupational exposure, 54 (78 percent) developed AIDS. This is why **universal precautions** should be recognized as a vital routine for all health professionals. Universal precautions serve a dual function: to protect the health professional from exposure in the workplace, and, second and equally important, to protect the patient against infection from the health care provider. The patient with HIV is at a greater risk of contracting a pathogen from the staff, than the staff is of contracting HIV from the patient (Marcil, 1992). Table 16-1 outlines the universal precaution guidelines, which require that all bodily fluids from all persons be treated as potentially contaminated.

The late 1970s to 1985 was a period in U.S. medical history when infection from blood transfusions was a primary concern. During this time individuals

Table 16-1. Universal Precautions

- Wear barrier precaution items with all patients whenever there is a potential for exposure to bodily fluids and discard items after treating each patient.
- Wash hands immediately and thoroughly after removing gloves or if skin has come in contact with bodily fluids.
- Do not bend or recap needles or sharps after use. Do dispose of them in a red plastic "sharps" container bearing the biohazard label.
- When performing cardiopulmonary resuscitation (CPR), use a mouthpiece or resuscitation bag.
- Medical personnel with skin lesions should refrain from direct patient care until lesions have healed. All minor skin breaks should be covered (cuts, hangnails, etc.).

requiring a blood transfusion were exposed to a contaminated blood supply because blood-screening procedures had not yet been developed. The number of reported incidences in the United States of infection from recent blood transfusions are on the decline due to the development and constant improvement of blood-screening methods (Gonzales-Aviles, 1992). However, this is not the case for many nonindustrialized countries, where the number of reported cases of HIV infection as a result of a blood transfusion indicates that this continues to be a high-risk procedure.

It is often innacurately thought that to test HIV positive automatically means that the individual has AIDS, whereas in reality, HIV disease is best viewed and managed on a continuum involving a four-stage process (Gonzales-Aviles, 1992; Weinstein, 1990):

- Stage one: HIV infection—can include flu-like symptoms such as fever, rashes, and joint pain
- Stage two: seroconversion and asymptomatic reduction in immunity
- Stage three: noticeable reduction in immunity as evidenced by opportunistic infections with some functional deficits
- Stage Four: "classic AIDS"—drastic impairments of the immune system resulting in symptoms such as night sweats, diarrhea, infections, secondary cancers, and neurological diseases

As recently as 1992, the term *AIDS* was scrutinized for its vague description and horrifying connotations. The current definition and classification system used by the CDC focuses heavily on the CD4+ (T cell) count and the presence of **opportunistic infection**. It is suggested that a more accurate diagnostic term is *HIV disease* by allowing the term *AIDS* to be revised to include persons with CD4+ count of 200 or less. These counts are especially used as indicators for medication management in treating or even preventing AIDS-related diseases (Ungvarski, 1992).

CASE ILLUSTRATION: SHARON—HIV TRANSMISSION

Sharon is a 19-year-old African-American female. She presented herself at the community health clinic for an HIV test approximately two years ago; at the time, she was three months pregnant. A television program educating teens about safe sex prompted Sharon to get tested. From the television show she knew that she had two options for testing. She could either go to her family physician, where the results would become part of her permanent medical record, or she could go to a local clinic for anonymous testing, where she would be issued a number to protect her identity.

Sharon opted for anonymous testing at a women's clinic, where the public health nurse counseled her on the procedure, drew her blood, and two weeks later called her to come back to the clinic to receive her results. She was informed at this time that her test had come back positive. Her blood was drawn again for retesting to insure that the result was not a false positive. The second test confirmed the diagnosis: she was HIV positive. Sharon states that despite having had unprotected sex, she was shocked by the news that she had tested HIV positive. The public health nurse counseled Sharon after the diagnosis and gave her several referrals to clinics and support groups; however, Sharon felt too overwhelmed to make contact with any of the agencies. At her next obstetrics appointment, she considered not telling her doctor about her HIV status because of stories she had seen on the news about how "people refuse to treat anyone with AIDS." However, Sharon ultimately decided to tell her doctor after she read one of the pamphlets that she was given at the clinic about pregnant women with HIV which described how early intervention with the drug AZT can reduce the risk of fetal infection without serious short term side effects to mother or infant. Her obstetrician explained that by taking azidothymidine (AZT), the odds of infecting her fetus dropped 25.5 percent to 8.3 percent (Fackelmann, 1994). Sharon chose to take the AZT, but unfortunately, her daughter was discovered to be HIV positive as well.

PSYCHOPATHOLOGY OF HIV

HIV disease can contribute to psychiatric symptoms via physical (organic) changes in the brain or because of psychosocial issues (defined further in this section). Although the functional deficits associated with HIV are variable, in general, impairment in functioning related to behavior, activities of daily living (ADLs), or physical or mental status cause the patient or the patient's family to seek medical treatment.

Depression

Depressed HIV positive patients generally have two disorders: HIV disease and depression. In most cases the mood disorder precedes the onset of HIV infection (Markowitz, Rabkin, & Perry, 1994). Like organic mania secondary to HIV (discussed later in this section), depression can be the result of advanced HIV disease through the development of HIV organic depression. However, when organic factors are omitted, the risk factors for depression in HIV positive individuals are similar to those for HIV negative patients (Markowitz et al., 1994). The risk factors for depression in HIV positive individuals include the following:

- history or family history of depression
- alcohol or other drug use
- loss of social supports
- isolation
- multiple losses
- advanced HIV infection (possibly organic mood syndrome)

Markowitz et al. (1994) report that recent studies of nonpatient samples have found similar rates of depressive disorders among HIV positive and HIV negative subjects. The vast majority of people with HIV infection are not clinically depressed; however, learning that one is HIV positive is a major life stressor, which can contribute to suicidal ideation or attempts. Whether the depression is caused by the knowledge of a change in HIV status or some other factors, it is very important to treat the depression, as patients do respond to pharmacological treatment. Since most HIV positive people are not clinically depressed, occupational therapists who encounter depressed HIV positive patients need to be careful lest they dismiss hopelessness and depression as normal reactions to HIV infection, thereby failing to treat a patient's psychiatric depression.

Psychosocial stressors (i.e., multiple losses) are risk factors for depression. For example, a patient with HIV disease may find him- or herself on an inpatient psychiatric unit after becoming intoxicated and making a suicide attempt. The initial knowledge of a positive HIV test result may put an individual at risk for a suicide attempt (Williams, 1990). Patients often report a variety of recent stressors, such as the death of friends or partners secondary to AIDS, testing HIV positive, the progressive and unpredictable nature of HIV disease, fear and stigma associated with HIV, all of which lead to isolation, financial burdens because of medical care, changing appearance and body image, and difficulty adjusting to changing levels of functioning (Karasic & Dilley, 1994).

Decreased appetite, weight loss, insomnia, and fatigue may be symptoms of HIV disease or depression. Experienced physicians and psychologists can usually distinguish the symptoms and diagnoses, possibly assisted by neuropsychiatric tests. When using antidepressant therapy, HIV infection may impact the dosage, duration, and type of medication prescribed (Markowitz et al., 1994). The possible reaction of a psychiatric medication with other medicines the patient may be taking for HIV disease also needs to be considered. Some antidepressants are chosen because of their additional effect of relieving pain associated with neuropathy (i.e., amitryptyline hydrochloride).

Mania

Secondary manic syndromes, such as HIV-related mania, are distinct from bipolar mood disorder and can be caused by a variety of organic factors. Manic syndromes have been described in people with HIV disease, suggesting that HIV may cause organic mood syndromes. Between 15 and 20 percent of people with AIDS dementia develop manic syndromes, which is far greater than the .5 to 2.0 percent risk of having a manic episode among the general population (Kieburtz, Zeltelmaler, Ketonen, Tuite, & Caine, 1991). These figures support the conclusion that HIV infection causes manic syndromes, but at this time it is not known exactly how this occurs. Other HIV-related findings in individuals displaying a manic syndrome include an abnormal brain scan from magnetic resonance imaging (MRI), a three-dimensional scan used in diagnostic procedures, and some types of cognitive impairment (Kieburtz et al., 1991). It is unusual for HIV-related mania to develop unless there is significant immunosuppression; however, more research is needed to determine the link between the degree of cognitive impairment and the development of HIV-related mania.

HIV mania has some distinctive characteristics that distinguish it from bipolar mood disorder. Table 16-2 outlines the distinguishing symptoms of HIV mania and bipolar 1 disorder. Manic symptoms often respond to treatment, but the organically derived cognitive deficits remain, posing challenges concerning disposition.

Table 16-2. Symptoms Distinguishing HIV-Related Mania from Bipolar 1 Disorder

HIV-Related Mania	*Bipolar 1 Disorder*
No prior history of bipolar disorder	Recurrent disorder, with more than 90 percent of people with manic episodes going on to have future episodes
Person displays confusion	Person may be distractible but is not confused
May have concurrent HIV-associated dementia	Symptoms are not due to direct physiological effects of a medical condition.
Abnormal brain MRI	Normal brain MRI
Negative family history for the disorder	First-degree biological relatives have increased incidence of bipolar 1 disorder (4–24 percent), bipolar 2 disorder (1–5 percent), and major depressive disorder (4–24 percent)

CASE ILLUSTRATION: ANDREW—HIV MANIC SYNDROME

Andrew is a 29-year-old, bisexual, African-American man with AIDS and no prior psychiatric history. Prior to admission, the patient had been spending increased amounts of money on clothing and had been ringing neighbor's doorbells at night and singing. When he was picked up by the police, the patient stated that he was "auditioning for a musical." Upon admission to the unit, he was irritable and confused and had grandiose delusions regarding being a film star and having a record contract. Initially the patient was combative and required seclusion for a short period of time for his own safety and that of the staff. Medications (valproic acid and perphenazine) were started, and clear expectations for behavior were conveyed.

The occupational therapist first made contact with Andrew during grooming sessions. The patient was social regarding hair styles and remarked upon the therapist's hair as well as his own. The patient and the occupational therapist collaboratively set a goal to work on hair care and grooming. Andrew used multiple supplies and used them excessively. He said he was a hairstylist, claimed the supplies were his, and became angry when the therapist attempted to retrieve them. The occupational therapist decided to work with Andrew one-on-one to limit the number of supplies, provide structure, and decrease environmental distractions. These adaptations assisted Andrew to follow through on tasks. Through this interaction a rapport developed and Andrew began attending other occupational therapy treatment groups. In a cooking group, he displayed impaired safety awareness when using the stove and impulsively added extra ingredients into the recipe. The occupational therapist reported to the rest of the treatment team this information regarding judgment and safety, which was considered critical information for determining the level of care Andrew would need upon discharge. After being in the hospital for two weeks, Andrew was discharged to a supervised living situation.

HIV Dementia

HIV dementia—also called AIDS dementia complex or HIV encephalopathy—is caused by HIV infection of the brain, which causes motor, cognitive, and affective symptoms that significantly impair social and occupational functioning. HIV enters the brain shortly after initial infection when macrophages harboring the HIV virus cross the blood-brain barrier (Perry, 1990). There is a great range in the progression of HIV-induced organic disorders. In some patients, the mental decline can be quite rapid, while others may have a very prolonged course with transient periods of recovery (Perry, 1990). Some people will have signs of dementia as an early symptom of HIV infection rather than an end stage symptom of AIDS. Often people with beginning cognitive changes will first notice the problem themselves (e.g., they start forgetting phone numbers). HIV dementia can cause a wide range of behavioral, cognitive, and affective impairments leading to a slowing and loss of precision in cognitive and motor control (Polan, 1991). Table 16-3 outlines the symptoms and deficits that may be found in HIV dementia. Although these conditions are not yet curable, they are treatable (treatment issues will be addressed later in this chapter).

Common behaviors or functional symptoms of HIV-related cognitive impairment that an occupational therapist may observe during group or individual treatment include the following: rummaging through supplies, wandering, incontinence, social withdrawal, passivity, impaired grooming and hygiene, and limited attention span. Patients may demonstrate symptoms of HIV dementia and HIV mania concurrently. Other behaviors may have already been evident in the community and facilitated the person's contact with treatment providers.

CASE ILLUSTRATION: JIM—HIV DEMENTIA

Jim is a 44-year-old Caucasian male who uses intravenous drugs and has a long history of alcohol use. He has had an AIDS diagnosis for one year after having had pneumocystis carinii pneumonia (PCP). Jim lives in a general assistance hotel and has worked with his case manager, an occupational therapist, for six months. Jim reports being easily fatigued; he has episodes of disorientation and complains of memory problems. He frequently misses his medical appointments because of forgetfulness, and states that he would like "help to remember things." His occupational therapist has noticed increasing periods of disorientation and confusion and describes Jim's appearance as apathetic, with deteriorating grooming. Jim recently accidentally caused a fire in his room after forgetting to put out a cigarette. He cannot remember his address or his therapist's name. The occupational therapist met with Jim for short treatment sessions every day at the same time to assist with memory compensation strategies (writing down appointments), environmental adaptation (checking smoke detectors, encouraging smoking outdoors, and reducing clutter), and the promotion of daily bathing and dressing. Jim's medical doctor was contacted because of Jim's worsening symptoms of confusion, and the visiting nurses association was contacted to do an assessment. The occupational therapist arranged other support services such as meal delivery, a "support buddy" to assist with household chores, and social day treatment two times a week to promote a routine in a safe environment.

HIV dementia can be viewed as having distinct stages, with orientation, memory, motor, behavioral, problem solving, and activities of daily living affected to varying degrees. The stages are classified as mild, moderate, severe, and end stage HIV associated dementia (HAD). Some patients may display minor memory problems, slightly slowed motor movements, and slight mental slowing, which

Table 16-3. HIV Dementia Symtoms and Deficits	
Appearance	*Motor Skills*
Personal grooming and hygiene	Psychomotor retardation
Inappropriate clothing choices for	Ataxic gait
the weather or situation	Tremor
Food on clothes or face after eating	Slowed speech
Incontinence (late stage)	Slowed response time
	Bilateral leg weakness
	Impaired handwriting
Thought Process	*Cognition*
Difficulty answering questions	Memory
directly (circumstantial)	Short-term memory
Difficulty shifting to new topics	Visual-spatial memory
Talking self through tasks in a	Concentration
step-by-step manner	Complex sentencing
	Receptive speech
Affect	*Insight and Judgment*
Apathy, blunting, or withdrawal	Unaware of limitations
Vacant stare or indifference to	Impulsivity
surroundings	Poor safety awareness
Agitation or confusion	Unaware of need for assistance
Irritability or euphoria (with	Denial of cognitive problems
concurrent HIV mania)	

Note: Impairments may be observed in one or more of the six areas listed here.

is indicative of HIV associated minor cognitive/motor disorder (HACMD) (Boccellari & Dilley, 1992). Asymptomatic HIV positive patients (those without opportunistic infections or other clinical symptoms related to immune system compromise) have the same risk of cognitive impairment as HIV negative controls. However, patients with HIV disease who are immune compromised as measured by elevated beta 2 microglobulin (an immune system protein), even while asymptomatic, have an increased risk of cognitive impairment. It appears that immune compromise must exist first (not just HIV infection) for cognitive impairment to develop (Boccellari et al., 1993). The Neuropsychiatric AIDS Rating Scale (NARS) presented in Figure 16-2 is one tool to diagnose and conceptualize the range of cognitive, motor, and behavioral changes that are associated with HIV infection (Boccellari and Dilley, 1992).

Occupational therapists can help to structure the environment to assist in orienting confused patients with late-stage HIV dementia. Examples of techniques include posting patients' names on bedroom doors and displaying an orientation board with the day, date, and address of the facility. Creating a

(NARS)*

NARS Staging	Cognitive/Behavioral Domains					
	Orientation	Memory	Motor	Behavioral	Problem Solving	Activities of Daily Living
0 (Normal)	Fully oriented	Normal	Normal	Normal	Can solve everyday problems	Fully capable of self care
.5 (Minor) HACMD	Fully oriented	Complains of memory problems	Fully ambulatory; slightly slowed movements	Normal	Has slight mental slowing	Slight impairment in business dealings
1 (Mild) HAD	Fully oriented but may have brief periods of "spaciness"	Mild memory problems	Balance, coordination, and handwriting difficulties	More irritable, labile; or apathetic and withdrawn	Difficulty planning and completing work	Can do simple daily activities, may need prompting
2 (Moderate) HAD	Some dis-orientation	Memory moderately impaired; new learning	Ambulatory but may require a cane	Some impulsivity or agitated behavior	Severe impairment poor social judgment; gets lost easily	Needs assistance with ADL's
3 (Severe) HAD	Frequent dis-orientation	Severe memory loss; only fragments of memory remain	Ambulatory with assistance	May have an organic psychosis	Judgment very poor	Cannot live independently
4 (End Stage) HAD	Confused and disoriented	Virtually no memory	Bedridden	Mute and unresponsive	No problem-solving ability	Nearly vegetative

*NARS developed by A. Boccellari, Ph.D., J.W. Dilley, M.D., and I. Barlow, M.D., Department of Psychiatry, San Francisco General Hospital in collaboration with S. Hernandez and B. Haskell, San Francisco Department of Public Health

Adapted from: Price RW, Brew BJ: The AIDS Dementia Complex. *J Infect Dis.* 158(5):1079-1083, 1988; Hughes CP, Berg I., Donziger WI., et al: A New Clinical Scale for the Staging of Dementia. *British Journal of Psychiatry* 140:566-592, 1982; Criteria for diagnosis of HIV-I Associated Dementia Complex from the Working Group of the American Academy of Neurology AIDS Task Force: Nomenclature and research case definitions for neurologic manifestations of human immunodeficiency virus-type I (HIV-I) infection. *Neurology,* 1991, 41:778-784.

Revised 6/22/92

Figure 16-2.　Neuropsychiatric AIDS Rating Scale (NARS)

consistent structure and daily routine can help patients to feel less anxious. Always keeping belongings in the same place and exhibiting familiar objects such as photographs can be comforting. These patients are very sensitive to the level of stimulation in the environment, and either too much or too little stimulation can lead to confusion, agitation, and fearfulness (Leary & Zeifert, 1994).

Preexisting Psychiatric Diagnosis and HIV Disease

People with mental illness may have impaired judgment or impulsive tendencies, which may lead to behavior that puts them at risk for HIV infection (Steiner, Lussier, & Rosenblatt, 1992). The abuse of alcohol and other drugs also creates opportunities for exposure to the HIV virus via impaired judgment, intravenous drug use involving shared needles, and victimization in higher-risk sexual behavior (Goisman, Kent, Montgomery, Cheevers, & Goldfinger, 1991). HIV infection is found in men and women with every type of psychiatric diagnosis and of every race, ethnic group, and class. In treatment, especially in an acute inpatient setting, the psychiatric symptoms are generally more prominent and require the more acute treatment. Then, as the patient stabilizes psychiatrically, more dialogue regarding the HIV status and resultant concerns can occur. Of course, the HIV disease also needs complete treatment, which is often provided on the inpatient unit as well through medical consults and collaboration with outpatient AIDS care providers.

A wide variety of responses to HIV infection and coping strategies are employed by people with mental health disorders. Some patients will be in a state of denial and refuse to address HIV issues in any manner, while others will have basic information and a general understanding of the chronic nature of the illness and a few patients are well connected with HIV supports and information. Any level of HIV infection can be combined with any mental health disorder and level of concern. For example, a man with HIV mania and severe AIDS dementia may be able to accurately name his AIDS medications (including dapsone, fluconazole, ketoconazole, clofazimine, and cipofloxicine) but omits his psychiatric medications. Consequently, it might be inferred that for this patient the HIV disease is the most prominent health issue. In contrast, a 25-year-old man with a diagnosis of schizoaffective disorder and asymptomatic HIV infection may insist that he does not have HIV and complain of people poisoning him. He may also complain of hearing voices and may work on strategies to decrease their volume (i.e., listening to music with headphones, playing basketball), which indicates his readiness to address his psychiatric symptoms but not his HIV disease at this time.

HIV Psychosocial Issues

In addition to the specific diagnostic issues already discussed, HIV disease has a far-reaching psychosocial impact. This is understandable considering the potentially life-threatening nature of the disease and its progressive and unpredictable course. The stigma associated with HIV and the lack of a unified strategy in attempting to find a cure—and even the prejudicial opinions that some people "deserve" to be infected—point to the division in beliefs and the various strong feelings that come up in relation to this illness (Falk-Kessler, Barnowski, & Salvant, 1994; Hansen, 1990). Societal stigma may add to guilty feelings about being, or recently having become, HIV positive, and patients may also feel guilty over possibly infecting others (Williams, 1990). Systems of social support may be lost or fragmented, leading to feelings of isolation because of the fears and stigma associated with HIV disease (Piemme & Bolle, 1990).

Often people feel angry upon initial diagnosis, and feelings of frustration may build as they attempt to access various health care services with limited insurance resources (Schaffner, 1990). Some HIV positive people will feel shocked and deeply sad when they first learn they are infected (Williams, 1990). Other typical feelings may range from a sense of disbelief and feeling stunned or shocked to feeling paralyzed with fear.

People with HIV disease may worry about transmitting the virus to others, avoiding opportunistic infections, and informing friends and family that they are HIV positive (Schindler, 1992). Some may respond to their HIV positive status by acting out sexually, while others may feel they must give up all sexual behavior. Concerns about being a burden to one's family or no longer being able to work and having to disclose one's status to colleagues are common issues facing people with HIV disease. The loss of occupational roles secondary to physical fatigue can be devastating, and many patients feel too sick to continue to carry out former roles such as a worker, parent, artist, or community volunteer (Schindler, 1992). HIV disease can cause "wasting syndrome," in which patients lose muscle bulk and body mass; this, too, may generate self-esteem and body image issues (Piemme & Bolle, 1990).

New information about HIV becomes available frequently, and some patients are experts on the many new treatments available, but remaining informed may also be a stressor, as the recommended treatments keep changing and patients must be quite savvy to keep up with the new options (i.e., clinical trials of new medicines or alternative therapies). For example, even within the approved treatments for HIV disease, such as the use of Retrovir (zidovudine, or ZDV), there is a wide range of conflicting beliefs among patients, treatment advocacy groups, and health care providers concerning its efficacy. Political decisions keep HIV in the national spotlight (i.e., immigration policies and HIV funding decisions) and may influence the emotional state of people with HIV disease. The multitude of unknowns, the use of medical language, and the specific criteria for different treatments are difficult topics for anyone to keep abreast of and must be even more difficult for someone with HIV disease, who may feel fatigued and be anxious to get answers.

People with HIV disease experience a variety of feelings, such as sadness, shock, anger, fear, worry, and guilt, which are appropriate responses to the stress that accompanies the disease. Occupational therapists can help validate these feelings by listening attentively and allowing feelings to be expressed in a nonjudgmental arena. A knowledge of psychosocial issues may give therapists the information they need to create a safe and open place where patients can express themselves.

ETHICS, STIGMA, AND HIV DISEASE

Unlike many other potentially life-threatening illnesses, such as cancer, upon its first appearance, HIV and the groups who were initially infected were already stigmatized by society (Plumeri, 1984). As the CDC became more aware that a disease was causing Kaposi's sarcoma among homosexual males, there was little information available other than which groups were being affected. The first groups of people affected, intravenous drug users and male homosexuals, were already stigmatized by society, causing many people to devalue the seriousness of the epidemic (Falk-Kessler et al., 1994). As the infected population has grown and diversified, there has been a gradual lessening of the shame associated with HIV, although it may still be argued that people remain curious about how a person was exposed to the virus and some tend to place blame or minimize it. The fact that the HIV virus can be spread via sexual contact in which body fluids are shared also contributes to the stigma associated with the disease. Many HIV positive people are **outed** regarding their sexual orientation, sexual practices, or drug use, which contributes to their fears. This phenomenon was especially prevalent at the beginning of the epidemic.

Fear

A fear of contagion has followed HIV disease because of the lack of a cure, the multitude of manifestations of the disease, the groups that were first infected, and the initial lack of information regarding routes of transmission (Peloquin, 1990). Initially, people with the virus were isolated and caregivers wore masks, goggles, and gowns when approaching the patient. Now that the ways in which the virus is transmitted are known, universal precautions are employed with all patients, regardless of their demographic group or whether they are perceived as highly contagious.

Self-Reflection

It is up to all clinicians to be self-reflective regarding their feelings regarding HIV disease, the population affected, and one's feelings regarding the possible risk of occupational exposure. The onus is on clinicians to spend time with this internal process (e.g., developing self-awareness and exploring personal values) in order to improve the awareness of what they bring to the treatment of patients with HIV infection. This process can be challenging, but it should help clinicians provide the best service to patients with HIV disease. Table 16-4 suggests questions the clinician can use to guide the self-reflection process.

Ethics

Occupational therapists are directed to provide services to patients that need them, regardless of diagnosis. The American Medical Association (AMA) policy states that physicians have a duty to treat the sick, which prevails even if the patient has AIDS (AMA, 1987). The Occupational Therapy Code of Ethics outlines practitioner's ethics as they relate to patients, professional competence, colleagues, employers, and the profession (American Occupational Therapy Association [AOTA], 1994). The code of ethics states:

> Members are committed to furthering people's ability to function within their total environment. To this end, occupational therapy personnel provide services for individuals in any stage of health and illness, to institutions, to other professionals . . . and to the general public. (AOTA, 1994, p. 1037)

The refusal to treat a patient with HIV or AIDS because of fear or prejudice is an ethical violation, as are other forms of discrimination such as premature discharge or referral to avoid physical contact with the patient (Hansen, 1990). Hansen further states, "Although the decision to treat a person infected with HIV and AIDS is a personal one, we must also consider our moral responsibility and professional accountability and must understand that very little personal risk is involved" (Hansen, 1990, p. 242).

Maintaining confidentiality regarding patients receiving mental health treatment and their HIV status is very important in order to protect the patient's

---

Table 16-4.   Self-Reflection Questions for Clinicians

- What frightens you about HIV disease?
- How do you feel about people infected with HIV?
- What are the current facts on HIV transmission?
- What aspects of treating a person with HIV disease make you feel differently than you do when treating someone with another potentially life-threatening illness?
- What is it about HIV disease that may make it more difficult for your patients than having another potentially life-threatening illness?
- How do your religious or spiritual beliefs impact your feelings about treating patients with HIV disease?
- How do you feel about homosexuals and intravenous drug users (the initial groups infected by the HIV virus)?
- How are your feelings about a person with HIV disease impacted based upon the route of HIV transmission (such as through blood via a needle stick, sexual contact, or intravenous drug use)?

privacy, particularly because a patient's HIV status may have ramifications for insurance coverage and, consequently, access to health care (Charrel et al., 1991). For example, upon seeing in the community a person whom you treated on an inpatient psychiatric unit, it is common practice to wait for your former patient to acknowledge you first or opt to ignore you. This allows him or her the option of maintaining confidentiality and avoiding having to explain to someone else where you met. In the case of an HIV diagnosis, care should also be taken to preserve the patient's confidentiality. Information such as lab results, HIV-specific dispositions, and, of course, the patient's full name should not be discussed with people who are not part of that patient's treatment team. Special care should be taken in elevators, lobbies, and other public areas in which one's conversation may be heard. The Occupational Therapy Code of Ethics addresses the issue of confidentiality as follows: "Occupational therapy personnel shall protect the confidential nature of information gained from educational, practice, research, and investigational activities" (AOTA, 1994, p. 1037). As clinicians working in an ever-changing health care arena, it is likely that ethical dilemmas will freqeuntly be presented to occupational therapists. Therefore, an awareness of the profession's ethical principles is essential for guiding practice.

Education

Education is a tool that can help therapists feel knowledgeable about the disease process and their own needs in treating people with HIV disease. Occupational therapists are encouraged to seek support and information as needed, apply the ethical treatment principles in practice, be a patient advocate in accessing services, be well-versed and consistent in the use of universal precautions, and challenge placement issues, which may be difficult because of discrimination based on the diagnosis of HIV. The Occupational Therapy Code of Ethics states, "Occupational therapy personnel shall take responsibility for maintaining competence by participating in professional development and educational activities and occupational therapy personnel shall perform their duties on the basis of accurate and current information" (AOTA, 1994, p. 1037). Keeping informed via current continuing education classes is especially important given the constant emergence of new information regarding HIV and the multitude of symptoms the disease can manifest.

INTERDISCIPLINARY TREATMENT OF HIV DISEASE

The importance of an interdisciplinary approach has been discussed throughout this book. In the case of HIV treatment, the interdisciplinary team may be exceptionally large due to the complexity of the disease process. Not all professionals will be treating patients concurrently, but all team members should be aware of all services potentially available to their patients. It is also important that all team members explain their roles to the patient.

CASE ILLUSTRATION: ELAINE— INTERDISCIPLINARY TREATMENT

Elaine is a 16-year-old, HIV-positive, Caucasian woman who was admitted to a psychiatric hospital following a suicide attempt. Upon admission to the psychiatric unit, a psychiatrist was assigned to oversee Elaine's care as well as to act as the team leader during her stay in the hospital. A few days into her hospital stay Elaine met with a neuropsychologist, who administered and interpreted a battery of tests to determine what, if any, organic neurological changes had occurred. A phlebotomist was responsible for drawing Elaine's blood, while the pharmacist issued and tracked all the medications she was taking and alerted her doctor of any potentially harmful drug interactions. A pulmonary consult was requested after Elaine complained of chest pain, a cough, and fever. The dietician was also consulted to address Elaine's poor nutritional intake. Nursing staff on the unit provided constant supervision in addition to ongoing assessment and education for her medical and psychiatric issues. The team social worker met with Elaine to discuss options for ongoing individual psychotherapy, peer support groups, and day treatment programs, as well as the need for placement in a supervised living environment should she decide not to return to her mother's home. It was agreed by the patient and her mother that she would return home for the time being but would consider the information offered by the social worker regarding attendant care, skilled nursing facilities, home health care, and hospice. Elaine later reported a sense of relief that she had been able to talk to her mother about these issues and that they would be able to plan for the future together now that she knew what options were available.

Much of Elaine's time on the unit was spent in therapeutic groups. In occupational therapy she attended life skills groups that provided opportunities to learn stress management, time management, relaxation, coping skills, and assertiveness training, and in recreation therapy she explored drama, art, movement, and music groups. Just prior to her discharge from the hospital, Elaine commented perceptively in the community meeting, "At first I really didn't think I needed to be here [on a psychiatric unit], but then I realized that all of the things I've learned here have not only helped me right now, but are going to help me even more down the road."

The treatment team conducted daily meetings to discuss Elaine's progress and share information regarding her response to treatment and readiness for discharge. The team considered discharge after Elaine reported, and demonstrated, a decrease in depressive symptoms and an absence of suicidal ideation and was medically stable. After an eight-day hospital stay, Elaine was discharged to her mother's home with a follow-up appointment with the community mental health clinic, where she would be seen once a week by a psychologist or psychiatric social worker who would also act as her case manager.

Continuum of Care

The continuum of care is a key concept for the HIV-infected client. As demonstrated in the case study, it is important that the patient receive information about community clinics and resources as well as available housing. Many HIV-infected persons have a strong support network, which allows them to remain at home throughout the course of the disease continuum with the assistance of day treatment, outpatient care, support groups, attendant care, home health care, community food projects, and hospice. However, many others either lack a supportive network or choose not to become dependent on friends and family. In any case, all patients should understand the options for skilled nursing care and assisted living facilities. No matter what their choice, all clients should be informed of the available options and resources so that an educated decision can be made well before the need for services arises.

Care for the Caregiver

As the HIV pandemic enters its second decade, there has been increasing acknowledgment of the needs of caregivers who attend to those with the disease. *Caregivers* is an umbrella term, which can apply to health care professionals, family members, attendants, and occupational therapists. The fact that the disease has infected mostly middle-aged to younger adults and that there is not yet a cure poses special challenges for health care providers (Piemme & Bolle, 1990). The sadness associated with HIV disease and the toll it has taken affects many, whether they work with people with HIV; have friends, family, or colleagues with HIV; or themselves have HIV.

Education is a primary defense against caregiver burnout as it provides new information, hope for a cure, and occupational therapy tools and treatment techniques. Clinicians may want to give themselves a "time-out" period in the form of a vacation or by rotating through different patient groups (for example, inpatient work versus case management) if they begin to feel overwhelmed (Donohue & McCreedy, 1990). In-house seminars that address related issues, such as managing grief and loss, can help clinicians manage their own feelings of loss in treating patients who often die or weaken progressively in the course of treatment.

In-service trainings and workshops that directly address HIV disease and related issues, such as the "AIDS Annual Update," a yearly conference of the newest developments in HIV disease treatment and research, can help clinicians feel informed and knowledgeable. Being in an environment that specifically addresses information related to HIV disease can also provide occupational therapists an opportunity to network and share information with other people in an environment where they can trust that their work with patients with HIV disease will not be stigmatized.

Support and discussion groups can be helpful in exploring feelings related to this work; providing a safe, nonjudgmental place to "vent" feelings; creating a sense of solidarity and support; and learning coping strategies to deal with the stresses related to treating people with HIV disease. Peer support groups may be held monthly or biweekly at the workplace, possibly facilitated by a mental health professional (Piemme & Bolle, 1990). Often a challenging situation will be discussed among staff informally as an opportunity to express feelings, provide support for one another, and increase collaboration among disciplines. Many urban communities have HIV and AIDS councils that sponsor groups, discussions, and hot lines to provide information and support.

San Francisco is fortunate to have a caregiver center, called Kairos House, that addresses the needs of professionals, volunteers, friends, and family involved with people suffering from HIV disease. This center offers support groups, counseling, resource materials, newsletters, consultation, outreach, and workshops on issues related to stress management and the prevention of burnout. These services are provided so that those with HIV infection will continue to receive treatment from people who are invested in their well-being and whose own level of well-being is such that they can provide quality care.

OCCUPATIONAL THERAPY INTERVENTION

Treatment for people with HIV disease can be provided through both inpatient and outpatient therapy, day treatment, and peer support groups, as well as in supportive living situations such as a halfway house, attendant care, or a hospice. Treatment may vary given the treatment setting, the length of stay, and the different psychological and functional issues confronting the person with HIV disease at different stages of the disease process. The section on treatment that follows can be modified to fit the given environment and the particular patient's needs.

Assessments

Assessments can be completed through observation during groups or in a one-on-one setting. If the patient is very fatigued and feeling physically ill, the assessment may need to be abbreviated and be completed at bedside. The Kohlman Evaluation of Living Skills (KELS) is an assessment that evaluates community living skills and is especially helpful in determining disposition plans and the level of care that will best suit the patient (Thomson, 1992). The KELS assesses self-care, judgment and safety (especially relevant for patients with dementia or mania), money management, community mobility, and social supports. The cognitive deficits seen with HIV dementia may be assessed and documented using Allen's Cognitive Levels (ACL) (Allen, 1985).

It is important that the therapist be flexible during all the steps (assessment, collaboration, and treatment), as the patient needs and abilities will vary within the group and also within the course of an individual's treatment. It is common with HIV disease to see a "waxing and waning" of symptoms and endurance, and the therapist needs to provide adaptations to the assessment process to allow the patient to participate at the highest possible level of functioning (Pizzi, 1994). The occupational therapy initial assessment may include the patient's physical skills (endurance, gait and mobility, vision, fine and gross motor skills, and hearing), psychological skills (initiation, time management, coping skills, socialization, and self-concept), cognitive skills (attention span, problem solving, and memory), activities of daily living (ADL) (feeding, dressing, bathing, and grooming/hygiene), the patient's goals for treatment, and the occupational therapy treatment plan to meet those goals. In setting treatment goals, the therapist should help patients determine their own priorities and give reality-based feedback about what occupational therapy can offer them. Even the sickest patients are usually quite clear about what is important to them, and even if they cannot completely meet their goal in occupational therapy, it can serve as a basis for treatment. For example, if a hospice-bound patient states that his goal is to open a catering company and he has done this type of work in the past, this interest and strength can be explored by the therapist and an adapted goal may be developed (i.e., acting as coleader during cooking group, choosing what the group will make, and reading the recipe to his peers). Denial and a limited acknowledgment of one's deficits can actually serve as positive coping strategies. A careful consideration of the patient's goals and level of functioning, combined with an assessment of the available resources, needs to occur before deciding whether to confront a patient's denial. Coping mechanisms should not be weakened or challenged unless there is an alternate method of coping to replace them. Ideally, the assessment of skills, patient's goals, and the occupational therapy plan are shared with the patient in a clear manner and the patient is provided with a copy of the initial assessment.

Treatment

After the assessment has been completed and treatment goals have been generated with the patient, the therapist determines whether group, individual, or a combination of treatment formats is warranted. One-on-one treatment is indicated if the patient has limited endurance or is bedridden, feels fearful, or is very confused due to dementia. Generally, treatment provides choices for the patient, provides successful experiences (not too challenging or irrelevant), and allows a format through which a patient can leave early without disrupting the group and without "losing face" or feeling as if he or she has failed.

In treating someone with HIV disease and depression, nurturing activities may be helpful, such as caring for fish or other animals, tending plants, or gardening (Dillard et al., 1992). The wellness model emphasizes the need for people with HIV disease to contribute to society and other people in order to improve their own wellness, which can occur through any volunteer work or contribution to others (Pizzi, 1994). For example, toys can be made and donated to a pediatrics ward or community agency. Expressive art activities allow patients to express themselves nonverbally and may also help with values clarification, depending on the theme (i.e., depicting how one sees oneself on half the page and how others see one on the other half). A movement group can help stretch tight muscles, improve body awareness, and elevate the patient's mood. Journal writing may be used as a more private method of self-expression, by helping with self-reflection and creating a safe place for the expression of feelings, concerns, and questions. Psychoeducational groups on topics such as goal setting, stress management, communication skills, and accessing community resources may also be relevant for this group. Gutterman suggests using health promotion groups that "(a) support clients physically, emotionally, and spiritually; (b) facilitate adaptive behavior; and (c) act as a catalyst for change where there is receptivity and motivation" (1990, p. 235).

In treating someone with HIV-related mania, treatment may include using an exercise bike or other exercises, doing outdoor activities, or painting. Supplies should be nontoxic, the environment should be free of clutter, and the focus of the activity should be on the process rather than the product. Patients may do best when only one step of the activity is presented at a time. Crafts activities such as woodworking or a previously learned craft are also suitable.

In treating someone with HIV dementia, relaxing music, magazines, and coloring activities can be used. Patients may enjoy cooking although increased impulsivity can sometimes lead to extra items landing in the bowl or difficulty in waiting for the finished product before tasting. Patients may enjoy stringing large beads, collage, or other activities that do not require fine motor coordination or sustained concentration. Sensory input can be provided with different textures of materials (i.e., making a collage of felt, flannel, yarn, and feathers) or through petting animals, working with clay, or repotting plants. A small notebook for writing down appointments and other information to compensate for memory difficulties is often useful. Occupational therapists are trained in grading activities and breaking them down into their component parts, a skill that is particularly applicable with these individuals, who do best when given one step of a task at a time. Similarly, it is preferable to ask questions that can be answered with a "yes" or "no" or to give the patient a choice of two items rather than asking an open-ended question.

Group treatment may include only HIV positive patients or may involve a mixed population. Occupational therapists facilitate the exchange of information related to HIV as it comes up and model appropriate responses while providing an environment and structure that will help patients to feel secure. Some individuals may be comfortable in readily disclosing their HIV status as it relates to group topics, while others may not share their HIV status with the group but may choose to speak about their concerns one-on-one with the therapist. In a mixed diagnosis group, patients are generally quite accepting of one another; however, it is important for the therapist to ensure a safe environment for all participants, so if name calling or slurs are uttered by a group member, limits should be set quickly, clearly, and calmly. The therapist helps create an environment that provides peer and social supports for the patients. Often, more able patients will assist those who need help (i.e., pushing wheelchairs, providing verbal encouragement), and some patients will make lasting connections with one another. Table 16-5 outlines a wide variety of groups that can address the needs of patients with HIV disease.

Psychotherapeutic treatment may involve educating patients about HIV, encouraging them to maintain a healthy balance of work, play, and self-care,

Table 16-5. Occupational Therapy Group Treatment for Patients with HIV Disease

GROUP	PURPOSE
Goal setting	Teaches how to set goals as a way of making changes in one's life
Stress management	Teaches stress reduction techniques and recognize the symptoms of stress
Relaxation	Provides a restful opportunity to unwind–may include self-massage
Anger management	Teaches ways to express and manage anger appropriately
Movement or exercise	Promotes body awareness, endurance, and agility
Task or workshop	Provides multiple choices to promote a sense of control and assist in developing leisure interests, work skills, and socialization with others
Animal-assisted therapy	Offers the opportunity to nurture an animal and provide sensory input
Expressive art	Offers a primarily nonverbal way to express thoughts and feelings and serves as an outlet for self-expression
Crafts	Promotes task focus and self-esteem through task completion; helps in developing hobbies
Community resources	Teaches about community resources for food, shelter, entertainment, support, money management, and transportation
Safer sex discussion	Teaches how HIV is transmitted, assertiveness skills (may include role-play), and safer sex techniques to reduce the likelihood of infection or reinfection (if already HIV positive)
Money management	Teaches ways to budget money, shopping skills, and financial resources
Focus group	Provides practice in focusing attention in the present and exploring thoughts and feelings related to a particular topic
Grooming	Promotes good hygiene in order to improve self-esteem and socialization opportunities
Cooking	Promotes safety awareness, knowledge of nutrition, and the ability to work with others
Social skills	Provides practice in communicating with others, meeting people, and expressing needs clearly
Diversity awareness	Teaches about difference as it relates to race, ethnicity, gender, sexual orientation, and culture through music, art, food, language, festivals, and literature.

discussions about safer sex, teaching skills to handle grief and loss, and teaching ways to cope with changing roles at home, in relationships, at work, and with family. It is important for occupational therapists to help these patients feel understood, provide alternatives for their view of the future as hopeless, and examine their own feelings to consider how they may impact the treatment provided. Treatment usually addresses some of the issues inherent in coping with a potentially life-threatening illness such as HIV. Occupational therapists can help patients learn effective coping strategies (i.e., stress management), adapt to changing abilities (i.e., energy conservation techniques and values clarification), and access supports (individual, group, and community).

Occupational therapists may also help educate family and caregivers regarding how to adapt activities and the environment so as to promote patient independence as well as providing other information regarding HIV disease and available resources. A patient's adaptation to HIV will often be predicted by his or her history and past responses to stresses and challenges (Luber, 1991). Developing coping skills and accessing a support system are important. Exploring issues related to death and dying, grief, and loss and establishing goals and priorities throughout the stages of the disease can be done through individual discussions, in peer support groups, or with health care providers (Schindler, 1992).

Treatment addressing activities of daily living (ADLs) can include grooming, hygiene, dressing, bathing, and feeding. The therapist should provide gentle, concrete feedback (i.e., by using a mirror) and approach the patient at the appropriate time of day for the given activity (i.e., for feeding, during mealtime; for dressing, early in the morning). Grooming is often impaired in patients with HIV dementia, and they should be given visual and physical cues (i.e., putting a hairbrush into hand) rather than relying on verbal information, which can be difficult for them to follow. In some cases, a team-based behavioral plan with clear expectations and rewards may be employed to motivate patients to attend to ADLs.

Grooming is often an area of concern for families and caregivers, especially if the patient lives at, or is returning, home. Family teaching can include breaking down an activity into simple steps, presenting one item at a time, and allowing the patient some choices. A broad definition of family includes partners, friends, and lovers as well as the family of origin, children, and spouses. The patient's support system should be enlisted in treatment if available, as these individuals will often be the ones to help follow through on the skills developed in occupational therapy.

Summary

The HIV pandemic is constantly changing as the disease progresses and new information is generated. The face profile of the typical sufferer has shifted as the group undergoing the fastest rate of new HIV infection is that of heterosexual women; however, this may shift again as the pandemic continues (Pizzi, 1994). Occupational therapists will probably continued to treat patients with HIV disease regardless of the setting in which they work. HIV disease has a multitude of ramifications, including physical, psychiatric, and psychological symptoms. Occupational therapists are an integral part of the treatment team for this population and provide a range of assessment skills and treatment interventions. Caregivers also have needs that must be addressed in order to enable the continued provision of quality care for people with HIV disease. Occupational therapists need to take responsibility to stay current on the HIV literature as new information may impact occupational therapy treatment and the services that are provided. Treatments are continually being developed, and the occupational therapist should be aware of any potential side effects they may create. Occupational therapy publications, other health care literature, colleagues, and well-informed patients can all help the occupational therapist stay abreast of the multitude of issues regarding the symptoms, treatments, research, and ethics of HIV disease.

Review Questions

1. What factors impact the rapid rise in HIV infection among women aged 25 to 44 years old? What possible factors lead to decreased life expectancy for women initially diagnosed with HIV infection compared to their male counterparts?
2. Develop a treatment plan for the case illustration subject named Sharon based on the information given in the chapter. Include occupational therapy modalities, assessments to be used, and treatment goals.
3. Define the unique role of the occupational therapist on an interdisciplinary treatment team in working with the case illustration subject named Jim, who suffers from HIV dementia.
4. Think of a case example of an ethical issue involving an occupational therapist and a patient with HIV disease. What are the occupational therapist's rights, duties, and ethical responsibilities? What are the patient's rights, duties, and ethical responsibilities? How are they the same and how do they differ?
5. Describe two different scenarios involving patients and identify the different methods of employing universal precautions that would apply to the two situations. Develop three methods to explain the need for universal precautions to patients in a manner that is educational, honest, and concise.

Learning Activities

1. Read five newspaper or magazine articles and determine if the reporter's slant differs according to the method of HIV transmission (e.g., drug use versus perinatally).

2. Determine the HIV disease–related community resources in your area that assist with meals, peer support, legal aid, access to health care, and anonymous HIV testing.
3. Volunteer at an HIV-related community organization and determine the population it serves, the services provided, and what clients like best and least about the care they receive there.
4. Read Randy Shilts's book, *And the Band Played On*. Compare the current state of U.S. government and public response to the HIV epidemic with that depicted in this nonfiction account, which was published in 1988.
5. Visit an exhibit displaying panels from the AIDS Memorial Quilt. For location of displays contact local Names Project chapters or:
   Names Project Foundation
   310 Townsend Street
   San Francisco, California 94107
   415-882-5500

References

Allen, C. (1985). *Measurement and management of cognitive disabilities*. Boston: Little, Brown.

American Medical Association. (1987). *Report of the Council on Ethical and Judicial Affairs: Ethical issues involved in the growing AIDS crisis*. Chicago: Author.

American Occupational Therapy Association (AOTA). (1994). Occupational therapy code of ethics. *American Journal of Occupational Therapy, 48,* 1037–1038.

Boccellari, A., & Dilley, J. (1992). Management and residential placement problems of patients with HIV related cognitive impairment. *Hospital and Community Psychiatry, 43,* 32–37.

Boccellari, A., Dilley, J., Chambers, D., Yingling, C., Tauber, M., Moss, A., & Osmond, D. (1993). Immune function and neurological performance in HIV-1 infected homosexual men. *Journal of Acquired Immune Deficiency Syndrome, 6,* 592–601.

Charrel, J., Larher, M., Manuel, C., Enel, P., Reviron, D., & San Marco, J. (1991). AIDS: The rights of patients. *AIDS and Public Policy Journal, 6,* 41–45.

Chorba, T. L., Holman, R. C., & Evatt, B. L. (1993). Heterosexual and mother-to-child transmission of AIDS in the hemophilia community. *Public Health Records, 108* (1), 99–104

Dillard, M., Andonian, L., Flores, O., Lai, L., MacRae, A., & Shakir, M. (1992). Culturally competent occupational therapy in a diversely populated mental health setting. *American Journal of Occupational Therapy, 46*(8), 721–726.

Donohue, M., & McCreedy, P. (1990, May). *Supervising students and staff who treat persons with AIDS.* Paper presented at the AOTA Annual Conference, New Orleans, LA.

Fackelmann, K. A. (1994). AZT lowers maternal HIV transmission rate. *Science News, 145,* 134.

Falk-Kessler, J., Barnowski, C., & Salvant, S. (1994). Mandatory HIV testing and occupational therapy. *American Journal of Occupational Therapy, 48,* 27–37.

Flaskerud, J. H. (1992). Overview: HIV disease and nursing. In J. H. Flaskerud & P. J. Ungvarski (Eds.), *HIV/AIDS: A guide to nursing care* (2nd ed., pp. 1–29). Philadelphia: W. B. Saunders.

Goisman, R., Kent, A, Montgomery, E., Cheevers, M., & Goldfinger, S. (1991). AIDS education for patients with chronic mental illness. *Community Mental Health Journal, 27,* 189–197.

Gonzales-Aviles, A. (1992). The medical aspects of AIDS. In W. M. Marcil & K. N. Tigges (Eds.), *The person with AIDS: A personal and professional perspective* (pp. 73–86). Thorofare, NJ: Slack.

Gutterman, L. (1990). A day treatment program for persons with AIDS. *American Journal of Occupational Therapy, 44,* 234-237..

Hansen, R. A. (1990). The ethics of caring for patients with HIV or AIDS. *American Journal of Occupational Therapy, 44,* 239–242.

Karasic, D., & Dilley, J. (1994). HIV associated psychiatric disorders: Clinical syndromes. In P. T. Cohen, M. Sande, & P. Volberding (Eds.), *The AIDS knowledge base* (pp. 5.30-1–5.30-5). Boston: Little, Brown.

Kieburtz, K., Zeltelmaler, A., Ketonen, L., Tuite, M., & Caine, E. (1991). Manic syndrome in AIDS. *American Journal of Psychiatry, 148*(8), 1068–1070.

Leary, M., & Zeifert, P. (1994). Clinical education and management of HIV dementia. In P. T. Cohen, M. Sarde, & P. Volberding (Eds.), *The AIDS knowledge base* (pp. 5.30-1–5.30-10). Boston: Little, Brown.

Le Cocq, L., Bonck, J., & MacRae, A. (1995). The role of rehabilitation after human immunodeficiency virus (HIV) infection. In D. A. Umphred (Ed.), *Neurological rehabilitation* (3rd ed., pp. 556–570). St. Louis: Mosby.

Luber, P. (1991, May). *Neuropsychiatry of HIV for primary care practitioners, Part one.* Paper presented at the meeting of the HIV Primary Care Education Project, New York, NY.

Marcil, M. M. (1992). AIDS and the human dimension. In W. M. Marcil & K. N. Tigges (Eds.), *The person with AIDS: A personal and professional perspective* (pp. 3–10). Thorofare, NJ: Slack.

Markowitz, J., Rabkin, J., & Perry, S. (1994). Treating depression in HIV positive patients. *AIDS, 8,* 403–412.

Peloquin, S. (1990). AIDS: Toward a compassionate response. *American Journal of Occupational Therapy, 44,* 271–278.

Perry, S. W. (1990). Organic mental disorders caused by HIV: Update on early diagnosis and treatment. *American Journal of Psychiatry, 147,* 696–710.

Piemme, J., & Bolle, J. (1990). Coping with grief in response to caring for persons with AIDS. *American Journal of Occupational Therapy, 44,* 266–269.

Pizzi, M. (1994). *HIV infection and AIDS: A professional's guide to wellness, health and productive living.* Silver Springs, MD: Positive Images & Wellness.

Plumeri, P. A. (1984). The refusal to treat: Abandonment and AIDS. *Journal of Clinical Gastroenterology, 6,* 281–284.

Polan, J. (1991, May). *Neuropsychiatry of HIV for primary care practitioners, Part two.* Paper presented at the meeting of the HIV Primary Care Education Project, New York, NY.

Schaffner, B. (1990). Psychotherapy with HIV infected persons. In S. Goldfinger (Ed.), *Psychiatric aspects of AIDS and HIV infection.* San Francisco: Jossey-Bass.

Schindler, V. (1992). The psychosocial issues of AIDS. In W. M. Marcil & K. N. Tigges (Eds.), *The person with AIDS: A personal and professional perspective* (pp. 9–23). Thorofare, NJ: Slack.

Segal, M. (1993). Women and AIDS. *FDA Consumer, 27*(8), 9–13.

Shilts, R. (1988). *And the band played on: Politics, people and the AIDS epidemic.* New York: Springer.

Steiner, J., Lussier, R., & Rosenblatt, W. (1992). Knowledge about and risk factors for AIDS in a day hospital population. *Hospital and Community Psychiatry, 43,* 734–736.

Surveillance for occupationally acquired HIV infection—United States, 1981–1992. (1992). *Journal of the American Medical Association, 268*(23), 3294.

Thomson, L. (1992). *The Kohlman Evaluation for Living Skills* (3rd ed.). Rockville, MD: American Occupational Therapy Association.

Ungvarski, P. J. (1992). Clinical manifestations of AIDS. In J. H. Flaskerud & P. J. Ungvarski (Eds.), *HIV/AIDS: A guide to nursing care* (2nd ed., pp. 54–145). Philadelphia: W. B. Saunders.

Weinstein, B. D. (1990). Assessing the impact of HIV disease. *American Journal of Occupational Therapy, 44*(3), 220–226.

Williams, J. (1990). Values and life goals: Clinical intervention for people with AIDS. In M. Pizzi (Ed.), *Productive living strategies for people with AIDS.* New York: Hayworth Press, pp. 55–68.

Suggested Reading

Boccellari, A. (1990). *AIDS dementia training manual.* San Francisco: Family Survival Project.

Grady, C. (1992). HIV disease: Pathogenesis and treatment. In J. H. Flaskerud & P. J. Ungvarski (Eds.), *HIV/AIDS: A guide to nursing care* (2nd ed., pp. 30–53). Philadelphia: W. B. Saunders.

HIV targets young adults. (1993). *Patient Care, 27*, pp. 14–15.

Hollander, H., Loveless, M. O., & Montauk, S. L. (1993). The HIV-infected patient: Early stage care. *Patient Care, 27*(15), 21–35.

Ross, J. W. (1986). Ethics and the language of AIDS. *Federation Review, 9*, 15–19.

Sacks, M., Burtoin, W., Dermatis, H., Looser-Ott, S., & Perry, S. (1995). HIV-related cases among 2,094 admissions to a psychiatric hospital. *Psychiatric Services, 46*, 131–135.

Sitzman, B. T., Burch, E., Bartlett, L., & Urrutia, G. (1995). Rates of sexually transmitted diseases among patients in a psychiatric emergency service. *Psychiatric Services, 46*, 136–140.

Occupational Therapy in the Criminal Justice System

Jane Dressler, MS, OTR
Occupational Therapist
San Francisco General Hospital
Adjunct Assistant Professor
Samuel Merritt College, Oakland, California

Fred Snively, OTR
Senior Occupational Therapist
California Medical Center at Vacaville

Key Terms

adjudication

commitment

forensics

incarceration

jail

prison

Chapter Outline

Introduction
Criminal Justice Settings
    Jails
    Prisons
    Forensic State Hospitals
    Community Programs
Clinical Competencies in a Criminal Justice Setting
    Analyzing the Environment
    Maintaining Safety and Security
    Overcoming Obstacles
    Developing Team Relationships
    Building Therapeutic Alliances
    Recognizing Malingering
    Documenting Accurately
    Knowing the Criminal Justice Language
Summary

Introduction

An understanding of the criminal justice system is mandatory for all occupational therapists working in mental health. The mental health and criminal justice systems overlap, and the boundaries between the two systems have become more blurred in the last 10 years. The number of people with mental illness in America's jails and prisons is significant and rising. The estimated prevalence of mental illness in jails and prisons is as follows (Jemelka, Trupin, & Chiles, 1989; National Alliance for the Mentally Ill [NAMI] and the Public Citizen's Health Research Group [PCHRG], 1992):

- 7.2 percent of **jail** inmates in most states have a serious psychiatric illness.

- 25 percent of jail inmates in eight selected states (California, New York, Virginia, Florida, North Carolina, Alaska, and Nebraska) have a serious psychiatric illness.

- 8 percent of state **prison** populations have a serious psychiatric illness.

- 17 percent of state prison populations have a psychiatric disorder that requires periodic attention.

- 66 percent of state prison populations require psychiatric treatment at some point in their incarceration.

Conversely, many people receiving mental health treatment in traditional, noncriminal justice settings have a history of contact with the criminal justice system. At any point in their **incarceration**, individuals from criminal justice institutions may be referred to traditional mental health settings for special services. The blurring of these systems will surely continue as trends such as rising unemployment, homelessness, cuts in community based mental health services, hospital closures, and legislation that favors stiffer criminal sentences persist. Criminal justice institutions will continue to be faced with growing mental health needs.

The role of the occupational therapist in the criminal justice system is as varied as in other mental health settings. Occupational therapy facilities, referral procedures, the institution's physical settings, frames of reference, modalities used, and goals of programs differ widely across the country. Occupational therapists may work in an administrative and consultation role or offer a range of services directly, including evaluation, group and individual treatment, program development, case management, and student supervision. They work with patients in high-security correctional facilities such as jails, prisons, and forensic state hospitals, as well as with outpatients in the community.

Occupational therapy evaluation and treatment procedures in the criminal justice system rely on the same principles and procedures that are applied in traditional, non–criminal justice settings. Occupational therapists work as part of an interdisciplinary team, evaluate functional abilities, and use structured, graded therapeutic activities with individuals and groups to achieve specific goals. They facilitate skill development in order to help patients function at their maximum potential within their current institutional environment and be more productive and successful when they reintegrate into the community.

CRIMINAL JUSTICE SETTINGS

There are several different criminal justice settings, each of which has potentially different populations and treatment issues. For the purposes of this chapter, the discussion will focus on jails, prisons, forensic state hospitals, and community programs.

Jails

As depicted in Figure 17-1, jails are the entry points of the criminal justice system. They are city or county funded and operated, and serve as holding facilities for arrested individuals awaiting arraignment, trial, or transfer to another facility. They also function as the institution in which people found guilty of a crime and given a sentence of under one year serve out their time.

Jails are stressful. In large populated areas they tend to be cramped and overcrowded. The **adjudication** process is often complicated, filled with delays, and misunderstood by the accused, and the environment is noisy and chaotic; individuals are separated from their social networks, and many choices and freedoms are taken away, as is their privacy. Most American jails have minimal outdoor recreational opportunities and limited rehabilitation programs of any type (NAMI & PCHRG, 1992).

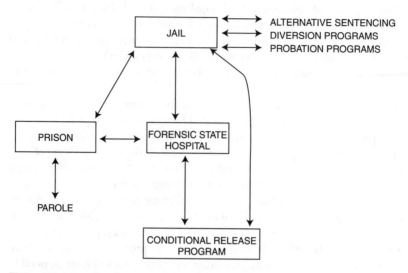

Figure 17-1. Jail Is the Entry Point of the Criminal Justice System

Adjusting to jail is difficult. Depression, suicidal ideation, confusion, and a sense of total loss of life control are frequent reactions among newly arrested individuals. People with a history of a major psychiatric disorder are vulnerable to decompensation in jail. Decompensation typically includes an increase in symptoms such as suicidal ideation, mutilation attempts, assaultive or violent behavior, auditory and visual hallucinations, delusional beliefs, loss of appetite, change in sleep patterns, and change in grooming and hygiene.

The availability of high-quality, comprehensive psychiatric treatment in jails varies widely across the country. All jails are required to have an operational plan that includes psychiatric screening and evaluation, crisis intervention, treatment, and discharge and transfer planning (American Psychiatric Association Task Force, 1989); however, the extent of these services may be limited to the on-call availability of a single mental health professional. The most effective and complete programs offer an array of services that include separate housing for people with mental illness with seven days per week clinical coverage, day treatment programs, training in community living skills, and an acute hospital unit for emergencies.

Occupational therapists are most likely to be found as part of the acute hospital program, which may be located at the jail or at a nearby hospital. The length of stay at these facilities is usually under two weeks. A wide variety of diagnoses are seen, but a majority of the hospitalized inmates have a chronic history of mental illness, and frequently their crimes are a manifestation of this condition (NAMI & PCHRG, 1992). Some typical arrest scenarios are described in Table 17-1. The occupational therapist in the acute hospital setting focuses on functional assessment, stabilization, treatment, and

Table 17-1. Typical Arrest Scenarios

- A woman with schizoaffective disorder is arrested for assault after she entered a department store and began rearranging the shelves because of a delusion that she worked there. When asked to leave, she struck a store manager.
- A man with schizophrenia who was behaving in a bizarre manner on the street is arrested for assault after striking a teenager who was making fun of him.
- A man with bipolar disorder–manic is arrested for theft after he impulsively stole a yacht at a dock and then drove it around until it ran out of gas.
- A homeless man with chronic schizophrenia and a substance abuse problem is arrested for defrauding an innkeeper after running out without paying at the end of a meal because he was very hungry and had no money.
- A woman with schizophrenia is arrested for trespassing after she refused to leave a building due to having the delusional belief that she owned it.

discharge planning. Treatment programs are designed to create a safe, non-threatening environment that emphasizes patient strengths and engages the patients in activities at the appropriate cognitive level to allow for success. Initially, self-care and social skills training are a main focus. Discharge planning involves assessing when the patient is stable enough to return to jail or choosing the right community placement based on his or her skill level. Stability to return to jail usually involves the patient being able to eat and perform basic hygiene routines independently, to safely tolerate and/or cooperate with others, and to adequately control self-injurious behavior.

The occupational therapist working in a jail setting may have a limited amount of time in which to devise and implement a meaningful treatment plan, and security restrictions may substantially limit patient access to traditional occupational therapy materials such as wood, leather crafts, or even cooking utensils. Jails do, however, offer a fast-paced environment with a varied caseload and the opportunity to provide a positive, supportive therapeutic program for individuals experiencing multiple problems.

San Francisco General Hospital, a public hospital in California, utilizes occupational therapy on its 12-bed, acute, inpatient psychiatric jail unit. Patients are referred to the unit by jail psychiatric workers if they meet the criteria for involuntary psychiatric hospitalization (danger to self, danger to others, or grave disability). Typical admission scenarios involve patients assaulting cell mates; attempting to cut or hang themselves; not eating, sleeping, or washing; or being totally unable to communicate with others due to psychosis.

Most patients have a psychiatric and/or substance abuse history that predates their legal problems. A full range of diagnoses are seen, but the most common are schizophrenia, bipolar disorder–manic, schizoaffective disorder, cognitive disorders, delusional disorder, and (jail) adjustment disorder. Legal charges vary from minor offenses like trespassing to more serious charges, including murder. The typical length of stay is five days, but occasionally a patient stays as long as two weeks.

The occupational therapist works as part of an interdisciplinary team consisting of nurses, psychiatrists, and social workers. Deputy sheriffs guard the unit and attend selected patient treatment–planning sessions. When first admitted, patients are often agitated, physically aggressive, and verbally abusive, and they may require seclusion and/or physical restraints. Patients are carefully evaluated for behavioral control and only begin to attend programming after they can reliably agree, as assessed by the treatment team, not to hurt themselves or others. Once exerting behavioral self-control, all patients attend community meetings, discussion groups, and two occupational therapy groups a day.

Patients are evaluated by the occupational therapist with the Allen Cognitive Level Test (a screening tool that detects the presence of cognitive disability) (Allen, 1985), a brief interview and observation in groups. The Kohlman Evaluation of Living Skills Assessment (interview and task observation of living skills) (Kohlman Thomson, 1992) may be used to further assess functional level. These assessments provide unique and vital information regarding patients' current and baseline functioning, specific assets and limitations when coping in the jail environment, and readiness to return to jail or another facility.

The overall goal of treatment is the stabilization of acute symptoms and an improvement in jail-coping skills. Groups are planned daily according to the patients' needs and abilities. Patients are generally appreciative of the opportunity for productive therapeutic activity and a respite from the jail environment, and patient cooperation with treatment activities tends to be high. Task skills groups, including crafts, light work, and gardening are very effective for increasing organizational skills, problem solving, and the ability to concentrate. For safety reasons, no sharp tools are allowed and patients are not allowed to keep projects of any type. Consequently, all work is donated to other parts of the hospital or to charity. Games and physical activities are used for stress management, the productive channeling of excessive or aggressive energy, and improving basic social and communication skills. Focus and art expression groups create a sense of a safe, cohesive community and provide an opportunity for patients to express themselves. Focus groups typically explore subjects such as frustration, respect, and living in close quarters. Cooking provides an opportunity to explore the knowledge of basic nutrition and issues surrounding caring for oneself. Psychoeducational groups on goal setting, anger management, leisure time management, stress management, and journal writing are used in higher-functioning groups.

Prisons

Prisons are state or federally operated facilities that house people found guilty of felonies or other crimes that carry a sentence of greater than one year. Prison environments tend to be more stable than jail environments. The inmates have been sentenced and the adjudication process is behind them. However, there are many stressors in this environment, including violence, victimization, and a highly controlled, but unpredictable, system where inmates are frequently cited and reprimanded for infractions of prison rules. Prison inmates frequently describe their experience as a daily "struggle for survival." As high as two-thirds of prison inmates are in need of some form of psychiatric care at one time or another during their incarceration (Jemelka et al., 1989).

Like jails, prisons have mandated requirements for providing psychiatric services. Mental health services can be provided by either the state mental health system, the state correctional system, or a combination of the two. The services provided vary widely from state to state and may include prison-based, acute, inpatient hospital units; prison-based, day treatment programs; "outpatient" (in prison, but out of the acute hospital phase) programs, and special, mental health program prisons (Mackain & Streveler, 1990).

Improving task and interactional skills is an important focus for prison-based occupational therapy programs. Many patients lack the basic skills to complete a task, such as the needed attention span, memory, cognitive skills, concentration, problem solving and sequencing abilities, the ability to follow instructions and to work with others, and frustration tolerance. Occupational therapy programs focus on these task skills as well as interpersonal and intrapersonal skills such as assertiveness, stress management, coping skills, and basic social skills. In order to function effectively and safely in prison, inmates must be hyper-alert to the environment and very cautious about how they present themselves to other individuals. Role-playing, videotaping, and structured communication exercises can be very helpful in developing necessary social skills.

Prison settings are challenging environments for the occupational therapist. Antisocial behavior and institutional blocks to program planning are prevalent, but the opportunity to help patients make real changes in their lives and develop new skills is genuine. In the prison setting, therapists can form positive, long-term relationships with their clients. The unique projects created in occupational therapy clinics seem to have increased significance to prison inmates, perhaps because so little else in their life is individualized. Figure 17-2 displays actual projects completed in a prison-based occupational therapy clinic.

The state correctional facility in Vacaville, California, utilizes occupational therapy. This is a 3,000-man prison housing physical medicine, psychiatric, and general population inmates. The focus of occupational therapy treatment is on the outpatient program servicing the 400-plus psychiatric inmates housed in the facility. This facility is the inmates' community, and the role of occupational therapy is to work with the pathology that restricts the inmates' productivity within their community.

By focusing on the inmates' abilities and capabilities, the occupational therapist helps individuals use their strengths for growth and stability through such modalities as an intake assessment (structured questionnaire and interview), structured activities, individual counseling, and task-oriented activities. The

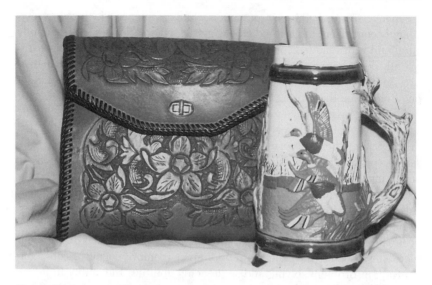

Figure 17-2.   Projects Completed in a Prison-based Occupational Therapy Clinic

treatment objectives are to explore the performance ability and capability of each patient; to maintain or improve reality awareness, concentration, self-esteem, self-image, social skills, and problem-solving abilities; and to develop tolerance and respect for individual needs and differences.

Occupational therapy services are provided in a central location for the various program units. Interdisciplinary treatment teams, which are comprised of a psychiatrist, psychologist, social worker, and psychiatric technician, provide referrals to occupational therapy services for reasons such as withdrawn and unfocused behavior, lethargy, poor motivation, anxiety, depression, inability to relate to others or express emotional needs, and acting-out behaviors that violate departmental rules and regulations.

Typical diagnoses seen are schizophrenia, polysubstance abuse, paranoia, depression and bipolar disorders. Diagnoses of borderline personality disorder, antisocial personality disorder, and mental retardation are also common. Many patients have been socially and culturally deprived.

Patients are initially interviewed by the occupational therapy staff to obtain a personal history of the individual; assess cognitive function, memory, and treatment needs; and set treatment goals. The observation of mood and body language is vital to this process, and these observations are often more valuable than the patient's direct statements. The interviewer must acquire the trust and confidence of the patient so as to reduce defensive behavior in an effort to obtain accurate, unguarded responses. The nonthreatening atmosphere of the occupational therapy clinic, which has arts and crafts projects displayed and music playing in the background, helps the patient to remove defensive barriers and talk freely.

Occupational therapy provides a highly structured program, with the average length of treatment being 4.5 months. The average patient has had a life of negative environments, negative behavior, and no positive reinforcement. He usually makes poor decisions and choices, feeling he is the victim of society with no power to change his life. Using the Allen Cognitive Levels frame of reference, patients are matched with activities exactly suited to their level of functioning in order to facilitate success. This process provides the patient with positive feedback and increases his self-esteem and sense of personal accomplishment. Learning that he can be successful builds confidence in the patient, who in turn will explore new directions and face challenges that he previously considered stumbling blocks. Mistakes are reframed, not as failures, as was their experience in the past, but as lessons in learning, growth, problem solving, and decision making.

Forensic State Hospitals

Forensic state hospitals are maximum security psychiatric hospitals, administered by state mental health systems, that serve jails and prisons. The laws vary from state to state, but generally, three categories of patients are treated at forensic state hospitals, consisting of individuals who are considered to be one of the following:

1. incompetent to stand trial
2. not guilty by reason of insanity/not criminally responsible
3. competent, criminally responsible, guilty, but mentally ill

Incompetent to stand trial.   The word *incompetent* has a specific legal meaning, which differs from the ordinary understanding of the word. *Incompetent to stand trial* means that:

a person, as the result of a mental disorder or mental retardation is unable to consult with a defense lawyer with a reasonable degree of rational understanding and otherwise assist in his or her own defense and/or does not have a rational, as well as factual, understanding of the criminal proceedings being conducted against him or her. (American Bar Association, 1989, pp. 167–168).

This means that an individual does not understand the criminal court proceedings. For example, he or she may not understand the role of the judge, jury, or attorneys or may not be able to communicate effectively or cooperate with a lawyer.

Individuals who are ruled incompetent to stand trial undergo **commitment** to a forensic state hospital for the specific intent of restoring them, through psychiatric treatment, to a sufficiently healthy mental state to permit an understanding of the nature of the criminal proceedings. Once this objective has been achieved, the individual is considered to have been returned to competence. The time frame for such restoration varies widely from case to case. The law then mandates that the competent person be returned to court for a reinstatement of the criminal proceedings (Donovan, 1991). The individual will then be returned from the forensic state hospital to jail in the county in which the alleged crime was committed and the adjudication process will continue.

Not guilty because of insanity/not legally responsible.   People who are considered not guilty because of insanity/not criminally responsible comprise another category of patients treated at forensic state hospitals. The terminology and criteria vary from state to state, but the key issue is:

> whether or not, a defendant, due to mental disease, disorder or defect at the time of the commission of an offense, was incapable of appreciating the criminality of his/her conduct and incapable of conforming that conduct to the requirements of the law. (American Bar Association, 1989, p. 294).

People may be found not guilty because of insanity/not criminally responsible if they are incapable of distinguishing right from wrong (Donovan, 1991). When individuals are found to be not guilty because of insanity/not criminally responsible, they are committed to a state forensic hospital.

Both those committed as incompetent to stand trial and those committed as not guilty because of insanity/not criminally responsible are reviewed carefully in court as mandated by state statutory requirements. Most patients are ultimately released back to the community, some with court-ordered close supervision.

Competent, criminally responsible, guilty, but mentally ill.   The third category of patients treated at forensic state hospitals is made up of individuals who are considered competent, criminally responsible, guilty, but mentally ill. These individuals are transferred from other criminal justice institutions because they are in need of mental health treatment. Some patients are acutely ill and are transferred to the forensic state hospital under emergency conditions; others may be more stable or chronic and are transferred for a specific type of treatment or training. Some patients are transferred specifically for preparation and training before being released into the community.

Forensic state hospital treatment programs and occupational therapy programs vary widely depending on patient and security needs and the state's resources. Some hospitals allow patients to wear their own street clothes, while others require uniforms. Some programs are sparse, while others are quite rich with services and opportunities. Some even provide outings (usually requiring court notification of approval), both on and off hospital grounds.

The forensic state hospitals with the most resources have large occupational therapy departments that offer comprehensive, specialized programming with multiple tracks for various categories of patients. Sensorimotor activities, living skills training, cooking, task groups, prevocational programming, and expressive arts are all typical of the offerings. These settings offer the advantage of the availability of a wide variety of modalities and have a clear institutional mission for treatment. A special challenge in this setting is combatting institutional dependence and motivating the more chronic patient.

A role for the occupational therapist that is unique to the forensic state hospital setting is leading a pretrial competency group for patients identified as incompetent to stand trial. This group uses role-playing and paper-and-pencil tasks to increase patients' understanding and appreciation of their current legal charges, their own social interaction styles, and the roles and procedures of a courtroom. The overall goal of the group is to facilitate the patient's return to competency. Specific group goals include increasing the abilities to verbally express charges, verbally express what charges mean, verbally identify the participants in a courtroom, verbally identify a range of possible criminal penalties, cooperate with others, and express both positive and negative feelings appropriately.

Community Programs

In the community, occupational therapists work with newly released individuals. There are a number of ways in which people can be released from custody while remaining under court-ordered supervision. Some states are experimenting with alternative sentencing for mentally ill individuals, which includes referrals to traditional, non–criminal justice, mental health programs and intensive case management. Individuals may also be placed in diversion programs, be put on probation or parole, or be referred to a conditional release program. Diversion programs typically mandate services such as structured, supervised living situations; volunteer community service time; mental health treatment; drug counseling; and participation in educational activities, work, and other meaningful daytime activity. Individuals may also leave custody on probation in lieu of jail time or on parole in lieu of prison time. Both involve a release from custody subject to conditions, and both require supervision by either a probation or parole officer. If a condition of release is violated, the individual's sentence is reinstated and he or she is sent back to jail or prison. Common conditions of probation and parole include required community service, testing for controlled substances, warrantless search conditions, restraints on certain types of employment, restraints on associations and activities, abstinence from the use of alcohol and drugs, involvement in educational activities, and mental health or substance abuse treatment (Mental Health and Forensic Task Force, 1989).

Newly released individuals may also be court-ordered to participate in formal conditional release programs, which are comprehensive psychiatric programs providing services such as individual therapy, case management, group therapy, skills training, family therapy, home visits, and screening for drug and alcohol use (California Department of Mental Health, 1991).

At the community level, criminal justice occupational therapists have a vital role in providing living and job skills training and activities that focus on self-confidence, accomplishment, goal setting, taking responsibility, and problem solving. They also have the very important function of focusing on skill development to facilitate compliance with release requirements and court-ordered conditions. For example, they may help individuals develop the transportation or telephone skills needed to contact their probation officer or facilitate the development of appropriate communication skills needed for court appearances. Occupational therapists also evaluate patients' level of function, information that may be used to help determine how long a patient will need to remain under close supervision.

Community programs offer the occupational therapist the advantage of working with a stable, motivated group of patients for whom medication compliance may be a condition for release. The potential exists in this community for drug and alcohol abuse, and therapists must be aware of this possibility and be skilled in substance abuse treatment methods and resources.

Riverside and San Bernadino Counties in California have a conditional release program that utilizes occupational therapy. The overall goal of the program is to prevent relapse and/or reoffense while stabilizing the patient in the community. Close observation, support, and immediate response to potential problems are provided. Supervision and support are then gradually reduced while promoting the patient's ability to function in the community. Skill building, symptom recognition, acceptance of mental illness, substance abuse prevention, social skills training, stress management, and building a sense of self-determination are all critical.

Before they are admitted to the program, patients sign a contract in which they agree to follow the rules, participate in treatment, take prescribed medication, and remain drug and alcohol free. Abiding by the contract is a condition of their court-ordered release into the community, and patients may be reincarcerated if they violate it. Most patients, at least initially, attend a highly structured day treatment program, although some participate in a less-structured program of outpatient visits.

Patients represent a wide range of ethnic and socioeconomic backgrounds. Many report a poor educational history and have been in the forensic state hospital for several years before release. The primary diagnoses cover a wide spectrum, but the most common are schizophrenia, bipolar disorder, and alcohol- or substance-induced psychosis. About half the patients carry a diagnosis of personality disorder. The average length of stay is 2.5 years. Discharge from the program is primarily dependent on an evaluation of the person's potential for relapse or reoffense.

The occupational therapist works with an interdisciplinary treatment team consisting of several clinicians (social workers, psychologists, or marriage, family, and child counselors), a program manager, and a psychiatrist. The occupational therapist screens new patients for day treatment using an interview and questionnaire adapted from the Occupational History (an interview protocol focusing on educational and occupational history and living skills). Once in day treatment, patients are evaluated with observation in a wide variety of groups as well as with specific evaluations, including the Kohlman Evaluation of Living Skills (Kohlman Thomson, 1992) as well as various educational and vocational assessment tools.

The occupational therapist addresses work skills, independent living skills and the development of social supports. Work skills are addressed on two levels, with role-play and psychoeducational groups for the higher-functioning patients and a token economy for the lower-functioning group. When appropriate, the occupational therapist will do in-depth prevocational evaluations. This is followed by making appropriate referrals to the state department of vocational rehabilitation and acting as the liaison throughout the vocational rehabilitation process. Training in independent living skills is approached through cooking groups, shopping groups, problem solving, and discussion groups. When needed, the occupational therapist can provide more intensive, one-on-one training in independent living skills, perhaps even working in the patient's own home. The occupational therapist addresses developing a support system within the community through engaging in altruistic activities, humor, crafts, games, expressive art, and community outings.

CLINICAL COMPETENCIES IN A CRIMINAL JUSTICE SETTING

Criminal justice settings provide a unique set of challenges requiring occupational therapists to refine their competency in a number of areas. They must be able to understand and adapt institutional environments, redefine the concept of independence in a confined setting, blend therapeutic practice with safety and security issues, and be creative problem solvers when they encounter difficult patients and institutional blocks to good treatment. These skills are required in all mental health settings, but they must be well developed to function effectively within the criminal justice system, particularly within the locked environments of jails, prisons, and forensic state hospitals.

Analyzing the Environment

Performance is greatly affected by environmental influences and how the patient interprets them (Spencer, 1978). Correctional facility environments vary between states, between facilities within states, and between housing units within facilities, but all have demanding and unique environments. Therapists in the criminal justice system must understand the specific demands of the various environments in which their patients function. They must also understand the difference between the institutional environment and the community (Michael, 1986).

Jails and prisons are closed societies, with their own rules and culture. They are, essentially, small cities providing all the services of a city while maintaining a high degree of security. Although there are a variety of positive roles that inmates may assume within these institutions (church member, volunteer, student, worker), many factors in the jail and prison environment reinforce maladaptive behavior. Victimization is common, and inmates may learn how to protect themselves by fighting or gathering support by joining a gang. While rigid institutional structures attempt to control inmate access to legal and illegal goods, underground economies controlled by the inmates themselves often flourish. Complicated systems develop for the distribution of extra food and the "good" work and housing assignments, as well as for contraband such as cigarettes, drugs, alcohol, and weapons. Inside the facility, inmates may learn ways of meeting their needs that foster continued criminal behavior. Occupational therapists are faced with the challenge of creating programs to improve individuals' coping skills, decision-making ability, and self-esteem and counseling inmates on how to develop alternative strategies for controlling and eliminating criminal behavior.

Forensic state hospital environments offer another set of demands. These hospitals tend to be highly structured and organized. Compliance and conformity to external controls are emphasized, which can foster dependence, passivity, and social withdrawal on the part of the patients. The structured environment of the hospital is in sharp contrast to the lack of structure encountered in the community. Occupational therapy programs in forensic state hospitals focus on increasing patients' sense of competency, autonomy, and productivity in an effort to combat the institution's tendency to create passivity and dependency.

All programming must keep the patients' current and future environments in mind. Therapists may be called on to help patients make the transition from mental health housing to mainstream prison housing, from prison to a forensic hospital, from prison or a forensic hospital to the community—and there are many other possibilities. Each of these environments is different and requires a different adaptive performance in order for patients to be successful.

Effective social skills, ways of expressing feelings, and communication skills may greatly differ from one criminal justice unit to another, one institution to another, and, certainly, from inside to outside this system of institutions. In jail, for example, it would be considered adaptive to develop a quiet interpersonal style whereby one keeps to oneself, does not initiate conversation or does not openly express emotion, and remains detached from other people's problems. In many community mental health programs, however, quite the opposite is considered adaptive. People are encouraged to form close personal relationships, make inquiries regarding each others' lives, openly express their feelings, and assist each other when needed. It is also considered adaptive in jail to develop a tolerance for long stretches of inactivity and engage in quiet, solitary interests like solitaire, journal writing, and reading, whereas most community settings expect tolerance for a more active, social, and productive schedule. Moreover, how one projects one's self-image is very different inside and outside of jail. On the outside, it is frequently considered good to have a realistic sense of one's assets and limitations, and be open about one's frailties, and be proud of one's accomplishments and material assets. In jail, however, adaptive functioning involves presenting a low-key, but confident, persona, with little said about personal assets (for fear of angering someone) or personal weaknesses (for fear of victimization). Thus, each area of patient functioning must be evaluated within the context of the particular environmental demands and norms.

Maintaining Safety and Security

Safety and security are the primary mission of all criminal justice settings. Correctional facilities usually have a number of security levels or classifications, ranging from light to moderate and, finally, to close custody status. Policies and procedures are outlined for each security level and must be adhered to without deviation. Automatically locking doors, increased awareness of danger, the presence of custody staff, clear emergency plans, high staffing ratios, security cameras, buzzer systems, emergency alarms, and restrictions on materials are vital to the security of an institution.

To maintain safety, occupational therapists must maintain close, continual communication with other staff members and avoid situations where they may be isolated or lack immediate staff support. Patients must be carefully assessed, especially those with a high violence potential or history of impulsive behavior. All clinical staff must be observant, sensitive to subtle changes in a patient's behavior and affect, and constantly alert to the surroundings. Treatment planning in these settings starts with the highest degree of structure and control, which lessen only as a patient demonstrates reliability and predictability.

Occupational therapists must be very careful with tools and supplies since quite a few of these items are considered contraband. They must also be aware of alternative, and potentially dangerous, uses of common materials, such as using chewing gum to jam locks or sharpening plastic and wooden items into weapons. Some glues are very flammable; some paints can be "sniffed" for an intoxicating effect. Because of the potential of misusing occupational therapy supplies and equipment, body searches and metal detectors are common in this system. Figure 17-3 reflects the policy and procedures for tool safety and security for one prison-based occupation therapy clinic; the photograph in Figure 17-4 illustrates this application.

General
- The OT tool room will be locked at all times and out of bounds to all inmates unless under the direct supervision of staff.
- All OT tools will be painted and engraved "OT Clinic" to denote origin.
- Periodic, unscheduled searches of the entire OT clinic will be made for safety and security.

Tool Accountability
- Tools are stored in locked rooms, secured inside cabinets and on shadow boards.
- Each morning tools are inventoried.
- Tools are accounted for at the end of each group before inmates are released to their housing areas. No one is allowed to leave until all tools are accounted for.
- All inmates will be given a clothed body search for contraband before leaving the OT clinic.

Use of Tools
- Inmates and OT staff are assigned a number with five corresponding numbered tags for checking out tools. For each tool used by an individual one tag assigned to that person is placed where the tool is stored. No one will be allowed to use more than five tools at a time.
- Large floor power tools will only be used under the direct supervision of an OTR.

Figure 17-3. Policy and Procedures for Tool Safety and Security in a Prison-based Occupational Therapy Clinic

Strict adherence to infection control policies is mandatory as tuberculosis, HIV infection, and hepatitis are common in correctional institutions. Groups, such as cooking and grooming, that involve eating communal food or close physical contact require adherence to universal precautions.

Professional and modest clothing is mandated. While most inmates' crimes are not of a sexual nature, incarceration deprives individuals of privacy and inhibits normal sexual outlets, creating a certain degree of sexual tension. Therapists will be more effective when their clothing does not act as a disruption or distraction to the therapeutic process. Fashionable clothing is quite acceptable, but short skirts and low-cut blouses, for example, are not.

Overcoming Obstacles

The safety and security policies for any given correctional facility may drastically alter the modalities and scope of occupational therapy that is provided. There may be policies to avoid "overfamiliarity" with patients that discourage one-to-one contacts or place restrictions on the types of materials patients can take out of the occupational therapy clinic. For example, sharp tools may be prohibited altogether. The occupational therapist must model positive problem-solving strategies. Each obstacle can serve as a creative opportunity for

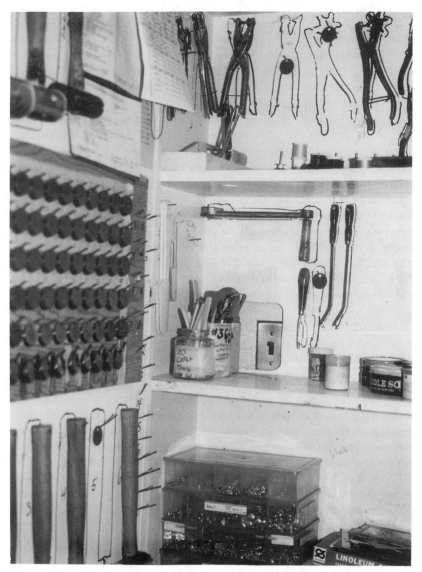

Figure 17-4. A Tool Closet Arranged as Required by Tool Safety Policies in Figure 17-3.

problem solving. For example, if sharp tools are not permitted, the occupational therapist can explore alternative, and perhaps more creative, novel, and meaningful, activities. Similarly, if patients cannot take finished projects out of the occupational therapy clinic, they can be encouraged to donate their work to charity or make a gift of it.

Developing Team Relationships

In any criminal justice setting, the occupational therapist will interface with the non–mental health, criminal justice staff, such as deputy sheriffs, prison or security guards, parole officers, and correctional case managers. These staff may be unfamiliar with mental health treatment philosophy and benefits and concerned instead with public safety and compliance with institutional rules. Some staff may feel that patients should be punished because of their criminal involvement and do not comprehend the benefits that the occupational therapist can provide. In other words, there is potential for conflict between mental health and criminal justice staff because of philosophical differences.

Occupational therapists can build alliances with all staff by clearly articulating the benefits of occupational therapy for the patient and the institution. Some of these "selling points" are listed in Figure 17-5. The occupational therapist must also try to understand the other staffs' perspective. Relationships can be developed by including other disciplines in decisions, program planning, and in-service training. Clear lines of communication, well-defined staff roles, and an attitude that promotes sharing ideas is beneficial for all staff. It is always recommended to use humor when appropriate, to be persistent, and, above all, to be flexible in meeting conflicts and working toward resolution.

Building Therapeutic Alliances

One challenge when working in the criminal justice system involves developing and maintaining relationships with patients who are impaired in their ability to trust and cooperate with others, find it difficult to express their thoughts and feelings, and are unable to interact in a socially acceptable manner. The general atmosphere of mistrust and suspicion typical of correctional facilities increases the difficulty of fostering therapeutic relationships.

Personality disorders, and antisocial personality disorder in particular, are quite common within the criminal justice setting (Jemelka et al., 1989). People with personality disorders typically exhibit problems with conflict resolution, delaying gratification, repressing impulses, forming stable relationships, and tolerating emotions. Internal feelings are often transformed into social

- Increases safety by providing productive, creative outlets for aggression.
- Increases safety by building cooperation and a sense of cohesiveness among inmates.
- Increases safety by reducing individuals' feelings of tension and stress.
- Provides unique evaluation material and a new view of inmates' abilities, deficits, and capabilities and how they best learn.
- Provides inmates with new skills that ultimately will help with productive integration into their community and decrease the possibility of reoffense.

Figure 17-5. Benefits of Occupational Therapy in Criminal Justice Settings

or somatic complaints or projected onto another person. These patients may have difficulty assuming responsibility for their actions. They frequently try to bend and break rules, divide the staff, and undermine authority. People with personality disorders tend to view themselves as tough, smart, entitled, and victimized by the legal system and may view the therapist as foolish and weak, ineffective, and easily manipulated (Hoyt, 1989). Such patients are likely to view situations with concrete thinking, with their ultimate goal a self-centered, self-serving one. They view conflicts in terms of right or wrong, seeing things in black and white rather than in shades of gray, and are unable to comprehend others' emotions.

Knowing this information about personality disorders, the therapist can be better prepared and avoid taking conflicts personally. This population can be very enjoyable and satisfying, and these problematic traits described are found in patients in traditional mental health settings as well. Guidelines for building effective therapeutic alliances include being assertive and honest and maintaining a healthy degree of suspicion, as the patient's word may not always be reliable. Occasionally, it is necessary to give firm, direct orders and set clear limits. The here-and-now approach, whereby the therapist only focuses on current, relevant factors, is quite helpful, as is the ability to communicate to patients exactly what is expected of them. Unacceptable patient behavior is best handled through immediate confrontation. Occupational therapists are most effective when they are fair, reliable, and consistent and when they use rational limits that apply to everyone, without deviation. All patients seem to respond to a genuine show of respect and concern.

Recognizing Malingering

Malingering is defined as the conscious, planned simulation of an illness for the sake of gain or the pretense of a slow recuperation from a disease once suffered; in either case, the intent is to receive benefits (Rogers, 1988). There are several reasons why patients within correctional institutions may want to feign or exaggerate psychiatric symptoms.

Malingerers may believe that being diagnosed with a mental illness will make them more sympathetic to a judge or a jury. Some individuals prefer mental health programs to mainstream jail or prison, as these programs are associated with fewer restrictions and work expectations. Some patients may also be "medication seeking," trying to obtain prescription drugs to "get high," alter consciousness, or ease the frustration and boredom associated with incarceration rather than for the intended purpose of reducing specific psychiatric symptoms.

Clinicians within the system need to share observations with other team members and carefully document suspicious or unlikely symptoms. The occupational therapist is often the first person to observe or confirm malingering as patients tend to relax and let their guard down in occupational therapy.

Malingerers become fully absorbed in their tasks during treatment sessions and forget to "act sick," thus revealing the inconsistencies in their functioning.

Documenting Accurately

Documentation must be clear, accurate, concise, and in accordance with professional guidelines. The focus, as in other mental health settings, is on functional ability, progress toward goals, and plans for future interventions. The occupational therapist's observations and documentation regarding cognitive and functional abilities can be instrumental in the treatment team's decisions regarding a patient's transfer and discharge and therefore are taken very seriously. In preadjudication settings, specific information regarding an individual's charges, the circumstances resulting in arrest, and the patient's beliefs regarding his or her innocence or guilt should be avoided. It is not the occupational therapist's responsibility to investigate a case or pass judgment regarding a crime.

Although the issue is becoming controversial, medical records tend to be more accessible to patients and their lawyers in the criminal justice system than in the traditional mental health system. In some prison systems, patients are allowed to review their charts by simply asking to see them. Criminal justice medical records are frequently subpoenaed, either in reference to an individual's criminal case or medical treatment or as part of a class action lawsuit concerning jail or prison conditions. Such class action lawsuits are not uncommon in these settings. Every therapist is ethically and legally obligated to inform patients of confidentiality guidelines within this system in order to maintain a therapeutic, trusting relationship.

Knowing the Criminal Justice Language

Having a knowledge of the basic terminology used in criminal law will increase the occupational therapist's credibility with staff and patients, who will frequently make reference to the adjudication process. The occupational therapist must understand this process to understand the stressors, demands, and decisions facing patients. Jail and prison slang words are also commonly used. Table 17-2 defines some of the basic legal terminology, and Table 17-3 describes slang vocabulary commonly used in this system.

Summary

An understanding of the criminal justice system is mandatory for all occupational therapists working in mental health, as it impacts many patients. The mental health and correctional systems overlap and will continue to blend in

Table 17-2.	Basic Criminal Law Vocabulary
TERM	*DESCRIPTION*
Arraignment	An initial step in the criminal process wherein the defendant is formally charged with an offense.
Bail	A monetary or other security given to insure the appearance of the defendant at every stage of the criminal proceedings.
Defendant	The accused.
District Attorney	The prosecuting attorney.
Felony	A class of criminal offenses that are considered more serious than misdemeanors and are usually punishable by imprisonment for more than a year (possibly death).
Misdemeanor	A class of criminal offenses that consists of offenses less serious than felonies, which are sanctioned by less severe penalties, usually including fines, community service, probation, or a sentence of under one year in jail.
Parole	A conditional release from imprisonment that entitles the person receiving parole to serve the remainder of the term outside the prison provided he or she satisfactorily complies with all the terms and conditions of the release and remains under the supervision of a parole officer.
Plea Bargaining	The process whereby the accused and the prosecutor negotiate a mutually satisfactory disposition of a case, thus avoiding a complete trial.
Probation	A procedure whereby a defendant found guilty of a crime upon verdict or pleas of guilty is released by the court to the community without imprisonment, subject to conditions imposed by the court, under the supervision of a probation officer.
Prosecute	To bring legal action against the accused.
Public Defender	A lawyer whose duty it is to defend accused persons who are unable to pay for legal assistance.
Revocation	To recall a power of authority previously conferred, as in revoking probation or parole if a condition of release is not met and requiring a return to jail or prison.
Sentence	The punishment ordered by the court to be inflicted on a person convicted of a crime.
Trial	An examination involving the offering of testimony before a judge and/or jury.

line with current trends of economic hardship, hospital closures, and the general decrease in mental health resources.

Occupational therapists in the criminal justice system may work in jails, where the treatment program focuses on evaluation, crisis intervention and symptom stabilization; in longer-term prisons and forensic state hospitals, where the focus is on improving task skills, interactional skills and on the opportunities for choices and decision making; or in the community where the

Table 17-3.   Jail and Prison Slang

TERM	DESCRIPTION
Beef	A written action against an inmate.
Behind the wall	Inside the prison.
Bunkie/cellie	Someone who sleeps above or below an inmate (in a bunk bed).
"Burn rubber"	"Get lost, leave, you're not wanted"
Canteen	A version of a store in which inmates are allowed to purchase needed and wanted items, based on how much money is available in their trust account.
Chrono	Information written about an inmate that is either negative or positive and becomes part of the inmate's "central" (permanent) record.
Clean time	Period of time for which an inmate has been infraction free.
Date	Prison release date.
Down	Amount of time in prison.
Gooner	Security and investigation prison task force.
Hang	Staying with someone to the end, no matter how tough the situation gets.
Hog	Tough guy, leader.
"Homes"	General greeting, refers to "homeboy" or someone from your hometown.
In the car	Refers to being in the in-group.
Jacket	Inmate's central file or record.
Mainline	Areas of prison accessible to inmates.
On the leg	Describes inmates who spend time with the staff to cultivate influence.
PC	Protective custody, where inmates are housed for their own safety when they need to be locked away from others.
Pruno	Prison-made alcohol.
Punk	Young, defenseless inmate who is forced into homosexual activity
Road dog	Friend who can be trusted for life.
Rolled up	To be locked up in a security housing unit.
Schooled	Inmate who has earned respect; someone who knows how to survive in prison.
Shakedown	What officers do when they search the work or living areas of the prison.
Take care of business	To do what is necessary for day-to-day living or to protect oneself.
To the house	Home, getting out on parole.
Yard	Outside space for recreational activity.

focus is living skills and vocational skills training. All programs must take the institutional environments and legal process into account.

The occupational therapist in the criminal justice system must possess expertise in certain areas to function effectively. These include a thorough knowledge of **forensics**, the ability to understand and adapt to institutional environments, the ability to blend therapeutic practice with safety and security issues, the ability to think flexibly and creatively to overcome obstacles, the ability to form strong team relationships with mental health and correctional staff alike, the ability to form therapeutic alliances with difficult patients, the ability to recognize malingering behavior, the ability to document occurrences in an unbiased manner, and a basic understanding of the legal system.

Occupational therapy provides professional diversity to the criminal justice environment. The profession's understanding of one's ability to adapt in different environments, its emphasis on problem solving strategies, and its commitment to treating people with dignity makes occupational therapy an asset to the criminal justice setting.

It is the authors' hope to demystify some of the myths related to the criminal justice system and to encourage increased involvement in it. There is currently a paucity of occupational therapists in the criminal justice system and a growing need. The population is compelling and opportunities are rewarding: The work is fascinating and satisfying.

Review Questions

1. How does the role of an occupational therapist in the criminal justice system differ from the role of an occupational therapist in a traditional mental health setting? What are the differences in assessments, treatment planning, treatment implementation, and documentation?
2. Use the Model of Human Occupation (Kielhofner, 1995) to identify how a prison environment may affect an inmate patient. Specifically, what effect may a prison environment have on a person's sense of personal causation, values, and interests? What effect might the environment have on his or her roles and habits?
3. How can the criminal justice occupational therapist work to maintain strong team relationships? What would you do if a criminal justice or mental health official posed a question to you such as: "How can you treat these people? They are guilty and do not deserve treatment."

Learning Activities

1. Visit a traditional psychiatric occupational therapy clinic. What adaptions would you make to insure safety and security if this clinic were in a criminal justice setting?

2. Arrange a tour of a local correctional facility. Note the environment. Inquire about the number of mentally ill inmates and ascertain what treatment, services, and programs are available?

3. Sit in on a criminal court proceeding. Do you comprehend the process? Do you understand the identity of all the players? What terms are unfamiliar to you? What are your emotional reactions? How would you imagine a psychotic individual would respond to this setting?

4. Divide your class into two groups. Take turns role-playing the therapist and a patient who is attempting to break the rules and undermine your authority. Practice setting limits and stating clear behavioral expectations.

5. Visit a halfway house that serves a postincarceration, postrelease population. What are the goals of this program? How is it different from other halfway houses? What would the role of the occupational therapist be?

6. View the videotape *Families and Law Enforcement* (available from the California Alliance for the Mentally Ill, 111 Howe Avenue, Suite 275, Sacramento, California, 95825).

References

Allen, C. (1985). *Measurement and management of cognitive disabilities*. Boston: Little, Brown.

American Bar Association. (1989). *Criminal justice mental health standards*. Washington, DC: Author.

American Psychiatric Association Task Force. (1989). *Psychiatric services in jails and prisons* (Task Force Report No. 29). Washington, DC: American Psychiatric Association.

California Department of Mental Health. Forensic Services Branch. Office of Forensic Services. (1991). *The Forensic Conditional Release Program: An orientation guide*. Sacramento, CA: Author.

Donovan, J. (1991). *Forensic Conditional Release Program: An overview of laws pertaining to Conrep*. Unpublished paper.

Jemelka, R. P., Trupin, E. W., & Chiles, J. A. (1989). The mentally ill and the prisons: A review. *Hospital and Community Psychiatry, 40*, 481–489.

Kohlman Thomson, L. (1992). *The Kohlman evaluation of living skills*. The American Occupational Therapy Association: Bethesda, MD.

Kielhofner, G. (1995). *A Model of Human Occupation: Theory and Application*. Second Edition. Baltimore, MD: Williams & Wilkins.

MacKain, S. J., & Streveler, A. (1990). Social and independent living skills for psychiatric patients in a prison setting. *Behavior Modification, 14*, 490–518.

Mental Health and Forensic Task Force (California). (1989). *Violence and treatment*. Unpublished paper.

National Alliance for the Mentally Ill (NAMI) and Public Citizen's Health Research Group (PCHRG). (1992). *Criminalizing the Seriously Mentally Ill.* Arlington, VA: Author.

Rogers, R. (1988). *Clinical assessment of malingering and deception.* New York: Guilford Press.

Spencer, E. A. (1978). *Willard and Spackman's occupational therapy* (5th ed.) Philadelphia, PA: Lippincott.

Suggested Reading

Chiles, J. A., Von Cleve, E., Jemelka, R. P., & Trupin, E. W. (1990). Substance abuse and psychiatric disorders in prison inmates. *Hospital and Community Psychiatry, 41,* 1132–1134.

Curran, W. J., McCarry, A. L., & Shah, S. A. (1988). *Forensic psychiatry and psychology.* Philadelphia: F. A. Davis.

Fansworth, L., Morgan, S., & Fernando, B. (1987). Prison based occupational therapy. *Australian Journal of Occupational Therapy, 34,* 40–46.

Fowles, G. P. (1988). Neuropsychologically impaired offenders: Considerations for assessment and treatment. *Psychiatric Annals, 18,* 692–697.

Freeman, M. (1982). Forensic psychiatry and related topics. *British Journal of Occupational Therapy, 45,* 191–194.

Green, N. S. (1984). OT Education Bulletin: Utilizing inmate populations in training occupational therapy assistants. *Occupational Therapy News, 38*(10), 9.

Halleck, L. S. (1986). *The mentally disordered offender.* Rockville, MD: National Institute for Mental Health.

Hamm, M. S., & Schrink, J. L. (1989). The conditions of effective implantation: A guide to accomplishing rehabilitative objectives in corrections. *Criminal Justice and Behavior, 16,* 166–182.

Jones, E. J., & McColl, M. A. (1991). Development and evaluation of an interactional life skills group for offenders. *Occupational Therapy Journal of Research, 11,* 80–92.

Lloyd, C. (1983). Forensic psychiatry and occupational therapy. *British Journal of Occupational Therapy, 46,* 348–350.

Lloyd, C. (1985). Evaluation and forensic psychiatric occupational therapy. *British Journal of Occupational Therapy, 48,* 137–140.

Lloyd, C. (1987a). The role of occupational therapy in the treatment of the forensic psychiatric patient. *Australian Journal of Occupational Therapy, 34,* 20–25.

Lloyd, C. (1987b). Working with the female offender. *British Journal of Occupational Therapy, 50,* 44–46.

Lloyd, C. (1988). Discharge preparation for the forensic psychiatric patient: A proposed model. *Journal of the New Zealand Association of Occupational Therapists, 39,* 12–14.

Lloyd, C., & Guerra, F. (1988). A vocational rehabilitation programme in forensic psychiatry. *British Journal of Occupational Therapy, 4*, 123–126.

Maier, G. J., & Miller, R. D. (1987). Models of mental health service delivery to correctional institutions. *Journal of Forensic Sciences, 32*, 225–232.

Michael, P. S. (1991). Occupational therapy in a prison? You must be kidding! *Mental Health Special Interest Section Newsletter 14*(2), 3–4.

Miller, R. K., Maier, G. J., Van Rybroek, G. J., & Widermann, J. A. (1989). Treating patients "doing time": A forensic perspective. *Hospital and Community Psychiatry, 40*, 960–962.

Morrison, E. F. (1991). Victimization in prison: Implications for mental health professionals. *Archives of Psychiatric Nursing, 5*(1), 17–24.

National Alliance for the Mentally Ill. (n.d.). *A guide to mental illness and the criminal justice system: A systems guide for families and consumers.* Arlington, VA: Author.

Nelson, S. H., & Berger, V. F. (1988). Current issues in state mental health forensic programs. *Bulletin of the American Academy of Psychiatry and the Law, 16*, 67–75.

Penner, D. A. (1978). Correctional institutions: An overview. *American Journal of Occupational Therapy, 32*, 517–524.

Platt, N. P. (1977). Level I field placement at a federal correctional institution. *American Journal of Occupational Therapy, 31*, 385–387.

Police Executive Research Forum. (1986). *Special care: Improving the police response to the mentally disabled.* New York, NY: Author.

Reed, K. L. (1991). *Quick reference to occupational therapy.* Gaithersburg, MD: Aspen.

Sadler, C. (1989). Held without help . . . Mentally ill offenders. *Nursing Times, 85*(4), 16–17.

Samarneh, G. (1993). Taking treatment behind bars. *OT Week, 7*(47), 20–22.

Samson, S. T. (1990). Occupational therapy in a forensic psychiatric unit. *Journal of the New Zealand Association of Occupational Therapists, 41*, 18–22.

Seek, N. (1989). The New Zealand prison system: The potential role of occupational therapy. *Journal of the New Zealand Association of Occupational Therapists, 40*,16–19.

Simon, R., & Aaronson, D. (1988). *The insanity defense: A critical assessment of law and policy in the post-Hinkley era.* New York: Praeger.

Smith, J. A., & Faubert, M. (1990). Programming and process in prisoner rehabilitation: A pison mental health center. *Journal of Offender Counseling Services and Rehabilitation, 15*, 131–153.

Sturm, H. V. (1988). OT gives new outlook to inmates of a Texas prison. *OT Week, 2*(22), 16–17.

CHAPTER 18

Vocational Programming

Glenda Jeong, MA, OTR
Director of Operations
Community Vocational Enterprises
San Francisco

Key Terms

Americans with Disabilities Act (1990)
consumer/client empowerment
job coaching
prevocational services

psychiatric rehabilitation
supported education
supported employment (SE)
work programming

Chapter Outline

Introduction
History of Work Programming in Occupational Therapy
Changing Roles of Occupational Therapists
    Knowing Your Customers—New Alliances
Implementation of Occupational Therapy Services
    Assessment
    Forms of Intervention
Summary

Introduction

A primary goal of occupational therapists working in community mental health is to support independent living. Assisting someone to enter or reenter the work force provides a real and meaningful context in which both the occupational therapist and the client can address issues of daily living. The work arena becomes the backdrop for occupational therapy interventions aimed at assisting an individual to reestablish his or her age-appropriate balance in work, play, and leisure.

Providing occupational therapy within a community context requires the recognition that one is truly operating in an open, dynamic system with many players. Maintaining sensitivity to the community context ensures that the activities pursued are both personally and socially meaningful. Figure 18-1 depicts the multiple levels of collaboration necessary when operating in a dynamic community context. The dynamic system depicted in this figure will be referred to throughout the chapter, which reflects my strong belief that the

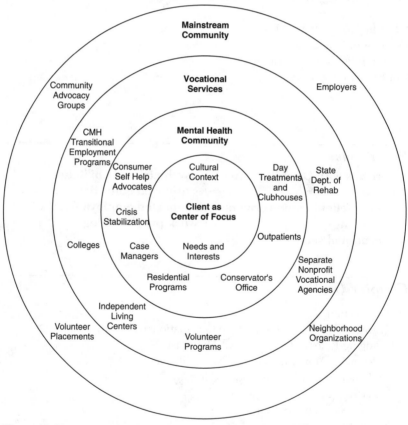

Figure 18-1. Levels of Collaboration

vocational approach advocated is the most useful and meaningful model for clients and therapists.

HISTORY OF WORK PROGRAMMING IN OCCUPATIONAL THERAPY

Occupation involves engaging with clear intent in activity that nourishes and sustains one's relationship to oneself (body, mind, and spirit) and one's relationship to the community. The value of work—that is, productive activity—has always been key to the philosophical basis of the profession. The roots of occupational therapy come from moral treatment, an approach that was used in the early 1900s for humane treatment of the mentally ill. During World War I, occupational therapy assisted disabled soldiers to regain their self-discipline, build their morale, and obtain training for reentering the civilian workforce. Operating from a holistic perspective, occupational therapy continued to be actively involved in the work adjustment of soldiers through the early 1900s during the immediate post–World War I period. During that same period, the Vocational Rehabilitation Act (Smith-Fess Act, Public Law 66-236) of 1920 established rehabilitation as a necessary service benefit for disabled individuals to enable them to return to remunerative employment (Flexor & Solomon, 1993). Occupational therapists actively developed **prevocational services** through the 1930s, and in 1943, and with the passage of the Vocational Rehabilitation Amendment (Barder-La Follete Act/Public Law 78-113), people with psychiatric and developmental disabilities became eligible for such benefits. During this time, occupational therapists, including those in mental health, were actively involved with work adjustment programming.

In spite of the clear need and opportunity for occupational therapists to continue and expand their roles within work programming during the post–World War II era, there was a decline in professional interest during the 1950s. However, during the 1960s the profession saw a resurgence in this area with the emergence of evaluation practices in industrial therapy.

Ironically, **work programming** is presently seen as a specialty within community mental health practice, and many occupational therapists do not see themselves involved with work. If occupational therapy began as a forerunner in this arena in clear alignment with rehabilitation, what happened to its clear view? With respect to work programming, some noteworthy occurrences during the 1950s and 1960s had a significant impact in shaping the direction of mental health occupational therapy and its predicament of today.

A phenomenon that was most prevalent in the decade of the 1950s was the adoption of the medical model of diagnosis and treatment that prevailed in all arenas of health care, including psychiatry. Occupational therapy was no exception. Embracing the medical model, occupational therapy shifted away from its holistic perspectives and adopted the more popular scientific, reductionist perspectives (Lang, 1991). This philosophical perspective viewed human behavior as purely a result of biological and physiological, mechanical function. Like a machine, the human could be dismantled and reduced and then understood by examining its structural parts. Hence, humans were considered separate from nature and the mind considered separate from the body. This perspective manifested itself in medicine as specialties in practice emerged. Emphasis was placed on developing expertise in specific modalities and techniques. While occupational therapists in physical disabilities became experts at adaptive equipment, occupational therapists in mental health became experts at craft modalities and projective techniques for supporting the psychoanalytic process.

Although the 1960s was also the era of deinstitutionalization, it was marked by greater focus on occupational therapy practice to assist the individual to "process" feelings through activity. The therapeutic focus was limited to a part of the client—the psyche—without a visibly meaningful link to the whole client as a center of focus for community function. That is not to say occupational therapy did not address function, but within the medical model, function had a biomechanical meaning. For instance, occupational therapeutic interventions were aimed at structuring medication management, with the end goal being to alleviate symptoms. Given the prevailing viewpoint of the era—that people with mental illness could never improve—achieving maintenance and stability of the condition was considered achieving function.

Ironically, while the medical model took precedence, the 1950s also saw the emergence of the psychosocial rehabilitation programs in community mental health. Hallmark agencies such as Fountainhouse and Thresholds (see resource list in "Learning Activities" at the end of this chapter) were established throughout the country with the mission of improving the lives of people with mental illness by providing a supportive environment for learning skills and encouraging mastery through community membership and activity.

Originally, two separate approaches, **psychiatric rehabilitation** and psychosocial rehabilitation (Cook & Hoffschmidt, 1993) (both terms are currently often used interchangeably), evolved into one model as medication management became recognized as being integral to optimal community function (Flexor & Solomon, 1993). Historically, psychiatric rehabilitation (Cook & Hoffschmidt, 1993), in alignment with the medical model, focused on deficits, symptom reduction, and pathology, in the belief that people with psychiatric illnesses had no hope for improved function.

Psychosocial rehabilitation originally differed from psychiatric rehabilitation due to its exclusion of medication management as a part of treatment, and this approach emerged as a separate movement in the 1950s (Anthony & Blanch, 1987). Psychosocial rehabilitation represented an effort to apply the principles of physical rehabilitation to mental illness in order to achieve independent functioning in the community. The emphasis was on changing environmental and social supports for individuals. Services were focused on helping people evaluate their strengths and weaknesses and setting their own goals for optimal function in the community. Commonsense and practical techniques were used to address vocational, social, recreational, and housing issues. The environment and interventions were deliberately kept informal to decrease the psychological distance between staff and clients in the program.

While occupational therapy in mental health focused on using activity to address the patient's intrapsychic process first and self-care maintenance second, psychosocial rehabilitation programs maintained a steady pace in addressing the person's function and relationship to the community, including work. It was not until the late 1960s that the occupational therapy profession expressed concern over the paucity of work programming in mental health, and it was not until the late 1970s and early 1980s that occupational therapy began to increase its involvement with work programming for people with psychiatric disabilities.

Occupational therapists began to recognize that the psychosocial rehabilitation perspective was similar philosophically to the perspective held by the profession of occupational therapy. Indeed, the following principles are common to both:

- There can be no health without meaningful occupation.
- People can change themselves by their own efforts, and they have the choice—and responsibility—to do so.
- To effect change requires enlisting client choice and engaging in activities that promote skill building, exploration, education, and community role development.

For the clients, this was a natural partnership. For occupational therapists, it was difficult to discover that mental health administrators and practitioners within the mental health field considered psychiatric rehabilitation, and not occupational therapy, to be the pioneer approach promoting independent living. Today, occupational therapists who choose to practice in vocational rehabilitation come into a practice arena in which psychiatric rehabilitation is widely accepted and recognized.

Given the flow of these historical events, many mental health occupational therapists find themselves in a position that necessitates redefining their roles in work programming as well as in mental health.

CHANGING ROLES OF OCCUPATIONAL THERAPISTS

The present trends in health care provide numerous opportunities for occupational therapists to creatively carve out new roles and perspectives. Health care is clearly shifting from the medical model toward a model of preventative care. This movement is driven by numerous factors, including the aging of the population, the increasing awareness of people regarding the mind-body link in health, and the uncontrollably rising costs of health care.

Managed care principles mandate a system of care designed to provide quality services that are customer driven, effective, and cost efficient. By necessity, community mental health services in some U.S. states are restructuring to become such systems of care. Consequently, occupational therapy practitioners may have to redefine their roles and strategies if they are to be regarded as necessary participants within the emerging systems of care. This period of transition represents both a crisis and an opportunity. The potential crisis for occupational therapy is that functional outcome is now everyone's business and not specialty specific. The opportunity is for occupational therapy to demonstrate the vital role occupational therapy services play in achieving functional client outcomes. For instance, Medi-Cal (the California Medicaid program) historically paid for mental health services only if they were provided within a designated site (clinic option). The adoption of the "Rehab-Option" (psychiatric rehabilitation coverage) under Medi-Cal now allows for the reimbursement of services provided outside a clinic. On a program level, occupational therapists can now provide direct services much more creatively within the community arena. On a systems level, they can not only become invaluable service providers to clients and family members, they can also take on diverse roles such as program development consultants and community-based advocates and educators. Figure 18-2 outlines the historical shifts in the occupational therapist's role and services.

Knowing Your Customers—New Alliances

In the current environment of managed care, high-quality, cost-effective service within the community is a priority. For the occupational therapist, providing service in a larger public arena can mean expanding one's definition of the customer. In this instance, customers include not only those who receive direct services, but also those who fund the services—and thus indirectly benefit. These customers can become important allies.

Clearly, the most important customers are the clients served and their family members and significant others. When clients value services, their message and active support carry weight in the clinic, community, and political arenas. Family members and significant others are also significant advocates (for further discussion see Chapter 2, "The Social and Personal Effects of Family Illness"), representing a powerful voice about which services are critical to the health of their loved ones.

Internal allies.   Intragency as well as interagency coordination often provides a vehicle for education within the provider community. Services that assist clients to attain functional outcomes, such as school or paid employment, demonstrate concretely to professional peers, administrators, policy makers, and community organizations the value of including occupational therapists in the multidisciplinary community team.

Community allies.   The needs and concerns of the business community are important quite simply because it is this community group that holds and

A. Therapeutic Relationship	Then	Now
The O.T. Role	Decision-Maker Authority	Facilitator Navigator
The Client Role	Recipient of Service	Pilot, Decision-Maker
Nature of Participation by Client	Passive	Active

IMPACT OF SHIFT: Ongoing collaborative dialogue. Greater opportunity for change, since momentum is coming from the client.

B. Arena of Service Provision	Then	Now
Location Site	Clinic Site	Community-Chosen Site
Achievement of Treatment Objectives	Unknown	Observable
Degree of Carry-Over of Skills to Community	Unknown	Immediate

IMPACT OF SHIFT: The activity becomes truly meaningful, because the what and where of the service is directed by the client. The service gains greater value.

C. Role of O.T. as Advocate Leader	Then	Now
Programming Planning and	Clinic Site Specific to Program	Systemwide Policy Level
Advocacy	Team Member in Clinic Arena	Community Arena

IMPACT OF SHIFT: The opportunity to promote independent living as well as understanding and appreciation of how occupational therapy equals function by DOING.

Figure 18-2. Historical Shifts in the Occupational Therapist's Role and Services

creates the jobs. Services provided can include information, education, and consultation in areas such as mental health, fears and misconceptions about people with mental illness and with the **Americans with Disabilities Act (1990)** compliance (e.g., reasonable accommodations, interviewing etiquette, job analyses, and identifying essential functions for jobs). These services are needed because the reality at present is not in accord with Title II of the Americans with Disabilities Act (ADA): (a) people with severe mental illness rarely choose to disclose and ask for reasonable accommodations due to the fear of stigma and discrimination, and (b) employers rank their level of comfort in working with the mentally ill second to last of all different disability groups (U.S. Congress, 1994).

IMPLEMENTATION OF OCCUPATIONAL THERAPY SERVICES

As depicted in Figure 18-2, the occupational therapist is a facilitator at all levels of occupational therapy service and all phases of service implementation. As a facilitator, the occupational therapist's action and goals are directed by the original needs and interests expressed by clients.

Assessment

The process of determining vocational interests begins simply by asking and listening to gauge how the assessment can be tailored to suit the individual's need. A basic interview procedure starts with the source; therefore, the therapist should ask, "What brings you here?"

Client choices drive therapeutic interventions from day one. The individual's self-report is the reference point for beginning the assessment, goal setting, and treatment planning needed to address any imbalances in work, leisure, and self-care. Hence, self-assessment is pivotal to obtaining the individual's view of his or her personal strengths and the obstacles that have blocked the desired goals.

An interview procedure gauges interests and insights; therefore, the therapist should ask, "What would you like to do and why?" With each identified vocational goal, the reasons behind the person's choice are explored to identify if the choice is based on previous work/volunteer experience, personal and/or cultural values, life roles, or interest. The individual's perception and fund of knowledge of how to attain the desired objectives is tapped by asking, "What do you think you need to do/learn to achieve that goal? What helps? What gets in the way?"

The interview reviews past and present work/role experiences, which enables the occupational therapist to ascertain the individual's level of insight, foresight, perceptions for goal achievement, and strategies. Having determined the desired goal and obtained a self-report on abilities and limitations, the occupational therapist engages the individual in assessment activities.

The interview ascertains skills. The therapist should suggest, "Let's take a look at some basic core skills you'll need to use in any job, for example, problem solving." Based on the individual's stated vocational goal, situational assessments and occupational therapy assessments are selected to note the level of match between the person's task performance, the self-report, observations, and the person's desired goal. The individual's self-care habits and daily living routines are also discussed to determine if, and how, these self-care patterns are productive or counterproductive to the desired goal. The assessment activities chosen are explained to the client to clarify how they relate to his or her desired goals. Feedback given throughout the process clarifies how the information gained is directly relevant to the person and the stated goal. The assessment is framed as a shared learning experience, and not a testing situation.

Occupational therapy assessments (cited in Asher, 1996) often used are:

- Allen's Cognitive Levels—to determine cognitive levels of functioning and accompanying levels of supervision and instruction.
- Jacobs Prevocational Skills Assessment—basic problem solving, sequencing, categorizing, and map reading.
- Cognitive Assessment of Minnesota—complex problem solving and memory retention.
- Bay Area Functional Performance Examination (BAFPE) Self Reports of Social Interaction—self-report regarding specific social components.

This is a sampling of assessments that can be used. Many other tools are available depending on whether the occupational therapist's purpose is to do career exploration (e.g., aptitude tests, vocational interests) or job-specific performance assessment. Assessment activities could include:

- work behaviors, problem-solving exercises
- clerical manual assembly
- restaurant assessments
- safety and coworker attitudes, judgment

The purpose of the assessment is to provide information so that the counselor can consider appropriate options to provide. The therapist can then say, "Given your strengths, experience, and needs, here are some options to consider and discuss with your vocational counselor." Depending on the setting, the depth, extent, and value of vocational assessment can often be tailored to meet the needs of consumers at various levels of care. The process is often determined by the consumer's level of focus and expressed desire to consider work activity. The occupational therapist may find that, at the very least, this expressed interest can be an opening for dialogue and short-term interventions. Dialogue can be particularly useful when the identified barriers to working are related to disability management issues (e.g., medication compliance, self-medication with substances).

Note that the vocational counselor may be same person as the occupational therapist. It is also likely that the occupational therapist may work in a consultative role. The choices and decisions made regarding the vocational plan of action are determined jointly by the client and the practitioner. The client can choose to adopt or reject the recommendations of the practitioner. Service options can include job-seeking skills groups, time management and stress management workshops, social security benefits workshops, volunteer experiences, transitional paid training experiences, individual counseling, and referral assistance to enter other employment training programs or educational programs, depending on the desired goal.

Once the client is engaged in training, situational assessments are done to evaluate progress. These are done on the work training sites while the person is performing the job. The work training sites are often paid transitional employment sites within the community. The following case illustration is an example of the evaluation process.

CASE ILLUSTRATION: CHARLOTTE— OCCUPATIONAL THERAPY EVALUATION

Charlotte is a 56-year-old female diagnosed with chronic paranoid schizophrenia who expressed interest in paid transitional work experience in the community. She was referred by a San Francisco mental health program to Community Vocational Enterprises/Keystone Vocational Services (CVE/KVS), a vocational rehabilitation agency in San Francisco. Charlotte was specifically interested in the CVE/KVS Clerical Program due to her previous work history in the secretarial field. After the CVE/KVS initial intake interview, Charlotte was referred by the CVE/KVS projects coordinator to occupational therapy for the CVE/KVS vocational evaluation and assessment. The client was administered a battery of tasks designed to assess performance in specific work-related areas. Cognitive abilities, learning styles, strengths and limitations with respect to employment, social and communication skills, safety awareness, and special needs with respect to ability and disability were evaluated. Functional activities of daily living (ADL) skills, sensory perception and motor functioning, physical endurance, self-concept, and judgment were also assessed. A baseline for understanding the client's current skill level and work readiness was established to assist Charlotte, the occupational therapist, and the vocational counselors in determining appropriate job placement in the community.

As a short-term goal, Charlotte wanted to receive clerical training and transitional work experience from the CVE/KVS Clerical Program for approximately three to four hours per day, three days per week. Her long-term educational and vocational goals were to learn computer skills for data entry and to find a part-time clerical job in the community.

From the assessment, it was determined that Charlotte had the following difficulties:

1. *poor problem-solving skills*
2. *poor short-term memory*
3. *difficulty making decisions and self-correcting work*
4. *difficulty planning with foresight and accurately*
5. *decreased activity tolerance (two hours)*
6. *need for increased time to learn new tasks*
7. *poor stress and frustration tolerance*

From the assessment, it was also determined that Charlotte had the following assets:

1. *very motivated to work and to learn computer skills*
2. *previous work experience*
3. *clear, legible penmanship*
4. *initiates questions when needs clarification of instruction*
5. *strong sorting and filing skills*
6. *excellent telephone-answering skills*
7. *good self-care habits*
8. *daily living routines consistent with desired goals*

From the results of the assessment, the following functional requirements were identified:
1. *a very structured environment*
2. *clearly defined tasks*
3. *increased time to learn new tasks*
4. *both written and verbal instruction*
5. *compensatory techniques (i.e., lists)*
6. *feedback from supervisors and coworkers regarding task performance and decision making*
7. *opportunities to practice problem-solving behavior in familiar settings with familiar people and with simple tasks in simple situations*
8. *a break every two hours until activity tolerance increases*

Charlotte began the CVE/KVS program in June 1994. After completing the Volunteer Clerical Program in November 1994, she was placed in a paid transitional secretarial position at a human service agency in San Francisco. She is currently doing very well in her secretarial position and will be referred to the job developer at the CVE/KVS in approximately two to three months to begin searching for permanent employment in the community.

Forms of Intervention

Client choices often determine the nature, timing, and context for occupational therapeutic interventions. The arena varies from the agency site to the community and the workplace. Regular assessment and/or intervention can occur at work-training sites. The occupational therapist can often work with the training supervisors to adapt the training process.

One-to-one.   Counseling takes the form of problem-solving as opposed to psychotherapeutic sessions. The stated objective is to support the individual in learning how to manage situations that arise within a day-to-day context. The focus is on the immediate situation, learning from the present moment, and developing personal resiliency for the future. The therapeutic value lies in **consumer/client empowerment**—empowering the client in his or her ability to make decisions, act on them, and learn from the experiences.

Problem solving occurs most often while assisting people to build interpersonal and communication skills. Often, uncertainty results from not knowing how to interpret an interaction. The cognitive stress from perceptions based on incomplete information or misinterpreted nonverbal cues is often the source of stress and difficulties in getting along with others.

Group. Problem-solving skills can also be developed in the psychoeducational contexts of health, education, and leisure activity workshops. In addition to providing a peer support environment in which to learn new skills, these workshops also reinforce the holistic viewpoint that health does not simply involve being able to work productively, but also being able to interact with others within the community.

People have greater motivation to take in new information and apply what they learn when they are concurrently engaged in either volunteer or paid training positions. The day-to-day issues can provide concrete incentives for coming to a workshop either to address specific issues or to learn something that relates directly to one's job or role. The occupational therapist often surveys the current CVE employee needs/interests and then uses a marketing strategy to promote workshops (e.g., mailing workshop announcements with paychecks). This approach is taken because most people report negative past associations with groups from day treatment milieus, wherein group attendance was expected, if not mandatory, with little clear benefit to the present identified client needs. One result of their reported experience is that group size tends to be very small.

CASE ILLUSTRATION: ROCHELLE— SUPPORTED EMPLOYMENT

*Rochelle is a 49-year-old female diagnosed with chronic paranoid schizophrenia who was interested in a paid transitional work experience in the community. She was referred by a San Francisco mental health day treatment program to Community Vocational Enterprises/Keystone Vocational Services (CVE/KVS) for vocational rehabilitation and **supported employment** and has been affiliated with the agency for almost one year now. Rochelle started working with the CVE/KVS Janitorial Program in March 1994. Since then, she has been promoted to janitorial supervisor, working approximately 12 hours per week at $6 per hour, and has completed a Certificate for Custodial Programs from San Francisco Community College. Rochelle is fully responsible for three work sites and describes her job as follows: "I train new employees. I visit and work with employees on the job. I do training evaluations and I substitute when employees are sick."*

Rochelle had a few basic goals when she came to the program. She wanted to increase her work tolerance and further develop her ability to work with others harmoniously and patiently. She wanted to receive paid transitional work experience from the CVE/KVS Janitorial Program because she was not satisfied with depending on her social security entitlement as a means of in-

come, wanted to be financially independent, and wanted to lead a more active life.

Prior to enrolling in CVE/KVS, Rochelle had utilized services at various other vocational rehabilitation agencies. However, she commented that other facilities were unable to provide her with services that suited her needs. At CVE/KVS, she attended job-seeking skills workshops, supplemental security income (SSI)/supplemental security disability income (SSDI) benefits workshops, and work support groups and utilized additional services, including job development/placement assistance, **job coaching**, individual vocational counseling, referral to education programs, and work-related funding from the CVE/KVS and the state department of rehabilitation cooperative program. Rochelle stated that all of these services have been very beneficial to her recovery, especially the weekly work support groups. She reported that the group has a comfortable family atmosphere that makes her feel relaxed. In the group, she is able to discuss current work issues, both positive and negative, among peers and the CVE/KVS staff members. She commented that unless it conflicted with a doctor's appointment, she would never miss a group session because the group made her excited about the upcoming work week. At this point in time, Rochelle has successfully held a community-based job for approximately one year and has accomplished all her self-reported vocational goals.

Management skills.   As individuals begin earning wages, money management and decision-making skills are developed concretely through learning how to calculate social security withholdings, report earnings, maintain records, and make decisions about increasing hours and jobs. Counseling and support are given throughout to assist the person to address the fears surrounding the loss of cash and medical benefits. Given the confusing nature of social security work incentives, it is only through continuous review of the information, support, and actual experience over time that a person can learn and gain confidence over their money management.

When an individual on supplemental security income (SSI) reaches a point when he or she has set a specific employment objective and determined the specific equipment or training needs to achieve that goal, the occupational therapist can assist in developing a Plan for Achieving Self-Support (PASS) to set aside income funds for the long-term goal. An example of a PASS plan is setting aside 100 percent of one's wages to pay for a rehabilitation counseling degree program over a three year-period. Again, the responsibility of decision making and choice returns to the client and is directly experienced as such.

Applying the skills in the community.   There are numerous opportunities to assist the client to practice communication skills, stress management, and organizational skills when the practitioner accompanies the client to outside community offices such as the local social security office. Through **supported education**, the occupational therapist can assist the client to anticipate questions and role-play the situation beforehand. After the visit, reviewing what happened reinforces learning and the client's sense of mastery. The occupational therapist also reinforces the fact that the learning was a shared experience between the therapist and client. Regardless of the type of community-based activity, learning and adaptation are stressed as arising from every instance. Failure is reframed as a lesson learned to be added to one's stock of experience, reminding individuals that they are gaining their vocational maturity much in the same way that others have.

Interventions with the community.   As an advocate, educator, or consultant, the occupational therapist often works with several types of communities and groups. Such groups may include the business community, the mental health provider community, the consumer advocate community, and the rehabilitation provider community. The therapist can also practice the same concept of learning and adaptation for him- or herself when planning to work with community agencies, employers, and the local community at large.

It is often to the occupational therapist's benefit to research and identify the community or group audience with regard to values, attitudes, and culture. This can be part of a needs assessment done before the occupational therapist goes in to present information or education at a particular site. For instance, when working with an employment site, the workplace culture and practices can be identified and explored with the employees to facilitate the new employees' integration on the job as well as provide support services within or outside the workplace context (see Figure 18-3).

Interventions when the employer is involved.   Understanding the workplace culture assists to establish a dialogue with employers. One of the desired outcomes is that employers become receptive to being educated about mental illness and/or hiring qualified workers who have psychiatric disabilities. Many employers are unaware of how the Americans with Disabilities Act applies to such individuals. For an occupational therapist, adaptations made at the worksite are then considered reasonable accommodations for a qualified individual who can perform the essential functions of the job with certain modifications in either the job, the environment, or the supervisory process (Marcuso, 1993) (see Figure 18-4). Support is given to the employer throughout to address work issues that may arise. In the best-case scenario, an employer can appreciate certain accommodations as making good business sense for *all* employees. However, this does not always serve to eliminate the discrimination and stigma that an individual may fear or experience from others.

Interventions when the employer is not involved.   When clients choose not to disclose their diagnoses, the decision must be respected and occupational therapeutic interventions are done very much "behind the scenes." Coaching occurs in the preparation before and after the job interview, on the telephone during working hours while on break, before or after work, and/or

Community Mental Health	Local Community	Business Community
Consult/Educate Mental Health Providers Regarding:	Educate/Inform Members of the Community:	Consult/Educate Employers, Supervisors, Employees:
•Work readiness •Program planning	•Mental illness •Supervising volunteers with mental illness	•ADA •Mental illness
•ADA		•Supervising employees with mental illness
•System policy and service design •Supervision of consumer staff	•Stigma	•Staff education •Diversity awareness
Types of forums for these interventions can be as follows:		
Consult/Educate Mental Health Providers Regarding:	Educate/Inform Members of the Community:	Consult/Educate Employers, Supervisors, Employees:
•In-service presentations	•Outreach	•Educational
•Outreach	•Community service education	•Sensitivity training
		•Community outreach

Figure 18-3. Types of Interventions within Different Communities

during lunch. Accommodations are rarely explicitly presented and often are worked out by the employee independently or with coaching.

Support takes whatever form the client perceives would be helpful, whether a peer support group, a peer counselor, a community group affiliation, or mental health agency affiliation for therapeutic or socialization purposes.

The context of services. Thus far, the nature of occupational therapeutic interventions has been described within the context of a vocational service setting founded on a psychosocial rehabilitation philosophy. It is important to acknowledge that the extent, nature, and depth of occupational therapeutic intervention are driven, not only by customer choices and needs, but also by the setting in which the occupational therapist works. The variety of settings where occupational therapists work offer opportunities to develop programming to address varying levels of vocational and self-care needs of clients. Depending on the setting, the occupational therapist may focus on skills learning and building, skills application, or skills refinement and/or adaptation (see Figure 18-5).

TYPES OF REASONABLE ACCOMMODATIONS

Modifications can be made to:

The Job	•Job sharing, trading duties between workers
Physical Environment	•Partitions
	•Rearranging/positioning location of work area in office
	•Changing fluorescent lighting
Assistive Aids or Technology	•Tape recorders
	•Day organizers
	•Handheld organizers
Schedule Modifications	•Change break times
	•Shift scheduled hours earlier/later
	•Work or paid/unpaid leave
Supervising Structure	•Additions or adaptations of supervision schedule/style
	•Mentor/buddy
	•Adapting mode of instruction/training
Policy and Work Culture	•Diversity training and education
	•Mental health days/paper days

Figure 18-4. Reasonable Accommodations

Instrumental Activities of Daily Living Addressed Include:

- •Money Management
- •Transportation
- •Stress Management
- •Time Management
- •Physical Health Self Care
- •Communication Skills

Skills Learning and Building Can Begin within the Mental Health Community	Skills Application Can Occur in Vocational Settings	Skills Refinement Can Be Ongoing within the Mainstream Community
•Partial Hospitalization	•Vocational Programs	•Community-based Employment
•Day Treatment	•Volunteering	•Education
•Clubhouse Programs	•Transitional Employment Programs	

Figure 18-5. Continuum for Occupational Therapy Assistance with Skills

CASE ILLUSTRATION: CHUI—
VOCATIONAL PROGRAMMING

Chui is a 31-year-old male diagnosed with chronic paranoid schizophrenia who was interested in paid transitional work experience in the community through either the janitorial program or the cafe program. After the initial intake interview, Chui was referred by the vocational counselor to occupational therapy for the vocational evaluation and assessment. The client was administered a battery of tasks to assess performance in specific work-related areas. Chui's cognitive abilities, learning styles, strengths and limitations with respect to employment, social and communication skills, safety awareness, and special needs with respect to ability and disability were evaluated. His functional ADL skills, sensory perception and motor functioning, physical endurance, self-concept, and judgment were also assessed. A situational assessment was performed by the occupational therapist to provide additional baseline information for understanding the client's current skill level and work readiness.

As a short-term goal, Chui wanted to receive paid transitional work experience from the vocational janitorial (first choice) or cafe (second choice) program for two hours per day, five days per week. His long-term vocational goals were to work at least four hours per day, five days per week, and to live in his own apartment in the community.

From the assessment, it was determined that Chui had difficulties in the following areas:
1. paying attention to detail
2. concentrating on task
3. following verbal and written directions
4. pacing a task appropriately
5. quickly processing new information
6. problem-solving skills
7. planning with foresight and accurately
8. judgment
9. body mechanics
10. stability—bilaterally tremulous (does not interfere with job performance)

From the assessment, it was determined that Chui had the following assets:
1. good visual accuracy
2. learns well by demonstration
3. increased performance with familiarity of job
4. strong willingness and ability to adapt to supervisor feedback
5. good attention span
6. motivated to learn
7. initiates questions when needs clarification of instruction
8. looks for what needs to be done instead of waiting for supervisor to direct him

From the results of the assessment, the following functional implications were identified:

1. *works too quickly initially and requires pacing for accuracy and safety*
2. *needs verbal cues to pace task appropriately until the routine becomes more familiar*
3. *needs verbal cues to wear hearing aid at work until familiarizes self with job and coworkers*
4. *needs structured environment*
5. *needs clearly defined and routine tasks*
6. *requires demonstration to learn new tasks*
7. *needs to work on one task at a time (i.e., one customer)*

The plan for Chui was as follows:

1. *expose to more work situations to assess flexibility and work skills in different areas*
2. *engage in problem solving exercises on the job*
3. *educate regarding proper body mechanics*
4. *refer to Janitorial and Cafe supervisors for an interview*

The client began the program in October 1990. After undergoing occupational therapy assessment and participating in an educational workshop dealing with values clarification, personal strengths, and weaknesses, Chui was offered a position in the cafe. After four months of work, however, Chui was hospitalized, but before entering the hospital that day, he called his supervisor to inform him and tell him he covered his shifts (as is required of all employees) at the cafe. In return he was assured that there would be a position in the cafe when he was ready to return to work. In January 1992, when Chui moved into a board and care home in the community, he informed the agency that he was now living in the community and would be interested in going back to work in the future. In April 1992, he returned for an interview with the cafe supervisor and then, in May, began working one shift per week. Five months later, Chui began working two shifts per week (3 hours per day, two days per week). Over a two-year period, he gradually increased his time to five days per week. In January 1995, Chui successfully completed his transitional employment in the cafe program and was offered outside employment at a residential treatment program. He started work as a kitchen assistant at the program in February 1995 and worked a total of 10 hours a week. Three months later, he was offered extended hours (to 35 hours per week) and is now successfully working full time (40 hours per week).

The occupational therapist has played an extended role in Chui's supported employment environment by working closely with him to assist with his future independence by reporting his work hours to the social security office. Chui has progressed from not reporting work hours at all to independently calculating, documenting, and reporting deductions consistently.

Prior to entering the vocational program, Chui held one other job (at McDonald's restaurant, for a duration of three months); however, after receiving *vocational rehabilitation services, he has held a community-based job for approximately four years, has moved out of the board and care home into his own apartment, receives full medical coverage from his employer, and has exceeded his original, self-reported, long-term goal of working 20 hours per week.*

Summary

Occupational therapists who work in vocational rehabilitation may find themselves operating simultaneously within multiple arenas of service provision. Rather than considering it as a specialty, occupational therapy can be reframed to identify how services can directly contribute to a person's functional goals. Regardless of the number of arenas and where one stands in the system of care (see Figure 18-1), client choice can become both the central driving force and the compass for all aspects of service. The occupational therapist becomes primarily the navigator and facilitator.

Operating in a system of care requires continuous communication, negotiation, and adaptation. Such an arena is rich with experiences in which, much like the clients, occupational therapists can constantly challenge themselves to learn and adapt professionally in order to fully participate in the changing health provider community.

To practice effectively in the community, many occupational therapists want to understand the total picture of health care and the community at large. Occupational therapy in work programming is not so much a specialty as it is a different, and perhaps renewed, expression of how occupational therapy can and may be practiced.

Review Questions

1. Distinguish prevocational services, supported employment, and job coaching.
2. Identify the levels of collaboration necessary in the overall picture of community vocational programming. Who are the players at each level in your community?
3. What is the history of occupational therapy within the psychiatric and psychosocial rehabilitation movements? How do the two movements differ?
4. Who are allies of the client and therapist in vocational programming?
5. Briefly outline the assessment and intervention process in vocational programming. How does it resemble or differ from other occupational therapy assessment and intervention?

Learning Activities

1. Use the following resources to plan a vocational program in your school, community, or agency.

Bazelon Center for Mental Health Law
1101 Fifteenth Street, NW, Suite 1212
Washington, DC 20005
(202) 467-5730 (voice); (202) 467-4232
   (Telecommunications Device for the Deaf [TDD])

Center for Mental Health Services
Community Support Program
Substance Abuse and Mental Health Services Administration
U.S. Department of Health and Human Services
Parklawn Building, Room 11C-22
5600 Fishers Lane
Rockville, MD 20857
(301) 443-3653

Center for Psychiatric Rehabilitation
Reasonable Workplace Accommodation Research Project
Boston University
730 Commonwealth Avenue, Second Floor
Boston, MA 02215
(617) 353-3550

Disability Rights Education and Defense Fund
2212 Sixth Street
Berkeley, CA 94710
(510) 644-2555 (voice); (510) 644-2625 (TDD)

Fountainhouse
425 West 47th Street
New York City, NY 10036
(202) 582-0340

Job Accommodation Network
918 Chestnut Ridge Road, Suite 1
Morgantown, WV 26506-6080
(800) ADA-WORK (voice/TDD)

National Alliance for the Mentally Ill
2101 Wilson Boulevard, Suite 302
Arlington, VA 22201
(703) 524-7600

National Association of Psychiatric Survivors
P.O. Box 618
Sioux Falls, SD 57101-0618
(605) 332-9124

National Association of State Mental Health Program Directors
66 Canal Center Plaza, Suite 302
Alexandria, VA 22314
(703) 739-9333

National Council on Disability
800 Independence Avenue, SW, Suite 814
Washington, DC 20591
(202) 267-3846 (voice); (202) 267-3232 (TDD)

National Depressive and Manic-Depressive Association
730 N. Franklin Street, Suite 501
Chicago, IL 60610
(312) 642-0049

National Empowerment Center
130 Parker Street
Lawrence, MA 01843
(800) POWER-2-U (769-3728)

National Institute on Disability and Rehabilitation Research (NIDRR)
U.S. Department of Education
400 Maryland Avenue, SW
Washington, DC 20202-2572
(202) 205-8801 (voice); (202) 205-5516 (TDD)

National Mental Health Consumers Association
4401-A Connecticut Avenue, NW, Suite 308
Washington, DC 20008
(216) 621-5883

National Mental Health Association
1021 Prince Street
Alexandria, VA 22314
(703) 684-7722

National Mental Health Consumer Self-Help Clearinghouse
311 S. Juniper Street, Room 902
Philadelphia, PA 19107
(800) 553-4539

President's Committee on Employment of People with Disabilities
1331 F Street, NW
Washington, DC 20004
(202) 376-6200 (voice); (202) 376-6205 (TDD)

Reasonable Accommodations Report (Mancuso)
California Department of Mental Health
1600 Ninth Street, Room 120
Sacramento, CA 95814
(916) 654-2657

Regional Disability and Business Accommodation Centers
ADA Information Hotline (connects caller
   to the appropriate regional center)
(800) 949-4232 (voice/TDD)

Thresholds National Research and Training Center
   on Rehabilitation and Mental Illness
2001 N. Clayburn Avenue, Suite 302
Chicago, IL 60614
(312) 348-5522

U.S. Equal Employment Opportunity Commission (U.S. EEOC)
1801 L Street, NW
Washington, DC 20507
U.S. EEOC Publications Center
(800) 669-3362
U.S. EEOC ADA Helpline
(800) 669-4000 (voice); (800) 800-3302 (TDD)

U.S. Department of Justice (DOJ)
Civil Rights Division
Office on the Americans with Disabilities Act
P.O. Box 66118
Washington, DC 20035-6118
U.S. DOJ ADA Information Line
(202) 514-0301 (voice); (202) 514-0381 (TDD)

Washington Business Group on Health
Employer's Resource Center on the ADA
   and Workers with Psychiatric Disabilities
777 N. Capitol Street, NE, Suite 800
Washington, DC 20002
(202) 408-9320 (voice); (202) 408-9333 (TDD)

2. Think about the client empowered philosophy and program discussed in
   this chapter. Think about your approach to clients. Would you be able to
   follow, not direct their lead? Would you be able to work in a program
   with this model?

3. Visit any vocational program in your community. Does the program use a client empowered model? If so, what makes it work? If not, what are some barriers to implementing the model? How can occupational therapy make a difference in the program?

4. Do you have a committee sponsored by the mayor for employment for people with disabilities? How can you become a member? How can one be started? Call the President's Committee on Employment of People with Disabilities (see item 1).

References

Anthony, W. A., & Blanch, A. (1987). Supported employment for persons who are psychiatrically disabled: A historical and conceptual perspective. *Psychosocial Rehabilitation Journal, 11*(2), 5–23.

Asher, I. E. (1996). *Occupational therapy evaluation tools: An annotated index* (2nd ed.). Bethesda, MD: American Occupational Therapy Association.

Cook, J. A., & Hoffschmidt, S. J. (1993). Comprehensive models of psychosocial rehabilitation. In R. W. Flexor & P. L. Solomon (Eds.), *Psychiatric rehabilitation in practice* (pp. 81–97). Boston: Andover.

U. S. Department of Justice, Civil Rights Division, Office on the Americans with Disabilities Act (1990). *The Americans with Disabilities Act: Questions and Answers.*

Flexor, R. W., & Solomon, P. L. (1993). Introduction to psychiatric rehabilitation in practice. In R. W. Flexor & P. L. Solomon (Eds.), *Psychiatric rehabilitation in practice* (pp. xiii–xvii). Boston: Andover.

Lang, S. (1991). Perspectives—Work for psychiatrically disabled clients. In K. Jacobs (Ed.), *Work: A journal of prevention, assessment, and rehabilitation* (pp. 6–10). Boston: Andover.

Marcuso, L. (1993). *Case studies on reasonable accommodations for workers with psychiatric disabilities.* Study funded by the Community Support Program at the Center for Mental Health Services of the U.S. Department of Health and Human Services, Substance Abuse and Mental Health Administration.

U.S. Congress. (1994, March). *Psychiatric disabilities, employment, and the Americans with Disabilities Act* (Office of Technology Assessment Report). Technology Assessment Board of the 103rd U.S. Congress.

Suggested Reading

Anthony, W. A. (1994). Characteristics of people with psychiatric disabilities that are predictive of entry into the rehabilitation process and successful employment. *Psychosocial Rehabilitation Journal, 17*(13), 3–13.

Crist, P., & Stoffel, V. (1992). The Americans with Disabilities Act of 1990 and employees with mental impairments: Personal efficacy and the environment. *American Journal of Occupational Therapy, 46*(5), 434–443.

Danley, K. S., Scriarappa, K., & MacDonald-Wilson, K. (1992). Choose-Get-Keep: A psychiatric rehabilitation approach to supported employment. In R. P. Liberman (Ed.), *Effective psychiatric rehabilitation* (pp. 87–96). San Francisco: Jossey-Bass.

Harvey-Krefting, L. (1985). The concept of work in occupational therapy: A historical review. *American Journal of Occupational Therapy, 39*, 301–307.

Lang, S., & Cara, E. (1989). Vocational integration for the psychiatrically disabled. *Hospital and Community Psychiatry, 40*(9), 890–892.

Stauffer, D. (1986). Predicting successful employment in the community for people with a history of chronic mental illness. *Occupational Therapy in Mental Health, 6*(2), 31–49.

Case Management

Nancy Cooper, MS, OTR/L
Occupational Therapist
Swedish Medical Center Home Health and Hospice
Seattle, Washington

Key Terms

advocacy
conservator
deinstitutionalization

in vivo
Medicaid
prodromal symptoms

Chapter Outline

Introduction

The traditional practice arena of most occupational therapists working with persons with serious mental illness has been the short-term, acute or long-term, locked institution. Day treatment, partial hospitalization, and prevocational training programs have provided additional domains as the **deinstitutionalization** movement of the 1950s set the stage for a new era of community practice. Since that time, treatment in the community has evolved from mirroring the medical model of the institution, with a focus on diagnosis and symptom reduction, to the development of innovative psychosocial rehabilitation programs. Case management, a model previously well established in nursing and social work with other needy populations, is one of these innovations. Occupational therapists facilitate adaptation through evaluation and training in functional living skill performance, which are "the very needs of a chronically mentally ill population" (Klasson, 1989, p. 85). With an emphasis on strengths and abilities and a focus on skill building, occupational therapists bring a unique and valuable perspective to case management for persons with serious mental illness in the community.

HISTORY OF CASE MANAGEMENT

In the mid-1950s, the development of phenothiazines, along with a new collective social conscience and concern for patients' civil rights and treatment costs, led to the release of large numbers of people with serious mental illness from state institutions into the community and to the expansion of community treatment programs. Initially, community treatment centers focused on, and adequately served, higher-functioning and less seriously ill individuals, but they were inadequate in both number and scope to address the needs of those with chronic serious mental illness. Significant numbers of treatment dropouts, with no mechanism or mandate for follow-up intervention, resulted in the "revolving door syndrome." The revolving door represents repeated returns to the hospital, as well as the formation in communities of the "mental health ghetto" (Platman, Dorgan, Gerhard, Mallam, & Spiliadis, 1982) as an alternative to the state hospital.

Recognizing the inadequacy of the response to these clients' needs and the fragmentation of services in the community, the U.S. Congress enacted the Community Mental Health Act of 1963. This act made continuous and coordinated service delivery in federally funded community mental health centers (CMHCs) a requirement. Services did become better coordinated at the CMHC level, but the responsibility for negotiating the service system and complying with treatment remained with the client. Moreover, the services continued to be directed toward persons with less severe illnesses and not toward those who had been released from the state hospitals. It was not until 1977, when the National Institute of Mental Health established the Community Support Program, that the needs of the most seriously mentally ill became an established focus of concern. Case management was introduced in the Community Support Program as one of the essential services required for this population. It was described as a way to facilitate access to the service system by designating a single individual or a team to be responsible for helping the client and for coordinating services to meet the client's needs and goals. In 1978, the Task Panel on Deinstitutionalization, Rehabilitation, and Long-Term Care of the President's Commission on Mental Health affirmed the use of individualized case management services in its recommendations (Robinson & Toff-Bergman, 1989).

Federal funding for case management became available in 1985 when the Omnibus Budget Reconciliation Act (OBRA) designated it as an optional benefit under **Medicaid**. OBRA defined case management as a service for assisting eligible persons to gain access to needed social, educational, medical, and other services. The act gave broad flexibility to individual states in determining how and to whom these services would be provided. The Consolidated Omnibus Reconciliation Act of 1986 (COBRA) designated individuals with severe mental illness as a target population under Medicaid. Later that same year, the U.S. Congress passed Public Law 99-660 requiring states to develop and implement comprehensive mental health plans. This law mandated the provision of case management services to all individuals with serious mental illness who receive substantial amounts of public funds or services and stipulated that implementation of case management services commence during fiscal year 1989. Because the vast majority of persons with serious mental illness are insured under Medicaid, Public Law 99-660 thus made case management services available to large numbers of seriously mentally ill persons who had previously had little appropriate or accessible community care.

CASE MANAGEMENT SERVICES

Specific case management service guidelines vary somewhat as the individual states' interpretation and implementation of federal mandates differ. The needs and resources of a large inner-city population vary considerably from those of a rural community. A clear and consistent service definition has not been reached, and there is no consensus on what does and does not constitute case management. Some people describe case management as purely a brokering or linkage function, while others include comprehensive skill teaching and support in addition to service linkage. Controversy also exists regarding who can best provide the service: nonprofessionals, specified mental health professionals, or a combination of both in a team approach. Consumer case management, in which clients or consumers in the mental health system act as case manager aides for those with less functional ability, is also being undertaken (Porter & Sherman, 1988).

Generally, case management is understood to be a mental health treatment intervention that seeks to facilitate a client's adaptation to the community by identifying, coordinating, and insuring access to the services and resources needed for stable functioning. Characteristics common to the various types of case management are:

1. Services are provided **in vivo**.
2. Goals are to reduce hospitalization, maintain the client in the least restrictive community setting possible, and maintain quality of life.
3. A team or an individual case manager serves as a fixed point of responsibility.
4. Service is of unlimited duration.
5. Service will provide continuity of care over time and across referral agencies.

One of the best known and most widely studied programs of community mental health treatment that includes case management is the Program for Assertive Community Treatment (PACT) in Madison, Wisconsin (Thompson, Griffith, & Leaf, 1990). Established in 1970 in response to the failure of existing community mental health centers to adequately serve mentally ill persons in that community, PACT created innovative and progressive community supports to respond to the identified needs of those individuals. Multidisciplinary teams comprise a case management project known as Training in Community Living (TCL), which has been widely replicated in other communities across the United States because of its documented effectiveness.

Case management service components typically include evaluation, service plan development, placement services, linkage and consultation, assistance in daily living skills, and emergency intervention. **Advocacy** is usually not a distinct service in itself but is frequently done in the course of a case manager's routine duties in the other areas.

Evaluation

The initial case management evaluation period is typically 30 days, during which it is desirable to gain as complete a picture as possible of the client's past and current functioning. The case manager must evaluate the client's status, needs, and goals in each of the following areas: mental health, physical health, financial status, housing, living skills, leisure, vocational and educational activities, and availability of a support system. Table 19-1 lists relevant topics to evaluate in each of these areas.

Because case management is designed to address the broad range of a client's needs for maintaining satisfactory and stable community living, the initial evaluation phase is critical in identifying existing resources, skills, and strengths, as well as service and support needs and skill deficits. Evaluation forms and procedures will vary with each facility. The overall goal of case man-

Table 19-1. Evaluation Data

Mental Health
- brief psychiatric history: frequency and approximate number of hospitalizations, suicide ideation or attempts, assaultiveness, documented stressors or prodromal symptoms, typical patterns of decompensation, past treatment or services and results
- current psychiatrist
- current medication regimen
- compliance with medication and appointments or need for assistance
- current or past alcohol or drug use, drug of choice, pattern of use

Physical Health
- medical history, childhood illnesses or serious injury, learning disability
- last physical examination and results, including tuberculosis test
- ongoing medical problems requiring follow-up care or treatment
- any indication of a current medical problem
- date of last dental examination and results
- date of last eye examination and results

Financial
- amount and the source of income
- need for assistance to receive the appropriate entitlements
- name of representative payee, if any
- bank accounts
- current debts and monthly expenses

Housing
- current place of residence and how long there
- condition of living space
- satisfaction with current housing
- housing history, including successes and failures; client's preferences
- frequency and/or pattern of housing changes

Living Skills
- money management
- transportation
- social and communication skills and habits
- self care and hygiene
- time management
- parenting
- housekeeping and home management
- community resource awareness
- understanding of mental illness and relapse prevention
- current leisure interests and activities, past sources of enjoyable activities
- highest level of education completed
- current educational goals
- current and past volunteer or paid work experience
- goals for work or vocational training

Support System
- family available in local area
- nature of involvement with family members, frequency and type of contact
- availability and relationship with friends
- use of organized supports in the community such as a religious group or Alcoholics Anonymous

agement is to help maintain the client's quality of life in the least restrictive community environment possible; therefore, evaluation data should assist the case manager in identifying factors that may have resulted in either the client's successes or failures in the past.

Information should be gathered from a review of past records, interview and observation of the client, and interview of significant others in the client's environment, such as residential care operators, conservators, family members, and former treatment providers. Strict adherence to confidentiality laws is essential when seeking information from persons or facilities outside of the case manager's service agency.

Occupational therapists as case managers have a variety of pertinent assessment tools to supplement the evaluation process, particularly in the area of living skills. The Kohlman Evaluation of Living Skills, Bay Area Functional Performance Evaluation, Scorable Self-Care Evaluation, Activity Configuration, and the Allen Cognitive Level Evaluation are examples of instruments that may be helpful in gathering data on functional ability (Asher, 1996). Because case management services are provided in vivo, there are many opportunities to observe the client, either formally or informally, functioning in his or her own environment. Interactions with retail clerks, roommates, and family or residential care staff; decoration and condition of living space; and the ability to perform housekeeping or money management tasks all provide direct feedback regarding social engagement and functional task performance. The Comprehensive Occupational Therapy Evaluation Scale is useful in organizing data gathered from these observations.

In most states, case management is a client-directed service, which means that interventions are made and service is provided primarily according to the client's stated needs and desires. Evaluation data provide information with which to help identify appropriate services, skills, and assistance for the client, but the case manager does not "do to" or "do for" him or her. Rather, the emphasis in case management is on "doing with" the client. Rather than being the problem solver, the case manager helps the client solve problems and seek solutions, thus helping him or her to gain skill as well as a sense of self-efficacy.

A component of the evaluation that underscores the client-directed nature of case management is the requirement for determining and documenting the client's level of satisfaction with various areas in his or her life. Client satisfaction is a subjective issue and must be considered in order to respect the client's individual choice and facilitate a successful outcome. It is important for the case manager to be aware of his or her own values and beliefs and not impose these on the client. For example, if the evaluation data indicates that a client has the living skills to function in his or her own apartment and has income sufficient for an available studio apartment or shared housing, it is nonetheless important to respect that client's wish should he or she choose to remain in a residential care facility (RCF). For many clients the RCF offers safety, socialization, and freedom from the stresses of homemaking responsibilities. Similarly, if a client is missing some teeth and Medicaid would pay for a bridge which would enhance his or her appearance and ability to eat a greater variety of foods, it is still essential to accept the client's decision to refuse that treatment. Reasons may range from delusions involving government implants in the bridgework to impatience with previously ill-fitting or repeatedly lost dental work. The case manager's role is to provide evaluation results to the client and to significant others, as appropriate. He or she should then discuss options and offer resources, which the client may choose to accept or decline. Exceptions to this are cases of the compromised health or safety of the client or others in his or her environment that may result in crisis intervention and emergency situations.

Concurrent with the initial evaluation phase is the period of engaging the client in case management services and beginning to establish trust. It is important that the client view case management as a help, and not a hindrance, and understand that it is a process through which to gain, and not lose, control over events and decisions in life. Depending on the client, this engagement process may be difficult and the development of trust may take months or never fully manifest. This is particularly true in the case of a client with a paranoid disorder. Similarly, an individual accustomed to the remote presence of a clinic-based therapist may not welcome a mobile, community-bound case manager. At its best, case management is a service that the client will welcome and he or she will be forthright in providing access to his or her life. Among the most challenging cases, however, is the client who appears paranoid, withdrawn, in denial of a mental illness, and resentful at what is perceived as an intrusion. Exercising clinical judgment is essential in these circumstances, and knowing when to terminate an interview or interaction can help establish trust. It is very important to respect the client's pace of interaction and gather as much information as possible without jeopardizing the relationship. A client is much more likely to allow access in the future to a case manager who is sensitive to his or her wishes and need for space and privacy from the beginning. Case management, by definition, is a long process, and evaluation is ongoing. Information not obtained within the first 30-day period may be accumulated later, as the relationship develops and as services are provided. Some guidelines for engaging the resistant client in case management services are:

- Make initial contacts brief.
- Meet with the client informally, for example, at his or her home or in a local coffee shop or park.
- Be clear about what case management is and how it will benefit the client.
- Be sure the client knows why and from whom you are obtaining information and that proper consent forms have been signed.
- Make it clear that you value the client's opinions and that he or she has input into the services received. Be sure to identify at least one issue of importance to the client.

- Respect the client's other activities and try to avoid scheduling visits that conflict with them.
- Allow the client to help determine future meeting times and places.

CASE ILLUSTRATION: ARTURO—INITIAL CONTACT

Arturo is a 23-year-old male of Filipino descent who was referred to case management by the psychiatric hospital treatment staff because of a history of medication noncompliance and recent repeated hospitalizations. He was first hospitalized at age 18, during what was diagnosed as a manic episode, while he was a community college student: Arturo had parked his car on the freeway one night when he ran out of gas, and walked several miles to the airport. He was taken to the hospital by the police, who had been called by airport security to respond to Arturo's bizarre behavior in the airport terminal (involving kung fu–like moves, during which he claimed to be fighter Bruce Lee). Arturo has been on medication since that time, and he has been seeing a psychiatrist at a county outpatient mental health clinic. His diagnosis is bipolar affective disorder, mixed, with psychotic features. He has not resumed community college attendance. He lives with his parents and three older siblings in a single-family home. His parents have been reluctant to permit the intervention of mental health professionals. They tend not to seek help until Arturo becomes unmanageable, at which time his behavior often attracts the attention of the police.

Arturo was very engaging during the initial interview at his home. He signed consent forms to enable the case manager to obtain information from his father and sister Meg, who have assumed the primary liaison roles with mental health professionals. (Arturo's mother does not speak English.) The case manager observes Arturo's interactions with family members, talks with Arturo about his interests, and briefly discusses the effect of his illness on himself and his family. Arturo demonstrates no insight into his problems. He is unable to relate what led to his most recent hospitalization, and states that people "overreact" to him. He cannot name his current medications or dosages. When asked about specific past incidents leading to police involvement and hospitalization, Arturo laughs and says, "But I was only acting!" He does not associate stopping his medications with requiring hospitalization.

Arturo's medications are stored in a cabinet in the kitchen, where several outdated bottles are mixed in with current prescriptions. With the case manager's assistance and instruction, Arturo sorts through the bottles and safely disposes of the old medications by flushing the pills down the toilet. The case manager provides a pill organizer and helps Arturo distribute his medication into the individual compartments by daily dosages for a full week. This will lessen Arturo's confusion about the correct dosages and enable the case manager to monitor compliance by counting what remains of the current supply. In Arturo's presence, Meg provides the case manager with additional infor-

mation about her brother's current and past functioning, including his occasional uncontrolled spending sprees. (Arturo's father is currently trying to clear up bills for expensive gold jewelry and a health club membership purchased by his son.) Arturo does not know his monthly income and cannot name any expenses he has other than buying an occasional soda from the local market. Arturo states that his father gives him small amounts of money "whenever I ask for it." Most of the excessive spending has been the result of Arturo obtaining instant credit for purchases.

Service Plan Development

The service plan is the case management equivalent of the treatment plan as used in traditional inpatient or outpatient settings. It identifies the client's goals and objectives for a specified time period, typically a six-month time period, and it must be updated at least that often, or as necessary, as goals are achieved or are deemed inappropriate or unrealistic at any point during that period.

The format of the service plan varies, but generally it identifies the client's goals and the case management objectives and service activities for achieving each one. Because services are individualized, the number of goals appearing on the plan at any one time will vary. It is important to be realistic and set no more goals than can be accomplished within a given time period. It is preferable to state the client's goals in his or her own words. Objectives must be measurable, have projected time frames, and be consistent with evaluation results and client goals. They should be realistic and broken down as necessary into tasks deemed achievable for the particular client.

Client service needs determined via the evaluation process may fall into two distinct categories: needs as a result of a skill deficit and those resulting from a resource deficit. For example, a client whose housing is jeopardized due to interpersonal conflicts may have limited available options for housing or may need to learn skills in communication and conflict resolution. Often a combination of both skill and resource deficits impedes a client's functioning, and it is the case manager's responsibility to help set goals and objectives to address the deficits.

In case management there is a great emphasis placed on the client's involvement in the goal-setting process. It is preferable, and often required, to have the client's signature on the completed plan to indicate acknowledgment of, and agreement with, the stated goals. This process is designed to insure that the services are client directed and to promote individualized service planning. In this way an individual may experience a greater sense of responsibility for him- or herself, and participate actively in "doing" rather than "being done to."

In addition to involving the client in the planning process, it is advisable to identify appropriate family members or significant others to assist or support in achieving particular goals. Assigning appropriate responsibilities and facilitating healthy relationships with clearly defined boundaries and tasks promotes the development of an extended support system in the community. The development and maintenance of a comprehensive social support system in the community is often difficult for people with mental illness, and case managers may provide valuable assistance with support network expansion (Biegel, Tracy, & Corvo, 1994; Walsh, 1994). Adherence to confidentiality issues is crucial when actively enlisting others in the care of the client. The client must approve of the person's assistance or support, and the proper release forms must be signed and placed in the client's records. Table 19-2 contains examples of case management goals and objectives, accompanying service activities, and the involvement needed from significant others.

CASE ILLUSTRATION: ARTURO—SERVICE PLAN

Having gathered sufficient data from various sources to complete an initial evaluation, the case manager scheduled a meeting with Arturo to discuss his goals for the next six months. Arturo's sister Meg was present for the planning meeting, which was held at their home. Arturo expressed a desire to resume his education in computer-assisted design at the local community college. The case manager additionally introduced the issues of medication noncompliance, and poor money management. Arturo was agreeable to having assistance with medication compliance but was offended by the case manager's characteriza-

Table 19-2. Sample Service Plan Components

Client's Goal	Measurable Objective	Service Activities	Significant Others' Assistance
"I want to live in my own apartment."	Lee will participate in living skills evaluation and training twice weekly for six months; he will also perform at least one task per week at home.	The case manager will provide living skills evaluation and training and monitor home task performance.	Lee's mother will remind him of training appointments, monitor home task performance, and provide feedback to the case manager.
"I need something to do with my time."	Juanita will volunteer at the Senior Center 10 hours per week for six months	The case manager will link Juanita with the senior center and monitor attendance weekly via contact with the client and/or the volunteer coordinator.	The volunteer coordinator will train Juanita, meet with her weekly to provide feedback, and contact the case manager as needed.

tion of his spending problem. He was initially unwilling to include the second item in the service plan but stated he was open to learning more about his income and expenses since his father currently handled all his money. The goal was written to address his lack of knowledge rather than his lack of control, a focus of which Arturo approved. Arturo also stated that he wanted to work on getting his own apartment. Although this was a reasonable and age-appropriate goal to the case manager, Meg explained that this is unacceptable in the Filipino culture, where "you stay with the family until you get married." For this reason, and because of the case manager's desire to gain the family's trust and cooperation, this goal was deferred. The case manager explained to Arturo that this might be a consideration for the future, after the current objectives had been achieved .

A service plan was developed, with Arturo and Meg's input and concurrence, to address the following objectives: community college attendance, medication compliance, and money management training.

Placement Services

Case management placement assistance may be defined as any support provided to the client in locating, obtaining, and maintaining a satisfactory living environment. This may include preplacement visits, negotiation of contracts and agreements, actual placement, and follow-up visits and monitoring.

Obtaining and maintaining stable, satisfactory community housing is a common goal for persons with serious mental illness. Unfortunately, unstable housing is often a chronic problem and is repeatedly addressed on service plans. Several factors that contribute to the disruption of housing are rehospitalization and the resultant loss of housing, a client's desire to move, eviction, lack of affordable housing alternatives in the community, a relapse that necessitates a move to a higher level of care, or progress that indicates a move to a lower level of care.

If a client is hospitalized for a brief, acute stay, housing usually is not disrupted, but long-term hospitalization (greater than 30 days) usually results in a loss of housing unless the client has the financial resources to pay for both rent and a hospital stay. Client entitlements are not adequate to provide for this, so most people are unable to retain housing during a serious relapse.

Clients obviously make decisions to move for many of the same reasons that persons without a mental illness decide to move. However, some of the reasons are related to difficulties resulting from their mental illness, such as unmanageable conflict with roommates, landlords, board and care staff, or neighbors; refusal or inability to accept and abide by established rules; and discomfort in the environment due to paranoia. A case manager may be able to intervene in all these situations and prevent the client's need to relocate.

A thorough knowledge and understanding of the available resources, including what a specific environment offers to the client and what it demands in return, is essential in order to assist with housing decisions and make appropriate placement referrals. Housing resources are usually identified by the amount and type of structure and support provided. Table 19-3 lists commonly available community housing options and gives a brief description of each. The table ranks resources from most to least restrictive, although there may be slight individual variations among programs in different geographic areas. Each program is a voluntary community placement and requires the client's concurrence with the decision, except in the case of placement decisions made by a **conservator**, who frequently has the authority to mandate placement and override the wishes of the client and the mental health treatment provider (although in some locales this authority is given to the treatment provider). Ideally, all individuals work together to reach agreement regarding placement decisions.

Placement issues may arise in several different ways, ranging from routine hospital discharge planning and placement to unexpected evictions. Routine or anticipated placements often follow a predictable pattern of assisting the client with identifying and exploring potential resources and then narrowing the choices to determine the best available. Whether dealing with the result of a hospital discharge back into the community or a client's voluntary decision to move from one community placement to another, the case manager usually follows these eight basic steps to secure alternative housing:

1. Discuss with the client which type of housing (of those types identified in Table 19-3) is desired or appropriate. Historical and current evalua-

Table 19-3. Common Community Housing Options

Type of Facility	Meals Provided	Medication Administered	On-Site Programming	On-Site Staff
Intermediate Care Facility	yes	yes	yes	yes
Residential Treatment Program	yes, with client participation	yes	yes	yes
Residential Care Facility	yes	yes	varies	yes
Boarding House	yes	no	no	manager
Homeless Shelter	varies	varies	varies	yes
Independent Living	no°	no°	no	no
Single-Room Occupancy (SRO) Hotel	no°°	no°	no	manager

°May be monitored by case manager via routine home visits.
°°May be set up by case manager or representative payee via voucher or charge account system at a local restaurant.

tion data, in conjunction with client preference, will guide this decision. Hopefully there will be concurrence on this issue and the client will be amenable to the case manager's suggestions based on the former's level of functioning. If the client is not amenable, discussion will need to focus on reaching agreement by providing the client with facts to support the case manager's recommendation.

2. Obtain or develop a list of local housing resources of that particular type. Depending on the type selected and the particular community, there may be several or very few from which to choose.

3. Assist the client with decision-making regarding characteristics of places on that list. Desired geographic area, physical environment and surroundings, coed versus single-sex, house rules and restrictions, cultural or ethnic background of owners or staff, cost, and current vacancy all must be considered. A case manager's familiarity with resources and sensitivity to client's needs and preferences are invaluable in this phase. Some clients may want to reside with people of a common cultural background, while others may want to avoid a particular race or culture due to personal biases or delusional beliefs. Alternately, a client may place great emphasis on food and the quality of the meals provided, and a case manager's awareness of a facility's reputation in that regard is helpful. Some clients may want to be near family members, which may rule out certain geographic areas. Others may want to live close to parks, shopping areas, day treatment or vocational programs, or specific bus lines.

4. Determine which of the available resources fits the criteria that are important to the client.

5. Select two or three places to visit and schedule interviews.

6. Assist the client with the interview if needed or desired and with evaluating the pros and cons of each facility in order to promote decision making skills. Clients have varying abilities and methods of approaching decisions. Some are very impulsive and will accept the first placement opportunity presented; others will be ambivalent about all options and have difficulty settling upon any placement decision. The amount and type of assistance the case manager provides will vary depending on the client's needs and skills. Some clients are quite familiar with community resources and procedures for obtaining housing, while others will need guidance and support through each step of the process. As a way to encourage independence, the case manager may provide a client with a selected list of residential care facilities and assign him or her the task of scheduling two interviews. Training in how to use the classified ads to find an apartment and assistance in identifying appropriate questions to ask by telephone and during the interview are other ways of building skills and promoting autonomy. It is often helpful to role-play the interview and application process, either in a group setting or on a one-to-one basis.

7. Once a decision has been reached, the case manager or client must notify the facility landlord or manager and insure that all follow-up requirements of the application process are completed.
8. Assist the client with making the move or securing the resources necessary to move personal possessions into the new residence.

Engaging in routine follow-up and monitoring of a new placement allows the case manager to be proactive, dealing with issues as they arise in order to avoid potential problems. The frequency and type of monitoring is highly individualized. A client with a long history of placement failures who is newly discharged to a residential care facility after a lengthy period of hospitalization may benefit from daily contact initially. This contact may be either face-to-face or by telephone and may include an additional weekly check-in with facility staff. Clients who have been stable in the community for some time may require weekly or monthly monitoring with the frequency to be increased or decreased as changing situations warrant.

If two or more of the case manager's clients share housing, particularly in a supported independent living situation, house meetings are an effective and efficient way of monitoring placement. A house meeting gives the case manager an opportunity to address any current issues among the roommates as well as to provide living skills training, assess the living environment, and facilitate social gatherings. It is also an opportunity to organize and perform major group chores such as yard work or spring cleaning. Common issues that arise in shared housing situations are interpersonal conflicts, inequitable sharing of household chores, and difficulties in dealing with roommates' psychiatric symptoms. In many supported independent living situations, house meetings are led by facility staff and the case manager then acts as a liaison to the staff and to the individual client in addressing these issues.

Sudden evictions and other housing emergencies can be stressful for the client, and in these instances, a knowledge of housing regulations and tenants' rights is essential. State and federal housing regulations protect persons from sudden eviction without cause. For example, in California there must be a minimum of 3 days' notice provided with just cause, which must include an option for correction of the violation, which would then enable the tenant to remain. A 30-day notice is required for an eviction without cause. State and federal laws also protect an individual from discrimination based on mental illness or source of income. However, depending on the severity of the threat and the precipitating factors, an eviction due to verbal or physical assaultiveness by the client may necessitate immediate removal from the environment and referral to intermediate care or acute hospitalization.

The key to successful placement is finding a good match between client and housing. Factors that enhance the likelihood of successful client placement and housing stability include the following:

1. familiarity with the client's placement history and coping skills
2. thorough knowledge of community housing resources

3. a trusting relationship with the client and respect for client choice
4. knowledge of housing laws pertaining to people with disability
5. skills in crisis intervention, conflict resolution, negotiation, and advocacy
6. routine monitoring of placement

CASE ILLUSTRATION: JANICE—PLACEMENT

Janice is a 34-year-old female, diagnosed with schizophrenia, paranoid type, currently staying at an intermediate care facility (ICF) after a two-week acute hospitalization. Prior to her hospitalization, Janice had been living with a roommate in a two-bedroom, supported, independent living situation. Her case manager had been addressing medication compliance and living skills training through weekly home visits. Janice had recently been refusing her medication, with a resulting deterioration in self-care skills and increasing psychotic symptoms. Janice was hospitalized one afternoon after the police were called to her apartment complex. She had been at home watching a soap opera when she became convinced that she was involved in the television events and ran outside, agitated and crying that she had just committed a murder on a carousel. Neighbors called the police, who took Janice to emergency psychiatric services, where she was subsequently hospitalized.

A conference was held to coordinate plans prior to Janice's discharge from the ICF. Janice became angry when told by her case manager that she could not return to her apartment and blamed the problems she encountered on her former roommate. She did not recall her behavior or the events prior to her acute hospitalization and demonstrated no insight into her difficulties in maintaining independent living despite receiving ongoing support and assistance from the case manager. Janice insisted on getting her own apartment, despite the ICF staff and case manager's recommendation of a residential care facility placement. Janice does not have a conservator.

With further discussion among Janice, her case manager, and the ICF treatment staff, a compromise was reached whereby Janice agreed to enter a three-month residential treatment program to focus on independent living skills, with the ultimate goal of obtaining her own apartment upon successful completion of the program.

Linkage and Consultation

Linkage and consultation in case management may be defined as the identification and pursuit of community resources necessary and appropriate to implement the service plan. This includes, but is not limited to, interagency and intraagency consultation and referral, and communication with the client's family and significant others. The purpose of linkage and consultation activities (as shown in Figure 19-1) is to coordinate and monitor service delivery to insure the client's access and to facilitate continuity of care. These activi-

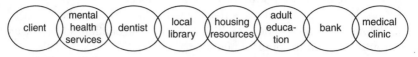

Figure 19-1.   Linkage with Community Resources

ties help prevent the client from "falling through the cracks," which was characteristic of traditional community mental health services.

The case manager links a client or consults with another resource whenever information or a service is needed outside what the former has or can directly provide. A case manager also provides linkage whenever there is information to relay that may facilitate service delivery or enhance continuity of care for the client. Linkage or consultation may be done in the client's presence or on behalf of the client.

As a member of a multidisciplinary team, a case manager may perform intraagency linkage by scheduling an appointment for the client with the team psychiatrist (for medication problems) or the psychotherapist (for counseling). A client may be referred to a weekly substance abuse group facilitated by another team member. Likewise, the case manager may consult with other team members to gain or provide information regarding any of these issues if direct client linkage is not deemed necessary.

Interagency linkage and consultation and communication outside of the case management agency require a consideration of confidentiality laws if the client is identified by name as a recipient of mental health services. Often, however, information can be obtained or referrals can be made without such identification. For example, making a dentist appointment for a client or inquiring about volunteer opportunities available at a local museum does not require that the client be identified as mentally ill. Referral to a program specifically targeted for persons with mental illness will identify the client as mentally ill, so in this case the case manager must have the client sign the appropriate consent forms before the referral is made. A case manager may also make direct referrals to the client for independent follow-up, such as a recommendation to attend a local Alcoholics Anonymous meeting.

Making appropriate and timely referral depends on accurate and ongoing assessment and planning with the client as well as a clear understanding of the services provided by a particular agency. A client who states that he or she wants a job may or may not have realistic ideas about what he or she is able to do. Prevocational evaluation and training by the case manager may help the client identify areas of strength and weakness, gain needed skills, and identify interests in preparation for employment. Based on those results, a decision may be made to seek volunteer work, a sheltered workshop, a vocational training program, or competitive employment.

Knowing the purpose and the parameters of an agency is essential in determining its suitability for a client's needs. For example, a vocational rehabilitation program designed for a client's placement in competitive community employment would not be a suitable referral for a client whose goal is to work in a sheltered workshop. Community resources need not be targeted specifically for the mentally ill in order to be useful and appropriate for a client's needs. When using resources available to the general population, a client may or may not choose to disclose his or her diagnosis of mental illness. The case manager may assist with this decision, discussing and role-playing the range of potential consequences of this disclosure and how to deal with them. Individuals or agencies unfamiliar with mental illness or the mental health system may require or request specific information. This is usually a good opportunity to advocate and enhance awareness of the needs and potential contributions of persons with mental illness in the community. Table 19-4 lists some possible community resources and suggested indications for referral or consultation with them.

Once a resource has been identified as potentially appropriate, a client will need varying degrees of assistance to be linked with that resource. It is important to allow the client as much freedom and autonomy as possible, providing support as needed and withdrawing it as tolerated to promote client empowerment and ensure a successful referral. For some clients, merely providing the agency name and phone number or address will be sufficient for them to follow through and make the contact successfully. Other clients may require that the referral be made on their behalf and that they then be accompanied and assisted with an application and intake process or a doctor's visit or lab test. For example, a client with a strong fear of having blood drawn may benefit from the comforting presence of a trusted case manager. A client making an initial visit to a doctor's office may have difficulty filling out the nec-

Table 19-4. Community Resources for Linkage and Consultation

Resource	Available Services
Churches, religious organizations	Support, volunteer work opportunities
Visiting Nurses Association, American Diabetes Association, Planned Parenthood, services for the deaf or blind, psychologists	Medical support, consultation, education, and testing; peer support; volunteer work opportunities
Adult education, community college, YMCA	Low-cost educational opportunities
Alcoholics Anonymous, cultural centers, gay community centers	Peer support and education
Food bank, beauty college	Low-cost products and services
Senior center, nursing home	Volunteer opportunities
State department of rehabilitation	Vocational evaluation and training
County housing authority, Housing for Independent People	Low-cost housing opportunities

essary intake forms without assistance due to reading problems or an inability to accurately recall medical history. Some programs or facilities may want to limit a case manager's involvement, particularly if it is a mental health program designed for client independence. The usual steps in making a referral to link a client with services are shown in Figure 19-2.

Once a referral has been made, it is important to facilitate continuity of care via regular contact with the appropriate resource person or agency. As with monitoring after-placement, the frequency and type of consultation and communication will depend on the client and the resource to which referral has been made. Some agencies will want close communication to share information; others will want to be more autonomous. For example, a probation officer may want weekly telephone or written contact to verify a client's court-mandated compliance with mental health treatment, but it would probably not be advisable to make weekly contact with a client's supervisor in competitive employment unless a previous agreement had been made, among the supervisor, client, and case manager, to do so. For a client placed in an inpatient program, important information can be mutually shared about medication history, compliance with the program, family issues, and discharge plans.

It is helpful to develop a resource book, keeping notes or a log of particularly helpful or knowledgeable resources in the community. Developing a positive working relationship with other agencies helps ensure open lines of communication regarding your client, provides good-role modeling for the client, and enhances the probability of success of future referrals. The case manager will encounter particularly sensitive dentists, doctors, and agencies and want to recommend them. Likewise, insensitive or otherwise inappropriate resources may be encountered, to which the case manager will want to avoid further referrals. It is important to get the client's feedback regarding the referral experience, such as how he or she was treated. The client and case manager may identify stigma, unresponsiveness, poor communication, and resultant poor continuity of care. Accompanying the client whenever necessary or appropriate helps the case manager obtain direct experience with the program staff. Some staff will be more openly communicative with the case manager than others, and more willing to assist the client. Encountering undesirable situations provides an opportunity for the case manager to intervene to attempt to rectify a situation, offer in-service education, advocate for the client as needed to obtain service, or seek another resource if these efforts are not effective.

CASE ILLUSTRATION: ROBERT—LINKAGE

Robert is a 34-year-old male with a diagnosis of schizophrenia, undifferentiated type, who lives in a residential care facility. Robert had been complaining of vomiting after meals but described no other symptoms. He was not disturbed about his condition but rather accepted it as a consequence, he explained, of being "still connected to my mother's womb." The case manager

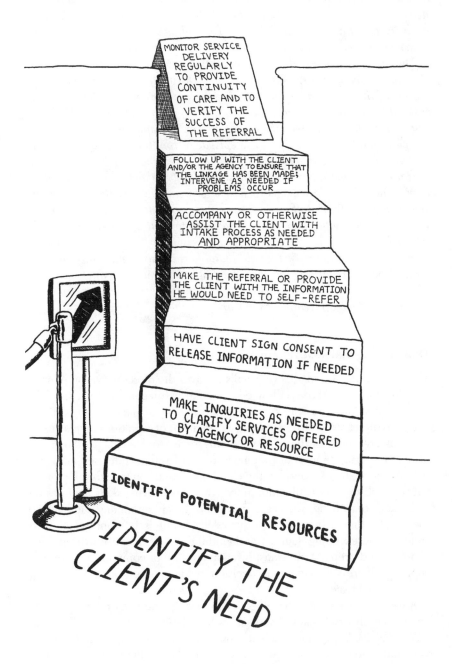

Figure 19-2. Steps in Making a Referral

consulted with staff at the RCF, who confirmed that Robert occasionally vomited after meals and that no other signs of illness are present. Despite his nonchalance about his symptoms, Robert was willing to see a doctor at his case manager's recommendation.

The case manager scheduled an appointment with a family practice physician and accompanied Robert to the clinic. During the interview and examination in the physician's office, Robert became annoyed as he agitatedly insisted to the physician that "there's a piece of my mother's womb in there." The case manager informed the doctor of Robert's rapid eating habits, ongoing pattern of experiencing a single episode of vomiting shortly after meals, and previous report to her that "it feels like something's stuck in there." The doctor ordered an upper gastrointestinal (GI) series and scheduled a return appointment. The case manager reviewed the preexamination instructions with Robert and the RCF staff and left a written copy with them. She accompanied Robert to the hospital x-ray department to ensure compliance with the test and then accompanied him back to the clinic for the follow-up appointment. The doctor diagnosed a mild hiatal hernia, prescribed Tagamet, and advised Robert regarding his pace of eating and positioning after mealtime. The case manager discussed the results with the RCF staff and monitored adherence to follow-up treatment to insure a resolution of the problem.

Daily Living Skills Development

The development of daily living skills involves the direct provision of assistance or training in those skills needed for successful community living. This is the occupational therapist's area of expertise. As case manager, the OT provides this direct service to clients and, as a member of a multidisciplinary team, serves as a resource for the provision of this service to other clients. The range of skills requiring support or training is as broad as that addressed in the initial evaluation, that is, any skill the client needs and wants to develop or enhance to aid in successful community living. Daily living skills includes the wide range of activities such as money management, grooming and hygiene, social skills, time management, leisure skills, health, safety, and relapse prevention, housekeeping, laundry and clothing management, nutrition, meal planning and preparation, transportation and use of community resources, coping and stress management, decision making and problem solving, and prevocational issues.

A case management service agency following strictly a brokerage model (acting merely as a broker of services rather than a direct provider) may not be as effective in promoting client growth and skill development as full-service, multidisciplinary teams, which provide brokerage in conjunction with direct service. Daily living skills training can be very effective at the case management level. Persons with serious mental illness often demonstrate concrete thought processes and extreme passivity, and they may have difficulty generalizing learning and transferring skills learned in one setting to another living environment (Morrison & Bellack, 1984). Recidivism from day treatment or other traditional outpatient settings is a common problem. Skills may not be adequately maintained over time, as periods of unstable functioning, possibly accompanied by acute hospitalization and a move to a higher level of care, often result in a deterioration in skill functioning. In addition, skills training in the client's own environment facilitates integration into the neighborhood. The case manager who works with the client over time in his or her own environment is ideally suited to train, reinforce, or support existing skills as applied to the current environment and to help monitor and maintain skill performance.

Occupational therapy principles and techniques of living skills training and assistance in the community do not differ from those used in a clinic or inpatient setting. The use of task analysis and graded activities enables the client to experience success at each level, and gradually decreasing the support and assistance empowers the client as he or she gains independence in a particular skill area. Skills training may be done on a one-to-one or group basis. Some activities are more conducive to groups, such as meal planning and preparation or nutrition; others are more effective with individual instruction and support, such as grocery shopping, money management, and laundry. Some tasks may initially be taught and discussed in a group setting and then practiced and monitored on an individual basis. It is often effective to encourage peer support and have more experienced clients provide support and assistance to those learning a new skill. This is a way of empowering and reinforcing higher-functioning clients while encouraging socialization and peer support-building.

Living skills training in the community does differ in some respects: the length of time available to work with a client is greater than in most institutional settings, there is more opportunity to work with clients on an individual basis, and the amount of control over the environment is less. For example, a case manager may be unprepared for a rude or impatient bank teller, the angry or fearful reactions of other shoppers to a client's delusional speech, or the client's slowness in writing out a check at the register. A cooking activity held in a well-stocked, readily accessible, and fully equipped OT clinic kitchen is much more predictable than one planned in a client's apartment, as a client living on a limited budget may consider items such as measuring spoons or a loaf pan to be an unnecessary extravagance. These situations offer the opportunity for creative adaptation and problem solving and give the therapist a glimpse of the obstacles encountered and values held by the client. It is important to make living skills training both culturally and economically relevant.

Daily living skills training and assistance in case management may range from initial task instruction to periodic monitoring of successful task performance. For example, the occupational therapist may begin living skills training by teaching a client to perform various housecleaning tasks. When the client is able to perform the tasks independently, case management support may then advance to helping the client develop a household chore checklist and monitoring adherence to that list. Tasks begun on a training level ideally will progress to maintenance and monitoring levels as competence increases and the client becomes empowered to assume more responsibility. In one-to-one training situations it is often effective to do a task with the client. This lessens the stress on the client of being watched while performing a new task and helps promote a relationship of trust and mutual problem solving. The photograph in Figure 19-3 shows a client doing a daily activity with a case manager.

CASE ILLUSTRATION: JIM—LIVING SKILL DEVELOPMENT

Jim is a 32-year-old male who has been stable in a residential care facility (RCF) in the community for almost one year. He was diagnosed with a schizophrenic disorder, paranoid type. His case manager has provided home visits to monitor placement and has worked with Jim to try to engage him in structured daily activity. Recently, Jim has expressed to his case manager a desire to live in his own apartment, complaining that the other residents in the home "are always asking me for money and cigarettes because they know I always have some."

Jim has many strengths that suggest he would be a good candidate for independent living, including good money management skills, family support, a one-year history of medication compliance, ability to keep his living space

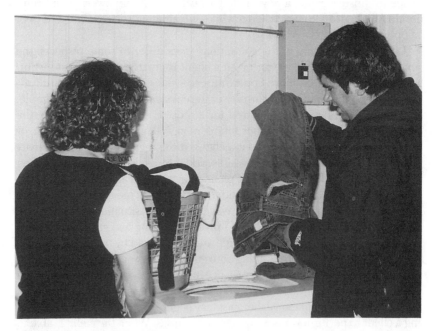

Figure 19-3. Living Skills Training in a Client's Home

clean and neat, an established routine for doing his own laundry, experience with the local bus system, and knowledge of community resources. However, interview, task observation, and administration of the Kohlman Evaluation of Living Skills test enables the case manager to identify several skill deficits: lack of skill in meal planning, shopping, and food preparation tasks; lack of skill in kitchen- and bathroom-cleaning tasks; lack of work or leisure activity involvement; difficulty setting limits; and limited social contact.

The case manager began Jim's living skills training with housecleaning, meal planning, nutrition, food storage, kitchen safety, and price comparison activities at the RCF and at a local supermarket. The RCF staff allowed Jim to help with some of the simple food preparation and cleaning tasks. The case manager arranged a "pot luck" lunch at the home of two other clients, and Jim participated in group meal planning, shopping, food preparation, and cleaning for that event.

Living skills training continued after Jim moved into a studio apartment. The case manager facilitated the transition by helping Jim explore local resources, such as the closest bank and supermarket, and by assisting him with using the new laundry facilities at the apartment complex. She also accompanied him on grocery shopping trips until he was able to complete the task on his own. Initially, home visits were made twice weekly to monitor and reinforce successful performance of housecleaning, meal planning, and preparation tasks.

Emergency Intervention

Emergency intervention may be defined as a quick, unplanned response at the onset of a crisis situation to solve a problem or facilitate the client's access to other needed services. The goal is to maintain, to the greatest possible extent, the client's status as a functioning community member. Often a crisis is determined by the severity of the client's response to an incident or situation. What is perceived as a threat or is stressful for one client may not be a stressor for another. Moreover, the crisis may be brought to the attention of the case manager by a telephone call from the client or a significant other person, or it may be discovered in the course of a routine case management appointment or home visit.

Clinical judgment guides the case manager's response to a crisis. An emergency related to the client's physical health and safety may require a trip to the hospital emergency room or doctor's office or the application of simple emergency first aid. A housing crisis may involve promoting conflict resolution among roommates, arranging a temporary respite placement, or obtaining the services of a repair person to see that emergency household maintenance is performed. A crisis in which the client shows signs of psychiatric relapse may be resolved by an unscheduled visit with the psychiatrist for medication adjustment along with close monitoring until the client restabilizes, or it may require an emergency hospitalization.

The case manager who works with a client over an extended period of time will become aware of stressors specific to that client and often be able to recognize **prodromal symptoms**. There are clients for whom any change in residence is stressful and therefore must be monitored carefully and provided with extra support during those transition periods. Some clients are vulnerable to environmental stressors such as storms, fires, and earthquakes. Some will react strongly to changes in a structured daily routine, money problems, changes in support staff, arguments with significant others in their lives, or a serious illness of their own, a family member, or their residential care operator. Drug or alcohol abuse, noncompliance with the prescribed medication regimen, or any change in the medication prescription may precipitate relapse. Prodromal symptoms include any alteration in the client's typical behavior, such as the rate, volume, or content of speech; style of dress; or sleep or activity pattern.

Clients have different ways of responding to a case manager's intervention during a period of relapse, which will depend on the relapse stage and on client-specific traits and patterns characteristic of relapse. Some individuals will welcome the support and comfort of a familiar and trusted person in a stressful and unstable period, but others will resent the intrusion, be suspicious of motives and intentions, and be resistant to any intervention, particularly if they suspect it will lead to hospitalization. It is always advantageous to recognize prodromal symptoms and intervene before a full-blown relapse occurs and hospitalization is required, which underscores the value of routine monitoring via regularly scheduled case management contacts.

As in any inpatient setting, it is important for the case manager to be aware of safety issues in the community. The case manager who feels that his or her safety or the safety of the client is jeopardized at any time during a community visit should leave the environment immediately to obtain adequate help. Because of the sensitivity and unpredictability of relapse situations, it is advisable to take another staff member or insure that others are around when making a contact in which you suspect the client may be unstable. In a particularly volatile situation, it may be appropriate or necessary to have the police make an initial check or meet the case manager at the client's home. Most police departments have a "welfare check" policy through which they will go to a home if there is concern regarding the well-being of a resident, and they will always respond to a report of potential danger in the community. Because of the long relationship a case manager will usually have established with a client, including prior experience with his or her specific relapse patterns, should the police need to be involved, the case manager should be available to advise them how best to approach and communicate with the client.

Agency policies and state regulations for hospitalizing a client against his or her will vary. Some clients will cooperate with the process and demonstrate insight, awareness of their need, and a willingness to be admitted, but others may need to be restrained for their own safety and must be transported via police car or ambulance.

CASE ILLUSTRATION: BETH— EMERGENCY INTERVENTION

Beth is a 35-year-old female, diagnosed with schizoaffective disorder, who lives with her boyfriend, Mark, and their two-year-old son, Jason. Beth's case manager received a telephone call one morning from Mark, who told her that Beth was "up all night changing clothes, and now she's mad at me and talking weird." When questioned, he reported that Beth has not eaten since the previous morning and that he had not seen her take her medication since that time. Beth's angry verbalizations were audible in the background. She refused to come to the telephone.

The case manager, who was familiar with Beth's pattern of rapid relapse, enlisted the assistance of another team member for a home visit involving a probable hospitalization. (Beth had never been assaultive, but an extra staff person is nonetheless helpful for support in a crisis situation.) At the home, the case manager found Beth dressed bizarrely, with heavier makeup than usual and black nail polish carelessly applied. She was agitated and pacing; her speech was rapid, pressured, and tangential and was coupled with hostile glares and accusations. She called Mark "Hitler" and shouted at the case manager, "You're all made of wax and you're going to die in the nuclear meltdown." She made no appropriate responses to her case manager's attempts to talk with her.

The case manager told Beth that she had to go to the hospital and reminded her that it was hard for her to take care of Jason when she was feeling like this. Beth made no verbal acknowledgment of the case manager's statements and rather continued her pacing, stopping occasionally to stare at the two staff members and make a bizarre accusation. While the case manager talked with Beth, her team member wrote a hold order for an involuntary 72-hour commitment to psychiatric emergency services, citing Beth as gravely disabled due to acute psychotic symptoms and her recent lack of sleep and food intake. Mark drove Beth to the hospital, accompanied by the case manager. Beth continued her tirade but offered no resistance. The other team member met them at the hospital, where the written hold order was given to the hospital staff and Beth was admitted for evaluation.

THE CLIENT–CASE MANAGER RELATIONSHIP

There has been considerable research and discussion regarding case management service provision, including its definition, its methods, and its effects. One aspect of this research is the case management relationship itself, as distinct from the service. This relationship may be a strong factor in the success

602 PART V—SPECIALIZED ROLES FOR OT IN MENTAL HEALTH

or failure of any particular intervention; it has been described as being as strong an effector of change as the intervention itself (Harris & Bergman, 1987).

In 1978, the Task Panel on Deinstitutionalization, Rehabilitation and Long-term Care of the President's Commission on Mental Health described the case manager as someone "remaining in extended contact with the individual and acting as friend and advocate if required and desired by him or her" (Platman et al., 1982, p. 308). Case managers have been described as "travel guides" (Kanter, 1989, p. 362) and "life coaches" (Robinson & Toff-Bergman, 1989, p. 42). In a study of case management support, Baker and Weiss (1984) found that case managers viewed their clients as "individuals to work with rather than individuals to treat" (p. 926). Clients participating in that study described their case managers as persons who provide advice and support similar to that of an older brother or sister. While their therapists and psychiatrists seemed distant, they felt that their case managers established a "peer-like friendliness" (p. 926). The relationship was described by the clients as comfortable, nonthreatening, and respectful. They felt they were taken seriously, were worthy of attention, and were less vulnerable because there was "someone to rely on when things get rocky" (p. 927).

A client-case manager relationship has challenges and benefits that may differ from those of a treatment relationship established in a hospital or traditional outpatient program. In these settings an individual is treated for a time-limited period in a specific environment with a focus on more narrowly defined objectives, while in case management, boundaries and roles are less clearly defined and contained as a case manager works with a client over time and across a spectrum of environments and experiences and through periods of crisis and stability.

There may be challenges in setting limits with a client who considers the case manager a friend and with family members who expect or want more from the case manager than is realistically possible. There are challenges in being consistent and continually modeling behavior that may encourage positive growth in the client. There are challenges in providing the needed assistance without creating excessive dependency and to intervening for the safety and well-being of a client at times when he or she may view the case manager's action as intrusive and controlling. There may be challenges to the case manager in attending to personal needs when the needs of the clients seem vaster and far more serious in comparison. Challenges such as these can be managed with time, experience, and awareness, as well as through open communication and problem solving with team members, peers, and supervisors. Lamb (1979, 1986) addressed many of these issues, and Carl Rogers's characteristics of a helping relationship are beneficial in establishing professional guidelines for authenticity, consistency, and facilitation of positive client growth (Rogers, 1989).

The challenges of being a case manager for persons with serious mental illness are balanced with the benefits. A case manager may derive a sense of professional pride in being able to establish and maintain a trusting relationship with individuals who have been slow to trust; and there is gratification in discovering that along with the dark side of mental illness, the sufferer usually has an enjoyable, bright side as well. There is a shared journey of discovery and joy as a determined case manager and client work together to help the client move into a first apartment, accomplish a new and difficult task, take a risk, or negotiate a bureaucratic system to get needs met. There will be a growing sense of competence as the case manager gets to know the clients and becomes able to recognize or even anticipate problems and to intervene successfully to prevent hospitalization. Case management services, when provided sensitively and effectively, can be the lifeline that helps a client remain a part of the larger community. By facilitating the gradual development of more effective habits of living and dealing with chronic illness, the case manager provides an opportunity for clients to finally feel at home in the community after years of rotating through the "revolving door."

Summary

Case management is a community treatment method designed to provide continuity of care for persons with serious and persistent mental illness. Its goals are to reduce hospitalization, maintain the client in the community in a minimally restrictive setting, and help maintain the client's quality of life. Unlike traditional mental health treatment, case management services are provided in vivo and are of unlimited duration.

Case management service components typically include evaluation, planning, placement, linkage and consultation, daily living skills assistance, and emergency intervention. Researchers who have studied the client–case manager relationship have described the unique qualities that make it a powerful effector of change, and which are distinct from the actual services provided. Working as case manager, with a professional focus on enhancing functional daily living skills and facilitating adaptation to disability, the occupational therapist plays a key role in achieving the goals of case management. With this support and assistance, individuals with serious and persistent mental illness can live far more satisfactory and meaningful lives in the community than were available in the institutions from which many of them came.

Review Questions

1. The following is a list of community mental health service activities. Indicate which are case management functions and explain your reasons.
   a. counselling a client regarding grief issues
   b. referring a client to Planned Parenthood for birth control education
   c. helping a client find a job
   d. evaluating a client's social skills
2. What are the three main goals of case management?

3. Discuss ways of engaging a treatment-resistant client in case management services.
4. What is meant by the phrase, *client-directed services*?
5. Discuss reasons why living skills training for people with serious mental illness may be particularly effective at the case management level. How does training in the community differ from training in the institution?
6. Discuss safety precautions that may be taken when dealing with a crisis situation in the community.
7. In the case illustration about Beth, what are some of her prodromal symptoms?

Learning Activities

1. Visit a residential care facility in your area. Describe the environment, including physical surroundings, staffing patterns, and activities provided onsite. Interview the operator regarding licensing requirements and the difficulties and the rewards of operating the facility. Talk with residents about their experiences in residential care.
2. Attend a conservatorship (evidentiary) hearing. In most counties these are open to the public. Call the county courthouse to find out where and when they occur in your jurisdiction.
3. Visit local community programs, including social/recreational, vocational, and residential treatment programs, in order to become familiar with the range of services provided. Interview staff regarding program goals and objectives, services provided, population served, average length of service provision per client, and success rate. Interview clients regarding their goals and participation in the program.
4. Attend a hospital discharge-planning case conference.
5. Spend one day "shadowing" an occupational therapist–case manager, or if none is available in your area, a case manager from another discipline.
6. Role-play the following scenarios. You are the case manager at a hospital discharge planning conference with the inpatient treatment staff and your client, who is resistant to their recommendation of placement in a residential care facility.
   a. Scenario 1: You want to advocate for your client and convince the staff that she does not require residential care placement.
   b. Scenario 2: You want to help the treatment staff convince your client that he currently needs residential care placement.

References

Asher, I. E. (1996). *Occupational therapy evaluation tools: An annotated index* (2nd ed.). Bethesda, MD: American Occupational Therapy Association.

Baker, F., & Weiss, R. S. (1984). The nature of case manager support. *Hospital and Community Psychiatry, 35,* 925-928.

Biegel, D. E., Tracy, E. M., & Corvo, K. N. (1994). Strengthening social networks: Intervention strategies for mental health case managers. *Health and Social Work, 19,* 206–216.

Harris, M., & Bergman, H. C. (1987). Case management with the chronically mentally ill: A clinical perspective. *American Journal of Orthopsychiatry, 57,* 296–302.

Kanter, J. (1989). Clinical case management: Definition, principles, components. *Hospital and Community Psychiatry, 40,* 361–368.

Klasson, E. M. (1989). A model of the occupational therapist as case manager: Two case studies of chronic schizophrenic patients living in the community. *Occupational Therapy in Mental Health, 9*(1), 63–90.

Lamb, H. R. (1979). Staff burnout in work with long-term patients. *Hospital and Community Psychiatry, 30,* 396–398.

Lamb, H. R. (1986). Some reflections on treating schizophrenics. *Archives of General Psychiatry, 43,* 1007–1011.

Morrison, R. L., & Bellack, A. S. (1984). Social skills training. In A. S. Bellack (Ed.), *Schizophrenia: Treatment, management, and rehabilitation* (pp. 247–279). New York: Grune & Stratton.

Platman, S. R., Dorgan, R. E., Gerhard, R. S., Mallam, K. E., & Spiliadis, S. S. (1982). Case management of the mentally disabled. *Journal of Public Health Policy, 3,* 302–314.

Porter, M., & Sherman, P. S. (1988). *The Denver Consumer Case Manager Project.* Unpublished manuscript, Denver, Colorado, Division of Mental Health.

Robinson, G., & Toff-Bergman, G. (1989). *Choices in case management: Current knowledge and practice for mental health programs.* Washington, DC: Mental Health Policy Research Center.

Rogers, C. R. (1989). The characteristics of a helping relationship. In H. Kirschenbaum & V. L. Henderson (Eds.), *The Carl Rogers reader* (pp. 108–126). New York: Houghton Mifflin.

Thompson, K. S., Griffith, E. E. H., & Leaf, P. J. (1990). A historical model of the Madison model of community care. *Hospital and Community Psychiatry, 41,* 625–634.

Walsh, J. (1994). The social networks of seriously mentally ill persons receiving case management services. *Journal of Case Management, 3,* 27–35.

Suggested Reading

Adams, R. (1990). The role of occupational therapists in community mental health. *Mental Health Special Interest Section Newsletter, 13* (1), 1–2.

Bachrach, L. L. (1989). Case management: Toward a shared definition. *Hospital and Community Psychiatry, 40,* 883–884.

Chamberlain, R., & Rapp, C. A. (1991). A decade of case management support: A methodological review of outcome research. *Community Mental Health Journal, 27,* 171–188.

Dass, R., & Gorman, P. (1985). *How can I help?* New York: Knopf.

Estroff, S. (1981). *Making it crazy: An ethnography of psychiatric clients in an American community.* Berkeley: University of California Press.

Lamb, H. R. (1980). Therapist–case managers: More than brokers of services. *Hospital and Community Psychiatry, 31,* 762–764.

McGurrin, M. C., & Worley, N. (1993). Evaluation of intensive case management for seriously and persistently mentally ill persons. *Journal of Case Management, 2,* 59–65.

Mercier, C., & Racine, G. (1995). Case management with homeless women: A descriptive study. *Community Mental Health Journal, 31,* 25–37.

Moeller, P. (1991). The occupational therapist as case manager in community mental health. *Mental Health Special Interest Section Newsletter, 14*(2), 4–5.

Olfson, M. (1990). Assertive community treatment: An evaluation of the experimental evidence. *Hospital and Community Psychiatry, 41,* 634–641.

Quinlivan, R., Hough, R., Crowell, A., Beach, C., Hofstetter, R., & Kenworthy, K. (1995). Service utilization and costs of care for severely mentally ill clients in an intensive management program. *Psychiatric Services, 46,* 365–371.

Skinner, P. C. (1995). The role of the family in the strengths model of psychiatric community case management. *Kansas Nurse, 70,* 3–4.

Stein, L. I., & Test, M. A. (1980). Alternative to mental hospital treatment. *Archives of General Psychiatry, 37,* 392–397.

Witheridge, T. F. (1989). The assertive community treatment worker: An emerging role and its implications for professional training. *Hospital and Community Psychiatry, 40,* 620–624.

PART VI

Clinically Related Roles

CHAPTER 20

Fieldwork Supervision in the Mental Health Setting

Elizabeth Cara

Key Terms

eclectic

interpersonal

intrapersonal

mode

parallel process

style

supervision

Chapter Outline

Introduction

This chapter focuses on the fieldwork experience and the process of **supervision** during fieldwork. Because it emphasizes the fieldwork experience, a discussion of how to supervise other employees in the mental health setting is not included. However, since the chapter delineates useful models and practical approaches, the information should also be useful for general supervision in the mental health setting.

    The American Occupational Therapy Association ([AOTA], 1988) states that the purpose of fieldwork is to provide the opportunity to integrate academic knowledge with applied skills at progressively higher levels of performance and responsibility. The student is able to test firsthand what was learned in school and to refine skills while interacting with clients and staff under the "supervision of qualified personnel." In Level II fieldwork, the qualified personnel must be a registered occupational therapist with at least one year of experience. The person responsible for the day-to-day training is considered a fieldwork educator (also known as a clinical educator, fieldwork supervisor, or student supervisor). In this chapter the terms are used interchangeably. All designate the person responsible for the day-to-day supervision of the student (as opposed to the person who may be the fieldwork coordinator and has primarily administrative duties).

The American Occupational Therapy Association defines supervision as:

> a process in which two or more people participate in a joint effort to promote, establish, maintain, and or elevate a level of performance and service. Supervision is a mutual undertaking between the supervisor and the supervisee that fosters growth and development; assures appropriate utilization of training and potential; encourages creativity and innovation; and provides guidance, support, encouragement, and respect while working toward a goal. (1994, p. 1045)

This chapter will discuss, for those new to the role, the tools needed to assume the role of fieldwork supervisor and ways in which the process can be made smoother for individuals in both the supervisor and supervisee positions. In an attempt to offer a comprehensive view of supervision, different models that address particular aspects of the supervision process in occupational therapy and other fields will be presented. It is hoped that supervisors and supervisees can adapt this broad view for their specific experience and mental health setting.

In occupational therapy as well as other professions, supervision is a valuable aspect of training. In most health professions, supervision is mandated and is recognized as a learning situation. A good relationship between the supervisor and supervisee is valued or, indeed, essential, and the emphasis is on the role, rather than the techniques, of the supervisor (Christie, Joyce, & Moeller, 1985; Loganbill, Hardy, & Delworth, 1982). Despite these common assumptions, there is little formal training given prior to promoting someone to the role of supervisor, and it is expected that:

- Training will be a somewhat smooth process.
- The supervisor will successfully guide the process.
- The supervisee will successfully become a competent occupational therapist.
- Quality occupational therapy will be promoted.
- Professional development of the involved individuals will be enhanced.

A supervisee may experience the same ups and downs and the same anxieties or worry about adequacy and competency that students experience during the academic process. A fieldwork educator may question her or his skills and competency to facilitate the training process and may also experience anxiety and confusion. However, ultimately both supervisor and supervisee expect that the "learner" will successfully "pass" through the training on the way to becoming a professional and that the supervisor will successfully guide the process.

Perhaps the practical fieldwork process can be viewed as similar to the academic process. Learning is acquired in a nonlinear manner and the course does not always seem smooth. Think back on your academic learning career, whether for the past four or more years or the last few years specifically in occupational therapy. Was the process as smooth as you expected? Was it linear or was it an up-and-down pattern of certainty and confusion? Did you approach graduation in a step-by-step process in which each step was clear or did you sometimes stumble, or miss a step—or take two at a time?

As you read this chapter keep in mind that fieldwork education and training, and supervision as one aspect of it, can be seen as a metaphor for the entire learning process. Thus, it is difficult to predict how each step will be taken.

SUPERVISION: DIFFERENT ELEMENTS FORM THE WHOLE

Supervision is an aspect of training that includes four elements: the supervisor, the supervisee, the relationship, and the context or environment (Frum & Opacich, 1987; Loganbill et al., 1982). Within the mental health arena specifically, supervision is "an intensive, interpersonal focused, one-to-one relationship in which one person is designated to facilitate the development of therapeutic competence in the other person . . . . [It is] a master apprentice approach" (Loganbill et al., 1982, p. 4).

The Supervisor

The supervisor is a licensed or registered professional with a minimum of one year of clinical experience who assumes authority for the student's education. The supervisor is responsible for setting, encouraging, and evaluating the standard of work performed by the supervisee (AOTA, 1994). The fieldwork supervisor's responsibilities include:

- providing an adequate orientation to the site and to its policies and procedures
- assigning patients to the student
- supervising the provision of services, including oral reports and documentation
- evaluating the skills and knowledge level of the student
- meeting with the student regularly to provide guidance and review performance
- using the fieldwork performance evaluation at midpoint and termination (AOTA, 1988)

In addition, the supervisor assumes responsibility for the supervisee's client caseload and is responsible, not only for the supervised person's development into a professional in clinical practice, but also for the outcome of client interventions. Therefore, the supervisor assumes multiple roles (Munroe, 1988), serving as a model, guide, teacher, organizer, and clinician all in one.

The Supervisee

The supervisee is the student who is learning to practice. The supervisee will assume a caseload and learn clinical practice, including the skills of relating therapeutically, choosing and applying interventions correctly, communicating and documenting information accurately, and becoming a team member. New standards (AOTA, 1988) ask that students experience roles of service management and research in addition to direct care. The supervisee thus learns the multiple roles of the professional. The assistance or guidance of another experienced professional is integral to the process of professionalization.

The Relationship

The interaction of the supervisee and supervisor constitutes a relationship. The relationship developed between the two is recognized as an important and influencing component of the supervision process. In occupational therapy, the relationship is not emphasized as much as in some other professions, such as psychotherapy. However, the nature of the relationship, participation therein, and the opportunity it affords to work out communication and personality differences are recognized by supervisors as an important element in learning. The students themselves place much importance on the supervisor's attractiveness and skill level (Christie et al., 1985; Kautzmann, 1987).

The Environment

The environment in which the supervision and training takes place is recognized as having an impact on the supervision process. The environment can include the physical setting, the people and rules of the organization, and the relationships of the staff. All these elements form the culture of the organization, which is the unique way in it operates.

The context in which the fieldwork is experienced also influences the process. The context of fieldwork is educational; in this case, learning how to apply knowledge in a practical setting. Therefore, educational goals and objectives for the experience defined by the fieldwork site, the academic institution of the student and the professional organization (AOTA) will necessarily delineate the broad parameters in which the experience occurs.

THEORETICAL MODELS OF SUPERVISION

Traditional psychotherapy professions have presented models for supervision that have been based in their theoretical orientation. However, concepts of supervision have an *eclectic* background, having been developed from various professions and theories. Concepts also have emerged in a trial-and-error way from the actual training of therapists. Each field has maintained a specific emphasis.

Psychoanalytic

The concept of supervision began to develop in the 1920s with the acceptance of psychoanalysis. Psychoanalysis, or psychoanalytic therapy, goes much further than other theoretical practices in emphasizing the **intrapersonal** aspects of training and supervision. In fact, the dynamics of supervision and therapy are considered a rich process akin to an artistic weaving, in which students learn how the process of therapy is intertwined with an individual's personality and tendencies to respond. A perspective from this theory that sheds light on the occupational therapy supervisory process is that of the supervisor as a master who joins the student therapist in a rite of passage (Meerlo, 1952, cited in Loganbill et al., 1982). Additionally, the psychoanalytic literature describes a developmental process of various stages through which the supervisee travels; hence the term **parallel process** (Hora, 1957) comes from this field. In the developmental process, the therapist identifies with the patient and then elicits emotions in the supervisor that he or she experienced with the patient. Although occupational therapy supervision is not often conducted utilizing this concept, it is applicable to the mental health setting.

Occupational therapy and psychoanalytic supervision differ in that psychoanalytic therapy does not allow for as much variability in, or emphasis on, learning style and developmental level of learning as occupational therapy supervision does.

Humanistic

"Facilitative" supervision (Leddick & Bernard, 1980) was originally addressed by Carl Rogers, who discussed a program of experiences that gave trainees an opportunity to model the empathy and unconditional positive regard of the therapist/supervisor. The supervisor was to provide a model of behavior so that supervisees could learn by example. The assumption was that the supervisor would be an excellent therapist/counselor. Later research was contradictory regarding which methods (modeling, personal growth, or didactic training) were more useful and whether the supervisory relationship was similar to, or different from, the counseling relationship.

Occupational therapy supervision is similar to humanistic supervision in that occupational therapy supervisors traditionally emphasize role modeling and positive reassurance.

Behavioral

Behavioral therapy stresses learning theory. Trainees learn behaviors from skilled therapists through role modeling and coaching. They learn goal setting—identifying and selecting appropriate learning techniques—in behavioral terms. That is, supervision includes instruction in various behavioral techniques.

Occupational therapy supervision is similar to behavioral therapy supervision in the sense that traditional supervision stresses instruction in techniques and goal setting and recognizes the supervisor role as that of a coach.

Developmental

Developmental models assume that development proceeds in a chronological, hierarchical, sequential pattern. Development proceeds through identifiable stages, each stage of learning increases in complexity, and each stage must be experienced prior to further development in the next stage. Developmental theories may describe development in a specific area, such as the cognitive, moral, intellectual, sexual, or personality aspects of a person. A knowledge of developmental levels can aid in designing and fostering learning experiences specific to each stage.

Supervision in the area of cognitive development has been explicated in the occupational therapy literature and will be described in the next section, "Practical Models and Methods of Supervison."

Consistencies in Supervision

Aspects of different models have been blended and represent what is commonly recognized by most professions as supervision. Some consistencies that cross boundaries are (Leddick & Bernard, 1980):

1. Supervision is seen as a learning, "professionalizing" situation.
2. A good relationship between supervisor and supervisee is valued.
3. The role of the supervisor as coach and competent person has been emphasized rather than specific supervisory techniques.

PRACTICAL MODELS AND METHODS OF SUPERVISION

Useful developmental approaches for supervision have been conceptualized in occupational therapy and in counseling psychology.

Occupational Therapy

Schwartz (1984) proposed a method of supervision based on a synthesis of developmental (meaning that skills and knowledge are acquired in a sequential and hierarchical manner) models of personality that are correlated with learning experiences. Her model emphasizes the supervisor (importance of the approach) and supervisee (particularly cognitive and personality style). Table 20-1 shows ego stages, or individuals' ways of knowing, that are pertinent to occupational therapy clinical education. Ways of knowing are then correlated to student behavior and perceptions and interventions are suggested according to developmental levels (see Table 20-2 for one method of supervision). In an effort to move away from negative images and convey the concept of strengths, potential problems have been conceptualized instead in terms of levels. Behavior that is typical of occupational therapy students in fieldwork, as well as student perceptions of the learning process and suggestions for supervisory interventions, are described for each level.

The observation of behavior in the clinic and in the supervision process enables the supervisor to discern the supervisee's stage of development. Expectations can then be established based on a student's **interpersonal** cognitive style and sense of self at each stage of development. Hypotheses can thus be formed and checked concerning the supervisee's view of the learning process.

Once the supervisor has gained some understanding of students' behavior or a reasonable expectation of what their behavior may mean, he or she can then plan and implement specific approaches. The supervisor's role is that of model and evaluator and involves teaching, counseling, and instruction. The student's role is to learn through doing and by analyzing and critiquing his or her behavior within the supervisory sessions.

Table 20-1. Loevinger's Ego Stages Pertinent to Occupational Therapy Clinical Education

Ego Stage	Character Development	Interpersonal Style	Cognitive Style	What is Knowledge	The Learning Process
Level 3	Conformity to external rules, guilt for breaking rules	Belonging, superficial niceness	Conceptual simplicity, stereotypes	Necessary information in order to achieve the desired end. Takes the form of right or wrong, good or bad	Revelation of truth by an expert authority; if conflict between ideas is perceived, one element is dismissed as incorrect
Level 3/4	Differentiation of norms, goals	Aware of relation to group, helping	Multiplicity	Information to be applied to situational problems, possibility of several correct solutions	Student questions information received from the expert authority and tries to align with own view.
Level 4	Self-evaluated standards, self-criticism, guilt for consequences, long-term goals and ideals	Intensive, responsible, mutual, concern for communication	Conceptual complexity	Skill in problem-solving	Discovery of solutions through logical analysis, multiple views acknowledged but simplicity sought

Source: Schwartz (1984), p. 395, Table 1.

Table 20-2.   A Method for Clinical Supervision

Student Group	Teaching Approach	Supervision Sessions	Administrative Instructions	Counseling Intervention
Conscientious (Stage Level 3)	Assume student sees supervisor as "authority" and expert. Present information; show how several solutions can work. Lead toward student identification of problems, solutions.	Structure, with clear description of expectations. Make assignments to think about, bring to next meeting.	Delineate rules. Expect student to follow. Show disapproval if student does not.	Student desires acceptance, wants things to go well. Student will be upset with problems and look to supervisor for answers. Lead student to join supervisor in seeking answers.
Explorer (Stage Level 3/4)	Assume student in process of developing own system of problem solving. Discuss how student's view is worthwhile, problematic. Lead student toward accepting multiple viewpoints. Encourage exploration with clearly-defined limits.	Negotiate: Explain supervisor expectations, seek student input. Lead, but allow some flexibility in goals.	Delineate rules. Expect student will not follow if rules conflict with own ideas. Discuss implications if student chooses to follow low own inclination.	Student will be dogmatic and upset when things do not work according to plan. Lead student to see several ways to be effective. Support student through confusion.
Achiever (Stage Level 4)	Assume student has developed systems of beliefs, problem solving. Challenge ideas. Discuss implications. Lead toward greater analytic competence in problem solving. Encourage exploration with feedback.	Discuss supervisor expectations and student's. Collaborate on discussing best method to achieve goals.	Delineate rules. Discuss origins where appropriate. Expect student to seek exceptions. Explain when supervisor can/cannot be flexible.	Student will be hypercritical of failures. Help student see when guilt is appropriate, when student is exceeding reasonable limit of responsibility.

Source: Schwartz (1984), p. 395, Table 2.

Analysis of cognitive levels and interventions.   The developmental levels are posited as guides and not as rigid classifications. An individual does not always fit neatly into one level, particularly since this represents a combination of areas of development. However, the developmental model suggests patterns of learning and, therefore, clear methods of clinical supervision. (The levels noted are most typical of supervisees. It is assumed that knowledge in previous levels has been acquired by the time individuals begin fieldwork.)

Level 3.   Conscientious students usually obey rules without questioning because they wish to belong to a group and to gain approval from peers and authority figures. They have limited self-awareness and find it difficult to entertain many solutions to a problem, so they may personalize criticism. This group views the supervisor as the expert, which means that students do not realize or trust their own ability to elicit solutions. They will need assurance and an understanding of the separation of personal from professional worth. Structured questioning should elicit successful problem solving, and follow-up assignments should be given.

Level 3/4.   In the explorer group, thinking becomes more complex. The individual is able to see more possibilities and alternatives, and self-reflective ability increases. There is a conflict between wanting to stand out yet not wanting to stand outside the group. Although thinking is more complex, beliefs are stated in a dogmatic way. Explorers may fail to incorporate feedback with which they do not agree, and they may challenge the rules. The supervisor should engage in comparing the student's own view with the professional judgment of others. The explorer group consists of students who are developing their own problem-solving techniques, which means that a discussion of alternative solutions may ensue. The discussion should be limited and not provide so much information as to overwhelm supervisees.

Level 4.   Achievers are able to accept and utilize multiple strategies. Students are able to follow standards of performance in an individualistic way yet may still be hypercritical. The achiever group can define problems and solutions; therefore, an approach that will critique and analyze the solutions is useful. An analytical discussion of why and how solutions were arrived at can be useful. Also indicated is instruction in how new information can be accommodated or assimilated with previous knowledge.

CASE ILLUSTRATION: DARREN, CORDELIA, AND TABETHA—THE DEVELOPMENTAL STAGES

Darren and Cordelia had started their internship at the same time. They came from the same school, where they had been friends and worked on group projects together. As interns, they were joined by Tabetha, a student from a different school. Darren was a conscientious (level 3) student. He was quiet and rarely asked questions, but he listened intently to his supervisor and took notes during the supervisory sessions. He initially observed his supervisor's treatment. After each session, his supervisor carefully broke down her treatment in a step-by-step fashion and, for each step, explained what she was doing and why. She regularly provided Darren with a list of questions posed as treatment hypotheses regarding the treatment sessions. Dareen then would return to the next session and discuss his understanding of the hypotheses. His supervisor provided specific answers regarding his hypotheses, reassured him that his reasoning was sound, and thanked him for his earnest work.

Cordelia preferred to try out treatment right away. She was an explorer (level 3/4), who was more comfortable discussing alternatives in which she was involved. Her supervisor began a treatment and invited Cordelia to assist. She then pointed out one or two steps she had observed and elicited alternative ways of treatment from Cordelia.

Tabetha was an achiever (level 4), who also preferred to experience treatment right away. In fact, she had arrived early to observe treatment before the formal internship began. In supervisory sessions, she reported what she had learned from her observations and what she might add to the treatment. She then reported how the treatment session had turned out, what her strengths and weaknesses were, what she might change, and the reasons why the session had turned out the way it had. She requested permission to do a research project that she had been thinking about before starting the internship. Darren, Cordelia, and Tabetha eventually designed their own peer supervision group. Although the interns were at different developmental levels, their supervisors were able to incorporate their levels of learning into the supervisory process. Moreover, the three were eventually able to help each other in the learning process.

Counseling Psychology Model

This model mainly addresses the supervisee and explains the process he or she may go through. It also emphasizes the relationship's ability to help the student progress successfully through the learning process. The model is explained in some length here because:

- Training in occupational therapy supervision is based on it (Frum & Opacich, 1987).
- It is the model most cited in the supervision process literature.
- It specifically focuses on affect and the emotional process that may occur in supervision.

The counseling psychology model was influenced by the developmental stage theorists (primarily Erik Erikson and Margaret Mahler). Both indicate optimism and trust in the adaptive capacities of human beings, and both encourage the emergence of qualities such as competence and a sense of personal and professional identity. Erikson discusses "potential crises," meaning periods of vulnerability and heightened potential. The supervisor can be aware of these crises in the supervisee's development and make appropriate interventions. In Erikson's developmental model, identity is central in development. The training process is one in which the central task of the student is to acquire a professional identity. Mahler emphasizes separation and autonomy. The supervisee not only is learning how to disengage from those on whom he or she has relied, such as teachers and classes, but is also learning how to become independent in thinking and behavior. Figure 20-1 shows a three-stage

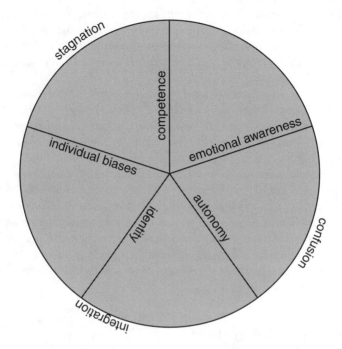

Figure 20-1. The Three-stage Developmental Model

Source: From Loganbill et al. (1992).

model of stagnation, confusion, and integration with key issues for each stage (Loganbill et al., 1982). It appears that students pass through and revisit different stages in the supervisory process. Moreover, they must grapple and struggle with the themes in each stage before reaching an emotional understanding that allows them to progress to the next stage. You will recognize some of the behavior, styles and thinking as similar to the occupational therapy model. An in-depth description of the stages of supervision can be found in Table 20-3.

Stage I—Stagnation.   In the stage of stagnation, the beginning supervisee is usually unaware, naively, of any difficulties or important issues in supervision. For the more experienced student, this is characterized more by feeling stuck or experiencing blind spots. Usually there is a naive sense of security and stability, and there may be some simplistic, black-and-white thinking or inability to define the nuances of interventions. The student may be particularly uninsightful regarding his or her skills in practice. Typically, supervisees overestimate their skills or, conversely, believe that they have none or have not learned enough to prepare them for this endeavor.

Attitudes toward the world and environment can be characterized by very narrow and/or rigid thinking. With the more experienced student, this may be

Table 20-3. Stages of Supervision

	Supervisee's Process	External Attitude	Internal Attitude	Attitude toward Supervisor
Stagnation	Unaware Stuck Blind spots Over- or under-estimates skills	Narrow, rigid, linear thinking and uncreative problem solving	Low self-concept or false sense of well-being	Idealizing or indifferent

Implications for practice: Caution against independence and responsibility, explain intricacies of practice, make few demands for advanced knowledge, give reassurance, show tolerance. Do not personalize.

	Supervisee's Process	External Attitude	Internal Attitude	Attitude toward Supervisor
Confusion	Erratic Confusion Conflict	Less rigid Inadequate problem solving	Unsure Fluctuate between incompetent and able	Disappointed and angry that supervisor does not have all the answers

Implications for practice: A nondefensive attitude and ability to identify problems and emotions and discuss them. Validate realistic portrait of the supervisee. Do not join in the turbulence.

	Supervisee's Process	External Attitude	Internal Attitude	Attitude toward Supervisor
Integration	Intellectual understanding Flexibility Stability	Understanding Acceptance of therapeutic situation	More realistic Acceptance of strengths and weaknesses, more confidence	More realistic and independent

Implications for practice: The supervisee can take much more responsibility for supervision, treatment, and learning. There is a consolidation of knowledge and probably less need for structured supervision. The supervisor, while still providing feedback, can enlist supervisees in reviewing what they find important in treatment, what they have learned, and what they must still develop.

confined to a specific issue in practice. Usually, thinking is linear and uncreative and problem solving is narrow. Often the supervisee may accurately recognize problems in practice but offer a solution that is too narrow to be realistic.

Attitudes toward the self are usually characterized by a low self-concept and dependency on the supervisor as the source of new learning or by a lack of awareness leading to a false sense of well-being that is not based on actual behavior. Usually the attitude toward the supervisor is one of idealizing him or her as an omniscient and omnipotent figure or being indifferent to the supervisor and considering him or her somewhat irrelevant. Although this stage may seem somewhat negative by the supervisor, it can be characterized as one in which the supervisee is passively learning and constituting an identity that will aid in the next, turbulent stages.

Implications for practice.   This is a difficult stage for the supervisor, who should resist the temptation to give the supervisee too much early independence and responsibility. This stage demands an explanation of the intricacies of practice without too many demands for advanced knowledge. The supervisor should provide reassurance and understanding concerning the student's positive interventions. To cope with a defiant attitude, the supervisor must understand and tolerate both the tendency to idealize and that to be indifferent. In other words, supervisors should enjoy being admired and not deny their knowledge. They must tolerate indifference and do not personalize behavior.

CASE ILLUSTRATION: DARREN, CORDELIA, AND TABETHA—STAGE 1, STAGNATION

After the initial two weeks, Darren and Tabetha showed indications that they were in the stagnation stage, though they expressed it differently. Darren wanted to continue to observe and discuss treatment and planned interventions that were just like his supervisor's. He felt that he could never know as much as she and he wondered if he could pass the internship. Tabetha asked if she could have her own caseload and did not think that she needed more than weekly supervision. She was not sure whether her supervisor really provided the best interventions.

Stage 2—Confusion.   Stage two is one of confusion. This represents a marked shift from the first stage, which can occur abruptly or gradually. It is often marked by instability; erratic fluctuations in emotions, thoughts, and practice; confusion; and, sometimes, conflict. The supervisee no longer is guided by, or guarded about, beliefs about the self, others, and solutions. His or her attitude toward treatment or the setting is less characterized by rigid thinking, though solutions to problems seem inadequate and may be impossible. However, the supervisee will recognize that something is amiss.

Generally, the attitude toward the self reflects the basis of this stage. Supervisees' attitudes fluctuate between a sense of self as inadequate and incompetent and a sense of being expert and able. The supervisee may know that she or he possesses some valuable skills or competencies yet be unsure that the skills will be useful in the context of practice. Students are also unsure whether their competencies are perceived by others.

Due to confusion and still-narrow thinking, the supervisee may continue to look to the supervisor for answers; however, the student will recognize that the supervisor does not have all the answers. Anger and disappointment may result. The supervisee may still idealize the supervisor and think he or she is deliberately withholding answers, or the supervisor may be viewed as incompetent or inadequate. Perhaps this is the source of the apparent contradiction in students' report that they perceive supervisors poorly while at the same time labeling their overall experience as good. Obviously, this stage may be difficult for the supervisor as well as the supervisee.

Implications for practice. The supervisor must recognize and understand the particular stage and the emotions that characterize it and not take any display of disappointment or anger personally. Naming the problem and emotions and being able to discuss them in a nondefensive way will go a long way toward helping a student move through this stage.

The supervisor should validate a realistic portrayal of the student and resist joining in the erratic self-evaluation. It is important to resist the temptation to overvalue yet nevertheless maintain a realistic, reassuring viewpoint of the supervisee as an occupational therapist. The value of this stage is in giving up former rigid, narrow beliefs and experiencing the opportunity to gain new ideas, perspectives, and skills. It is important for the supervisor to:

- remain objective
- remain unperturbed by the panic or turbulence that the supervisee may be experiencing
- be able to recognize and verbalize what is happening for the supervisee

The supervisor can help the student remain aware that out of confusion come knowledge and learning.

CASE ILLUSTRATION: DARREN, CORDELIA, AND TABETHA—STAGE 2, CONFUSION

After about five weeks, just prior to her midterm evaluation, Cordelia, who was usually talkative, became quiet and almost surly. She failed to attend two supervision sessions, claiming that her clients needed that treatment time. She revealed to Darren and Tabetha that she was not sure if any treatment in mental health was valuable or whether people really did get better. She was disappointed in her supervision and thought that her supervisor might be "testing" her before the midterm evaluation. A client who was paranoid and who, she believed, did not like her, stopped coming to Cordelia's vocational group. Cordelia began to feel better after her supervisor explained how students might feel at that stage and emphasized that her concerns were normal. She also became more aware of how her attitude affected her behavior with clients.

Stage 3—Integration. Stage three is characterized by integration, cognitive understanding, flexibility, and personal stability. The supervisee grasps and understands important issues for supervision. Usually supervisees can realistically assess their strengths and weakness without interference from their emotions and are able to grasp what skills need to be polished and integrated in treatment.

The supervisees' attitude toward the environment is less rigid and idealistic or extreme, and they now have a cognitive understanding of the therapeutic situation. There is acceptance and a sense of direction for the future. An individual's attitude toward the self is characterized by a more realistic view and an acceptance of both strengths and weakness. There is a sense of confidence that growth will continue, and the attitude toward the supervisor also becomes more realistic. The supervisor is now seen as a person who has strengths and weakness. The student is able to take more responsibility for the supervisory sessions and agenda, usually becoming more independent of the supervisor at this stage. This is a stable period with much flexibility and potential for further growth.

Implications for practice.   The supervisee can take much more responsibility for supervision, treatment, and learning. There is a consolidation and probably less need for structured supervision. The supervisor, while still providing feedback, can enlist the supervisee in reviewing what is finds important in treatment, what he or she has learned, and what can still be developed.

> ## CASE ILLUSTRATION: DARREN, CORDELIA, AND TABETHA—STAGE 3, INTEGRATION

In their peer supervision group held prior to their last weeks of the internship, Darren, Cordelia, and Tabetha discussed what they had learned and what they hoped for the future. They realized that their final project, in which they had developed a community outreach group that would be taken over by clients, was valued and desired by both staff and clients. They felt proud that they had been able to contribute.

The interns realized that although they were not sure whether they were advanced enough to work independently in mental health, they had acquired some good skills. They began to understand how their responses, attitudes, and behavior could affect clients; Cordelia had particularly learned this during stage 2. They appreciated what they had learned from their supervisor and other staff and were also able to differentiate what they could do best and less well. They realized that working in mental health is like an interesting dance between client and therapist; if they each listened to different music they would be unable to follow each other, but when they were hearing the same tune, treatment progressed more easily. They felt secure in their knowledge and identity as occupational therapists, and they had some ideas about the similarities and differences in their own and other mental health professions.

Themes in the stages. Within these stages, certain themes, or issues, of competence, emotional awareness, autonomy, identity, and respect for individual differences for beginning professionals may appear. The issues may not necessarily appear in sequential order, and they tend to continually resurface.

Competence. Competence means the ability to use skills and knowledge to carry out an appropriate treatment plan. Most often, this entails the students' ability to translate intellectual knowledge learned in a classroom to the practice or clinical situation. Usually, this is a core issue in stage 1, or in the beginning of training, because the supervisee does not have a repertoire of skills. In stage 2 she may realize that she does not yet have the adequate skills and may feel frustrated. In stage 3 the supervisee may have an understanding and integration of skills and techniques that she can use for a variety of clients and situations.

In the case illustration, Darren, Cordelia, and Tabetha displayed issues of competence in each stage. Darren was most questioning of his ability in stage 1, Cordelia felt frustrated in stage 2, and all three had realistically integrated their skills and knowledge during stage 3.

Emotional awareness. Emotional awareness is important in the psychosocial arena because it relates to an ability to be aware of how one affects, and is affected by, client responses, behavior, and style (see Chapter 1, for more information). This awareness of personal reactions and attitudes toward a patient are particularly useful for formulating impressions and directing interventions in the psychiatric arena.

In stage 1, supervisees may often be unaware of personal feelings toward clients or themselves. They may particularly deny anger, frustration, inadequacy, and attraction to, or from, clients. Supervisees finding their own way during the beginning of training most likely cannot risk revealing personal emotions. Moreover, beginning therapists may still carry the impression that they should always be "nice," thereby being unable to accept emotions considered "not nice" in either themselves or patients. The shunned feelings may then be expressed in inappropriate ways and at the wrong times in treatment. In stage 2, an awareness of feelings may occur but may be frightening or unacceptable. Stage 3 recognizes a newfound sense of acceptance and control that emotions and thoughts regarding clients can be distinguished from behavior.

The supervisor should name the feelings for the supervisee and accept them or explain their importance. Alternately, the supervisor should assure the supervisee they are natural feelings in this situation and that it would be unnatural not to have them.

While in stage 2, Cordelia had been most unaware of her feelings. After reassurance from her supervisor, however, she became able to accept them. In stage 3, she still wondered whether her feelings were important but was able to acknowledge and discuss with her supervisor concerns regarding her behavior toward clients.

Autonomy.   Students may have the sense that they are merely a reflection of all the books they have read, and the theories and teachers they have experienced. They may doubt that they can be effective. Supervisees may have a shaky self-concept and difficulty thinking of themselves as responsible occupational therapists.

In stage 1 the supervisee may be overdependent on the supervisor, seeing him or her as a magician who has all the right answers. The supervisee may want specific "how to" answers or to be told the "right way" to handle clients. Sometimes students are experiencing the unawareness characteristic of this period and so may disregard advice or information from the supervisor.

In stage 2, the supervisee may alternate between dependency and independence. This may be manifested by relying on the supervisor to have the right answer or, alternatively, countering suggestions or assuming that the supervisor's suggestions are one's own ideas. In stage 3, supervisees may recognize areas in which they are functioning autonomously and be able to realistically and unashamedly accept those areas in which they should rely on the supervisor for more assistance.

This issue will usually show up in the context of interpersonal supervision. The supervisor may be overburdened with the responsibility of providing the correct answer and may become annoyed with the pressure to do so, or he or she may feel unneeded by a student who naively feels too independent early in practice. The supervisor may feel chaotically pulled one way and then another. The supervisee may not be quite sure how to act in this tumultuous period of alternation between overreliance and no reliance. Again, the supervisor can weather these issues by not taking personally any actions by the supervisee and by naming and validating the behavior.

Darren initially displayed this issue in stage 1. However, by the middle of the fieldwork period he had become more confident in his ability to work independently. He thanked his supervisor for gently facilitating his independence through her concrete interventions and suggestions.

Identity.   The theme of identity may appear as the student struggles to assume a theoretical identity or discern which theory works best. The supervisee may be caught in a conflict of learning one theory while practicing with therapists who use another. In stage 1, the student may not understand how the theory relates to her or his practice and clients. In stage 2, there may be confusion and a sense of trying out different theories or a resistance to learning new theories. In stage 3, the supervisee usually has some sense of how theory relates to clients and which theory seems most appropriate.

Supervisors should consistently help the supervisee integrate theory with practice and explain how the theory relates specifically to clients and the occupational therapy department as a whole. Students may also benefit from projects in which they can research theories and their usefulness for the population with which they are working.

In the case illustration, Darren and Cordelia had learned a specific theory for mental health treatment. They were able to use it throughout the treatment, and were pleased that their supervisor followed the same theory. Tabetha had not learned a specific theory for mental health treatment and initially felt skeptical of having to follow one. However, she gradually came to appreciate its use in the mental health setting. Her final project discussed the theory more in depth.

Individual biases.   The theme of individual biases arises because of the negative stereotypes associated with many people with mental disabilities and because of the fear, on the part of society in general, of those stereotypes. Particularly in mental health, one must separate out behaviors that are maladaptive and need change from aspects of the person, which need to be respected.

In stage 1, bias may be manifested in cases where the supervisee criticizes clients yet is unaware of any disrespect. In stage 2, supervisees may find themselves avoiding or dreading contact with a client but be unaware why or, conversely, may find themselves overly controlling in their behavior toward clients and interacting in a demeaning, authoritative way that leaves little room for client autonomy. In the third stage, supervisees will be aware of their biases and prejudices and will hopefully strive, through self-education, to become familiar with different cultural patterns and the effect of symptoms on behavior.

Supervisors should remark on criticisms and authoritative interactions, elicit how the supervisee thinks and feels toward the clients, and discuss the fact that emotions experienced in this context are part of working with clients and thus are natural. Discussing client behavior as a result of, or in the context of, the mental illness rather than as behavior that is deliberately and willfully chosen is often helpful for the beginning therapist who is still learning the difference.

All three students initially were fearful of people with mental disabilities; specifically, they secretly believed them to be unpredictably violent, hopeless, and, maybe, lacking in discipline. They were able to discuss these attitudes with their supervisor, who tolerated the attitudes while at the same time questioning them. The students were shocked when they saw some of the symptoms of the different mental disorders about which they had read. At the same time, they were aware of how the people with whom they worked had thoughts, hopes, desires, dreams, frustrations, and struggles with many of the same issues as they had. Darren, Cordelia, and Tabetha finished their fieldwork with a new sense of respect for the clients' struggles to cope with their disorders and abilities to do many things independently in spite of the disorders.

Learning Styles Approach

A useful model in supervision is based on the experiential learning approach of Kolb (1976, 1984) and Kolb, Rubin, and McIntyre (1979). Experiential learning is considered a cyclical process perceiving and processing (Torrance & Rockenstein, 1988), and the effective learner relies equally on four different learning modes or strategies (Figure 20-2). For example, a **mode** could represent a style of clinical reasoning.

The effective learner is able to flexibly use all of these approaches and experiences for learning, but most people emphasize just one or two of the strategies and do not recognize that they use them exclusively. Consequently, they might not be able to learn effectively in situations or with people who do not include their modes or rely on a different **style**.

The Learning Style Inventory (LSI) (Kolb, 1976) measures relative emphasis on the four learning modes and provides two combination scores, or styles, that indicate the extent to which an individual emphasizes abstractness over concreteness (AC-CE) and active experimentation over reflection (AE-RO) (see Table 20-4 for a description of the various learning modes and styles). Divergers perceive information in a concrete manner, process it reflectively, and can generalize from it. Assimilators take in information abstractly, begin with an idea, and process it reflectively; they watch and think. Convergers take in information abstractly and actively process it through ex-

---

Learning Modes

Concrete Experience (CE) involving oneself fully, openly and without bias in new experiences

is the basis for

Reflection Observation (RO), the ability to reflect on and observe these experiences from many perspectives

these observations are assimilated into a "theory" using

Abstract Conceptualization (AC), the ability to create concepts that integrate observations into logically sound theories

and then to use these theories for

Active Experimentation(AE) or the ability to use hypotheses that serve as guides to create new experiences. (Kolb et al., 1979)

Learning Styles

Divergers (RO/CE) perceive information in a concrete manner, process it reflectively and can generalize from it.

Assimilators (AC/RO) take in information abstractly, begin with an idea and process it reflectively. They watch and think.

Convergers (AC/AE) take in information abstractly and actively process it through experimentation.

Accommodators (AE/CE) take in information concretely and process it actively through doing. (Torrance & Rockenstein, 1988)

Figure 20-2.   Experiential Learning Modes and Styles

Table 20-4. Learning Modes and Styles

Learning Modes

	Concrete Experience	Reflective Observation	Abstract Conceptualization	Active Experimentation
Approach to Learning	Experience-based approach to learning, relies on "feeling" judgments	Tentative, impartial, reflective approach to learning	Analytic approach to learning relies on logical thinking, rational evaluation	Active, "doing" approach to learning; relies on experimentation
Learn Best by	Specific examples in which can become involved. Treat each situation as unique case	Situation that allows for role of impartial observer rather than participant	Authority-directed, impersonal situations that emphasize theory and systematic analysis	Engagement with activities that test one's own knowledge and ability
Emphasize	People oriented	Introverts	Orientation toward things and symbols	Extroverts
Learn Least by	Theoretical approaches	Doing without thinking	Unstructured, or "discovery," approaches/ simulations	Passive learning situations

Learning Styles

Accommodator (AE/CE)	Diverger (RO/CE)	Assimilator (AC/RO)	Converger (AC/AE)
Ability to carry out plans, action oriented	Imaginative ability, good at generating ideas, brainstorming	Ability to create theoretical models	Good at practical application of ideas
Likes new experiences, "risk-taker," intuitive, trial-and-error style	Can view a situation from many perspectives	Inductive reasoning	Likes a single answer to a problem
Adapts to immediate circumstances	Emotional, interested in people	Concepts over people Less concerned with practical application of theory	Less emotional, less interested in people

perimentation. Accommodators take in information concretely and process it actively through doing (Torrance & Rockenstein, 1988).

Matching modes and styles.   For the supervisee, knowing the modes and style of learning that she or he emphasizes will provide an understanding of personal strengths and limitations. Modes and styles that are used can be emphasized in treatment, and less used modes and styles can be identified, learned, and practiced.

The setting and organization can be analyzed to assess the opportunities that exist for the supervisee's learning style; the supervisee can be placed in activities that match her or his style. Opportunities and learning experiences can be designed that appeal to specific styles.

An assessment of the supervisor's style offers an opportunity to match supervisory interactions. It provides an ongoing basis of mutual understanding that may consistently be referred to throughout a fieldwork experience. It also provides a safe and nonthreatening context in which to discuss more personal aspects of self.

CASE ILLUSTRATION: DARREN, CORDELIA, AND TABETHA—A LEARNING STYLES APPROACH

Modes

Concrete Experience (CE): involving oneself fully, openly, and without bias in new experiences.

Reflection Observation (RO): the ability to reflect on, and observe, experiences from many perspectives.

Abstract Conceptualization (AC): the ability to create concepts that integrate observations into logically sound theories.

Active Experimentation (AE): the ability to use hypotheses that serve as guides to create new experiences.

Styles

Accommodator (AE/CE): take in information concretely, process it actively through doing.

Diverger (RO/CE): take in information concretely, process it by reflection and generalizing.

Assimilator (AC/RO): take in information abstractly with an idea, process it by reflection. Watch and think.

Converger (AC/AE): take in information abstractly, process it actively through experimentation.

Darren's modes of learning were reflective observation (RO) and abstract conceptualization (AC). His style was that of the assimilator. Cordelia emphasized modes of abstract conceptualization (AC) and concrete experience (CE). Her style of learning was the accommodator. *Tabetha's preferred modes were abstract experimentation (AE) and concrete experience (CE). Her preferred style was as a* converger. *When they began their internship, all three interns filled out the LSI. They were then able to decide which groups and treatment approaches would most likely to interest them and which would most likely be difficult. With their supervisor's help, they were able to select which aspects of the program would match their styles, and therefore, where they would start. They also agreed on which aspects might be less of a match and therefore saved their involvement in these for later in the fieldwork.*

Their supervisor's learning style was diverger, *and her preferred modes were RO and CE. Since her preferred style was different than that of the students, all four anticipated how they might think or work differently and how the supervisor's expectations might evolve. She went through the Fieldwork Performance Evaluation (AOTA, 1988) to clarify specifically what behavior she expected. Whenever there were snags or confusion in their supervision, they were able to reflect back to their learning styles. They had fun throughout their fieldwork reflecting on their behavior and validating or disproving the validity of the learning styles for themselves. They appreciated that their supervisor made her expectations clear and at the same time listened to their thoughts and feelings before suggesting interventions.*

MAXIMIZING LEARNING—BENEFITING FROM SUPERVISION

As a fieldwork student, you can use different ways of learning to maximize your experience and to benefit most from supervision. Ways of maximizing learning during fieldwork are listed in Table 20-5 and elaborated in the following sections of this chapter.

Emotional Learning

Most individuals about to embark into fieldwork are excited, apprehensive, and willing to do all that they can to maximize the experience. Often the tendency is to find more academic texts or technical material to read. While seeking out information is always a good idea, certain information can be more useful for the fieldwork experience in mental health. Specifically, any texts that are personal stories or narratives that could broaden an understanding of people, of people with mental disabilities, or of oneself will help maximize the experience.

This chapter has highlighted a model that delineated emotional stages and issues, many of which will be encountered. A knowledge of the stages and understanding of the issues that might be most pertinent to yourself can help in anticipating potential personal "snags " in the process. Alerting the supervisor in advance to problems or anxieties that might arise will help both the supervisor and supervisee to flow through troublesome spots. This chapter

Table 20-5. Guidelines for Maximizing Learning during Fieldwork

Emotional	Intellectual	Interpersonal	Professional
Read narratives and personal stories of mental illness	Review academic material	Ask for help	Take initiative
Anticipate emotional issues and stages of fieldwork		Communicate expectations responsibly in supervision	Become familiar with your setting
Know your learning style	Plan a progressive program of involvement according to your learning style	Discuss learning style in supervision	Time management—plan a daily schedule and routine and use time effectively and flexibly
Self-reflection		Remain open and genuine and communicate with awareness	Schedule regular supervision time
Recorgnize when the work setting touches off personal issues		Communicate in supervision or with other staff when the work setting influences personal issues	Communicate in supervision when the work setting influences personal issues

also highlighted a model based on learning styles. Knowing your learning style in advance and alerting the supervisor to it may also anticipate, and possibly avoid, misunderstandings. You can anticipate in advance which experiences at your fieldwork site may match your learning style and therefore will be easiest to participate in, and which experiences will not match and therefore may be more difficult. Together, you and your supervisor could plan a step-by-step, progressive program starting with involvement in experiences that may be more comfortable and then attempting those that may be more difficult. Together, you and the supervisor can solve anticipated problems in advance.

Knowing yourself, your possible emotional stages, and your learning style will assist in maximizing a successful fieldwork experience. However, expressing your emotional interior and learning style in a direct, honest, and genuine manner with the ability to be self-reflective is also essential. In general, the more aware, open, and willing an individual is to communicate responsibly, the more the fieldwork and supervisory relationship will develop smoothly and the fewer problems will arise. With self-awareness and responsible communication, conflicts and disagreements can be avoided or resolved with mutual satisfaction.

Learning about Expectations

Fieldwork sites must clearly identify expectations of the fieldwork experience (AOTA, 1988). Therefore, students should be aware of, and ready to discuss, expectations at the outset of fieldwork. Expectations should be written and can be in the form of objectives specific to each category of the Fieldwork Performance Report (AOTA, 1988); guidelines outlining goals to be achieved during certain time periods; guidelines, dates, and formats of any assignments; and criteria for professional behavior at that center. The expectations should be verbally discussed and can be referred to during the experience. The early discussion of expectations is a good time to discuss strengths and weaknesses, interests, learning style, goals, and expectations.

Intellectual and Interpersonal Learning

Generally, now is the time to utilize material learned from academic classes, and to go back and look at it. Keep in mind a rule that never will fail—ask for help whenever there is the slightest doubt or question, provided taking the initiative to find the answer has failed. Take the time to familiarize yourself with your setting. This means finding out where things are kept, and what is available. Ask if you are unsure of the use of some equipment.

Plan a daily schedule and learn the day-to-day routine as quickly as possible. Observe other therapists to learn their successful treatment techniques and personal approach. Choose one whose style you can emulate. Make sure that regular time is scheduled with your supervisor and that appointments are always kept. If you are not getting enough feedback, or need to be observed more times, let your supervisor know.

Sometimes, how ideas and emotions are conveyed makes a difference. Take the time to read a few books concerning responsible communication. Remember that in mental health settings, issues and problems with which clients are dealing may touch off issues and problems that you are struggling with yourself. It is not normal in a mental health setting to deny emotions due to personal problems that may be uncovered or raised by client contact. It is normal to use your supervisory relationship to make sense of those emotions and plan the best way to personally handle them and use them in service of the client.

Professional Learning

Professional behaviors will be expected during the fieldwork experience. Behaviors of a professional are (AOTA, 1988):

- responsibility, such as initiative in learning and using resources, dependability in routine work, and punctuality;
- organizational skills, such as planning and carrying out daily responsibilities in a timely manner;
- flexibility, such as knowing how to use time effectively when changes in treatment or schedules occur;
- commitment to the department and profession

THE TRANSITION TO FIELDWORK EDUCATOR OR SUPERVISOR

The transition to fieldwork educator is an important change in professional identity. Although there has been much preparation for developing clinical skills, there is less preparation for using supervisory skills. In addition, there are no rituals or rites of passage, such as passing the registry exam that indicates the transition from student to professional, to facilitate the role transition from clinician to supervisor.

In spite of this, supervisors informally use different methods and experiences to assume their new role. *As a trainee,* the supervisee has had "hands-on" experience in supervision. Trainees have had a variety of role models, and the orientation of previous supervisors will influence their own style. *As a clinician,* the new supervisor has developed clinical competence in assessing and treating patients' needs and judging when to intervene. These skills can be useful in a supervisor relationship. The new supervisor has experience as a *colleague,* responding to, and interacting with, other professionals. In classrooms, they have taken clinical seminars where they have nondefensively assessed their strengths and weaknesses, provided and received feedback. New supervisors can generalize from their rich experiences to support their transition.

Role of the Fieldwork Educator or Supervisor in Mental Health

The supervisor has multiple roles:

- maintaining a contract with the academic setting and communicating with the academic fieldwork supervisor,
- facilitating the development of clinical competence through skill and knowledge development,
- facilitating professional growth in attitude and performance in the supervisee,
- shepherding the supervisee through a training process that includes standards, expectations, and evaluation,

- introducing the supervisee to the people and culture of the department and the overall setting,
- being a role model of a professional and clinically competent occupational therapist,
- being alert to the differences and conflicts that may arise in the supervisory relationship.

The last role is important specifically in a mental health setting, where therapists emphasize being sensitive to the nuances of interpersonal relationships and often urge clients to be aware of emotions that may arise. Being able to openly discuss or focus on emotions and differences, and communicating expectations clearly may be crucial to patients needs (Frum & Opacich, 1987).

Hopefully, the new supervisor will use the models presented in this chapter to assess the supervisory process and each of its elements. For example, using the Learning Style Inventory will allow a supervisor and supervisee to recognize interpersonal differences in learning and expectations that may occur in the supervisory relationship. Knowing a student's learning style will enable both the supervisor and supervisee to assess the opportunities for learning that exist at the setting and perhaps to anticipate how the setting may be lacking in experiences that match the student's learning style. Knowing the counseling psychology developmental stages may enable the supervisor to better understand and to validate the student's emotions and behavior as they relate to the stages and critical issues. The supervisor and student can both learn and anticipate the ebb and flow of the fieldwork experience. Knowing the cognitive developmental model may enable the supervisor to design specific interventions and to use specific language in the supervision process.

Tasks of the Fieldwork Educator or Supervisor

The tasks of supervision in a mental health setting are: (1) prearrival responsibilities, (2) orientation, (3) on-site assignments, (4) evaluating student performance, (5) developing fieldwork objectives, and (6) conducting supervision (Kolodner, Wiener & Frum, 1989). The fieldwork tasks can be adapted for any supervision process. (The roles and tasks of the fieldwork educator are listed in Table 20-6).

Prearrival responsibilities.   The responsibilities of the fieldwork educator include:

- working with the academic fieldwork coordinator to coordinate scheduling and gathering relevant information concerning the student,
- developing fieldwork objectives,
- developing a fieldwork manual.

Table 20-6. Roles and Tasks of the Fieldwork Educator	
Roles	**Tasks**
Contract with academic setting	Coordinate scheduling, develop objectives and a manual
Facilitating clinical competence and professional growth	Ongoing observation and evaluation and supervision
Shepherding student through fieldwork	On-site assignments
Introducing student to setting	Orientation
Role model	Consistent clinical and professional behavior
Being alert to supervisory relationship	Ongoing observation and communication, ongoing training

Orientation. Orientation includes written and verbal information and orientation sessions during the beginning two weeks of the fieldwork experience. The information should orient the student to the facility, department, and community, if necessary, and explain how the facility and its separate elements and departments operate together. Different sessions conducted by different departments can be planned in advance.

On-site assignments. Many centers have a schedule of weekly assignments that taper off after the midpoint evaluation. Many have special onetime assignments such as case studies, literature reviews, and projects. Some require students to visit other sites and to assess other delivery systems. It is highly recommended that supervisors collaborate and develop an assignment with the student, and if any projects are assigned, that only one, comprehensive assignment be required. The purpose of fieldwork education is for the student to develop as a professional and apply knowledge that has been already learned. Weekly assignments (unless necessary for certain individuals) may have the effect of keeping the fieldwork learner in a "student" performance mode and derail him or her from the business of learning to be a clinician.

Student evaluations. The student's performance should be evaluated formally at least twice, usually at the midpoint and at the completion of the fieldwork, using the official AOTA Fieldwork Performance Report (FWPR). It is recommended that the supervisor carefully go through the form with the student during the beginning two weeks of the fieldwork. At that time the supervisor can delineate those areas that are emphasized, any biases that the supervisor maintains about the performance areas, and expectations regarding the specific behaviors that are evaluated. For example, I stress the importance of verbal communication skills and will acknowledge my bias of observing verbal communication skills while being less observant with written communication skills. The supervisor should inform the supervisee of what is considered to be ideal communication and the expectations for performance of those skills at different points in the fieldwork.

Ongoing evaluation should take place throughout the fieldwork experience. Specific instances should be cited in giving feedback to the student, and a representative sample of work behavior and performance should be gathered in order to evaluate. Regular observations are recommended, particularly observations that are made immediate to a situation or behavior (AOTA, 1988).

Fieldwork objectives.   These are written statements that specify the minimal level of performance that should be attained. Although these may be verbally communicated they should be written and available for current and potential students. Objectives usually specify competency in assessment and evaluation, implementing treatment, effective written and oral communication, and the demonstration of professional characteristics (AOTA, 1988).

Supervision.   Supervisory tasks are divided into categories of skill development, personal growth, and evaluation. Personal growth is crucial in a mental health setting. Recognizing one's own behavior and how it is influenced by patients' responses will assist supervisees to better deal with clients' own interpersonal and intrapersonal struggles. Supervisors' acceptance and interpretation of patient interactions and of a supervisee's reactions and behavior with patients facilitate both personal growth and clinical competence. Overall, the supervisor should have first-hand information about the student's strength and weaknesses that is compiled from frequent observations of performance. The first-hand knowledge should be communicated regularly to help the supervisee to learn. Feedback should be constructive, timed as close to the occurrence as possible, and based on behavior.

Supervisory training.   There are various methods of learning how to be a supervisor. In addition to the resources listed in this chapter, it is recommended that individuals attend workshops and training at state, regional, and national conferences, belong to fieldwork councils associated with university programs, and seek consultation and training from academics who specialize in fieldwork supervision training

---

Summary

Supervision is valued in most health professions, particularly mental health settings. Supervisors and supervisees often have different expectations of supervision. Students look more for instruction, while supervisors emphasize the interaction and relationship. The goal of the supervisee is often to learn techniques. The supervisor's goal is to help an individual become a professional.

There are four components influencing supervision—the supervisor, the supervisee, the relationship and the interaction of the two, and the environment or setting. Supervision is a dynamic process among these components. Theoretical models of supervision have been developed from the psychoanalytic, behavioral, humanistic, and developmental schools. Supervision usually involves an eclectic blend of techniques from all of these models. An occupational therapy developmental model emphasizes the supervisee and supervisor components. A counseling psychology model emphasizes the process the supervisee goes through and the supervisory relationship. A learning styles approach emphasizes the supervisee and the setting. The transition to the role of supervisor is supported by a variety of experiences.

Review Questions

1. Describe the elements or components of supervision.
2. What have the theoretical models contributed to supervision? Which has contributed most to occupational therapy?
3. What are the similarities of the developmental models?
4. How can the learning styles contribute to supervision?
5. Of the three students in the examples and case studies, with whom are you most similar, and why? What are experiences that might be easy and those that might be difficult for you during your fieldwork experience?

Learning Activities

1. Obtain the fieldwork experience manuals and supervisory training programs offered by the American Occupational Therapy Association (see References for complete information): American Occupational Therapy Association (1988, 1991); Frum and Opacich (1987); Kolodner, Wiener, and Frum (1989).
2. Attend supervisory training sessions at the annual American Occupational Therapy Conference or at state and regional conferences.
3. Attend clinical council meetings of supervising clinicians. If there is not one in your state, start one (Still, 1982).
4. Participate in the following role-plays with classmates.
   a. Break into two groups; one group will be the supervisors and the other, the supervisees.
      i. *Supervisors*: Select a member from your group and then help design the session based on what you have learned about the models.
      ii. *Students*: Select a member from your group and then help design the session based on what you have learned about your learning style and stages.
   b. The groups together decide on a specific setting, such as a community treatment center, residential center, inpatient hospital, home health agency, or vocational program.
   c. Role-play the following situations or design your own:

      i. your first meeting.

     ii. after a group observation.

    iii. midpoint evaluation.

    iv. telling the student that the contact she had in an individual or group session was done poorly and giving suggestions for further help.

     v. discussing how and why a student's sarcastic remarks are counterproductive in a mental health setting.

References

American Occupational Therapy Association (AOTA). (1991). *Self-Paced instruction for clinical education and supervision [SPICES]: An instructional guide for clinical educators and supervisors*. Rockville, MD: Author.

American Occupational Therapy Association. (1994). Guide for supervision of occupational therapy personnel. *American Journal of Occupational Therapy, 48*, 11.

American Occupational Therapy Association. Commission on Education. (1988). *Fieldwork experience manual for academic fieldwork coordinators, fieldwork supervisors and students*. Rockville, MD: Author.

Christie, B. A., Joyce, P., & Moeller, P. L. (1985). Fieldwork experience, Part II: The supervisor's dilemma. *American Journal of Occupational Therapy, 39*(10), 675–681.

Frum, D., & Opacich, K. (1987). *Supervision: Development of therapeutic competence*. Rockville, MD: AOTA.

Hora, T. (1957). Contribution to the phenomenology of the supervisory process. *American Journal of Psychotherapy, 11*, 769–773.

Kautzmann, L. N. (1987). Perceptions of the purpose of level I fieldwork. *American Journal of Occupational Therapy, 41*(9), 595–600.

Kolb, D. (1976). Learning Style Inventory technical manual. Boston: McBer.

Kolb, D. (1984). *Experiential learning: Experience as the source of learning and development*. Englewood Cliffs, NJ: Prentice-Hall.

Kolb, D., Rubin, I., & McIntyre, J. (Eds.). (1979). *Organizational psychology: An experiential approach* (3rd ed.). Englewood Cliffs, NJ: Prentice-Hall.

Kolodner, E., Wiener, W., & Frum, D. (1989). *Models for mental health fieldwork*. Rockville, MD: AOTA.

Leddick, G., & Bernard, J. (1980, March). The history of supervision: A critical review. *Counselor Education and Supervision*, pp. 187–196.

Loganbill, C. R., Hardy, E. V., & Delworth, U. (1982). Supervision: A conceptual model. *Counseling Psychologist, 10*(1), 3–42.

Meerlo, J. A. (1952). Some psychological processes in supervision of therapists. *American Journal of Psychotherapy, 6*, 467–470.

Munroe, H. (1988). Modes of operation in clinical supervision: How clinical supervisors perceive themselves. *British Journal of Occupational Therapy, 51*(10), 338–343.

Schwartz, K. B. (1984). An approach to supervision of occupational therapy students. *American Journal of Occupational Therapy, 38,* 1033–1037.

Still, J. R. (1982). Mini-councils: A solution to fieldwork supervision. *American Journal of Occupational Therapy, 36,* 390–394.

Torrance, E., & Rockenstein, Z. (1988). Styles of thinking and creativity. In R. Schmeck (Ed.), *Learning styles and learning strategies* (pp. 275–290). New York: Plenum Press.

Suggested Reading and Other Resources

Amerantes, J. (1994). *Supervisory styles of practicing occupational therapists.* Unpublished manuscript, San Jose State University.

Cara, E. (1994, May). *Ways of supervision: The Learning Styles Inventory.* Workshop presented at the San Jose State University Fieldwork Council.

Cara, E., & Schwartz, K. (1992, Oct.). *Reflections on clinical supervision: What works, what doesn't.* Workshop presented at the Occupational Therapy Association of California, Los Angeles.

Cohn, E., & Frum, D. (1988). The issue is: Fieldwork supervision: More education is warranted. *American Journal of Occupational Therapy, 42*(5), 325–327.

Mitchell, M., & Kampfe, C. (1990). Coping strategies used by occupational therapy students during fieldwork: An exploratory study. *American Journal of Occupational Therapy, 44*(6), 543–549.

Stafford, E. (1986). Relationship between occupational therapy student learning styles and clinic performance. *American Journal of Occupational Therapy, 40*(1), 34–39.

Swinehart, S., & Meyers, S. (1993). Level I fieldwork: Creating a positive experience. *American Journal of Occupational Therapy, 47*(1), 68–73.

CHAPTER 21

Demonstrating Effectiveness in Occupational Therapy

Anne MacRae

Key Terms

articulation
collaboration
efficacy

hypothesis
networking
research

Chapter Outline

Introduction

The **efficacy** of occupational therapy (OT) has not been fully explored. Occupational therapy is a relatively young profession and, therefore, needs all members of the field to contribute to its development. The philosophy of occupational therapy is, on the surface, so simple that it tends to be taken for granted. However, the relationship between occupation and health has profound significance, and it is our responsibility to fully explore all facets of occupational therapy. Figure 21-1 suggests a number of ways in which the demonstration of efficacy may occur. It also shows that each of the methods listed—**articulation**, documentation, research, promotion, and presentation and publication—are interrelated.

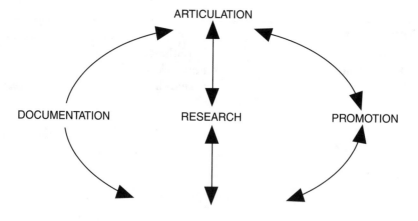

Figure 21-1. Ways of Demonstrating Efficacy in Occupational Therapy

All avenues of efficacy demonstration begin with the ability to articulate the philosophical principles and professional identity of occupational therapy. In other words, in order to show the effectiveness of OT, occupational therapists must be able to clearly express their beliefs and values in both oral and written communication. In their day-to-day lives, occupational therapists have many opportunities to share these principles. In a patient care setting, the occupational therapist will routinely represent the profession to patients, other health care professionals, administrators, and family members. This representation may be an informal conversation in a hallway or a presentation at a team or family meeting or case conference. However, in order for that sharing to be effective, the occupational therapist must have strong, confident communication skills and the ability to adapt the communication to the needs and level of understanding of others. Figure 21-2 suggests strategies for successful communication in these situations.

Descriptions of occupational therapy will vary depending on who is receiving the information and for what purpose. However, all descriptions should show a clear professional identity with identifiable goals. The recipient of the information should be able to identify the uniqueness of occupational therapy and what the occupational therapist has to offer.

Remember audience and purpose
  identify philosophical premise of treatment within the institution
  know expectations of meeting
  use shared, understandable language
Know yourself
  identify your own personal strengths and weaknesses as appropriate
  share desires for further development
  delegate and clarify roles within the OT department
Listen to others
  add, rather than duplicate, information
  be familiar with training and background of other professionals
  avoid "turf wars"
Structure Presentation
  use consistent format (based on predefined role)
  avoid repetitive or obvious information
  summarize data (technical competence and justification of services)
  interpret data (clinical competence)
Consult as needed
  refer audience to additional resources or documentation
  offer in-service education
  provide written protocols

Figure 21-2. Strategies for Successful Clinical Communication

DOCUMENTATION

Therapists often cite documentation as their least favorite job responsibility. Often it is considered a "waste of time" or meaningless paperwork. However, it serves several legal and ethical functions. Moreover, if documentation is done properly, it can be a valuable tool for increasing interdisciplinary communication and therapeutic effectiveness as well as provide a vehicle for patient and professional advocacy. According to the American Occupational Therapy Association (AOTA) (Kohlman Thompson & Foto, 1995), the purpose of documentation is:

1. provide a chronological record of the consumer's condition, which details the complete course of therapeutic intervention.
2. facilitate communication among professionals who contribute to consumer's care.
3. provide an objective basis to determine the appropriateness, effectiveness, and necessity of therapeutic intervention.
4. reflect the practitioner's reasoning.

Types of Documentation

There is tremendous variation in the forms and amount of documentation found in occupational therapy practice. However, recommended procedure includes an evaluation summary, a treatment plan, progress notes, and a discharge summary. This is typically, but not uniformly, required for reimbursement and/or institution accreditation.

Evaluation summary.   The evaluation summary can be as little as a few handwritten lines in a chart or a lengthy typed report sent to outside parties. Essentially, an evaluation summary should include an assessment of the patient's assets and deficits based on the overall evaluation process, including the results of any or all of the following: observation, interview, informal and formal assessments (nonstandardized and standardized tests), and previous chart history. Often, health care facilities have their own evaluation forms with information relevant to the treatment provided in the particular setting. In these cases, the summary is usually provided in a short narrative at the end of the form. The evaluation summary is crucial because it provides the baseline data by which the success or failure of treatment is measured.

Treatment plan.   Some treatment plans are written in the form of behavioral objectives, others are simply an added note to the evaluation form or first progress note. In some settings the actual treatment plan is only written on a form for reimbursement purposes. For example, Medicare requires a form known as a Plan of Treatment (POT). Regardless of format, all treatment plans should contain goals that realistically can be obtained in the particular setting and typical treatment time frame and should clearly represent the domain of occupational therapy. If treatment is to last for more than a couple of sessions, goals should be broken down into short and long term.

Long-term goals are developed by establishing with the patient the functional level he or she can achieve by discharge. However, in many cases, short-term goals are needed to reach the long-term goals. For example, the patient's long-term goal may be to "return home and participate independently in daily activities again." Two short-term goals, then, could be, "patient will shower and dress in clean clothing daily, independently, within one week"; and, "patient will plan and cook one meal of choice with minimum assistance from the occupational therapist within three treatment sessions." Long-term goals may be similar to major life changes, such as working in a paid job for 20 hours per week for two months, while short-term goals may be those steps in the process, such as exploring work options, participating in volunteer work or in vocational groups, and writing a resume.

Developing behavioral objectives for goals is desirable because the results are measurable and observable, thereby allowing the therapist to accurately document the outcome of treatment. Table 21-1 lists the elements of a behavioral objective and gives an example.

Progress notes. The various forms of progress notes include narratives (often called progress notes), Subjective-Objective-Assessment-Plan (SOAP) notes, Problem-Oriented Record (POR) notes, and checklists. It may be required, at least for reimbursement purposes, to chart a note following every treatment. Institutional protocol generally dictates the type of notes expected. Regardless of the type, it is expected that the professional service rendered will be stated and that an assessment of the individual's progress toward established goals will be noted.

Discharge summary. The purpose of the discharge summary is to assess the overall treatment process by stating the intervention provided, the goals met and not met (and rationale), and recommendations. Discharge summaries

Table 21-1. Elements and Sample of a Behavioral Objective

Example: Given participation in the daily grooming group, within one week, the patient will start to comb her hair without reminders prior to attending the group.

Element		
Performance (observable behavior)	Criterion (measure)	Condition (intervention)
Example		
independent hair combing	prior to group within one week	daily grooming group

are, all too often, a single line at the end of the last treatment note. This is unfortunate because if the patient goes on to receive other treatment, a well-written discharge summary can be invaluable to the new treatment team. Mechanisms should be established in every health care setting to facilitate the continuity of a patient's care by providing appropriate information. For example, it is not uncommon for a patient to transfer from an acute care hospital to a long-term facility or a day treatment center. If discharge summaries were provided at each stage of intervention, treatment could be more time efficient. Discharge summaries are often the only contact the occupational therapist may have with other professionals. Therefore, the summary can be a powerful tool for promoting occupational therapy services as well as providing input into a patient's long-term care.

Documentation Review

Skill in documentation comes primarily from practice, but even an experienced therapist can fall into bad habits. A consistent critique of documentation is necessary to insure quality. Furthermore, reviewing documentation (one's own and others) is a valuable learning tool for improving documentation skills. Documentation review is facilitated by asking the questions presented in Figure 21-3.

Treatment enhancement. Is the documentation enhancing treatment? Well-written documentation can help a therapist provide excellence in treatment as long as the descriptions are complete, with clearly stated objectives and an accurate representation of performance, strengths, and deficits. The data recorded should also follow a logical sequence, and it should be evident how a patient proceeded from point A to point B and what the next step should be. In other words, a new therapist should be able to take over treatment and proceed without repeating evaluations or treatments. In addition, documentation should not be laborious or redundant, as this robs valuable treatment time.

Understandable content. Is the content understandable to third-party readers? People who read (or should read) documentation include all members of the treatment team (medical doctors, nurses, other therapists), as well as quality assurance reviewers, clerks, and insurance providers. The content of the documentation must be clear to people with various levels and types of training. Most important, the written words must be able to tell a story on their own without the benefit of knowing the patient, setting, or situation.

Legibility. Is the document accessible and in a format that invites others to read it? Probably the most common mistake made in documentation is illegibility. However, even if one's penmanship is readable, it is of little value if the note is poorly organized or filled with grammar and spelling errors. Fur-

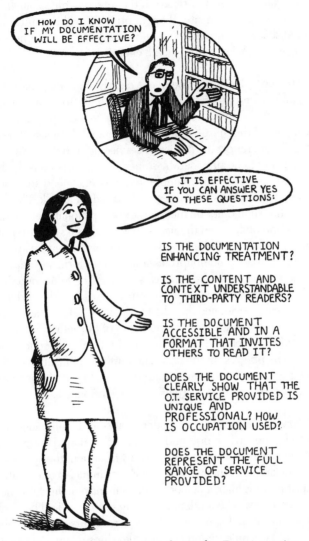

Figure 21-3.   Self-Review Questions for Quality Documentation

thermore, in this high-tech age, the format, or "packaging," is becoming more important. An evaluation or discharge summary that is well designed with clear subtitles and professional format is much more likely to be read. Another problem with notes is accessibility. That is, can the reader find the occupational therapy documentation? All charting should be placed in a clearly marked chart or subsection of a larger chart. Sometimes it is necessary to establish methods to call attention to documentation. For example, therapists may leave a note or phone message for a referring physicians, thanking them for the referral and stating that an evaluation has been completed and that they should refer to the appropriate section of the chart. If the referring physician or other interested professional is not on site, then an offer to mail the information (particularly the discharge summary) can be made, providing the necessary legal consent forms have been signed by the client.

Professional service.   Does the document clearly show that the OT service provided is unique and professional? Duplication of service and nonprofessional service are two common reasons for reimbursement denial and may lead to the occupational therapist being replaced in a job by a less expensive service. Charting should reflect the particular service offered. If the intervention is generic or likely to be provided by someone else, it is unlikely that it will be valued or reimbursed. For example, patients may need someone to give them a shower, write letters for them, or take them for a walk. These may be very real needs but should not be the focus of occupational therapy or the subsequent documentation. When the necessity of such tasks consistently interferes with meeting the established goals, the therapist can make appropriate professional referrals or train nonprofessionals to perform such tasks. On the other hand, there are situations when a task such as giving someone a shower with maximum assistance is a prelude for meeting a goal of independence in showering. In such cases, evidence that the treatment is rehabilitative rather than maintenance is required. A plan for gradation of the activity with a realistic timeline should be included in the documentation. Subsequent notes should also reflect the progress in the task. The best way to insure that documentation reflects a unique and professional service is for occupational therapists to have a clear concept of their roles and responsibilities.

Full range of service.   Does the document represent the full range of service provided? Occupational therapists perform many functions. However, therapists sometimes fall into the habit of charting only treatment they perceive as reimbursable and desirable to their employers. For example, in one treatment session, a therapist may evaluate a person's money management skills and explore new leisure activities. The tendency in many settings would be to chart only the evaluation because it is more likely to be reimbursed. The problem with this approach to documentation is that it devalues many important aspects of occupational therapy and confounds any research attempts made to determine the range, frequency, and effectiveness of OT. Certainly it is a professional responsibility to perform reimbursable service. However, it is not necessary to forfeit the integrity of occupational therapy in the process.

RESEARCH

Research is absolutely essential in the field of occupational therapy for several reasons. For one, all health care professionals, including occupational therapists, are currently being pressured by the economic market to "prove" the effectiveness of their techniques and interventions. While the need for outcome or efficacy studies is indisputable, occupational therapy also needs to continue developing its philosophical and theoretical basis, which usually implies a need for more exploratory methodologies. Both kinds of research should be encouraged in the field, and both have relevance to clinicians. Payton concurred:

> In all professions, and most especially in new and developing professions such as physical and occupational therapy, there is a continuous and urgent need to substantiate and further solidify the principles upon which clinical practice is built. There is an equally pressing need to organize those principles so that they assist the clinician in developing new principles that will improve practice. (1988, p. 207)

There appears to be a general consensus that occupational therapists should engage in clinically oriented research, especially outcome studies, and that the overall level of productivity in research must be increased (Baum, Boyle, & Edwards, 1984; Foto, 1996; Llorens & Gillette, 1985; Mann, 1985). However, occupational therapists still seem resistant to engaging in research. As more occupational therapists receive advanced degrees, the sophistication of the research and the willingness to engage in it are increasing, but it is still necessary to increase productivity in all occupational therapy clinicians. In a study conducted by Colborn, she concluded that "practitioners can be successfully involved in research given favorable conditions in the clinical work environment, as well as through a variety of educational and learning experiences" (1993, p. 699). It is important to remember that the basis of most clinical research is composed of the interview, treatment interventions, and observation, which are skills already incorporated into clinical practice. However, new technological trends may assist researchers. The most significant change in the production of research and collection of data is the advent of the computer. New technology can be tremendously useful in accessing literature and other resources, and it can be used to create a database for multipurpose analysis. However, the technology also requires that the researcher develop a whole new set of skills, including a knowledge of hardware and software, to manage the technology. As Renwick stated: "Computerized databases can facilitate several types of occupational therapy research. The value and usefulness of any database, however, is dependent on how well it has been designed" (1991, p. 827).

Another important tool for clinical research is the analysis of already existing literature. According to Bailey: "Research is any activity undertaken to increase our knowledge; it is the systematic investigation of a problem, issue, or question. This may mean reviewing all of the literature on a given topic and drawing new conclusions about that topic" (1997, p. xxi). An example of this technique is a study conducted by Henry and Coster (1996) in which the authors reviewed outcome studies in the psychiatric literature. Their purpose was to determine predictors of functional outcome among adolescents and young adults with psychotic disorders. The findings showed that premorbid functioning is the most consistent indicator of functional outcome. They therefore concluded that occupational therapists have a definitive role with this population especially in programs designed to "strengthen competence, coping skills, and social supports" (1996, p. 177).

Collaborative Research

Collaborative research is a common practice among experienced researchers, but it also has advantages for clinicians who feel they lack the necessary skills or resources to conduct research independently. **Collaboration** is especially helpful when an inexperienced researcher teams up with a mentor. A study conducted by Taylor and Mitchell "showed a strong belief in the importance of research in the profession, yet minimal involvement in research due to limited time, money, and skill. The role of collaborator with experienced researchers was rated as highly desirable" (1990, p. 350). DePoy and Gallagher (1990) suggest that an ideal collaborative team may consist of a clinician and an educator who is experienced in research methodology. Figure 21-4 presents DePoy and Gallagher's colleague model of collaborative investigation, which provides a blueprint for facilitating this kind of collaborative team. Bloomer (1995) further suggests that student fieldwork is an ideal time to engage in collaborative research, citing both the high educational value to the student and the importance of the already existing relationship between the university and the clinical community.

Another form of collaboration involves the recipient of services in the actual research design. Current day mental health practice is consumer oriented and there is a trend to include clients in the entire range of clinical, educational and research activities. Clark, Scott, and Krupa describe using this methodology in a study of client satisfaction. They concluded that "involving clients in all aspects of planning, including clinical decision-making, programme development and evaluation, and research must become a priority in order that occupational therapy remain meaningful to clients, and their treatment" (1993, p. 197).

In addition to collaboration between academics and clinicians and between clinicians and clients, there are several models of clinical team research available to occupational therapists that offer some of the same benefits as collaboration with educators.

Unidisciplinary research. Unidisciplinary research is undertaken by a team of people from the same field, such as occupational therapy, but may involve several different settings. This is an especially helpful design for occupational therapy outcome studies. Wilma West described this strategy and stated, "I feel strongly that our best hope for such documentation, with num-

Step No.	Definition	Aim	Outcome
1	Identifying a common research interest	To find a research partner	The beginning of a collaborative research relationship
2	Role taking	To enhance the collaborative relationship	An understanding of the partner's perspective
3	Planning and design	To plan clinical research to soothe clinical irritations	A carefully developed, systematic research plan
4	Negotiation	To meet individual needs and expectations and to use the skills of each collaborator efficiently	A detailed plan of the duties and payoffs for each collaborator
5	Implementation	To carry out the research plan, collect the data, and modify the plan to meet unforeseen obstacles	A completed data set for analysis
6	Completion	To analyze the data and create a format for dissemination	A publishable article, formal presentation of the findings, or both
7	Evaluation	To assess the project for strengths and weaknesses and to determine future research	A stronger collaborative research relationship

Figure 21-4. The Colleague Model of Collaborative Investigation

Source: Depoy and Gallagher (1990), p. 56.

bers that will have significance, lies in the collaborative studies that link together therapists using the same treatment strategies for patients with the same conditions" (1990, p. 10).

Multidisciplinary research. Multidisciplinary research is conducted with two or more representatives of different disciplines; however, each researcher retains his or her professional identity and generally collects data independently. An example of such a study may be a program evaluation wherein each discipline is responsible for collecting data for a certain piece of an overall program. This may include results of assessments from all the involved disciplines.

Interdisciplinary research.   Interdisciplinary research implies that researchers from different disciplines are studying the same phenomenon but each from a unique perspective. For example, researchers studying the social climate on a hospital unit or interactions within a group would use the same format for observation and record keeping, but the clinical insights would be based on the philosophy and training of each researcher. This type of study can yield a very rich description and understanding of the phenomenon, providing it is well coordinated. An added benefit of this type of study is that each member of the team has the opportunity to learn about each other's skills and perspectives.

Transdisciplinary research.   Transdisciplinary research involves multiple researchers studying the same topic and engaging in the same tasks with no regard to professional identity. For example, a group of researchers may all be interested in a single symptom, such as hallucinations, or a condition, such as homelessness. All the researchers use the same research tool. Although there is considerable role blurring in these situations and the research does not particularly show the efficacy of any single discipline, it may result in unique information about the phenomenon itself. In addition, the opportunity to work equally with an experienced team of researchers benefits occupational therapy by increasing the disciplines' knowledge base and increasing visibility of the profession in published reports. Another perceived benefit is that generally, while they are being conducted, these types of studies are viewed as client focused, whereby individual professional biases and attempts for the researcher to be self-serving are minimized.

Methods

There are many different methods used in clinical research, and it is not possible in the confines of this chapter to do justice to them. Table 21-2 provides examples of clinical research methods, but readers are also urged to explore them and other methods through additional sources (see the Suggested Reading list). Within each of these methods there are many variations. For example, life history and narrative research are specific types of case studies that have recently been introduced into the occupational therapy literature. These methods are significant for occupational therapy because they "provide the therapist with a view of the client's daily occupations, routines, family member relationships, sociocultural influences, and the effects of these factors on the delivery of occupational therapy services" (Larson & Fanchiang, 1996, p. 247).

Table 21-2. Examples of Clinical Research Methods	
Type	*Use*
Retrospective chart review and computerized databases	The basis of extensive data collection
Case studies	May be exploratory or used to examine clinical outcomes. Case studies have different designs such as descriptive or quantitatively analyzed, single subject
Specifically designed assessment tools	Clinical outcome studies or program review
Predetermined assessments	Clinical outcome studies or to establish reliability and validity of the assessment
Interview	May be transcribed and analyzed in different ways, using a phenomenological methodology or a more quantitative style, such as content analysis
Observation	The clinical basis for many types of data collection. Participant observation is usually used in ethnographic research

An example of a specifically designed assessment tool is goal attainment scaling, as described by Ottenbacher and Cusnick (1990). This tool is "a flexible evaluation methodology that can address the documentation and accountability concerns facing health care providers. Perhaps, most important, goal attainment scaling is a method that is practice based and practitioner oriented" (1990, p. 524).

Several recent research studies found in the occupational therapy literature related to mental health have focused on the reliability and validity of psychiatric OT assessment tools (Evans & Salim, 1992; Pan & Fisher, 1994; Penny, Mueser, & North, 1995). These are especially significant in this era when the profession must clearly demonstrate the value of occupational therapy in mental health care.

Although specific methods are not covered in this chapter, a discussion of general categories of methodologies is also in order. Typically, methodologies are considered either qualitative or quantitative in nature. However, many research designs can incorporate both quantitative and qualitative analysis.

Quantitative research.   Quantitative research involves many methods, but the most recognized form is the experimental method. In actuality, however, occupational therapy researchers rarely use a true experimental design. The limitations of the traditional experiment in clinical situations has been well documented in the OT literature (Campbell, 1988; Hacker, 1980a, 1980b; Ottenbacher, 1983; Ottenbacher & York, 1994). The limitations most often addressed include the difficulty of finding a suitable control group and the financial strain in a clinical environment. The researchers who support the use of quantitative methods generally seem to believe that true experiments are always desirable but not always feasible. Therefore, "recent efforts have been directed toward adaptation of traditional research models to methods suitable for the clinician with limited resources" (Hacker, 1980a, p. 103).

The most popular "adaptations" found in OT clinical research are the single-subject designs. Superficially, single-subject research is similar to the traditional case study approach. However, all data are quantified rather than described in narrative form. Furthermore, single-subject designs are considered to be an adaptation of the experimental method because "single subject research demands careful control of the variables, clearly delineated and reliable data collection and the introduction and manipulation of only one intervention at a time" (Hacker, 1980a, pp. 103–104).

There are a number of different designs used in single-study research, but "all single subject designs share features including (a) a dependent variable which will be measured repeatedly; and (b) an independent variable, which is the treatment approach that will be used" (Campbell, 1988, p. 732). In addition, most single-subject designs begin with a baseline phase where data is gathered on a subject's level of functioning without any treatment being provided.

Single-subject designs are more practical than traditional experiments for the clinician-researcher. They are less expensive to perform and generally require less time to complete. However, the limitations and concerns when using experimental methods with human beings as subjects also apply to single-subject designs. The most important consideration involves the ethical issues involved in withholding treatment during baseline periods (Hacker, 1980b). Another concern using experimental methods, including single-subject designs, is the level of therapist bias in data collection and interpretation. An automatic conflict will arise when a therapist attempts to use an experimental method, as the objectivity of the researcher is supposedly essential to the success of the method and "an essential component of occupational therapy is the use of self as therapeutic medium. This investment often brings a closeness to the client that makes maintaining objectivity difficult" (Hacker, 1980a, p. 105). Critics of the experimental method state that researcher objectivity is impossible, and all researchers must acknowledge this in their designs.

Qualitative research. Qualitative research differs philosophically from quantitative research. "The goal of quantitative methodology is to arrive at proof; therefore, it employs hypothesis testing. The goal of qualitative methodology is to provide evidence for an account of some aspect of the social world. Therefore, it employs a heuristic strategy of generating explanations, weighing evidence, and revising explanations to match new evidence" (Kielhofner,

1982, p. 71). Quantitative research is generally designed to test a specific **hypothesis**; qualitative research is meant to be a discovery or exploratory process in the development of theories (Merrill, 1985). Therefore, if the objective of clinical research in occupational therapy is to demonstrate the efficacy of specific treatment techniques, qualitative research is probably not appropriate. However, qualitative research does have its place in clinical research.

> Occupational therapy concepts generally are so nonspecific that the profession needs to give far greater emphasis to descriptive research than to experimental research at this stage. . . . Researchers cannot begin to manipulate variables until the important variables have been clearly defined and described. (Yerxa, 1988, p. 174)

Often what is needed in clinical studies is richer, more complete, clinical descriptions in order to refine and appropriately use quantitative studies at a later date.

Unlike in quantitative research, it is not necessary for a researcher to have a sophisticated knowledge of statistics in order to utilize any of the qualitative designs. However, it is a mistake to assume that qualitative research is less difficult.

> Most seasoned researchers agree that the methods and rules for qualitative research, if done well, are more difficult to follow than procedures for randomization of groups to treatments and controls, counterbalancing and blinding research designs, and some of the other techniques common to quantitative research. (Philips & Pierson, 1982, p. 168)

In summary, qualitative research is used to gather data for detailed descriptions of situations, events, people, and observed behavior (Merrill, 1985). It is especially appropriate for research into areas where little is known or understood about the phenomena to be studied or the concepts involved are not easily reduced to numerical values.

Both quantitative and qualitative research designs have their place in clinical settings, and each has specific benefits and limitations. Furthermore, it seems quite obvious that the choice of designs should be based on the particular subject to be studied. However, it is also obvious that researchers make decisions regarding design for a multitude of reasons having nothing to do with the research question. The considerations most often cited include ease of publication, prestige, funding, and (perceived) ease of analysis, as well as a simple lack of knowledge regarding possible research designs. In clinical professions, particularly developing ones such as occupational therapy, it is vitally important that the choice of research design be based on a thorough understanding of the characteristics of each design.

PROMOTION

Promotion is often negatively thought of as a self-serving mechanism of "selling" oneself. However, promotion is necessary to insure that significant contributions are known and available to the people who may benefit from the services. How this is accomplished is varied, but all occupational therapists share the responsibility of promoting the profession and should be versed in a variety of communication techniques, including multimedia.

At the 1992 AOTA National Conference in Houston, Texas, Lang, Kannenberg, and Brinson identified a number of ways in which occupational therapists can promote occupational therapy in mental health. Figure 21-5 is made up of suggestions based on their presentation. In addition to these suggestions, which are primarily geared toward practicing clinicians, it should be noted that the universities' programs and professional associations also have major roles in the promotion of occupational therapy in mental health.

A serious mistake often made by well-meaning promoters is attempting to undermine the integrity and skills of other professionals. The promotion of occupational therapy does not need to be accomplished by competition, and in fact, that approach is often counterproductive. Health care professionals quite often work in teams, and health care delivery improves significantly when the team has open lines of communication, is well coordinated, and is based on mutual respect and understanding of each other's roles. Interprofessional colleagues are an underutilized resource and can be powerful allies for promotion, providing we, as occupational therapists, are willing to advocate for them in a client-centered fashion.

If one keeps in mind that the purpose of promotion is ultimately to provide the best client service possible, then cooperation among the disciplines is optimum. One way to facilitate such cooperation is by forming interdisciplinary coalitions among service providers and agencies for the purposes of **networking**. According to Hurff, Lowe, Ho, and Hoffman, "the process of networking has extended and strengthened our individual professional efforts. A wealth of ideas has emerged from our relationships with one another" (1990, p. 430). Hurff and colleagues state that networking is especially needed in response to the trend towards community rather than hospital based treatment. They also report that through their networking efforts "they extended the role of occupational therapy into nontraditional settings" (1990, p. 424). Networks among mental health occupational therapists and interdisciplinary mental health coalitions are currently operating in several regions of the United States. Among them is the Psychiatric Occupational Therapy Action Coalition (POTAC) of the San Francisco Bay area in California. Members of this group are involved with projects such as lobbying for mental health resources, research and publication, advocacy, program development, education, and publicity (Dressler & MacRae, in press).

Communicate

Formulate a clear, simple definition of occupational therapy.
Write an article about occupational therapy for an agency newsletter.
Offer to hold an event sponsored by a nonprofit mental health agency.
Place visual media about the OT process and outcomes in the workplace.
Provide clients with pamphlets about OT in mental health.
Emphasize something about OT in business cards and stationery.

Educate others

Take a physician or other health care provider to lunch.
Volunteer to speak at a community center.
Mentor an OT student who shows a special interest in mental health.
Provide ongoing in-service training for new employees and interns.
Write letters to the editors of newspapers and magazines in response to health-related articles.
Write nondefensive, helpful letters to media personnel who misrepresent occupational therapy.
Speak at your local school district at a career day.

Educate yourself

Attend continuing education classes.
Tour other facilities that have occupational therapy.
Read the mental health professional literature, both within and outside occupational therapy.

Participate

Join your local, state, and national professional organizations.
Consider membership in non-OT organizations with shared interests.
Meet with representatives of the government, insurance companies, and legal agencies involved with mental health.
Collaborate with a consumer-oriented group on community-oriented projects.
Support and encourage occupational therapists who are pioneering programming in nontraditional areas.

Have a positive attitude

Make sure you are not talking down to people.
Convey enthusiasm about mental health to students and interns.
Remember that first impressions count.
Do not be defensive.
Display a positive, energetic, open, and nonjudgmental attitude.
Do not be apologetic about practicing psychiatric occupational therapy.

Figure 21-5. Simple Things You Can Do to Promote Occupational Therapy in Mental Health

Source: From Lang et al., 1992.

PRESENTATION AND PUBLICATION

The culmination of the demonstration of effectiveness involves disseminating the information that has been gathered and articulated. Without presentations and publications, any knowledge and insights gained through articulation, documentation, research, and promotion will, at best, only be meaningful on a local level. Too often, valuable clinical information does not get shared, creating a situation whereby occupational therapists are constantly "reinventing the wheel."

Presentations are typically given at conferences, which may be local, regional, national, or international. Formats also range from posters, papers, and workshops to symposiums, seminars, roundtables, and institutes. The choice of type of presentation depends on the level of skill and experience of the presenter, the depth of the information to be presented, and the type of information. For example, a poster can relay much visual information quickly but cannot provide a significant depth of process and theory. Posters are also limited in the scope of information that can be presented. Some presentations require an experiential or interactive component that does not fit well with a usual paper presentation format. These are more appropriate for workshops.

Another decision that applies to both presentations and publications is choosing the audience. There are advantages and disadvantages with each choice, and potential presenters should think carefully about their goals. Intraprofessional presentations and publications are essential to the growth and continuing education of occupational therapy, but there are also advantages to going outside the profession to share with others. Occupational therapists should consider publications and conferences of other related fields or interdisciplinary arenas. In the field of mental health, there is also an increasing number of journals and conferences sponsored by nonprofessional groups such as the Alliance for the Mentally Ill (AMI), which are geared toward client and family advocacy. These arenas provide excellent opportunities for occupational therapists to share their expertise and learn from others.

Publication can be an intimidating process for the novice. Many of the same suggestions for collaborative research apply to the publication process. It is especially helpful to have a mentor if this is a first attempt at publishing a paper. Figure 21-6 provides guidelines for the publication process.

Summary

Clear definitions and descriptions of occupational therapy services are essential for professional survival in these difficult times. This chapter provided guidelines for occupational therapists to articulate, document, research, and promote the profession of occupational therapy. In order to complete the process of demonstrating effectiveness, it is essential that occupational ther-

Getting Started
    pick a topic
    choose a journal
    determine authorship (single author versus joint authorship; primary and
        secondary authors)
    write an outline
    seek advice
    contact the editor

Clinically Oriented Topics
    evaluation procedures
    application of theory
    specific techniques of treatment
    unique aspects of a treatment setting
    OT role (traditional and nontraditional)
    peripheral topics (controversies and politics)

Components of Publishable Papers
    statement of the issue or problem
    background
    critical review of the literature
    data — statistical and descriptive
    case study and other types of examples
    graphics: tables, charts, figures, photographs
    discussion and recommendations

Article Submission
    author guidelines
    hard copy and computer disk (sometimes requested by editor)
    time line
    rejection, revision, acceptance

Figure 21-6. Guidelines for the Publication Process

apists present and publish the results of these efforts. Diligence is necessary to ensure that the unique and valuable contributions of occupational therapy to the field of mental health are recognized. Lela Llorens provided a synopsis of this diligence and a vision of the future for occupational therapy with the following statement (1984, p. 34):

- It is time for commitment to the science of occupational therapy and to the verification of occupational therapy theory.

- It is time for commitment to understanding and articulating the clinical reasoning process.

- It is time for commitment to the ownership of the meaning of occupation and activity, and the responsibility to explain the phenomena.

- It is time for commitment to unity of the profession.
- It is time for commitment to proactive professional management and publicly claiming the legacy of health through occupation.
- It is time for commitment to the habilitation and rehabilitation of clients in both clinical and community settings and to the quality of life beyond the role of medicine in the client's care.
- It is time for commitment to bridging the gap between the level of knowledge, theory, development, and practice as a vital part of our heritage.
- It is time for commitment to our belief in the poetry and value of the commonplace.

Review Questions

1. How does the articulation of occupational therapy demonstrate its efficacy?
2. How can occupational therapists enhance the effectiveness of their documentation?
3. What are the barriers for clinicians conducting research?
4. What skills does an occupational therapist need to effectively promote occupational therapy?
5. What are the pros and cons of collaboration in research and publication?

Learning Activities

1. This chapter mentioned the necessity of adapting the description of OT to fit the audience. Develop your own descriptions of OT based on what you would tell the following people and discuss methods of presentation that you would use in each situation.
   a. A patient with a some cognitive impairment in abstraction and memory.
   b. Parents who just recently began to understand the severity of their son's severe mental illness.
   c. A representative of a large insurance carrier questioning billing procedures of OT.
   d. A physician responsible for referrals to your agency.
   e. The administrator of a managed care health facility who is considering whether to fund an OT position.
2. For the situations described in question 1a and 1b, write a progress note describing your intervention.
3. Write a short information article describing an aspect of occupational therapy for one of the following publications:
   a. a special interest section newsletter of AOTA

b. a local OT publication such as a state association or chapter newsletter
c. A hospital newsletter
d. a neighborhood newspaper
4. Locate the author guidelines for at least one OT journal and one non-OT journal related to psychology or psychiatry. Think about how a chosen topic could be articulated using these guidelines and write an outline of a potential publishable paper.
5. Locate the guidelines for submission of a research grant and follow the same procedure as activity (4).
6. Locate a call for papers for a conference presentation and follow the same procedure as activity (4).

References

Bailey, D. (1997). *Research for the health professional* (2nd ed.). Philadelphia: F. A. Davis.

Baum, C., Boyle, M., & Edwards, D. (1984). Initiating occupational therapy clinical research. *American Journal of Occupational Therapy, 38*, 267–269.

Bloomer, J. (1995). Applied research during fieldwork: Interdisciplinary collaboration between universities and clinics. *American Journal of Occupational Therapy, 49*, 207–213.

Campbell, P. (1988). Using a single subject research design to evaluate the effectiveness of treatment. *American Journal of Occupational Therapy, 42*, 732–737.

Clark, C., Scott, E., & Krupa, T. (1993). Involving clients in programme evaluation and research: A new methodology for occupational therapy. *Canadian Journal of Occupational Therapy, 60*(4), 192–199.

Colborn, A. (1993). Combining practice and research. *American Journal of Occupational Therapy, 47*, 693–703.

Depoy, E., & Gallagher, C. (1990). Steps in collaborative research between clinicians and faculty. *American Journal of Occupational Therapy, 44*(1), 55–59.

Dressler, J., & MacRae, A. (In press). Advocacy, partnerships, and client centered practice. *Occupational Therapy in Mental Health*.

Evans, J., & Salim, A. (1992). A cross-cultural test of the validity of occupational therapy assessments with patients with schizophrenia. *American Journal of Occupational Therapy, 46*, 685–695.

Foto, M. (1996). Outcome studies: The what, why, how, and when. *American Journal of Occupational Therapy, 50*, 87–88.

Hacker, B. (1980a). Single subject research strategies in occupational therapy, Part I. *American Journal of Occupational Therapy, 34*, 103–108.

Hacker, B. (1980b). Single subject research strategies in occupational therapy, Part 2. *American Journal of Occupational Therapy, 34*, 169–175.

Henry, A., & Coster, W. (1996). Predictors of functional outcome among adolescents and young adults with psychotic disorders. *American Journal of Occupational Therapy, 50,* 171–181.

Hurff, J., Lowe, H., Ho, B., & Hoffman, N. (1990). Networking: A successful linkage for community occupational therapy. *American Journal of Occupational Therapy, 44,* 424–430.

Kielhofner, G. (1982). Qualitative research: Part I: Paradigmatic grounds and issues of reliability and validity. *Occupational Therapy Journal of Research,* 2 (2), 67–79.

Kohlman Thompson, L., & Foto, M. (1995). *Elements of clinical documentation.* Bethesda, MD: American Occupational Therapy Association (AOTA).

Lang, S., Kannenberg, K., & Brinson, M. (1992). *50 simple things you can do to promote occupational therapy in mental health.* American Occupational Therapy Association.

Larson, E., & Fanchiang, S. (1996). Nationally speaking—Life history and narrative research: Generating a humanistic knowledge base for occupational therapy. *American Journal of Occupational Therapy, 50,* 247–250.

Llorens, L. (1984). Changing balance: Environment and individual. *American Journal of Occupational Therapy, 38* (1), 29–34.

Llorens, L., & Gillette, N. (1985). Nationally speaking—The challenge for research in a practice based profession. *American Journal of Occupational Therapy, 39 (3),* 143–145.

Mann, W. (1985). Survey methods. *American Journal of Occupational Therapy, 39,* 640–648.

Merrill, S. (1985). Qualitative methods in occupational therapy research: An application. *Occupational Therapy Journal of Research, 5*(4), 209–221.

Ottenbacher, K. (1983). Quantitative reviewing: The literature review as scientific inquiry. *American Journal of Occupational Therapy, 37,* 313–319.

Ottenbacher, K., & Cusnick, A. (1990). Goal attainment scaling as a method of clinical service evaluation. *American Journal of Occupational Therapy, 44,* 519–525.

Ottenbacher, K., & York, J. (1984). Strategies for evaluating clinical change: Implication for practice and research. *American Journal of Occupational Therapy, 38,* 647–659.

Pan, A., & Fisher, A. (1994). The assessment of motor and process skills of persons with psychiatric disorders. *American Journal of Occupational Therapy, 48,* 775–782.

Payton, O. (1988). *Research: The validation of clinical practice* (2nd ed.). Philadelphia: F. A. Davis.

Penny, N., Mueser, C., & North, C. T. (1995). The Allen Cognitive Level Test and social competence in adult psychiatric patients. *American Journal of Occupational Therapy, 49,* 420–427.

Philips, B., & Pierson, W. (1982). Qualitative research on occupational therapy. *Occupational Therapy Journal of Research, 2*(3), 165–170.

Renwick, R. (1991). A model for database design. *American Journal of Occupational Therapy, 45*(9), 827–832.

Taylor, E., & Mitchell, M. (1990). Research attitudes and activities of occupational therapy clinicians. *American Journal of Occupational Therapy, 44*, 350–355.

West, W. (1990). Perspectives on the past and future, Part 2. *American Journal of Occupational Therapy, 44*(1), 9–10.

Yerxa, E. (1988). Research in occupational therapy. In H. Hopkins & H. Smith (Eds.), *Willard and Spackman's occupational therapy* (7th ed., pp. 171–177). Philadelphia: Lippincott.

Suggested Reading

Acquaviva, J. (1992). *Effective documentation for occupational therapy.* Rockville, MD: American Occupational Therapy Association (AOTA).

Cottrell, R. (Ed.). (1993). *Psychosocial occupational therapy: Proactive approaches.* Rockville, MD: AOTA.

Cottrell, R. (Ed.). (1996). *Perspectives on purposeful activity: Foundations and future of occupational therapy.* Bethesda, MD.: AOTA.

Denton, P. (1987). *Psychiatric occupational therapy: A workbook of practical skills.* Boston: Little, Brown.

Depoy, E., & Gitlin, L. N. (1994). *Introduction to research: Multiple strategies for health and human services.* St. Louis: Mosby–Year Book.

Frank, G. (1996). Life histories in occupational therapy clinical practice. *American Journal of Occupational Therapy, 50*, 251–264.

Kettenbach, G. (1990). *Writing SOAP notes.* Philadelphia: F. A. Davis.

Ostrow, P., & Kaplan, K. (Eds.). (1987). *Occupational therapy in mental health: A guide to outcomes research.* Rockville, MD: AOTA.

Polkinghorne, D. (1988). *Narrative knowing and the human sciences.* Albany, NY: State University of New York Press.

Weiss-Lambrou, R. (1989). *The health professional's guide to writing for publication.* Springfield, IL: Charles C. Thomas.

Glossary

Abreaction—an emotional release usually accompanied by vivid recall and the apparent reliving of a painful experience that had been repressed because it was consciously intolerable.

Accommodation—the process by which a pattern of behavior is altered to fit a new environmental reality or condition.

Acting out—expression of thoughts and feelings through maladaptive behavior instead of recognizing and verbalizing thoughts and feelings.

Activity group—one whose content focuses on activity, emphasizes occupation, and addresses occupational performance components or skills to aid in occupational performance.

Acute hospitalization—an admission to a hospital usually for a sudden and serious condition. The purpose of admission is for diagnosis and/or treatment of a medical condition which requires the attention of many health professionals and the use of equipment not available for home or office use.

Adaptive response—an effort to change behavior in response to a demand perceived as internal or from the environment; implies an adjustment or "course correction" in response to a stimulus that is different in some way from that previously encountered.

Adjudication—the multi-stepped process of coming to a judicial decision or sentence by going through criminal court proceedings.

Advocacy—speaking or writing in support of someone or something such as the rights of persons with mental illness.

Agnosia—failure of recognition that is not due to sensory loss. Often seen as an inability to identify objects and recognize familiar faces.

AIDS—Acquired Immune Deficiency Syndrome; the final stage of HIV infection, as evidenced by a positive HIV test, a T-cell count less than 200, and/or the presence of certain clinical syndromes or opportunistic infections.

Alliance for the Mentally Ill (AMI)—a grass-roots organization of families and significant others of people with serious mental illness. Members meet at the national (NAMI), state, and local levels, to provide education, support and advocacy.

Alter personality—an entity, sometimes described as a discrete state of consciousness, with a sense of self and a characteristic pattern of feelings and behavior, though not a separate person. (Used of a person with dissociative identity or multiple personality disorder.)

Americans with Disabilities Act (1990)—a federal law that provides for equal access and opportunity to all qualified individuals with disabilities in the areas of employment (Title I), equal access to public services (Title II), physical access to public facilities and transportation (Title III), and communications (Title IV) (EEOC, U.S. Dept. of Justice, 1991).

Apraxia—loss of ability to conceptualize, organize and execute complex learned motor tasks; one type may be seen as an inability to dress oneself.

Articulation—the process of conveying thoughts and meanings in a coherent and understandable form that can be applied to all forms of spoken and written communication.

Autogenic training—a relaxation program that teaches people to respond physically and mentally to their own verbal commands.

Autonomy—self-determination and independence. The process of becoming autonomous is characterized by a gradual reduction in dependency and steady movement toward ever-greater independence. The process of and timing for becoming autonomous are largely determined by the cultural context of the family.

Benzodiazapenes—a group of medications which act as sedatives and are commonly used for treatment of anxiety.

Biopsychosocial focus—the theoretical paradigm that aims to provide the most comprehensive understanding of the development of normal and abnormal behavior by exploring the interaction among biological, psychological, and social influences on behavior.

Caregiver—family member, health professional individual, attendant, or any other person who provides care to a dependent or partially dependent individual.

Client-driven services—coming from a social rehabilitation perspective. Services are often considered in the language of the client and what the client wants in terms of treatment and support. The goals of treatment are stated in the client's words, and treatment must meet these goals with relevant treatment and service plans. The client is the customer and drives the service sector.

Codependency—a set of unhealthy characteristics and coping styles that are often adopted by family members to deal with an addicted individual.

Cognitive deficits—a broad range of impairments, including but not limited to actual intelligence. In schizophrenia, the common cognitive deficits include poor judgment and reasoning, impulsivity, limited ability to abstract, and delayed processing time.

Collaboration—working together. This implies a greater amount of active interaction than cooperation, which may merely mean not interfering with each other. There is an expectation that people working in collaboration are helping each other produce an end or reach a common goal.

Commitment—court-ordered consignment to a mental institution.

Compulsions—repetitive and deliberate actions intended to diminish obsessions.

Conservator—the person legally designated to make decisions regarding medical issues, legal matters, housing and finances, for an individual who is impaired by a mental illness. The primary purpose of appointing a conservator is to protect the client from abuse or exploitation.

Consistency—the routine, reliable aspects of treatment that develop trust and reliance in the human and non-human environment.

Consumer/client empowerment—the client, not the service providers, makes all decisions and directs the process.

Consumers' movement—refers to patients/clients/consumers of mental health services who meet for support, education, and advocacy. They are organized in most communities and are advocates of research and humane treatment.

Crack babies—children whose development is adversely affected due to birth mother's use of cocaine during pregnancy.

Cross-dependency—the tendency of individuals who are addicted to or abusing one substance to abuse other substances, for example, alcohol to tranquilizers.

Culture—a conscious and unconscious internal process of identification with overt manifestations of traditions, beliefs, and values, often involving the use of objects, which guide human beings in organizing their lives.

Cyclothymia—a DSM-IV diagnosis that includes symptoms of mania, but is considered less severe than bipolar disorder.

Decompensation—the process whereby an individual with a mental illness loses the ability to maintain normal or appropriate compensatory functions; the individual loses touch with reality.

Defenses—unconscious mental strategy that psychologically protect the individual; for example, denial, rationalization, compliance.

Deinstitutionalization—the process which released large numbers of persons with mental illness from state institutions into the community.

Depersonalization—feelings of unreality.

Depression—a clinical term, ambiguous in general use; used to refer to a mood, a symptom, and a disease entity. As a symptom, it could be replaced with sadness. In Chapter 10 its use is restricted to a syndrome or disorder.

Derealization—feeling detached from one's surroundings.

Diagnosis—the result of a process of elimination in which a disorder is identified by meeting very specific criteria including demographic information such as age, as well as range, severity and duration of symptoms.

Dissociation—an alteration in a person's thoughts, feelings, sensations and actions, so that certain information is not consciously integrated.

DSM—the Diagnostic and Statistical Manual of Mental Disorders published by the American Psychiatric Association (APA). The third edition, known as DSM-III, was published in 1980 and contained a significantly different multiaxial format from earlier editions, allowing for more complete diagnostic descriptions. The current edition, the DSM-IV, was published in 1994 and continues to use a multiaxial format.

Dual diagnosis—a situation in which a person has two distinct diagnoses that require different treatment. Often applied to individuals diagnosed with both mental illness and substance abuse, but equally applicable as it is used in Chapter 7 to the presence of a psychiatric condition concurrent with a physical disability or illness.

Dynamic—a way of interacting between or among people; generally applied to a pattern of relating that is not explicitly or consciously acknowledged.

Dynamical systems theory—the view that new and unpredictable states of organization arise spontaneously within a system when sufficient energy flows through it.

Dysfunction—a deficit in the ability to perform tasks. It is often a result of effects of symptoms but there is not always a direct correlation. Occupational therapists view these deficits in a function/dysfunction continuum in the realm of occupational performance which includes work, leisure and self-care activities.

Dysthymia—a DSM-IV diagnosis that includes symptoms of major depression, but is considered less severe than major depression.

Eclectic—generally, made up of the best elements selected from a variety of sources. Used to refer to theorists and practitioners who do not adhere to any one system of beliefs, but who select and utilize what they consider to be the best elements of many different theories in their attempts to understand and treat aberrant behavior and psychological dysfunction.

Efficacy—effectiveness, or the power to produce effects or intended results.

Ego strength—a psychoanalytic term that has become a popular term for the ability to accurately and appropriately deal with reality adaptively, such as through the use of coping skills.

Ego-syntonic—not disturbing to the ego; generally applied to disordered traits or patterns that would usually be disturbing.

Enabling—behaviors, usually practiced by family and friends, that inadvertently reinforce the destructive habits of the substance abuser.

Executive functions—capacities that allow a person to engage in productive, self-serving and purposeful activities which include abilities to plan, sequence, manage time, initiate, think abstractly, monitor and control behavior.

Expectant treatment—the reliance on the natural healing process for improvement in a condition. The therapist selects routine tasks that are sensitive to the expected changes, observes the patient's behavior, and reports the observations.

Forensics—the science that deals with the interface between the practice of medicine and the law. In Chapter 17 the discussion of forensics is limited to the interface between mental illness and the criminal justice system.

General systems theory—the view that the universe is a whole composed of interconnected parts and that all phenomena belong to this larger whole and share similar properties.

Group—2 or more people who have a consciousness that they are a group. An intentional gathering of people for the purpose of change.

Group content—activity carried out in the group; what is said in the group. It can be verbal and non-verbal.

Group dynamics—the forces which influence the relationships of members and influence the group outcome (Cole, 1993).

Group process—how the work of the group is carried out, including how participants relate to each other, who talks to whom, how tasks are accomplished and how decisions are made and how therapy is undertaken; patterns or stages that groups usually go through.

Group protocol—a description of a group, including its purpose, goals, content, structure, logistics, who and who would not benefit by participation in it, and referral process.

Group structure—the way in which the activity is presented, the directions, procedures, techniques and time arrangements, and the way in which membership is organized.

"Hardwired"—an expression originating in computer science that designates an innate biological structure.

HIV—Human Immunodeficiency Virus; the causative agent of a syndrome characterized by a progressive, gradual, irreversible, and disabling deterioration of the human immune system, which renders the host susceptible to a wide range of opportunistic infections and other clinical syndromes. HIV disease is any stage of the disease caused by infection with HIV, including AIDS.

Host personality—the personality that has executive control of the body the greatest percentage of time (in a person with dissociative identity disorder).

Hypothesis—a logical assumption, reasonable guess or an educated conjecture that gives direction to research.

Identified patient (ip)—a term used to indicate the individual within the family system for whom the family is seeking treatment.

Incarceration—confinement in a jail, prison or a forensic state hospital.

Individuation—the process by which the developing child comes to recognize him- or herself as distinct from parent(s) and the surrounding environment; may also be used to refer to the process of becoming a unique individual.

Interpersonal—referring to external psychological processes, usually observable in an interaction between two or more people.

Intrapersonal—referring to the internal psychological processes and experience of a person. It is not observable and can be understood only through the explanation of the person.

In vivo—a Latin term referring to any treatment or intervention which occurs within a client's natural environment ("in real life"), rather than in the artificial or simulated environment of a hospital, clinic, or laboratory setting.

Jail—a correctional facility where individuals are confined while awaiting trial, or a correctional facility where those with a sentence of one year or less are confined.

Job coaching—a service whereby assistance is given in any or all of the phases of the supported employment (SE) approach; e.g., skills training, job modifications, employee/employer interventions, and ongoing support.

Latency age—between the ages of about five and twelve. In Freudian theory, the stage when both sexual and aggressive drives and impulses are latent, or hidden and subdued.

Limit—a boundary , restriction or rule that defines acceptable behavior.

Mania—a mood that is elevated, expansive, or irritable. Associated symptoms are hyperactivity, pressured speech, flight of ideas, diminished need for sleep, grandiosity, distractibility, short attention span, and extremely poor judgment in interpersonal and social areas.

Medicaid—the federal health insurance program for low-income United States residents.

Melancholia—as an emotional symptom, it is detachment, alienation, sadness, apathy, and dejection. Formerly used as a clinical term to describe the mental disorder of depression.

Memory—The ability to store and recall thoughts. This ability is crucial to acquiring new information and is highly influential on everyday functioning.

Mentor—a wise and trusted counselor, instructor, guide, coach, or advisor.

Meta-models—all-encompassing generic models that can be used in any area of practice or practice setting. They serve to unite a discipline with common language and purpose.

Mode—method, approach, strategy, or procedure for learning.

Mood—emotional state that usually colors one's whole psychological life.

Multiple personality disorder—the name for the clinical diagnosis of Dissociative Identity Disorder, prior to DSM-IV (APA, 1994). This is still a popularly used term.

Negative symptoms—absent or decreased emotional and behavioral repertoire. Includes flat affect, alogia (poverty of speech), avolition (poor initiation of activities and/or inability to sustain goal-directed activities), and anhedonia or hypohedonia (inability or decreased ability to experience pleasure).

Networking—the process by which individuals and agencies link together for the purposes of sharing information, providing support and working towards a common goal.

Obsessions—intrusive ideas, images, thoughts, and impulses that persist.

Occupation—the ordinary tasks of human existence in which people create their self-image and identity and organize their lives.

Occupational activity—a discrete activity that is occupational in that it is active, meaningful and process-oriented, with a tangible or intangible product.

Occupational readiness—characterizing skill-based activities and other such interventions that focus on change in the person in preparation for occupational activities. These include specific techniques, instruction, and assistive devices.

Open systems theory—the view that all living organisms maintain a constant interaction with the environment and are dynamic, self-organizing structures. (See General systems theory.)

Opportunistic infection—an infection or disease that proliferates in the presence of a compromised immune system (e.g.

pneumocystis carinii pneumonia, candidiasis, toxoplasmosis). The causal agents may exist naturally in the environment and/or body, but remain benign when governed by a healthy immune system.

Organizational abilities—taking all the steps necessary to establish and carry out a goal: setting priorities, scheduling time, arranging people and things, sequencing events, and identifying and gathering appropriate resources, tools and materials (Mosey, 1986).

Out—in dissociative identity disorder, when an alter has taken over the executive control of the body, or is present in the world as opposed to inside one's head, it is said to be "out".

Outed—having been made public; of the process by which private information about an individual of a potentially sensitive nature (usually sexual orientation and/or HIV status) becomes public knowledge without the individual's consent.

Paradigm—a theoretical framework or model that arises out of a specific set of basic assumptions.

Parallel process—of the dynamic between patient and therapist, and between therapist and clinical supervisor; the therapist identifies with the patient and then elicits emotions in the supervisor which he/she has experienced with the patient.

Parallel task group—one in which individuals work on individual tasks in the presence of others, but not necessarily with the others (Mosey, 1970, 1973).

Personality—style of relating, coping, behaving, thinking and feeling. A concept that represents a network of traits that persist over a lifetime. "A deeply embedded system of inclinations and psychological characteristics that are not easily altered" (Retzlaff, 1995, p. 25). The older term character includes a moral judgment.

Personhood skills—a term used by Corey and Corey (1992) to describe skills that depend on personal traits acquired through a combination of temperament and experience.

Positive symptoms—the active symptoms of psychotic disorders, including delusions and hallucinations as well as disorganized speech and behavior.

Preferred defense structure—those defenses preferred by a particular individual, in addition to other skills, abilities and strategies, to form the basis for psychological survival.

Prevocational services—services that provide structured activities which assist individuals to learn basic self-care skills, habits, and routines critical to developing work behaviors.

Prison—a correctional facility where sentences in excess of one year are served.

Prodromal symptoms—those which typically appear prior to onset of a psychiatric disorder or relapse.

Psychiatric rehabilitation—the use of various interdisciplinary interventions aimed at restoring function and role performance. The goal is to assist people with severe mental disabilities to function at their highest potential, in their environment of choice, with the least amount of professional support necessary. Interventions focus on changing environmental supports and/or skills within a framework that emphasizes personal assets, strengths, and the ability to change (Cook and Hoffschmidt, 1993); (Anthony and Blanch, 1987).

Psychodynamic—of a therapeutic process in which change is brought about primarily by talking and reflecting on one's thoughts and actions, and by a therapist's or group leader's interpretations. It assumes an unconscious process.

Psychoeducational—of a therapeutic process in which change is brought about by learning or through education, usually about a psychological topic. There is a clear objective to teach specific information or techniques.

Psychogenic—originating in the mind or in mental processes.

Psychopathology—from the Greek, meaning "the study of mind or brain disease." It refers to the study and classification of symptoms; can characterize a condition as a mental disorder.

Psychosis—significant impairment of reality testing and daily functioning due to the presence of positive symptoms.

Psychotropic—a descriptor for an agent, usually a prescribed drug, that directly affects the actions of the brain.

Recovery—a process of active sobriety maintenance through using support such as AA (Alcoholics Anonymous) groups, increasing awareness of use patterns, and active relapse prevention planning.

Referential thinking—ideas of reference, or the feeling that casual incidents and events have an unusual or particular meaning specific to the person (APA, 1994).

Relative mastery—the extent to which the person experiences the occupational response as efficient, effective, and satisfying to self and society.

Research—systematic and careful investigation that requires gathering and analyzing of data in order to establish facts and principles, or add to a general body of knowledge.

Respite care—Intermittent provision of services that provide temporary relief for the caregivers of a partially or completely incapacitated individual.

Roles—configurations of statuses, activities, expectations and responsibilities that persons hold in a particular social context. Occupational roles are distinct functions played by the individual; e.g., parent, student, sister, daughter.

Schizophrenogenic mother—now outdated term applied during the 1950s and 60s to mothers of children who had mental illness. It was thought that the environment and, more specifically, the parenting in which one grew up was the cause of mental illness.

Seroconversion—refers to an individual's change in status from HIV negative to HIV positive by the development of HIV antibodies in the blood.

Sobriety—abstinence from drugs and alcohol.

Splitting—a psychoanalytic concept, considered a defense, that causes an individual to perceive people as either all good or all bad and be unable to acknowledge both negative and positive features in one person. Resulting behavior may correlate with destabilizing relationships among staff members.

Structure—providing a form and design for treatment (Abramson, 1982).

Style—inclination to use the same adaptive strategies in various situations. A stable, consistent approach to attending, perceiving and thinking. Cognitive style or orientation.

Substance abuse—use of substances (usually drugs or alcohol) that have been harmful or are potentially harmful.

Substance addiction/dependence—the prolonged, chronic, excessive, compulsive use of a substance which is harmful and characterized by physical tolerance and psychological dependency.

Supervision—"a process in which two or more people participate in a joint effort to promote, establish, maintain and/or elevate a level of performance and service" (AOTA, 1994).

Supported education—similar to supported employment (SE), assisting a person to develop the community resources needed to pursue his or her educational and career goals.

Supported employment (SE)—an approach grounded in psychiatric/psychosocial rehabilitation that assists a person to choose, get, and keep a job. It is often referred to as the Choose, Get, Keep approach.

Switching—a term used to describe when a person with dissociative identity disorder changes from one personality to a different one, usually from the host to an alter personality.

Symptom—a subjective experience of the individual, such as what he or she may feel, do, or think. It is different from a sign, which is the objective finding of a medical practitioner.

Synthetic eclecticism—integrating concepts and principles from various theoretical paradigms to develop a more comprehensive understanding of a client's presenting problems.

Task environment—people, objects, and spaces that are external to the patient. The task environment may have a positive or negative effect on a patient's ability to regulate behavior.

Technical eclecticism—using therapeutic tools, techniques, and strategies from various theoretical paradigms in order to better meet the needs of individual clients.

Temporality—a sense of time, which is developed within a sociocultural context and can be influenced by many pathological and non-pathological means, including disease/dysfunction and developmental stage.

Third-party reimbursement—payment for health care services that is provided by private insurance or a governmental program rather than the patient or client.

Tic—any stereotyped movement or vocalization that is sudden, nonrhythmic, rapid, and repeated.

Time-out—a therapeutic intervention that is based on behavior modification involving a person's removal from a problematic situation and removal of positive reinforcers following the behavior that is to be extinguished.

Tolerance—the biological mechanism whereby greater amounts of an abused substance are required to produce the same/desired physiological and psychological effects of intoxication.

Traits—distinguishing characteristics of one's personal nature. A person can respond to a particular situation in a partic-ular way. When the response occurs in a variety of situations it becomes a habit. A group of response habits that form a repetitive way of psychological functioning or relating to the environment can be classified as a trait.

Treatment team—A team may be composed of some or all of the following: psychiatrist, psychologist, psychiatric nurse, social worker or therapist, case manager, occupational therapist, psychiatric technician, recreational therapist, and, more recently, family members.

Twelve step groups—refers to a self-help fellowship (modeled on Alcoholics Anonymous) offering individuals support for physical and spiritual recovery from alcoholism or other addictive substances. In meetings, the recovering individual is urged to "work the steps", each one focusing on a different aspect of recovery.

Universal Precautions—the mandate that treatment of blood and bodily fluids of all patients be considered potentially infectious with blood-borne pathogens. A set of protocols that includes barrier protections, hand washing, and disposal of contaminated or sharp materials that might be infected.

Work programming—the focused application of occupational therapy principles, knowledge, and skills to assist people to work productively and resume culturally valued roles in their community. Although paid employment is the reference point in Chapter 18, the term work is any productive activity, paid or nonpaid, that is valued and seen as contributing to the community.

Index